Ketsugo Goju-Ryu Karate-Do
Volume 2: Katas and Self-Defense

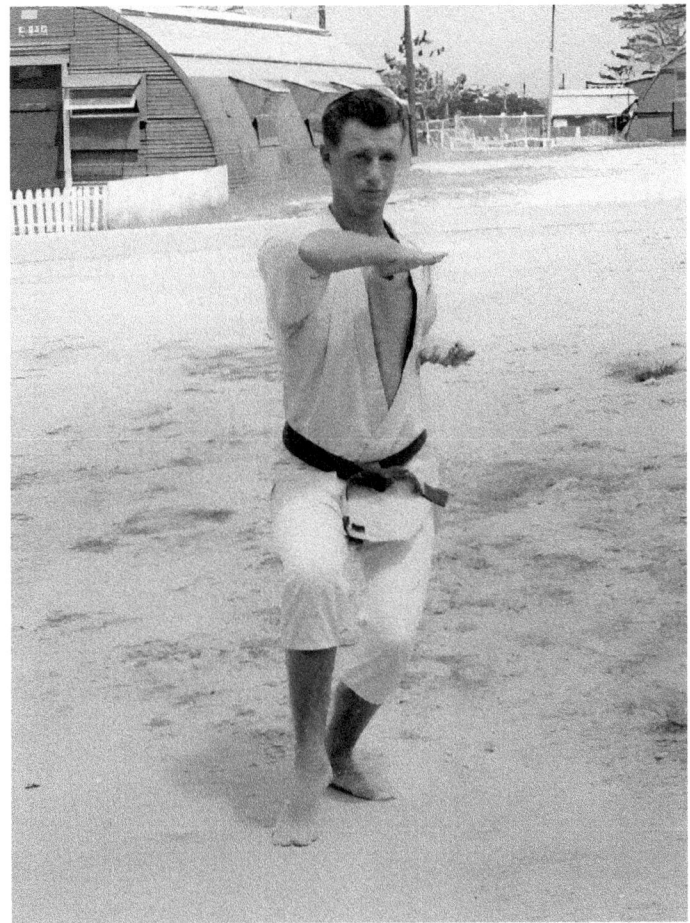

Shodai Jay Trombley, founder of Ketsugo Goju-Ryu Karate-Do, 1960

Ketsugo Goju-Ryu Karate-Do
Volume 2: Katas & Self-Defense
By Robert Oliver

Copyright © 2025 Robert Oliver
All rights reserved.
First Printing
ISBN: 979-8-9896402-5-6

WARNING

This book is presented only as a means of preserving a unique aspect of the heritage of martial arts. The author does not make any representation, warranty, or guarantee that the techniques described or illustrated in this book will be safe or effective in any self-defense situation or otherwise. You may be injured if you apply or train in the techniques of self-defense illustrated in this book, and the author is not responsible for any such injury that may result. It is essential that you consult a physician regarding whether to attempt any technique described in this book. Specific self-defense responses illustrated in this book may not be justified in any situation in view of all the circumstances or under the federal, state or local law. The author does not make any representation or warranty regarding the legality or appropriateness of any technique mentioned in this book.

DEDICATION

This book is dedicated to Shodai Jay Trombley, the visionary founder of Ketsugo Goju-Ryu Karate-Do who spent 61 years in the martial arts and will never be forgotten.

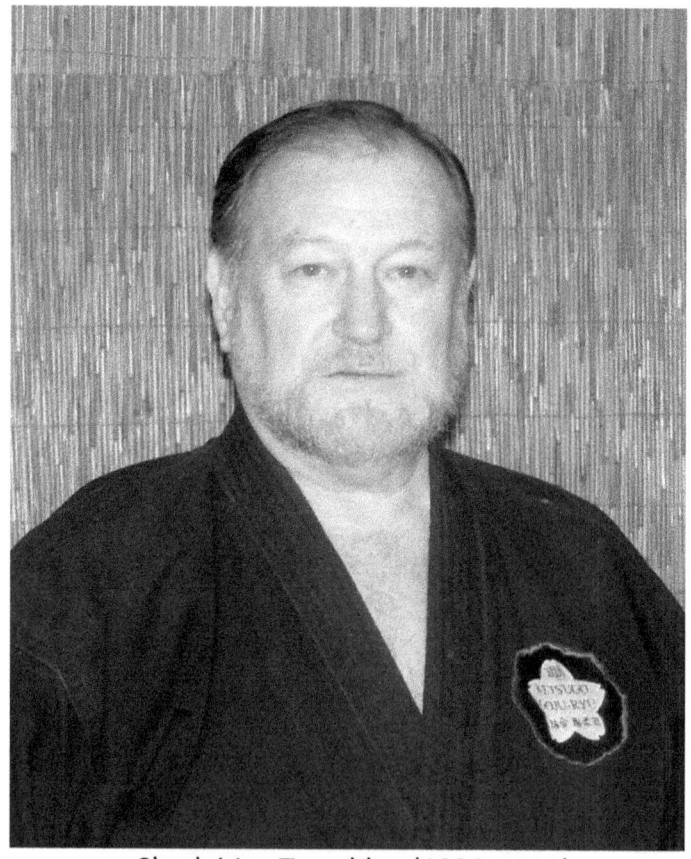

Shodai Jay Trombley (1938-2022)

ACKNOWLEDGMENTS

I want to thank my wife Ashley Oliver for helping me with the editing. Also, a big thanks to my cousin Rich Oliver, who graciously helped with some of the self-defense demonstrations. Finally, much thanks to everyone who purchased my first book, Shodai Jay Trombley, especially those who had no idea who he was or what karate means!

KGJKA Black Belts

Alyce Strickland | Tom Rieber | Rusty Fralia | Todd Kauffman | Lavada White | Shane Facemyer | David Griffin | Ken Johnson | Bob Loewenstein | Mark Ashraf | Sharon Griffin | Marshall Van Norden | Allen Crowley | Christine Landmon | Andrew Smith | Marvin Madison | Kyle Brown | Russell Dare | Chris Collins | Jared Smith | Kenneth Taliaferro | Alan Viengluang | Trent Boe | Mike Perry | Brodie Wolgamott | Ashley Oliver | Robert Oliver | George Eastlick | Cliff Knudson | Tim Bryant | Armando Navarro

FOREWORD

After cataloging many stories directly from Shodai Jay Trombley, talking to many of his prior students, friends, and of course his wife Karen, I was able to put together the first book about Ketsugo Goju-Ryu Karate-Do in December of 2023, approximately a year after Shodai's death. That book is about Shodai and his journey from childhood in Vermont to the Marine Corps, learning Shoreikan Goju-Ryu Karate in Okinawa, boxing and jiu jitsu in Florida, training and holding full contact fights in Texas, and of course creating his karate system, first called United Goju-Ryu, then Ketsugo Goju-Ryu. That book needed to be written simply because Shodai's story is such a unique one.

This second book and the ones to follow are about the karate system itself: the techniques, the kata, two-man training drills, self-defense, sparring, and the traditional weapons that make up Ketsugo Goju-Ryu Karate-Do. For those who have never taken martial arts before, this is an example of a truly mixed martial art which is still being taught today in both Colorado and Texas. For those familiar with karate already, you may enjoy reading about a system that came from Shoreikan Goju-Ryu (Seikichi Toguchi) in the 1950's, but with expanded techniques, additional kata, new variations of kiso and bunkai kumite, etc.

My goal with this book is to document the system that Shodai created in book form. Shodai was very protective of his system and did not like the idea of learning karate in any way except within a dojo. Once he told me about a dojo he visited where the instructor was literally teaching from a book. He never wanted that to happen to his system. With that in mind, this book and any subsequent book related to Shodai's karate system is not and will never be intended to directly teach or replace in any way training in an actual dojo. Karate should be learned in a dojo, but I have always found that reading about karate is a great way to spend time when you are not training.

- Author

TABLE OF CONTENTS

1 Techniques.. 13

Koryu Katas

2 Gekisai Ichi... 49

3 Gekisai Ni... 76

4 Saifa.. 109

5 Sanchin.. 127

6 Seiunchin... 151

7 Sepai... 182

Ketsugo Goju-Ryu Katas

8 Kihon Ichi.. 211

9 Gekisai San.. 226

10 Hon'nogeki.. 259

11 Genshin... 292

12 Isshoni San.. 335

13 Self-Defense 371

Appendix.. 406

Techniques

Techniques (waza) are the way a person does something, anything. Everything has technique, from how to sweep the floor, how to sit on a couch, and how to walk. In karate, there is a specific way to do everything, too. In karate we focus on different ways to stand, walk, punch, block, strike, kick, etc. Practicing technique is the bulk of martial arts training. Kata, which will be the focus on the rest of the book, is simply putting different techniques to use. Everything in karate, whether kata, self-defense, or sparring is made up of techniques, and they (techniques) all have purpose, even if it is not obvious at first. But the importance of practicing technique cannot be understated. No matter how strong a person may be, a bad technique means an ineffective strike at best, a clumsy injury at worst.

Karate starts with the feet. We work out barefoot and grip the floor with our feet as we strike or defend. The stance will give root to the strike, giving it power, and helping with balance. In Goju-Ryu Karate, we use the Sanchin crescent-style footwork. It is, however, different from sparring footwork because karate footwork is based on self-defense; a quick powerful movement to disable the attacker, not a timed sparring match.

Basic stances include heiko dachi (parallel stance), shiko dachi (sumo or horse stance), zenkutsu dachi (forward leaning stance), neko ashi dachi (cat leg stance), and the basic fighting stances. From these stances, basic punches and blocks are practiced. The benefits gained from learning and practicing stances vary, but at the very least will make the student's legs stronger. Legs are the foundation of the student and if the legs are in good, solid shape, the student will be harder to hit, kick, or take down and the muscles in the legs will react more effectively based on developing a stable base.

Punches, the most basic of all techniques, start with the feet (the stance), but extend all the way through the hips and up to the shoulders. This line of energy then goes past the shoulders, down the arm and ending with the first two knuckles of the fist. While that may seem academic, a person may only have one good opportunity for a punch, so the technique needs to be perfect.

When practicing strikes, the shoulders should be relaxed, the back should be straight, and the hips should be engaged to generate power in the punch through the core of the body. The starting point for the cross punch is called the chamber, which is the back hand, held about solar plexus height on the side of the body. When a hand is in chamber, the chambered forearm should be parallel to the floor and the wrist should be straight. The hand in chamber will be the one that either blocks or strikes for power. The chamber hand is typically palm up, and the punch itself should twist just before contact is made so the fist is palm down on contact, using the first two knuckles as the point of contact.

After learning the proper stances and how to punch and block, next comes footwork, half-circle steps, tracing the ground with the ball of the foot, keeping the center line balanced. Once the footwork is learned, it is put together with punches and blocks, but a new student will need to put focus on each thing separately at first: step, stop, then punch; or step, stop, then block. This pattern is important to focus on footwork independent of the strikes, so strikes are performed properly. Also, stopping just before the punch can help emphasize the power of each strike without hesitation, and with perfect balance. Obviously in a real confrontation or even when sparring, a student will step with a strike, but in the beginning, the student needs to focus on one thing at a time. Eventually, a student will be able to generate power without having to deliberately stop with rooted feet.

Basic techniques are an important foundation for karate. For most people it takes time to master the basics, but once mastered, it is far easier to learn intermediate and advanced moves. Something else to consider is that everything worth doing correctly starts with basics. And over time, the basics become as natural as breathing.

Goju-Ryu Karate footwork, for example, is designed to keep the feet rooted for balance and helps center the body. Eventually the student will be able to keep balance and center the body without thinking about crescent-style footwork. When first learning to punch, chambering the lead hand while punching with the rear hand helps to engage the body along with the strike, giving it more power. Over time, the student will be able to engage the body while keeping the back hand in a better defensive position. However, chambering the lead hand is not just for creating power in the punch. Chambering may also be used to pull an opponent in while striking with the other hand. Or perhaps the attacker may elbow someone directly behind while punching someone in front. Another example is blocking. In the beginning the hands are closed for blocks, but eventually open hands are used. Open hand blocks imply grabbing something, preparing to grab, or slapping something away, while closed hand blocks imply striking the attacker. But these are just a few examples, and the possibilities for usage are endless. With karate, there is usually a lot more going on than what we see.

In the next chapter, we will examine some of the Koryu Katas we train in Ketsugo Goju-Ryu. To prepare, this chapter of techniques will focus on some of the more frequent techniques used in those katas.

Stances

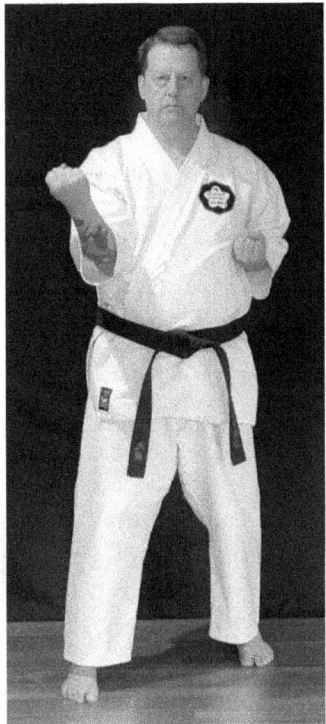

Kamae

Kamae (basic defensive posture). Kamae means "posture," but it is also a basic, forward-facing fighting stance, also referred to as the ready position. The feet are shoulder width apart; the front foot is a foot and a half in front of the back foot, and the trunk is centered. The back should be straight, and shoulders relaxed. The back fist (chamber position) is placed palm up on the ribs. The front arm is at a 90-degree angle, with the fist no higher than the shoulder and tilted just to the outside of the arm. The elbow should be a fist-width away from the ribs.

Heiko Dachi (parallel stance) is a relaxed position in which katas begin. The feet are parallel and a little wider than shoulder width.

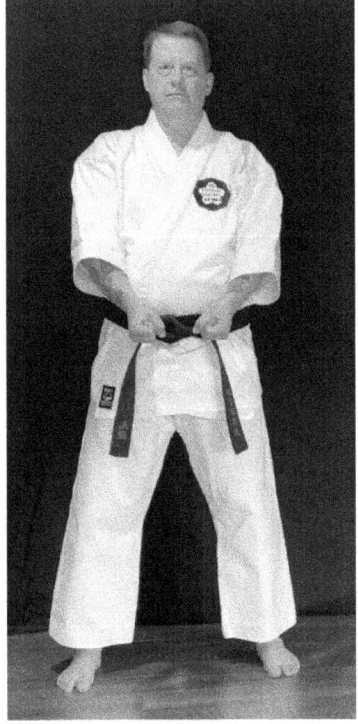

Heiko Dachi

Techniques

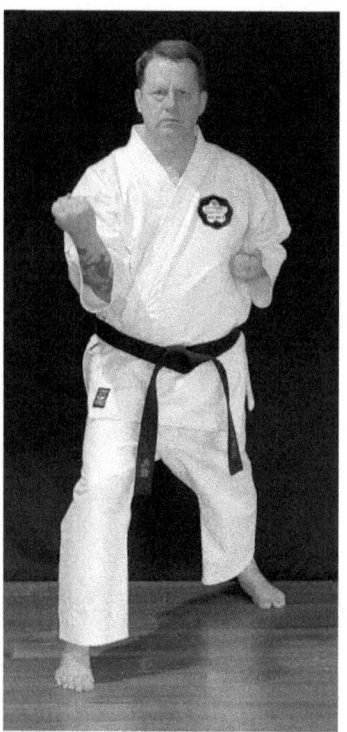

Zenkutsu Dachi

Zenkutsu Dachi (Forward leaning stance) From kamae, bring one foot forward about 2 ½ feet lengths from the back foot, and the trunk is centered. The front leg is bent at the knee until the foot is covered.

Neko Ashi Dachi (Cat leg stance) With neko ashi dachi, the back leg is bent, and the foot is at an angle, with the knee pointed in the same direction so it feels almost like sitting on an imaginary chair. Approximately 90% of the weight should be on the rear leg and the hip should come out a bit, drawing the groin area in. The front foot is on the ball of the foot with the knee directly over the ball. The angle of the front foot should be along the middle or heel of the back foot.

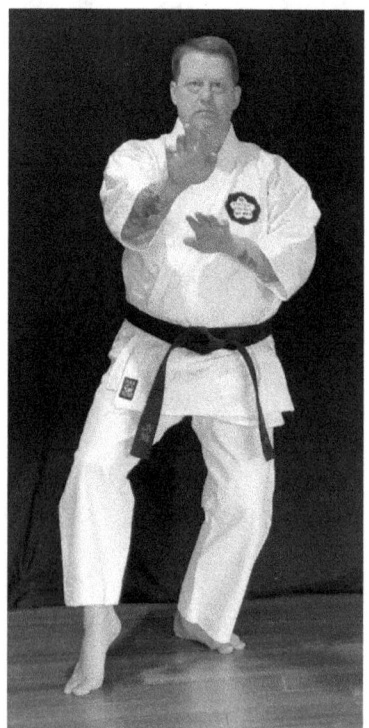

Neko Ashi Dachi

Techniques

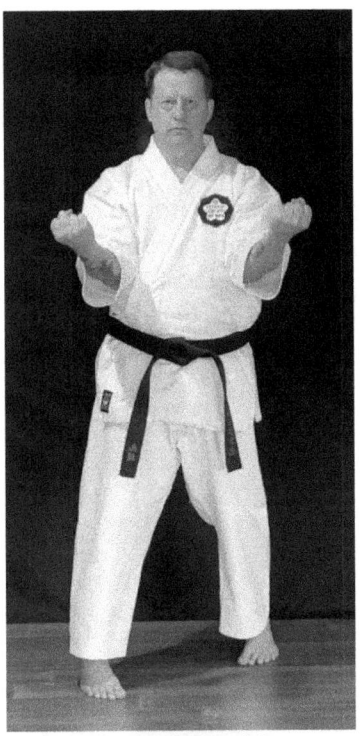

Sanchin Dachi

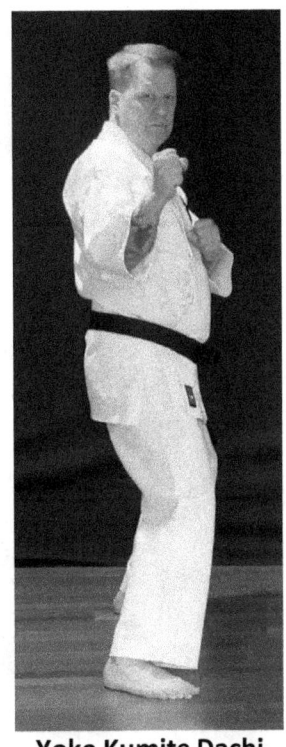

Yoko Kumite Dachi

Sanchin Dachi (Hourglass stance) Like kamae, except the feet are turned in slightly and grip the floor. Also, the pelvis should be tilted up, as if the belly is being pulled upward. This is to protect the groin.

Yoko Kumite Dachi (Sideways fighting stance) Like kamae, except the body is completely sideways and the chamber position is just below the solar plexus. Hands can be open or closed. The sideways fighting stance narrows the target for the opponent, and is useful if groin kicks are allowed, but leaves the fighter open to leg kicks.

Heisoku Dachi (Feet together stance) is very similar to Musubi Dachi. The difference is very minimal as the feet in Heisoku Dachi are together, while the feet in Musubi Dachi have open toes. Heisoku Dachi is the transitional stance while using half-moon footwork and used in some katas.

Musubi Dachi (Feet together, toes open stance) is used before bowing.

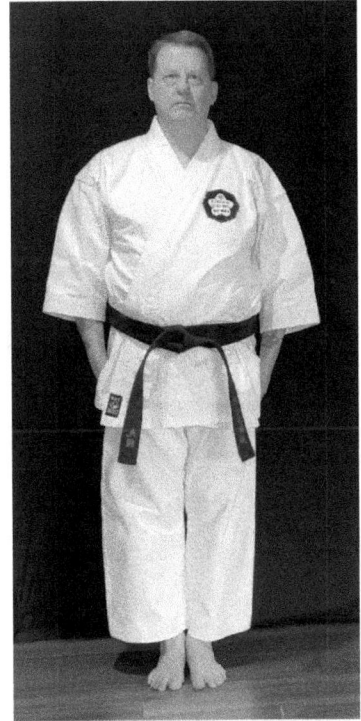

Heisoku Dachi

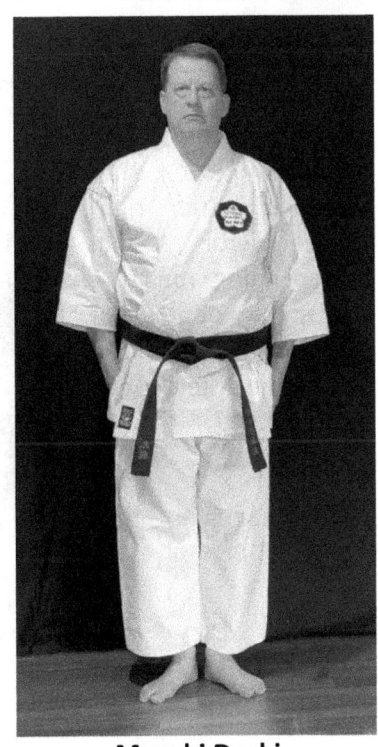

Musubi Dachi

Techniques

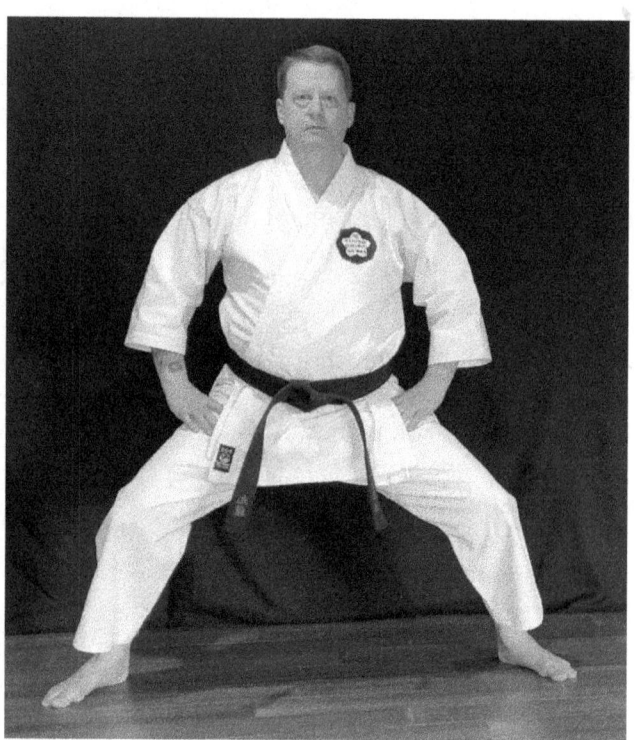

Shiko Dachi (straddle leg stance) is a low stance, feet wider than heiko dachi, going down until the student can touch his knees. Feet are pointed forty-five degrees in the same direction as the knees. The back should be straight, not leaning forward. The thighs should not be parallel to the floor.

Shiko Dachi

Kosa Dachi (Cross leg stance) Used in katas like Sanchin and Seiunchin to turn around. The right knee or shin (depending on the desired depth of stance) is stabilized by the left calf muscle.

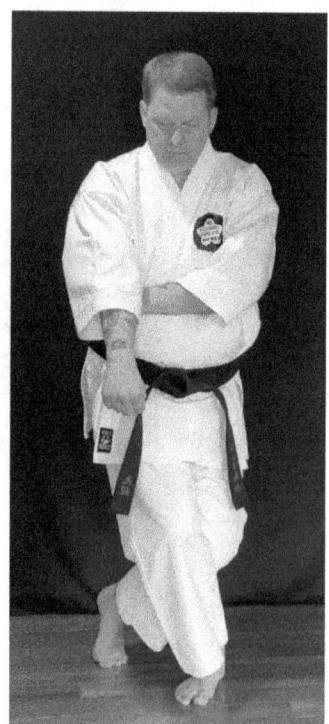 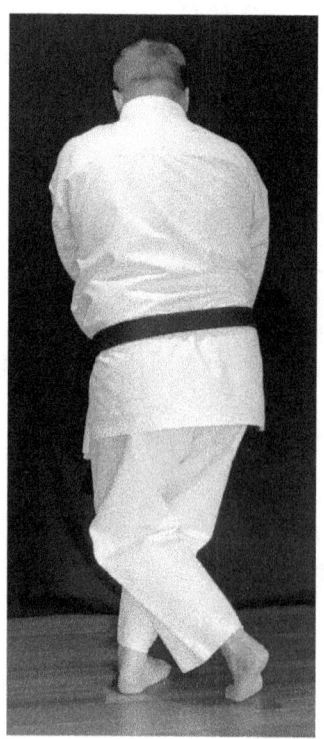

Kosa Dachi

Strikes, Punches (Tsuki/- Zuki, Uchi) & Blocks (Uke)

When training begins, punches and blocks are simple. Making a proper fist and learning how to generate power with the hips is an important foundation to build on after learning basic stances. Just learning how to use both hands independent of each other can be challenging, but with constant practice, it can become second nature. First, the fist must be tight enough that when punching something, it will stay strong. When punching, the wrist must be straight, and the fist must be held so the first two knuckles will strike the target. For basic punches, the targets are between the eyes for upper punches (jodan tsuki), to the solar plexus for middle punches (chudan tsuki), and below the belt for low punches (gedan tsuki).

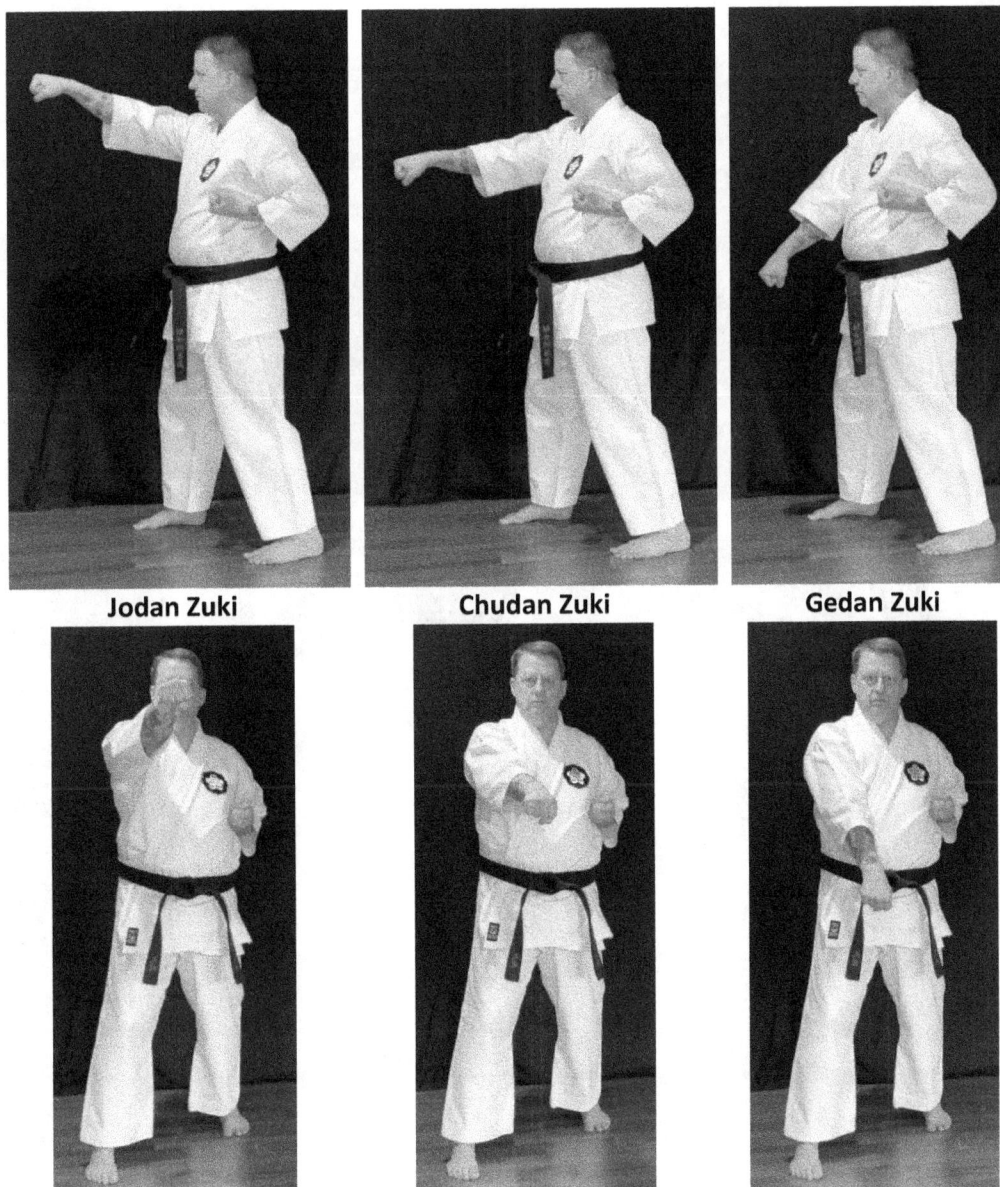

Jodan Zuki   **Chudan Zuki**   **Gedan Zuki**

Techniques

For forward facing basic blocks, use a rising block (age uke) for upper blocks (jodan uke), closed hands for middle blocks (chudan uke), and gedan barai (sweeping down block) for low blocks (gedan uke). Bear in mind a few things when doing these blocks: for head and chest blocks, circle the opposite elbow and then keep the forearm along the opposite arm when completing the block. This can function as a break from a hold as well as a block from a strike. For the down block, think of it as a low strike as much as a low block.

Jodan Uke (Age Uke)

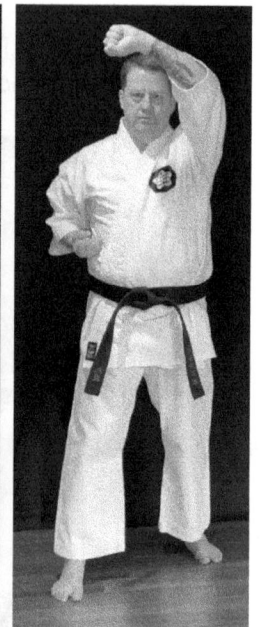

Chudan Uke

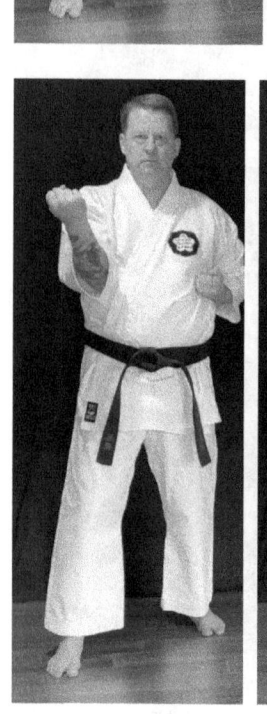
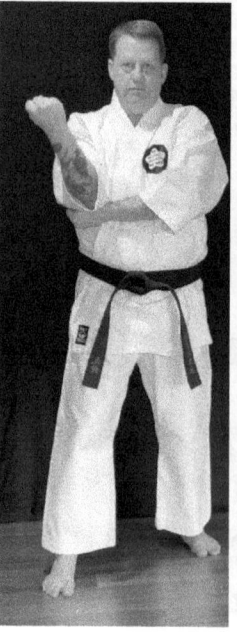
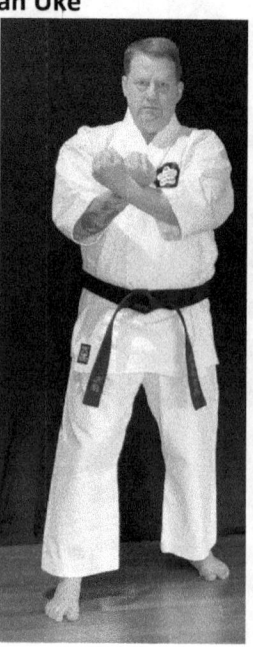
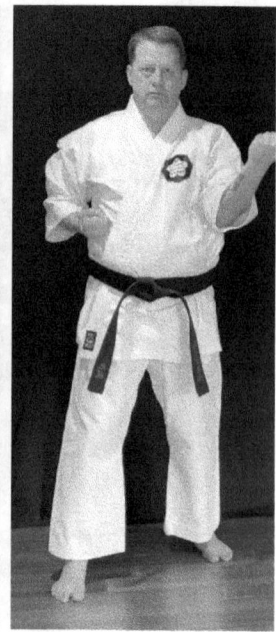

Techniques

Gedan Uke (Gedan Barai)

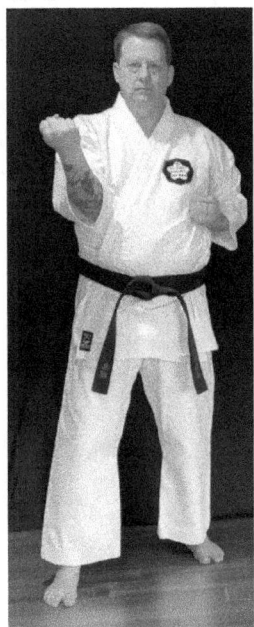 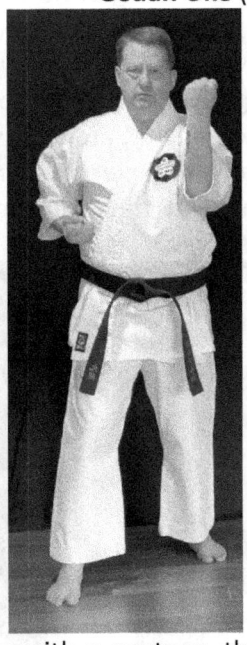 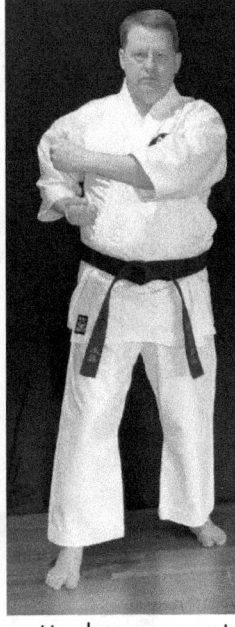 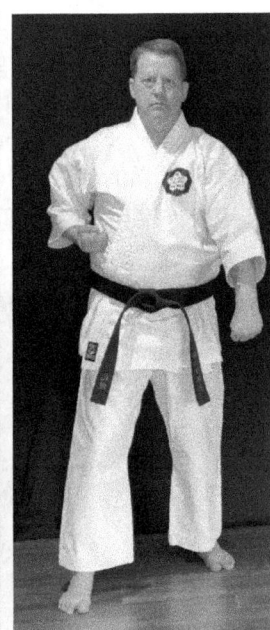

When working with a partner, the attacker concentrates on targeting. The attacker also dictates the distance, and the speed based on his stance and how fast he strikes. The defender will time his speed to the attacker. If the defender just tries to block as fast as possible, the block may happen before the punch, negating the defense. And if the defender moves with a longer step than the attacker, that eliminates the possibility for a counterpunch. This sequencing takes practice, but eventually the attacker should be striking close enough to contact the partner if he fails to block the strike. Finally, the two partners will strike and block with power. It should take effort to block a strike. The defender should aim just below the elbow when blocking to maximize leverage.

Jodan Zuki & Uke   **Chudan Zuki & Uke**   **Gedan Zuki & Uke**

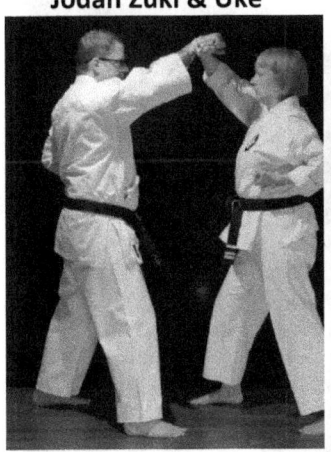 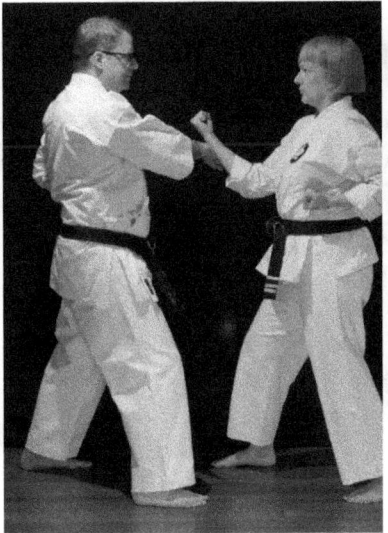 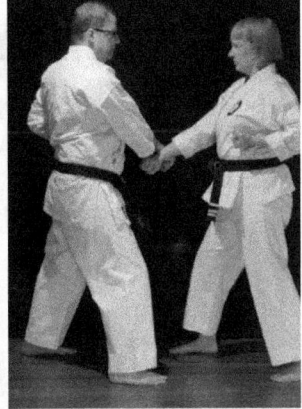

Techniques

For open hand versions of the forward facing basic blocks, use jodan ko uke (back of wrist) for upper blocks (jodan uke), a combination of chudan hari uke (palm up open hand) and chudan hiki uke (palm down open hand) for middle blocks (chudan uke), and shotei barai (palm heel sweeping down block) for low blocks (gedan uke). Once again, these "blocks" are as much strikes as they are blocks and can be used for a variety of purposes. The chest block, for example, can employ an elbow strike with the thumb side of the palm up block, following up with the pulling motion of the hiki uke.

Jodan Ko Uke

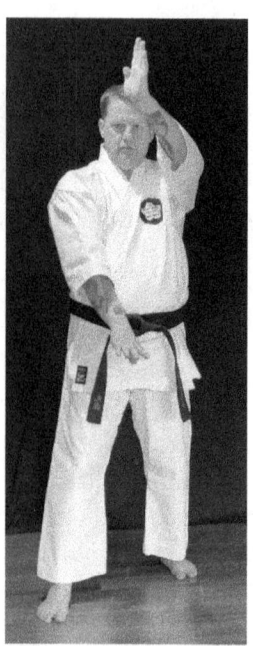
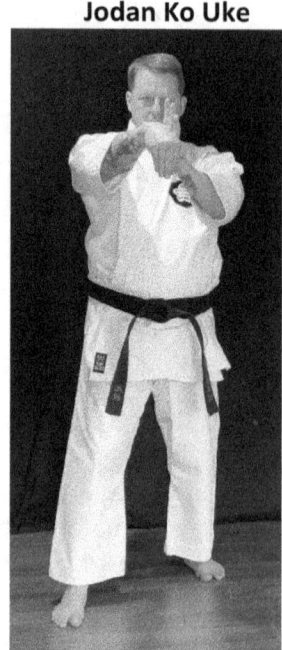
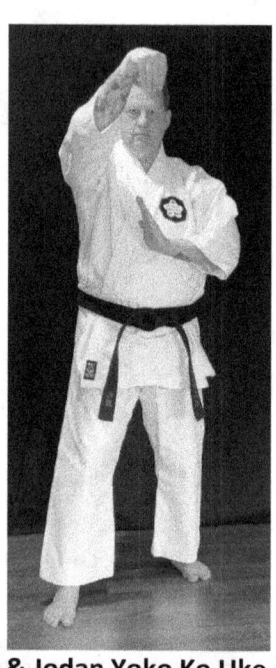

Jodan Zuki & Ko Uke   **Jodan Zuki & Jodan Yoko Ko Uke**

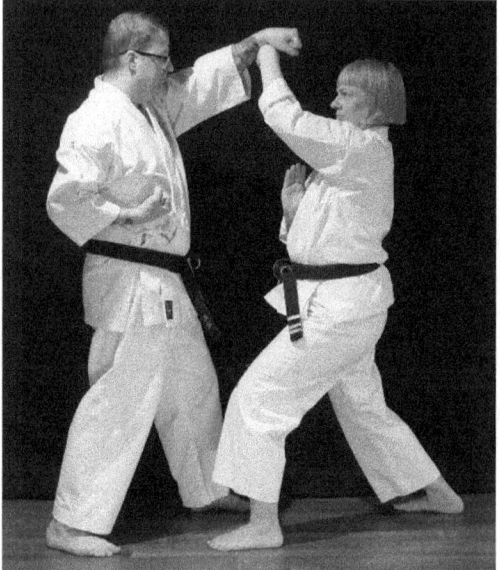
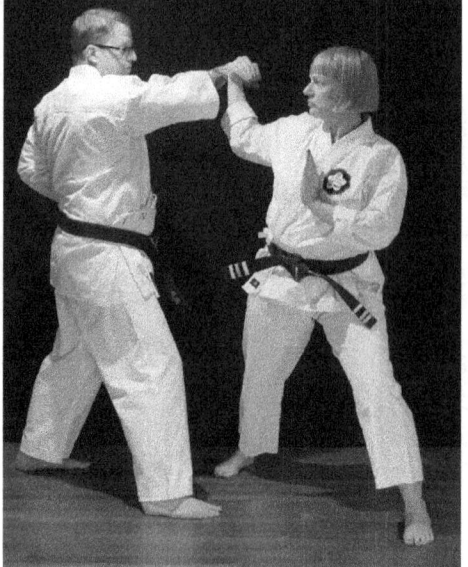

Techniques

Chudan Hari to Hiki Uke

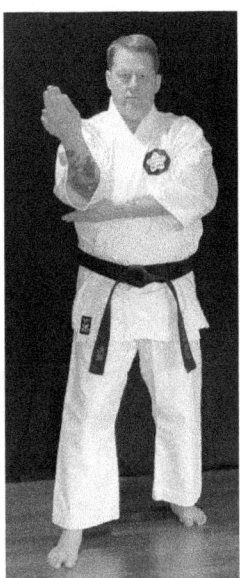 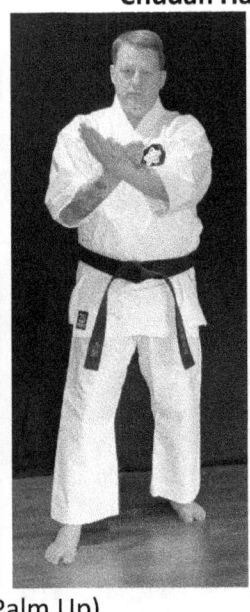 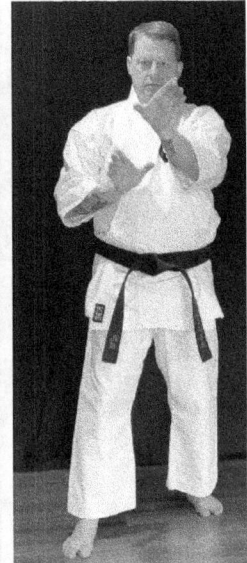 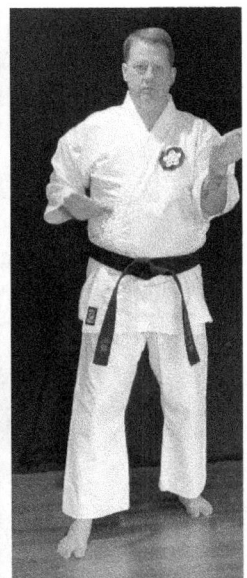

Hari Uke (Palm Up)   **Hiki Uke** (Palm Down)

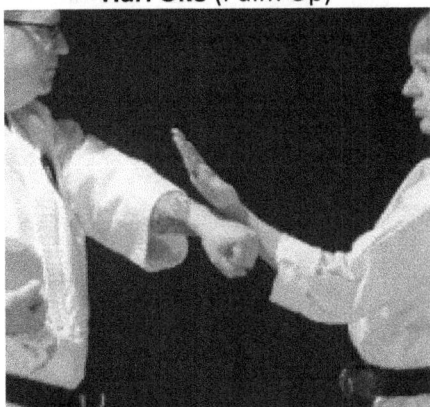 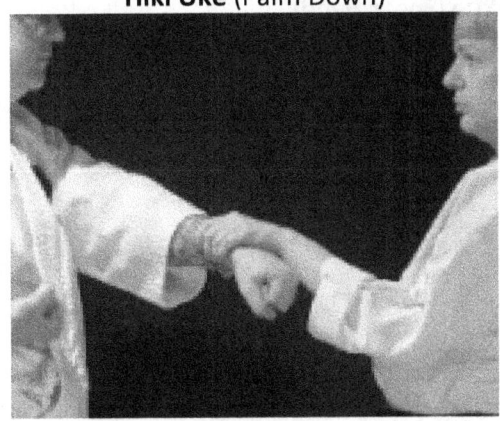

Gedan Shotei Barai

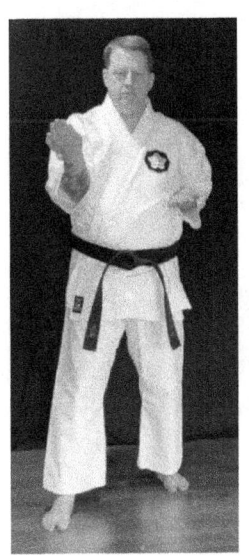 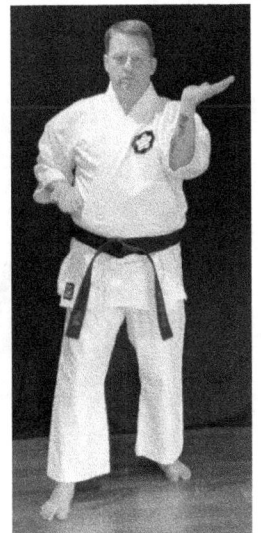 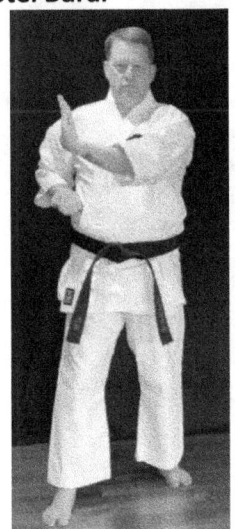 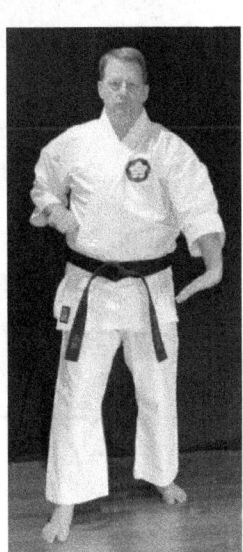

Hand Techniques

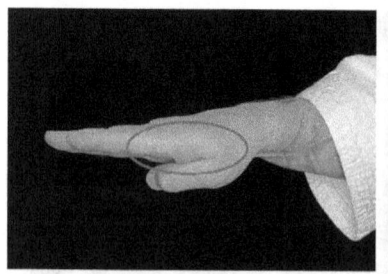
Haito (Ridge Hand)

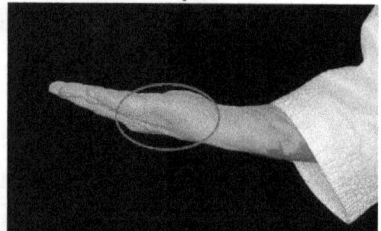
Shuto (Chop)

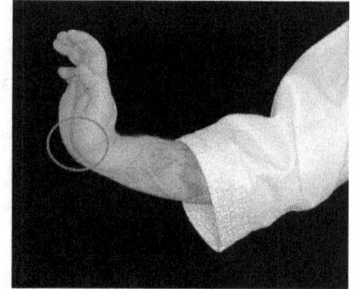
Shotei (Palm Heel)

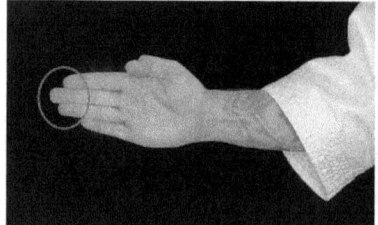
Nukite (Spear Hand)

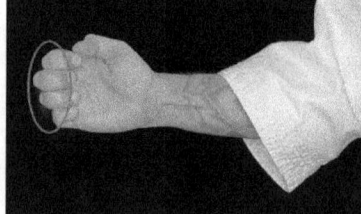
Kaiko Ken or Hiraken (Foreknuckle Fist)

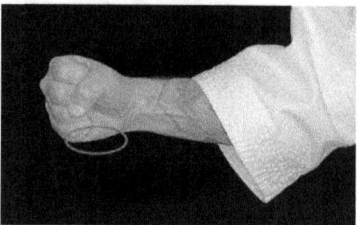
Tettsui (Hammer Fist)

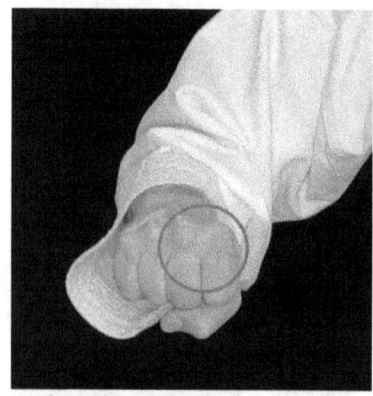
Seiken (Forefist)

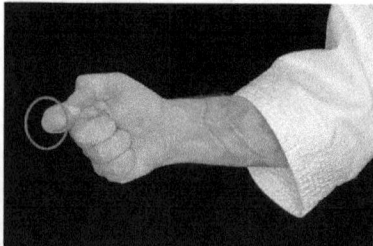
Ippon Ken (Single Knuckle Fist)

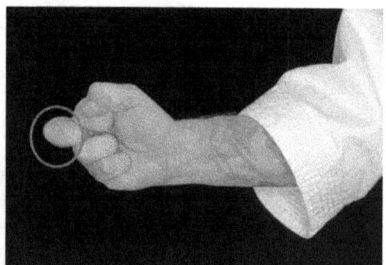
Nakadaka Ken (Middle Knuckle Fist)

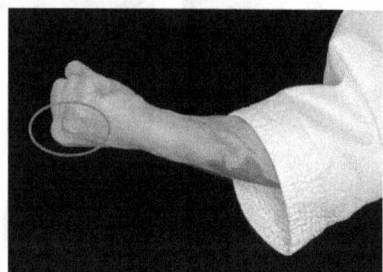
Soko Zuki (Undercut)

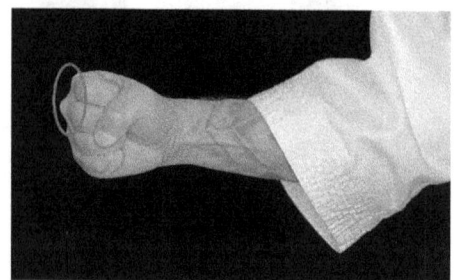
Tate Ken (Vertical Fist)

Mae Shuto Uchi (Forward Facing Chop Strike)

Shuto Uchi is a way to strike a narrow target, under the ear or the throat, as a few examples.

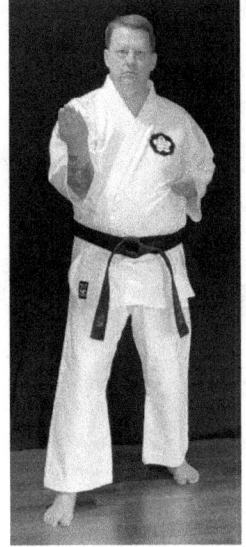
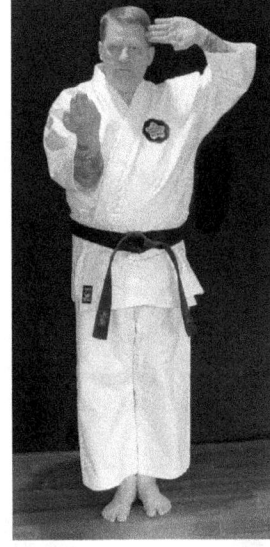
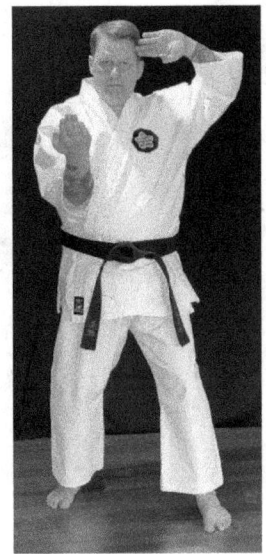
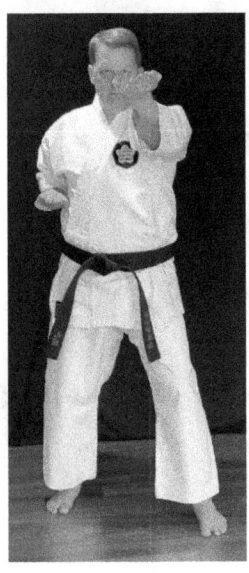
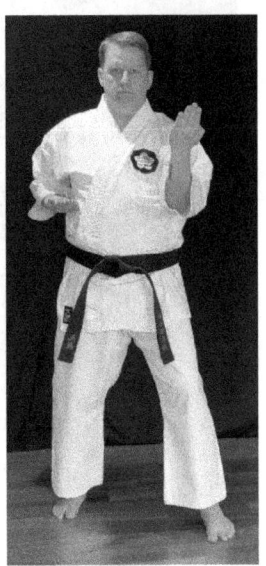

Techniques

Shuto Uke

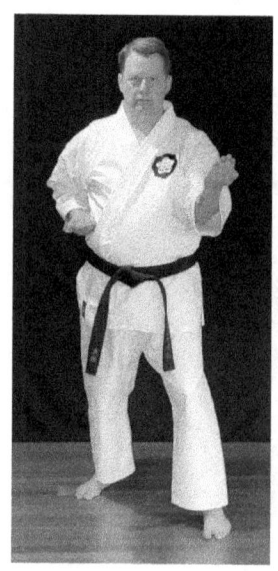 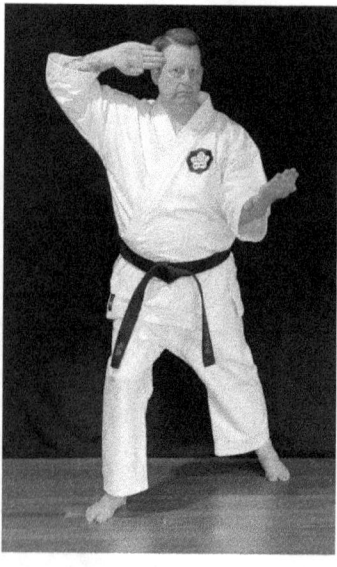 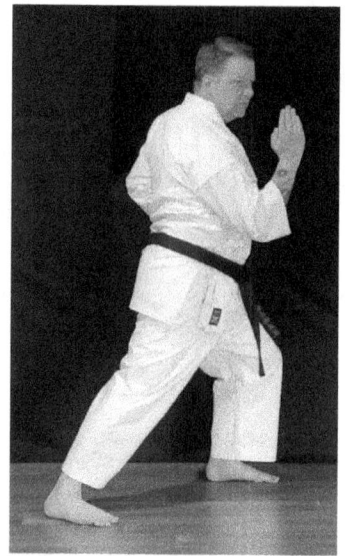

Yoko Shuto Uchi (Side Chop Strike)

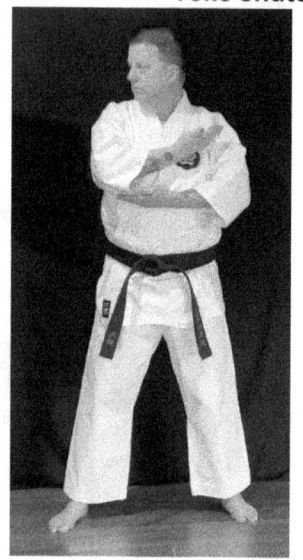 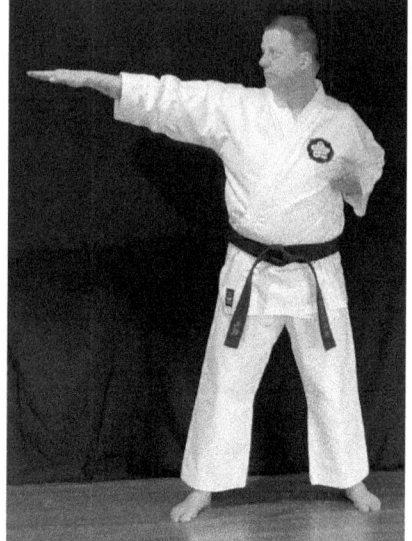

Techniques

Shuto Uchi (Chop Strike)

Mae Shuto Uchi **Yoku Shuto Uchi**

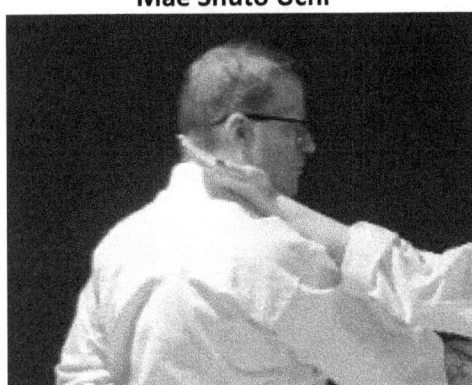 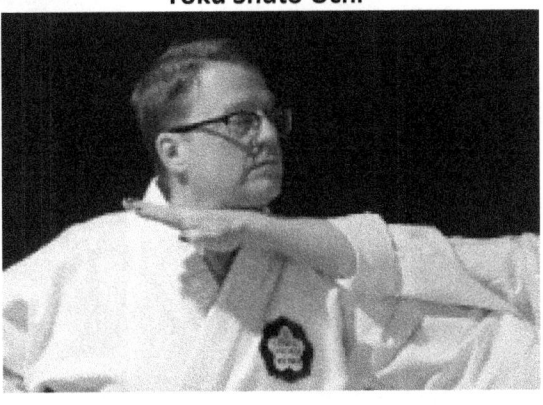

Mae Tettsui Uchi (Forward Facing Hammer Fist Strike)
Tettsui Uchi is a to strike a hard target, like the side of the head or the back.

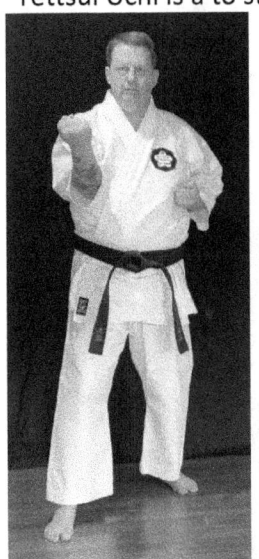 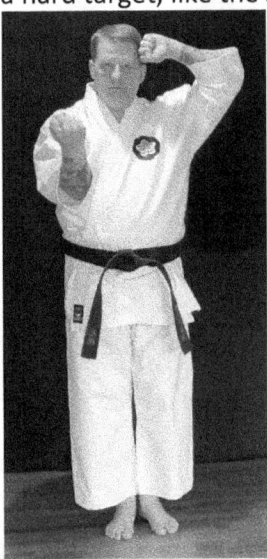 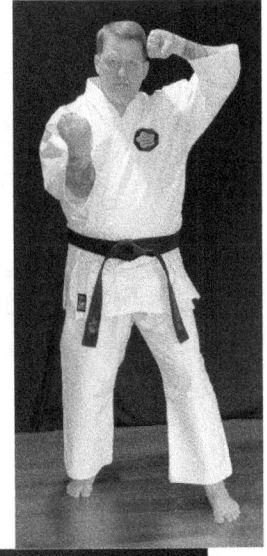

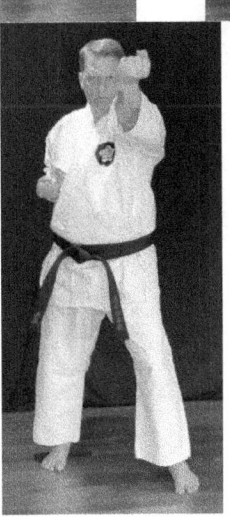 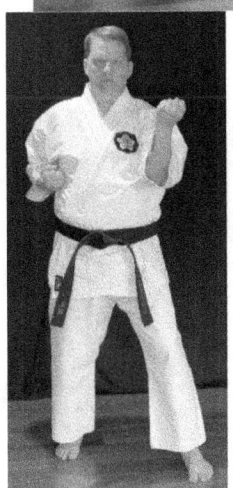

Techniques

Otoshi Tettsui Uchi (Downward Hammer Fist Strike)

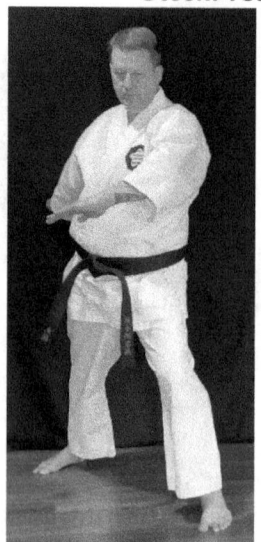
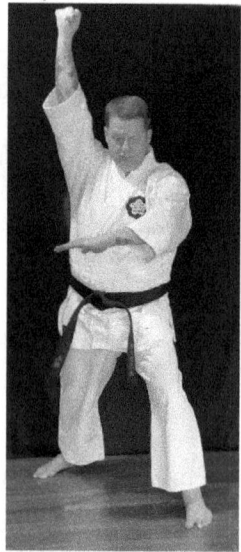
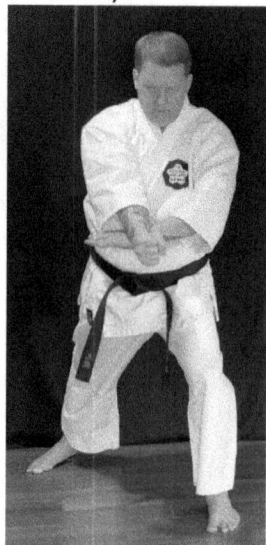

Yoko Tettsui Uchi (Side Hammer Fist Strike)

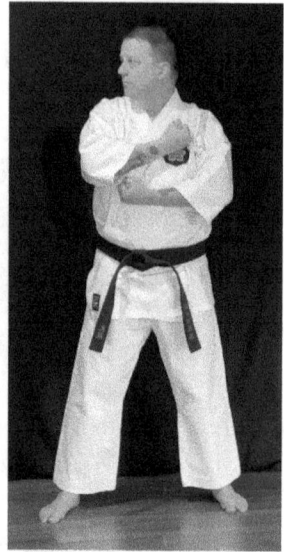
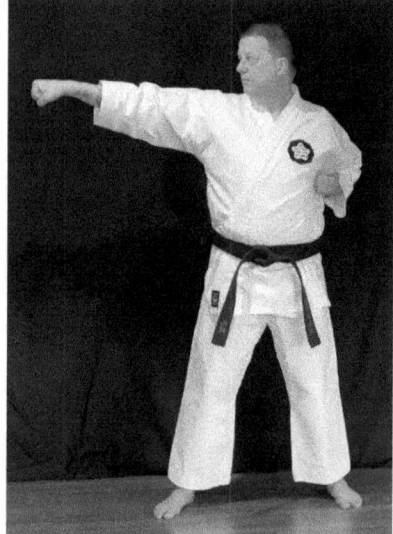

Mae Tettsui Uchi   **Yoko Tettsui Uchi**

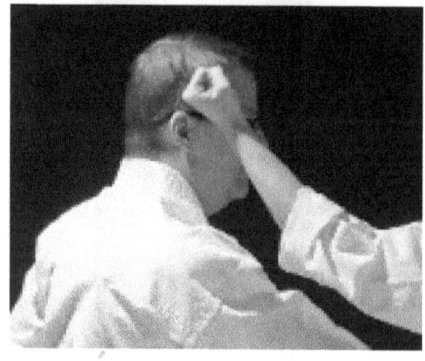
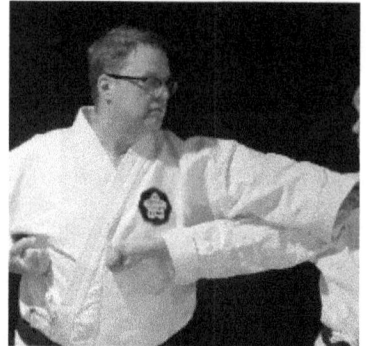

Techniques

Along with Shuto Uke, the following blocks use **Taihineri (Body Twisting)** movements to work off center to the opponent's strike.

Kake Uke (Hook Block)

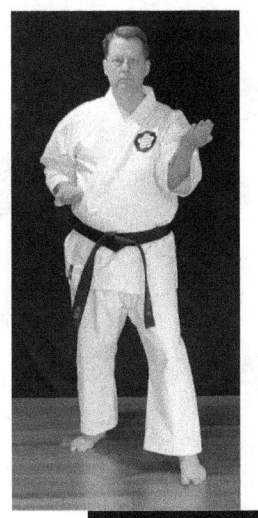
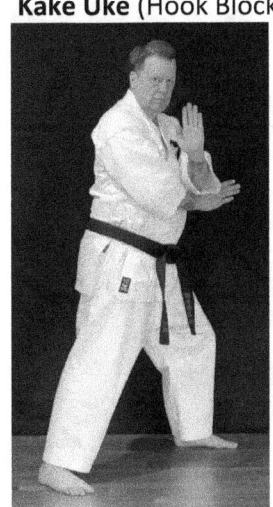
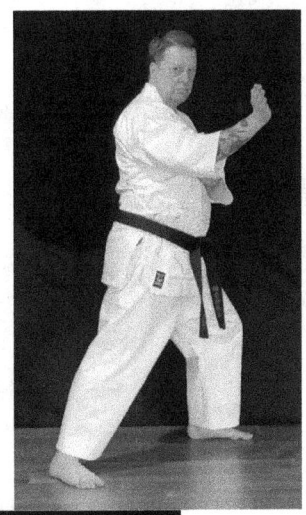

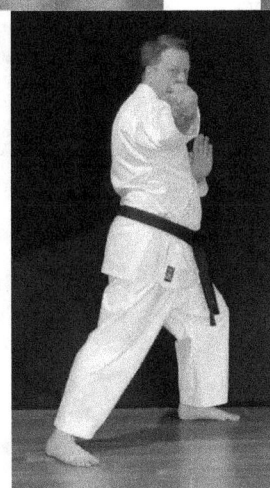
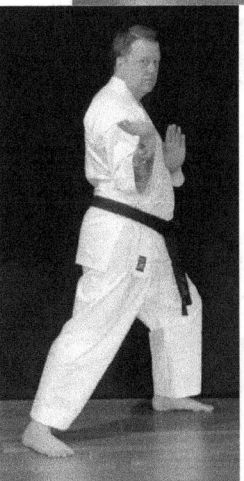

Kake Uke (Hook Block)　　　　**Shuto Uke** (Chop Block)

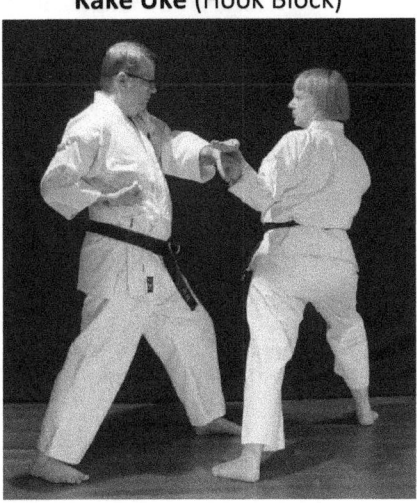
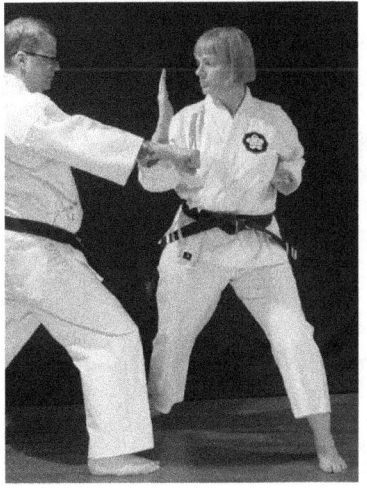

Techniques

Soto Uke (Outside Forearm Block)

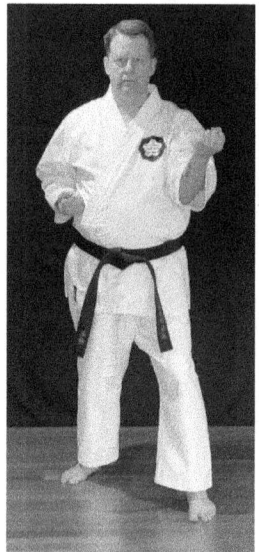 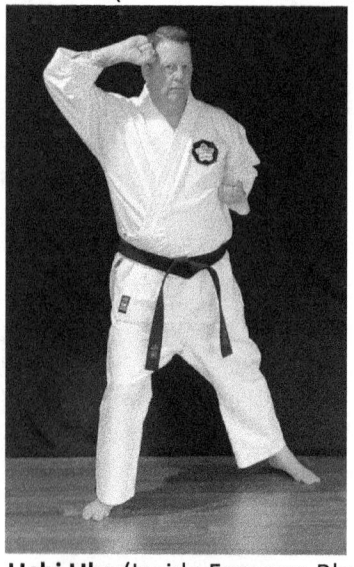 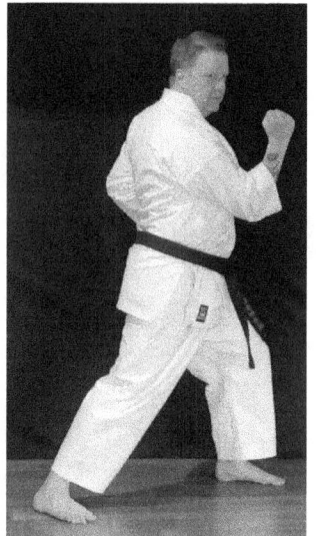

Uchi Uke (Inside Forearm Block)

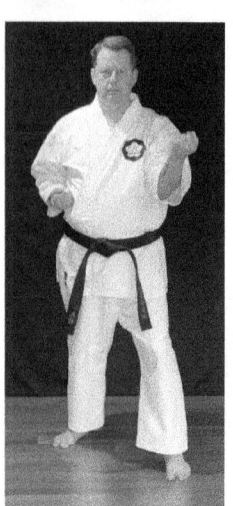 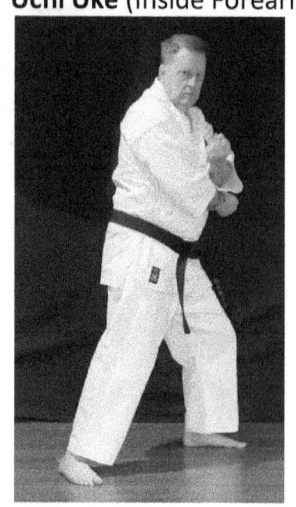 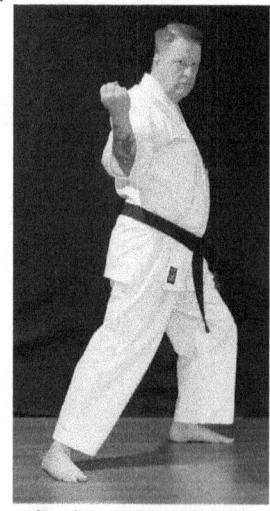

Uchi Uke (Inside Block)　　　**Soto Uke** (Outside Block)

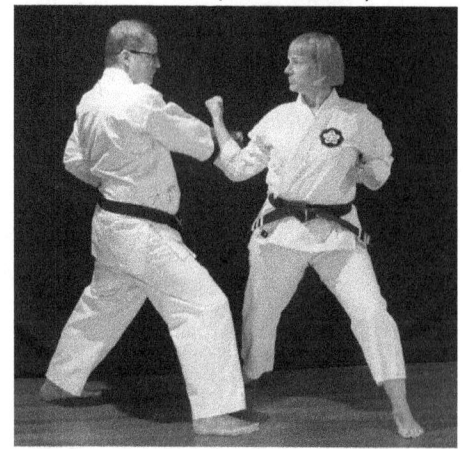 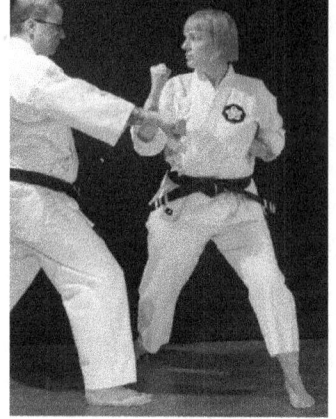

Techniques

Mae Uraken Uchi (Forward Facing Back Fist Strike)
Uraken Uchi utilizes the back of the hand and can be a quick and powerful strike.

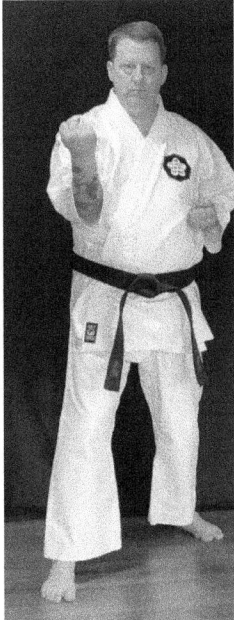 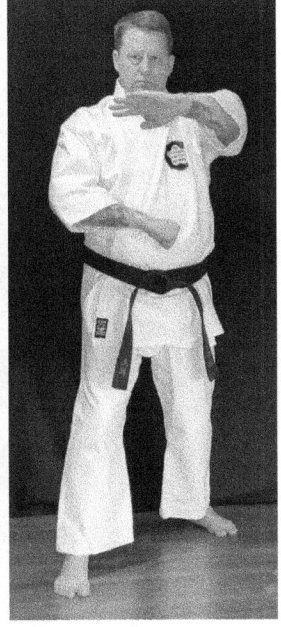 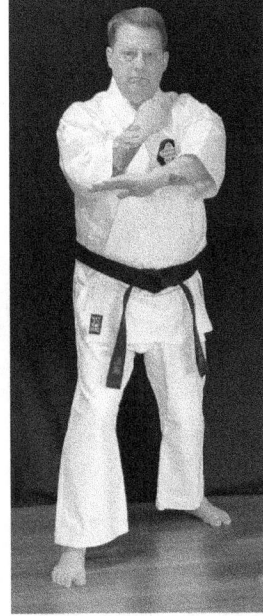 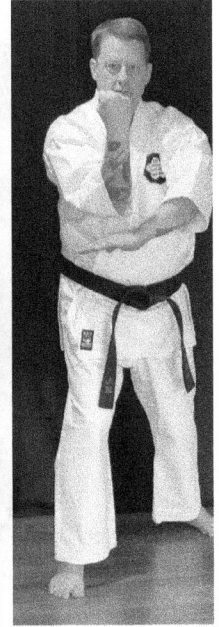

Mae Uraken Uchi

Yoko Uraken Uchi

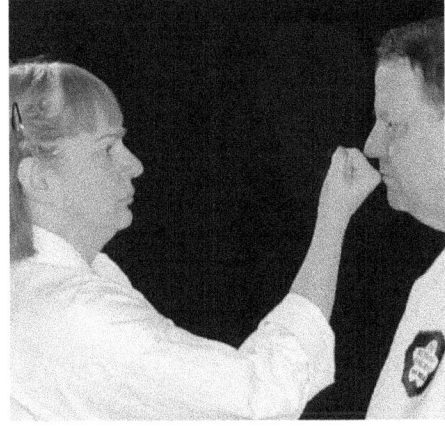 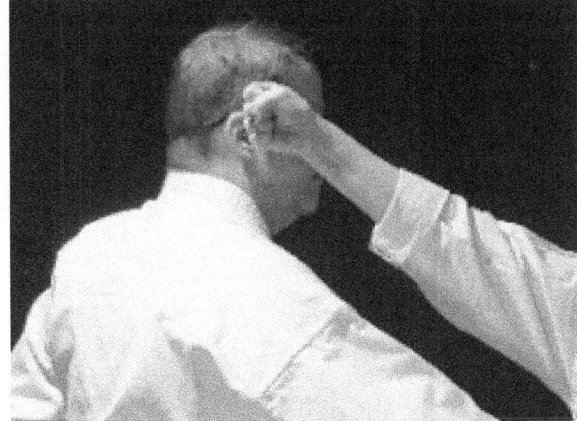

Techniques

Yoko Uraken Uchi (Side Back Fist Strike)

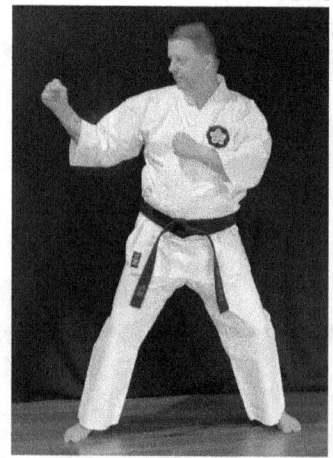
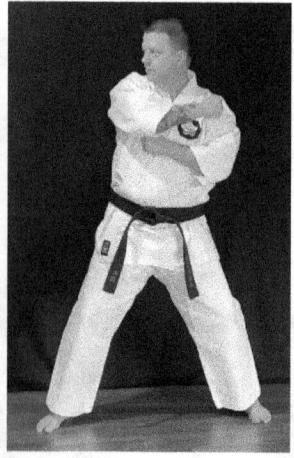
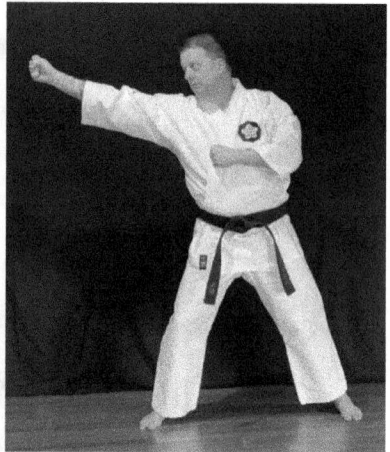
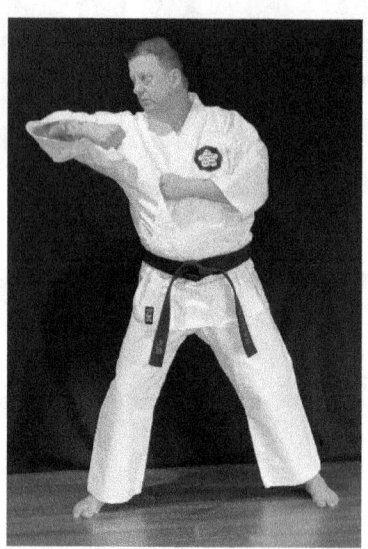
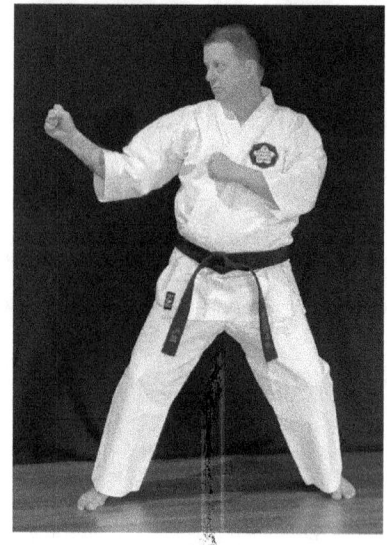

Techniques

Empi Uchi, elbow strikes, are effective at close range and can be used in any direction to any target in reach. The downward strike can be used on the back or the leg, the side strike to the face, head or ribs, the rear strike can be used to escape a grab, and the upward strike is effective to the chin.

Otoshi Empi Uchi (Downward Elbow Strike)

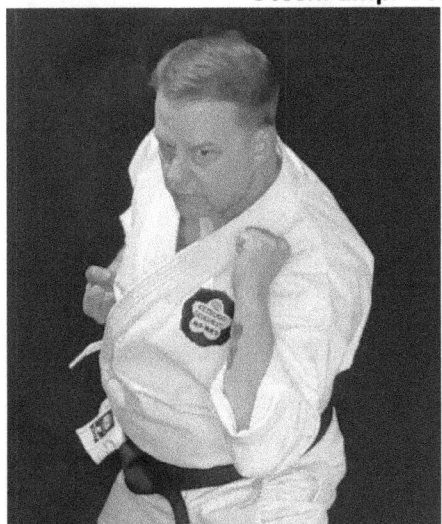 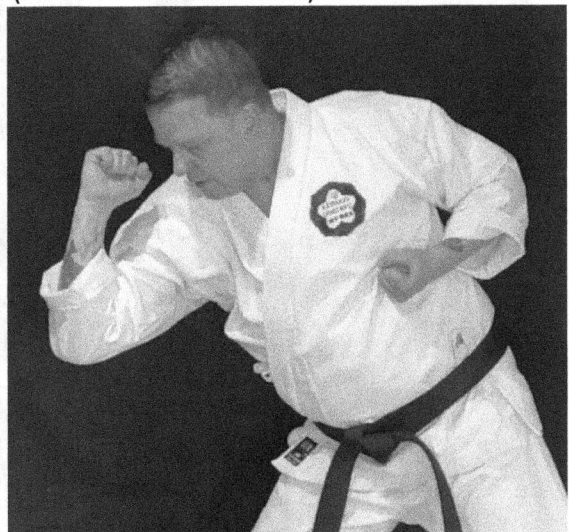

Yoko Empi Uchi (Side Elbow Strike)

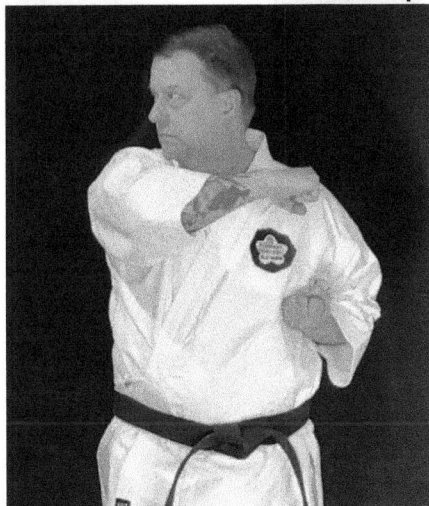 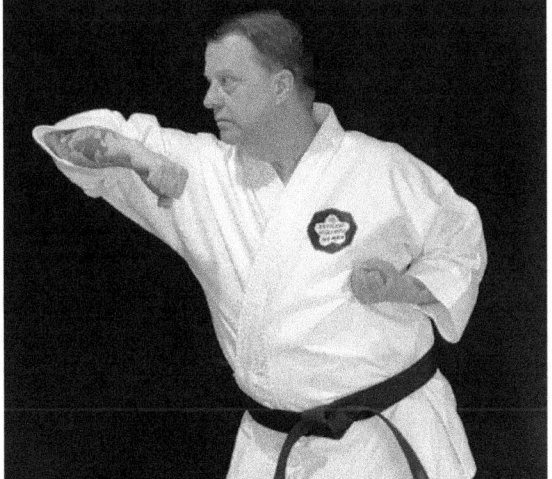

Techniques

Ushiro Empi Uchi (Rear Elbow Strike)

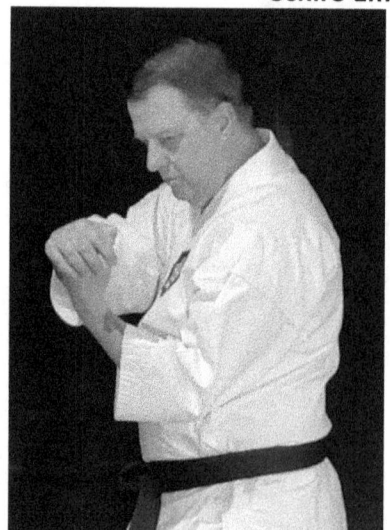
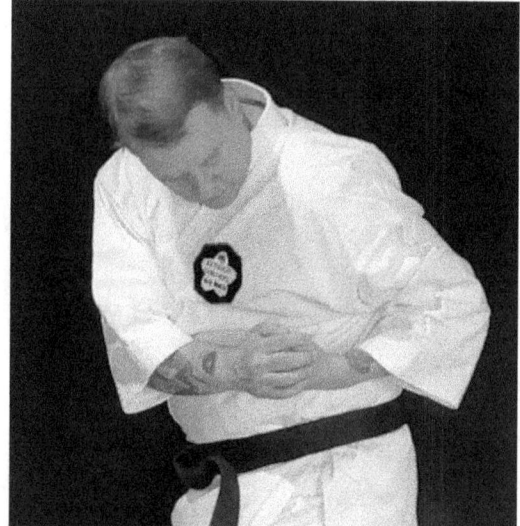

Otoshi Empi Uchi (Downward)

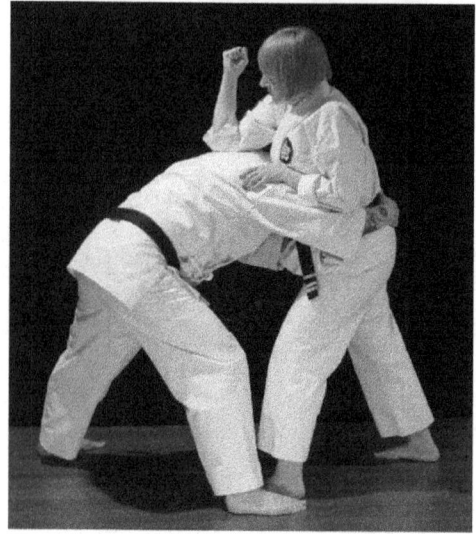

Yoko Empi Uchi (Side elbow strike)   **Tate Empi Uchi** (Upward)

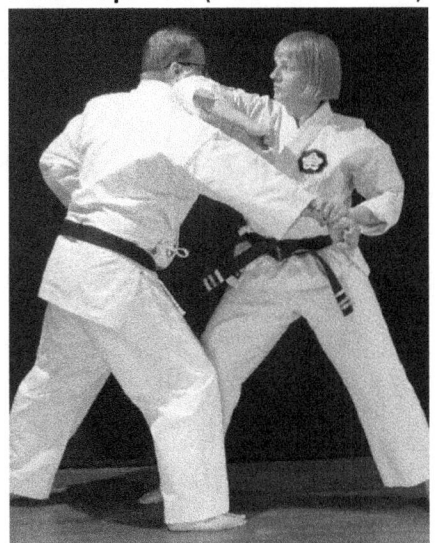
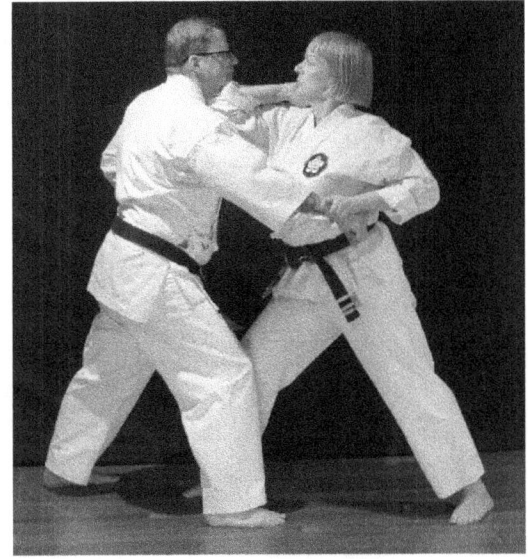

Kicks (Keri/- Geri)

While karate is mostly thought of as a striking art, kicks are used as well. When kicking, the stance is compromised, so balance and quickness is paramount. Originally, kicks were kept below the waist and only used to down the opponent. Full contact karate competition allowed participants to score points with head kicks and side stances were important in taking advantage of side kicks. Turn kicks also flourished with body shots in a system where a mandatory number of kicks were enforced. In self-defense, kicks below the waist are still the most important to learn, but high kicks help with developing balance, control, and overall fitness.

Techniques

Fumikomi Geri (Down Heel Kick)
The down heel, or stamping kick, is useful on a downed opponent.

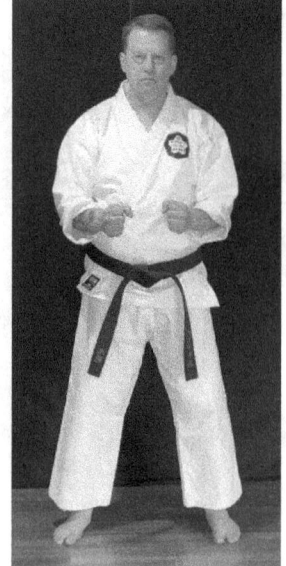
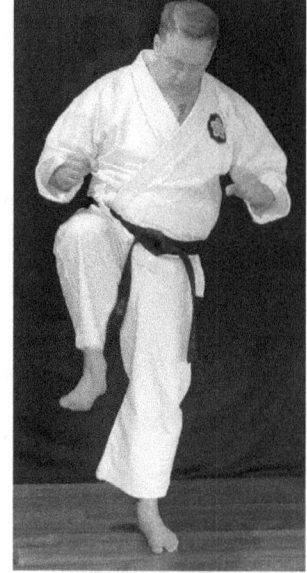
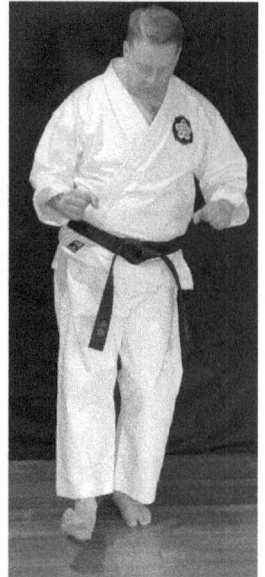
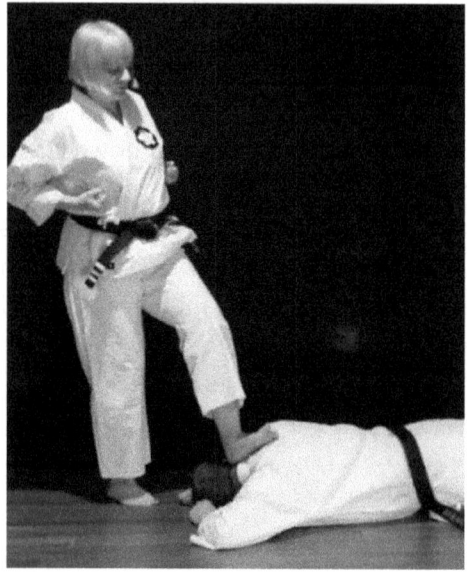

Gedan & Jodan Mae Keage Geri (Front Snap Kick to the Groin and Chin)
Kick with the Haisoku (instep), Josokutei (ball of foot), or Kakato (heel)
With the snap kick, after contact, the foot is brought back with a snapping motion.

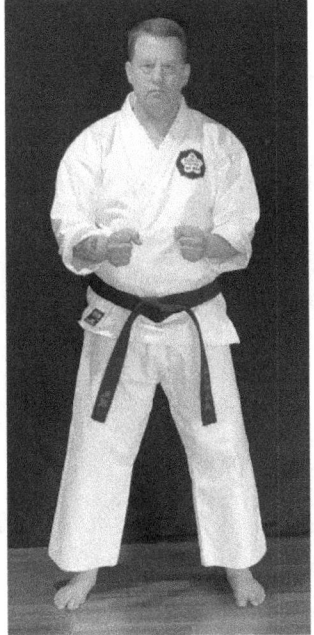
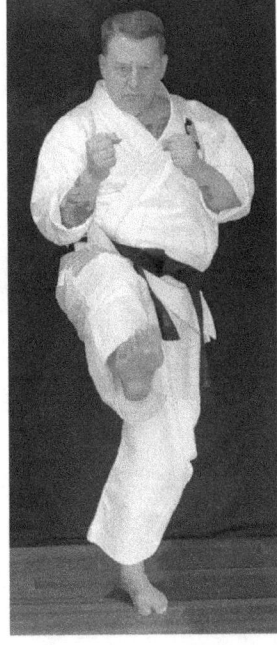
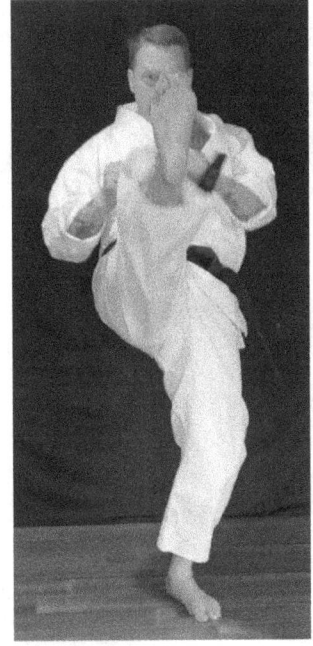

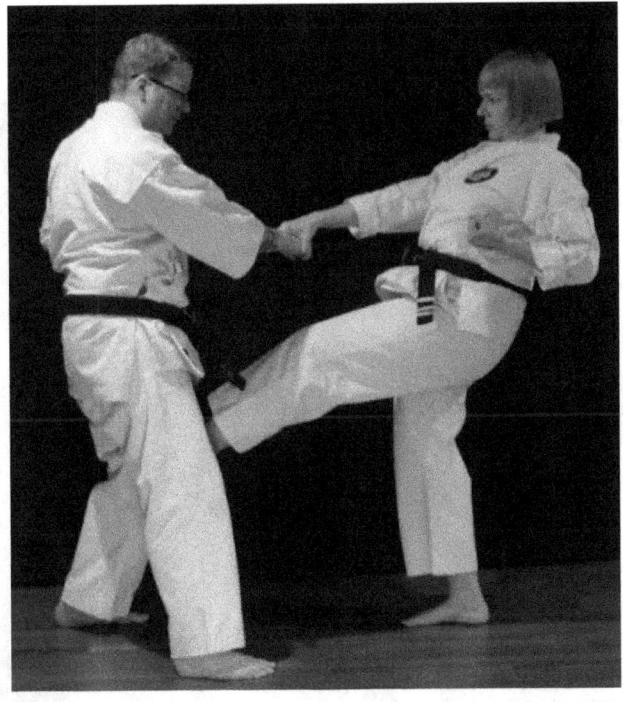

Techniques

Hiza Geri (Knee Joint Kick)
Knee and Ankle joint kicks are effective close range kicks for disabling an opponent.

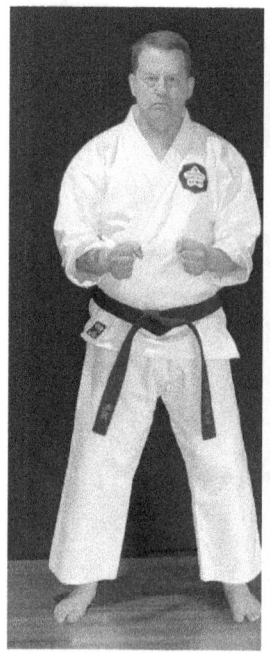
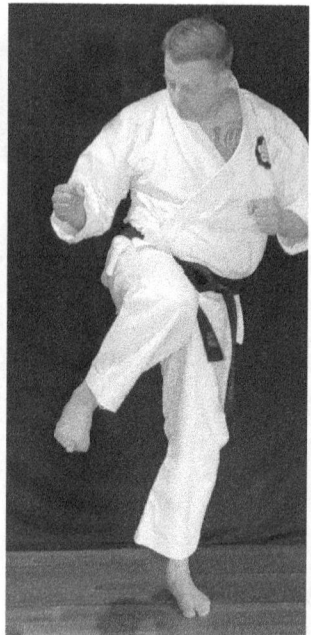
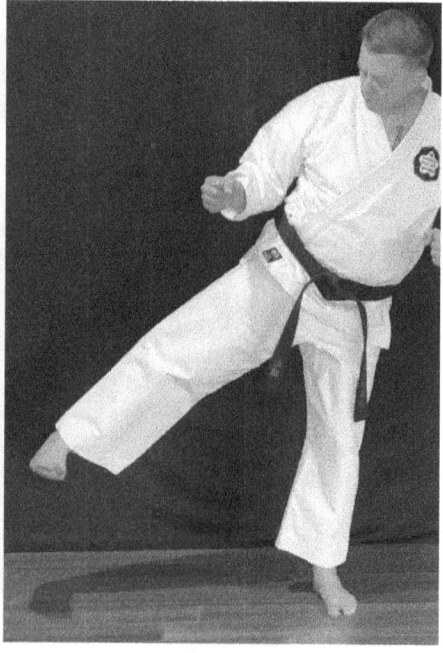

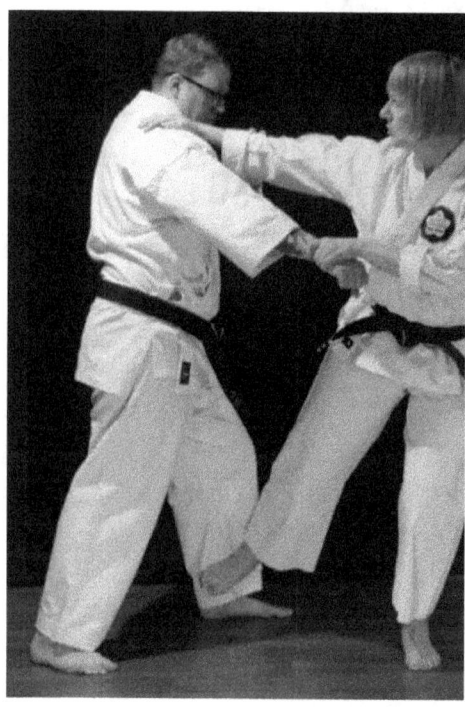
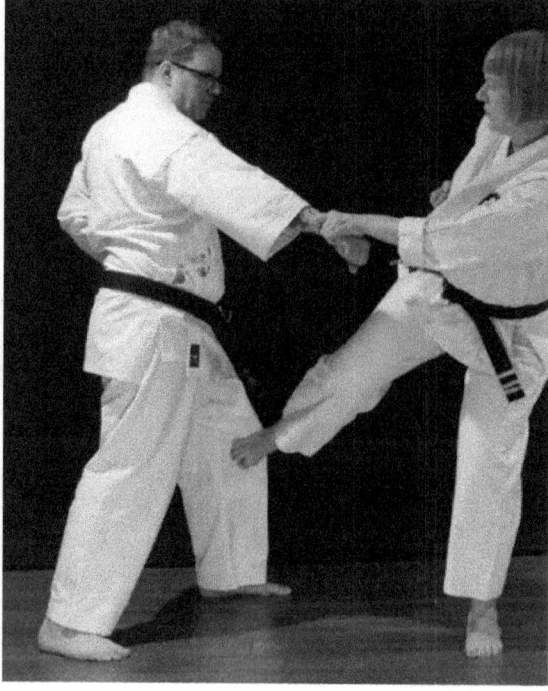

Techniques

Chudan Yoko Geri (Side Kick to the Ribs)
Yoko Geri are effective mid to long range kicks, particularly to the body.
Chamber the kick with the knee across the body for more power.

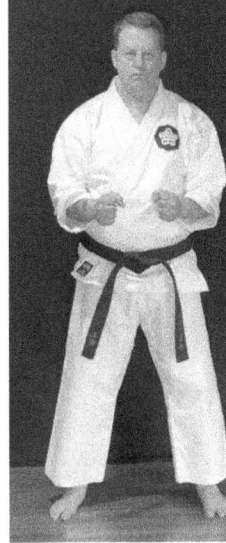
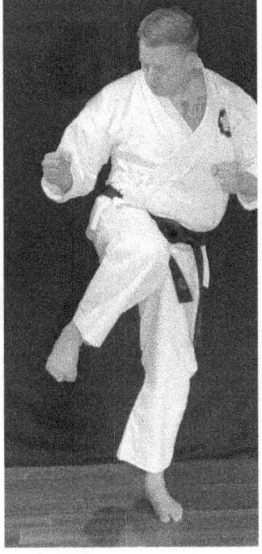
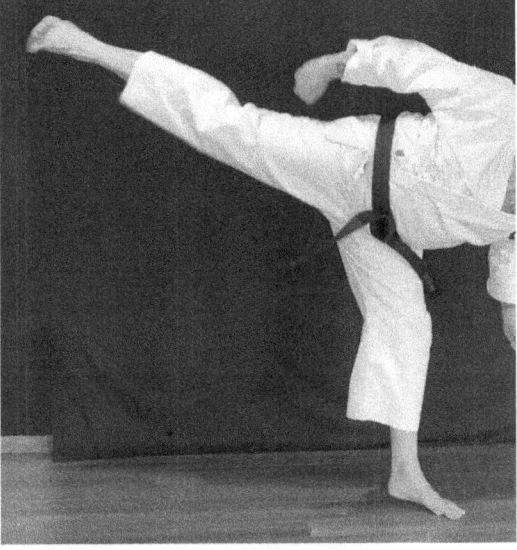
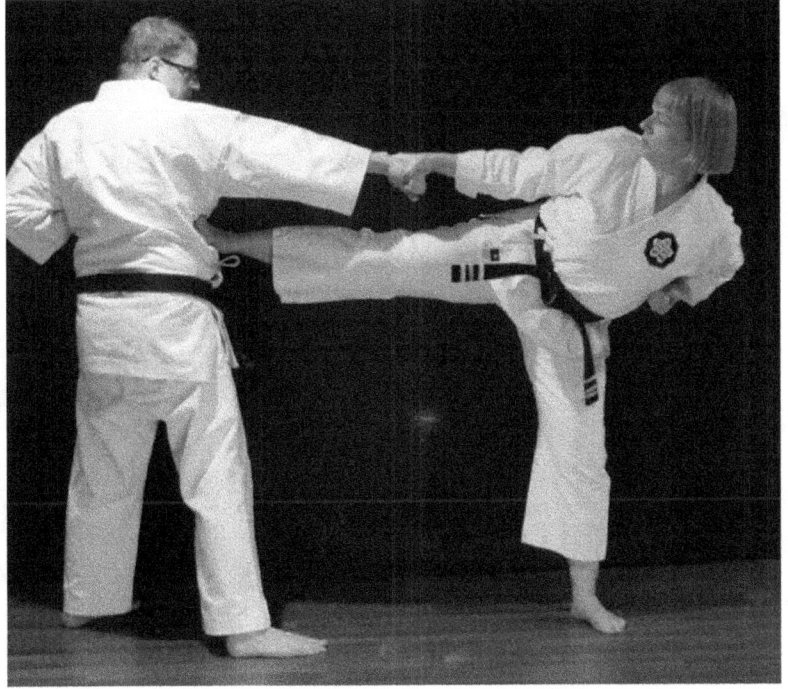

Techniques

Ushiro Geri (Back Kick)
Similar to Yoko Geri, Ushiro Geri is a good defensive kick with the knee pointed down.

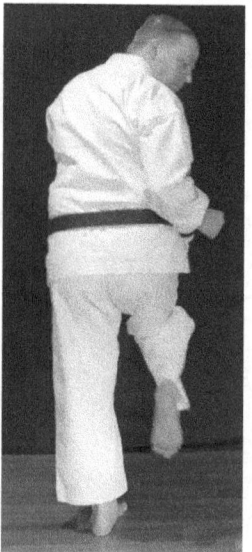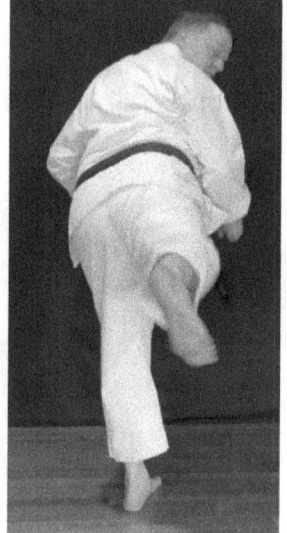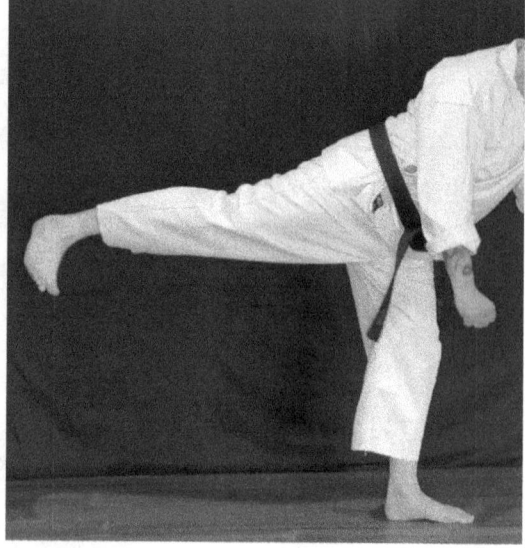

Mawashi Geri (Roundhouse Kick)
Chamber with foot behind the body and knee pointed at target, then kick with either the instep or ball of the foot. Mawashi Geri is generally a faster kick than the Yoko Geri, but less powerful.

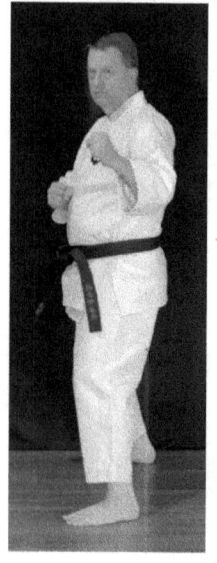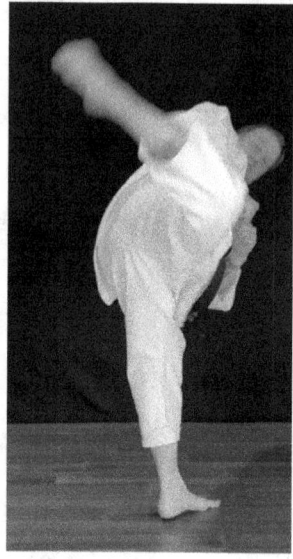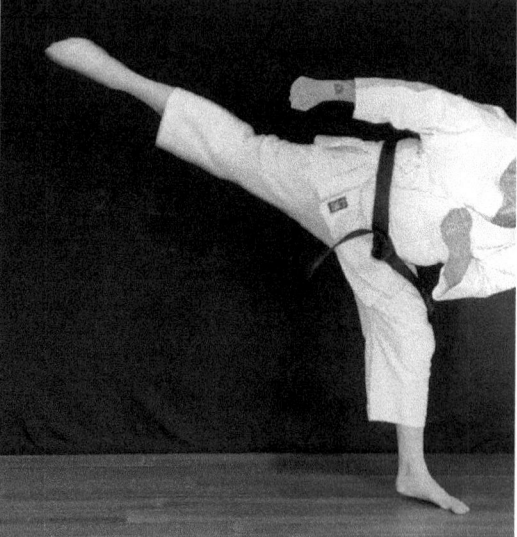

Techniques

Uchi Mikazuki Geri (Inside Crescent kick)
The shape of the kick is a crescent, starting on the inside and pushing out.

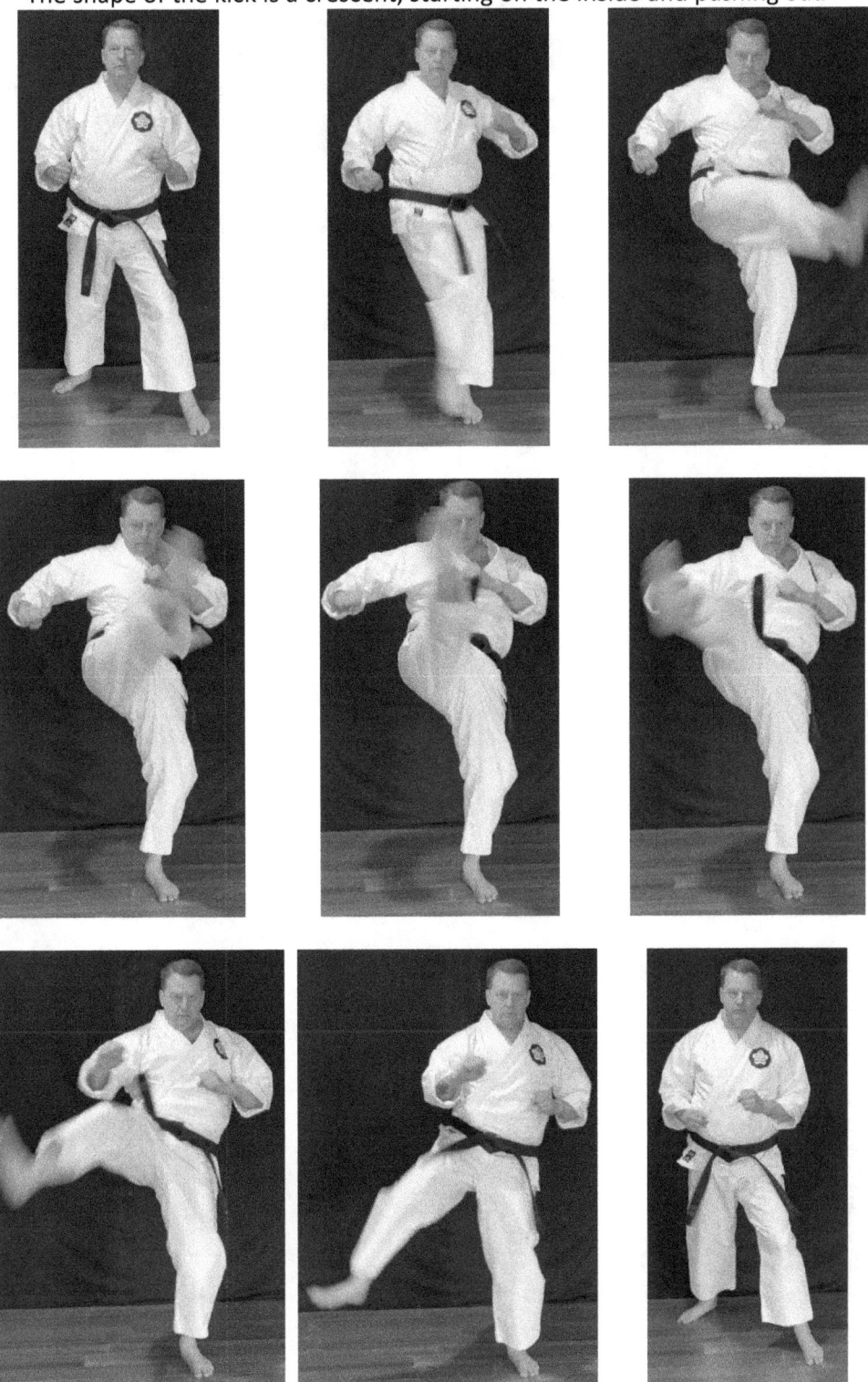

Techniques

Soto Mikazuki Geri (Outside Crescent kick)
The shape of the kick is a crescent, starting on the outside and pushing in.

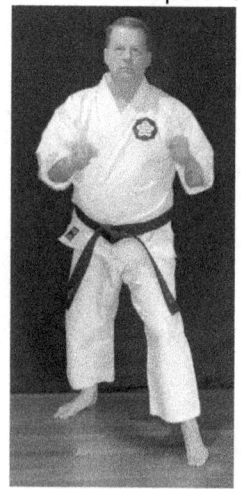
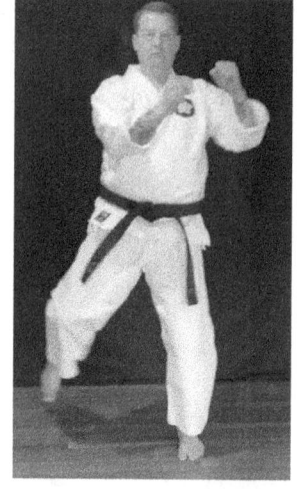
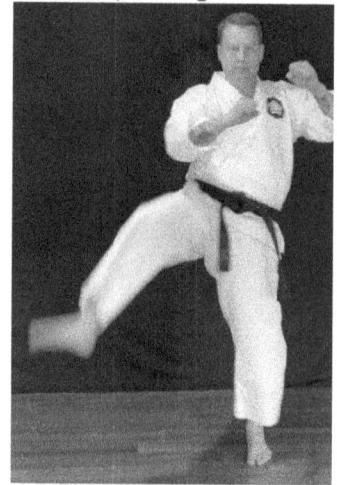
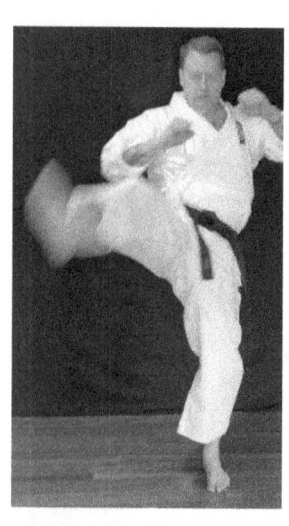
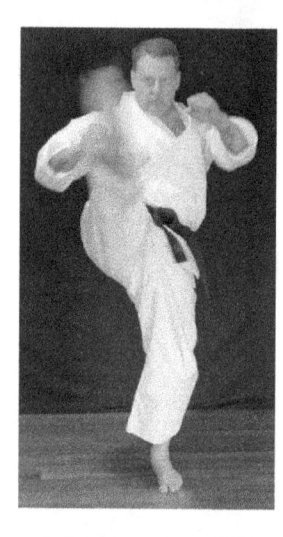
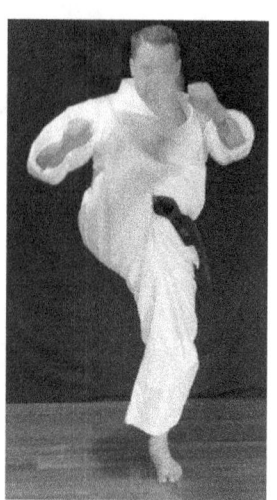
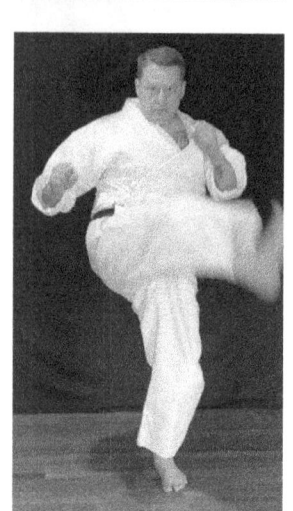
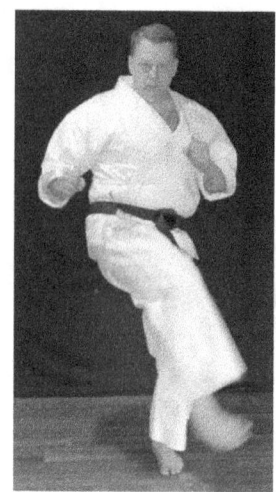
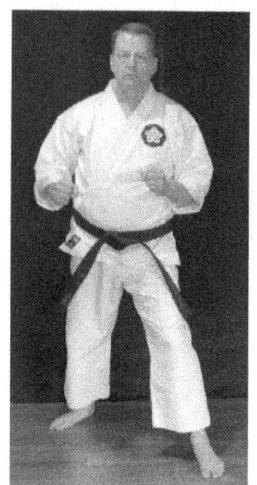

Uchi Mikazuki Geri (Inside crescent kick)
Use the edge of the foot to block the opponent's arms or legs.

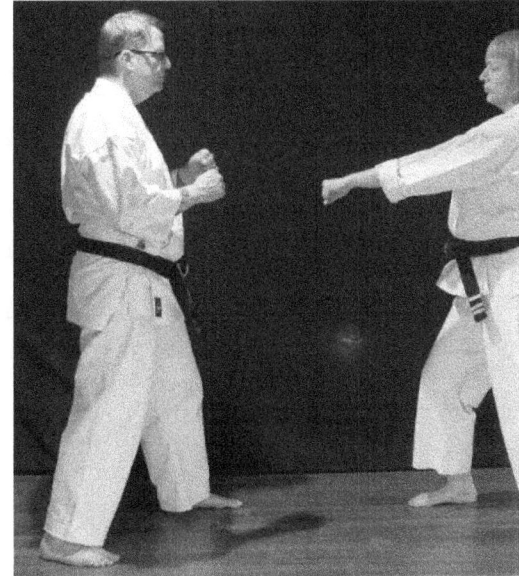
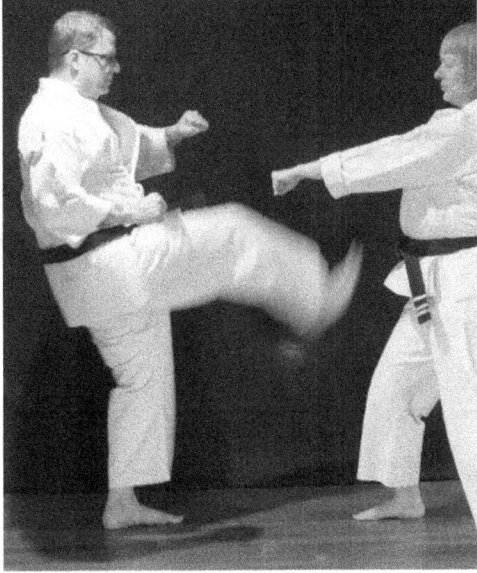
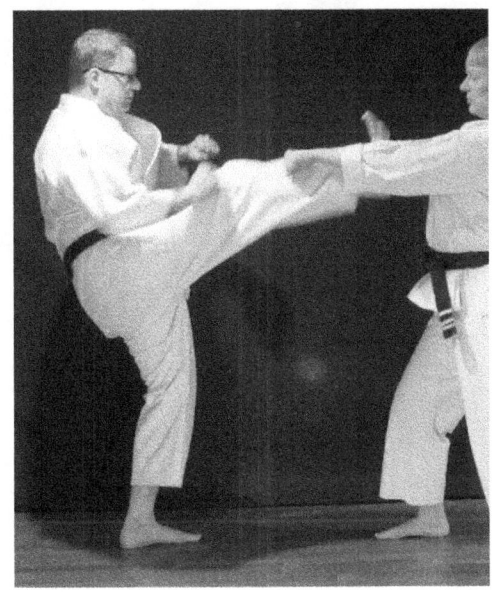

Techniques

Soto Mikazuki Geri (Outside crescent kick)
Use the sole of the foot to block the opponent's arms or hands.

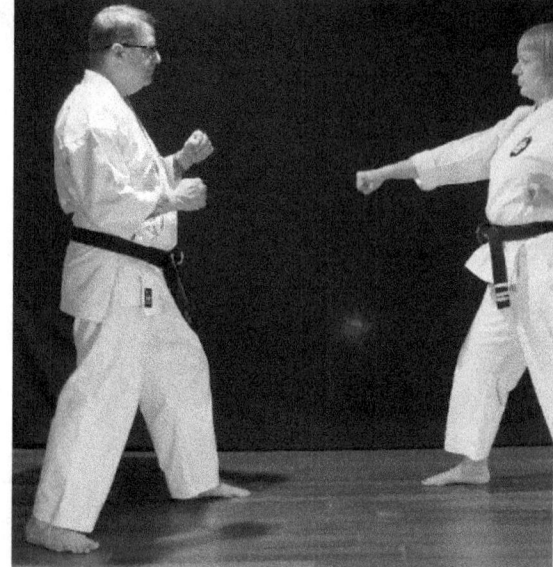
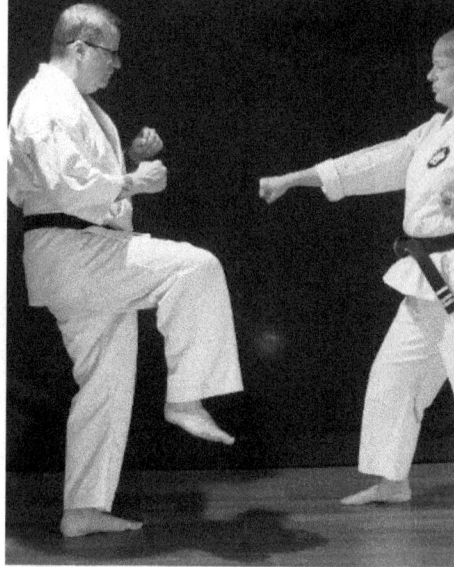
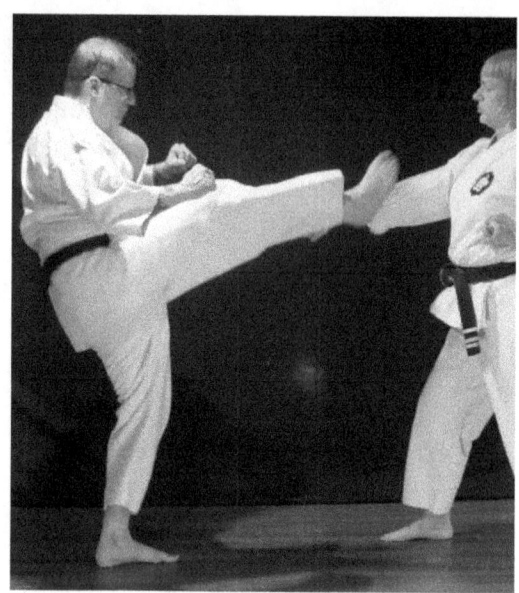

Koryu Kata

About Kata

The Japanese word *kata* means "form." Kata is one way a person can practice self-defense moves alone, and a way to commit these techniques to muscle memory. One might think of kata as learning a self-defense move, then linking it together with other self-defense moves, both offense and defense; that is basically kata. Historically, kata has been what sets apart one karate style from another. Each style has its own katas, some passed down from generation to generation. Outside of kata, most karate styles are basically the same. A punch is a punch, as is a kick, or a block, or a takedown. Kata and the way kata is trained are generally the distinguishing factors. It is a common belief that before karate went public in the beginning of the 20th Century, katas were performed in secret. This happened for a variety of reasons: officials disallowed organized martial arts and others just tried to protect their katas from other people, stealing moves. Whatever the reason, kata will oftentimes contain a vague idea of a self-defense move without fully committing to one interpretation. But this is not a bad thing. Situations and even body size can determine how to use certain techniques. Real life will never allow someone to use kata moves exactly as the kata is completed, but it can give the practitioner ideas that can be adapted to any situation. This is why kata should be studied, not just performed.

On the surface, kata can appear to be little more than performance art. In fact, the moves are taught with the choreographed precision of a dance. And like a dance, there is a rhythm to it, a cadence, and of course the all-over muscle development and cardio benefits are obvious. There are people who practice kata specifically for performance, and they train that way, not for self-defense. Perhaps if one gets a prize for a demonstration, entertainment may be the best way to describe it. Of course this is not the traditional meaning of kata. Kata has always been designed for self-defense, and the moves are meant to be analyzed to extract self-defense moves. The need for precision in kata is to discipline the mind and body together. In addition, there is a spiritual aspect to kata.

When one learns a kata, it is practiced in every manner possible: every direction, with a group, alone, wearing a weighted vest, in the dark, outside, etc. One might study a video of himself practicing a kata, or of other people, looking at every step, hand placement, and target. An instructor will watch the student practicing, critiquing every move until the kata is completed exactly the way it was taught. In kata, perfection is sought in every move, learning body control, yet always remembering that these moves are self-defense moves, not just exercise. And if one learns a kata and trains multiple times, multiple days, each time as intense as the last, always visualizing an opponent, always trying to complete each move with perfection, always with the same focus, only thinking of the kata, not even the whole kata but each sequence of moves and only those sequences of moves, ignoring everything else outside of the kata, then it will become part of the student's instinct or subconscious mind.

As for self-defense and the moves within a kata, it comes down to practice. For example, anyone can attend a self-defense workshop. At this workshop he can see most of the self-defense moves they would ever need in his lifetime. But will it occur to that person to practice what he has learned?

The only way to train technique properly is to practice it over and over until it cannot be done incorrectly. This takes a level of discipline that becomes the main by-product of karate, what many people are seeking, but have no idea how to achieve. It takes a certain passion for the art to perform these actions as many times as is really needed. Someone might learn kata from a book or video, but an instructor is critical for corrections and helping with the meaning of the moves. An instructor should know how much material to teach at any one time, how much to correct so as not to frustrate the student, and help the student maintain what he has learned. Human beings are inherently lazy, so an instructor can help keep a student on the right path. An instructor may assign supplementary exercises to do in addition to kata, which will not only make the kata easier to practice properly but give the body a break from the tedium. Of course, the "perfect method" to the moves of a kata is a matter of opinion and interpretation, but an instructor should have a uniform way the kata should be practiced. A move in the kata may seem unimportant, but keeping a standard to kata helps keep the mind sharp.

Various styles of martial arts have different numbers of kata with varying degree of difficulty and depth. Typically, a martial arts style begins with a somewhat easy kata and the last kata would be the hardest, or most important. Ketsugo Goju-Ryu currently has twenty-four katas including weapons katas (twelve traditional and twelve non-traditional). Regarding the specific bunkai, or analysis, for each kata, Shodai encouraged his students to come up with their own explanations. He said that his instructor, Seikichi Toguchi did not tell the students what every move meant. Toguchi preferred students to learn the movements of the kata first, then come up with ideas of what the moves mean. Shodai felt the same way. Learn the kata first, then open the mind to what a move could be, not regurgitate what someone says it means. Sometimes if Shodai was in the mood for it, he might tell a student what he thought a move was, or what he intended it to be in one of his own katas, but he also said, "if it works, then that's the meaning." If a student came up with an idea for a move, he would want that person to show him. If he liked it, he might agree with the possibilities, but he also might poke holes in it, testing how much the student really thought it out.

Beyond the bunkai, it will always be up to the student to achieve the value of kata. Some people cannot and will never see the benefits of kata, and for them it will always be a waste of time. The fact is that katas can be difficult, especially when a student is tired, forgetful, out of shape, or just not in the mood for it. An instructor will correct every move a student gets wrong so many times the student may feel like he will never do it properly. But if a student pushes through the difficulties of a kata until it clicks, if he accepts the fact that failure and correction is the basis for growth, it might even be enlightening.

In karate, one cannot overemphasize the importance of kata, and the tradition contained in so many of them. The changing of traditional katas, therefore, is a touchy subject, but I will contend that people have always changed moves in katas. Kanryo Higashionna changed Sanchin kata to closed fists instead of open hands, and towards the end of his life Chojun Miyagi took the three turns out of Sanchin because he did not think a student should turn his back on his teacher. His senior students put the turns back in after he died (explained in Seikichi Toguchi's book, *Okinawan Goju-Ryu II*). Variations on traditional katas exist, but as time goes on, kata within specific karate styles are getting more and more streamlined. Still, no one has a patent on a particular kata, so anyone can do Kururunfa, for example, any way he wants and still call it Kururunfa. The "standard" is only official according to the organization promoting it. The bottom line is that if a student practices kata seriously, he will benefit from it. I have never heard anyone say, "I would've won that fight if only I had practiced Seiunchin with a sliding step instead of a hard stomp."

When examining kata, position is important. The embusen of a kata is the line in which the kata moves. For the purposes of this book, when looking at the images of the kata, it may be obvious which way the kata moves, but other katas are more complex in terms of angles. Occasionally an actual degree of angle will be referenced. The angle will originate at the starting point, facing forward, called the Shomen. The direction (right or left) will be described from the student's point of view.

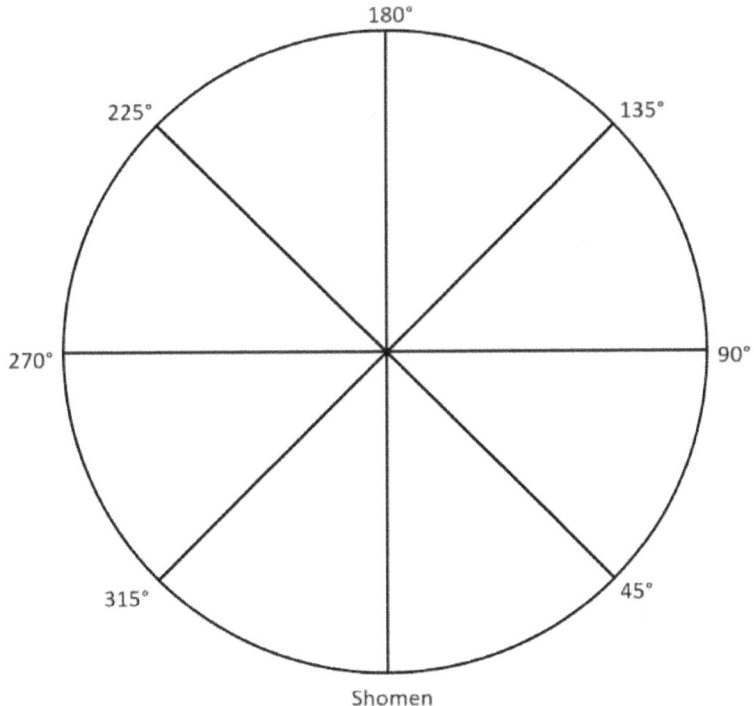

Koryu, or traditional kata in Goju-Ryu Karate are considered those created by or taught to Chojun Miyagi. Many of the traditional katas in Goju-Ryu have naming roots in Buddhism. For example, the kata Suparempei means one hundred and eight, Sanseru means thirty-six, Sepai means eighteen. The number one hundred and eight is prominent in Buddhism, made by multiplying smell, touch, taste, hearing, sight, and unconsciousness (six) by pain, pleasure, or neutral, (x three = eighteen) then by internal or external, (eighteen x two = thirty-six) then by past, present, and future (thirty-six x three = one hundred and eight). When designing katas, some of the moves represent these numbers. For example, in the kata Sanchin, the karateka steps three times while punching.

In this volume we will look at eleven katas, six traditional Goju-Ryu katas, and five katas unique to Ketsugo Goju-Ryu. The six traditional katas examined here are Gekisai Ichi, Gekisai Ni, Saifa, Sanchin, Seiunchin, and Sepai. The five Ketsugo Goju-Ryu katas examined here are Kihon Ichi, Gekisai San, Hon'nogeki, Genshin, and Isshoni San.

Gekisai Ichi

Gekisai Ichi and Gekisai Ni are traditional Goju-Ryu katas that translate respectively, "attack and smash one" and "attack and smash two." These katas were created around 1940 by Chojun Miyagi and Nagamine Shoshin[1] as beginner katas, to introduce the basic forms of karate (kihon) to middle school students in Okinawa, to help bring about the standardization of karate, and to teach a basic set of techniques for self-defense. Gekisai kata were strongly influenced by the Shuri-te techniques that Miyagi learned from Anko Itosu.

Below is the method by which Ketsugo Goju-Ryu performs Gekisai Ichi kata. Complete details about each move are not included, as this is simply a demonstration. This demonstration is not meant to imply that it is the only way to do it, but it is the way at Ketsugo Goju-Ryu.

These are the Japanese terms used for this kata. Bear in mind, karate terms are not completely streamlined. There are terms that were used in the middle of the 20th Century that are no longer used today. Oftentimes there are more than one term that can be used for the same technique. The important thing is not what it is called, but the technique itself.

Age Empi Uchi – Rising Elbow Strike	**Morote Zuki** – Double Punch
Age Uke - Rising Block	**Musubi Dachi** - Attention Stance, Toes Out
Barai - Sweeping Block	
Chudan - Middle	**Rei** – Bow (Respect)
Dachi – Stance	**Shiko Dachi** - Straddle Leg Stance
Fumikomi Geri – Stamping Kick	**Shuto Uchi** - Chop Strike
Gedan – Low	**Tettsui Uchi** - Hammer Fist Strike
Gyaku Zuki - Reverse Punch	**Tsuki/-Zuki** - Punch
Hajime – Command to Begin	**Uchi** – Strike
Heiko Dachi - Parallel Stance	**Uke** – Block (Receive)

Gekisai Ichi

Jodan - High	**Uraken Uchi** - Back Fist Strike
Mae Keage Geri – Front Snap Kick	**Yoi** – Ready Command
Morote Chudan Uke – Double Chest Block	**Yoko** - Side
Morote Sukui Uke – Augmented Scooping Block	**Zenkutsu Dachi** - Forward Leaning Stance

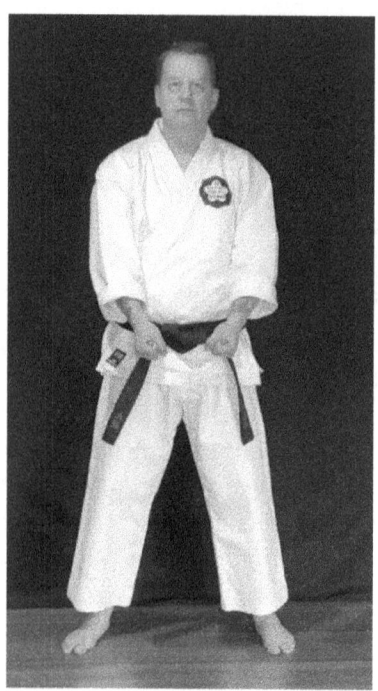

Heiko Dachi

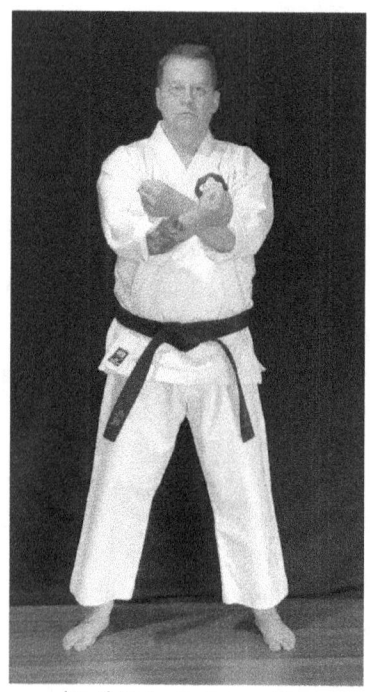

(Yoi) Brings Arms Up,
Crossed at the Wrist

Gekisai Ichi

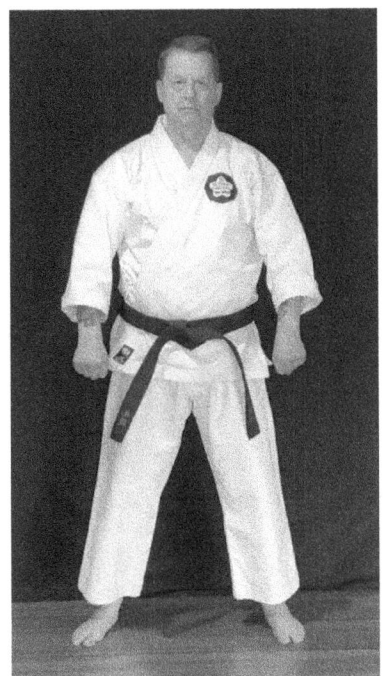
Brings Arms Down

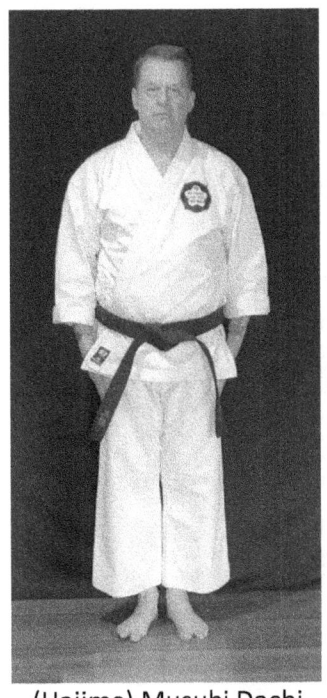
(Hajime) Musubi Dachi

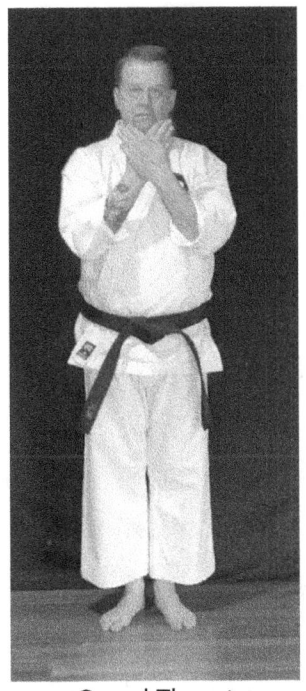
Guard Throat

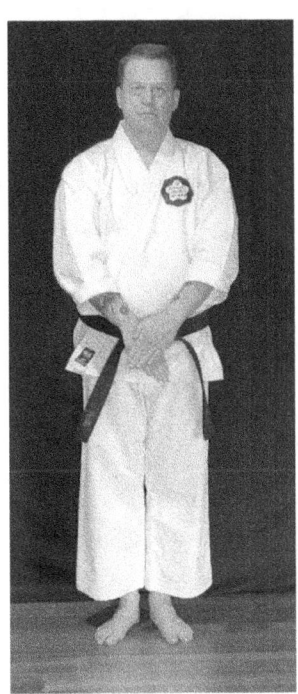
Turn Hands Down to Guard Groin

Gekisai Ichi

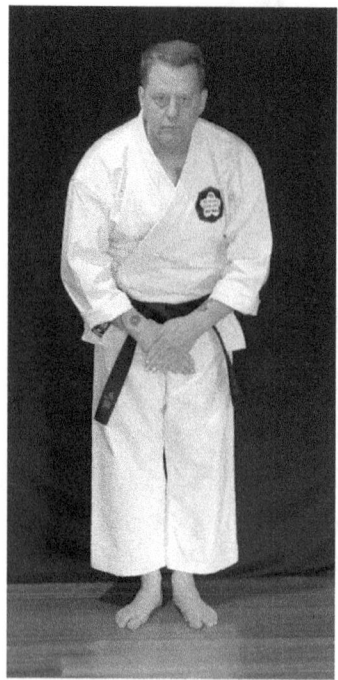
Rei

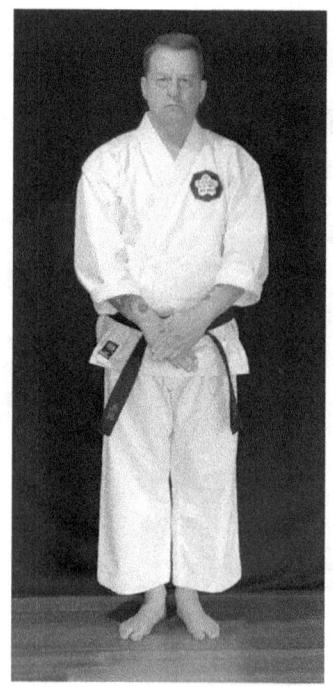
Musubi Dachi

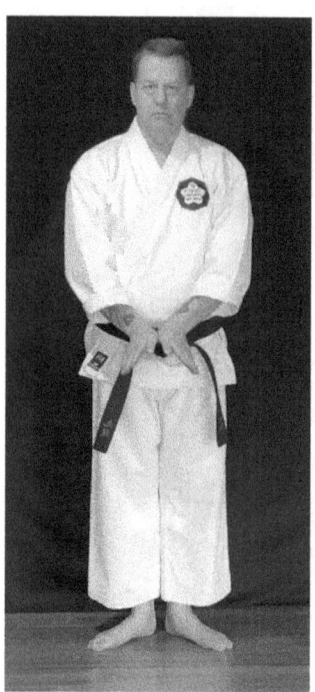
Open Hands at the Palm Heel and Feet at the Heel

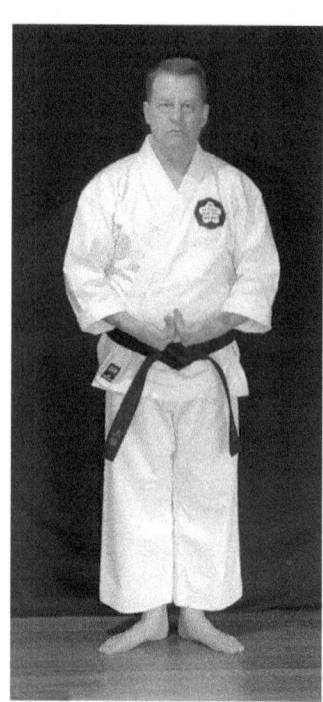
Complete Morote Sukui Uke, Bring Hands Up Against the Body, Keeping Back of Hands Together

Gekisai Ichi

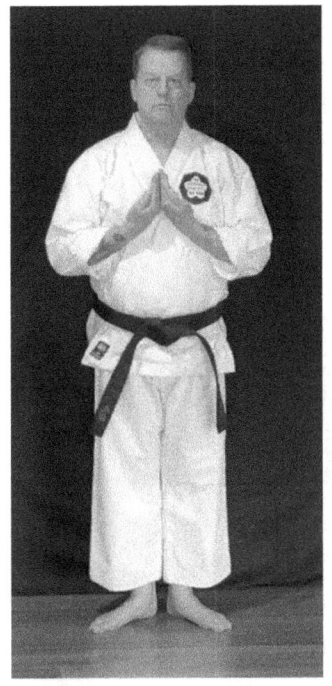 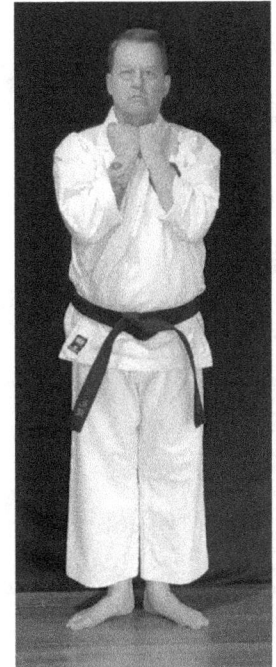

Close Hands Under Chin

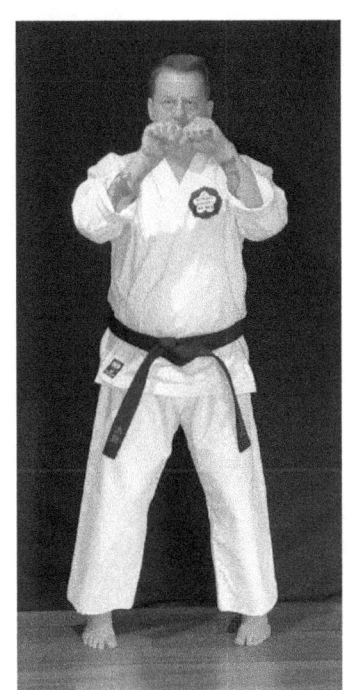 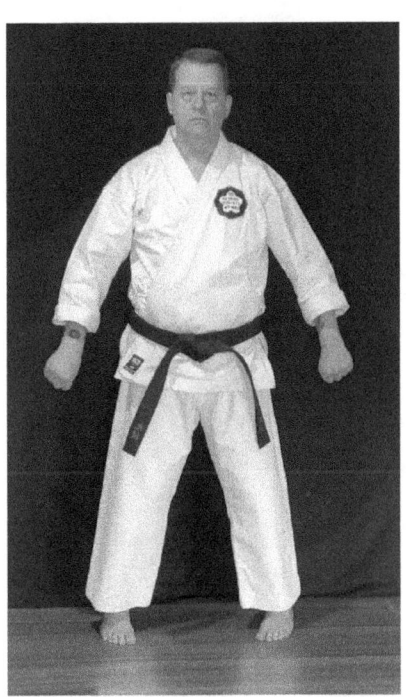

Arc Hands Out and Down While Moving Heels Out

Gekisai Ichi

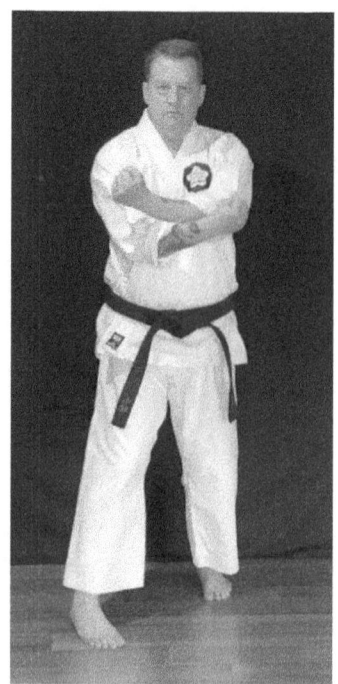 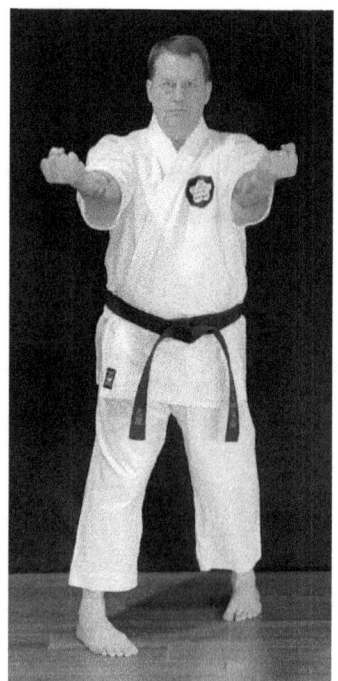

Complete Morote Chudan Uke

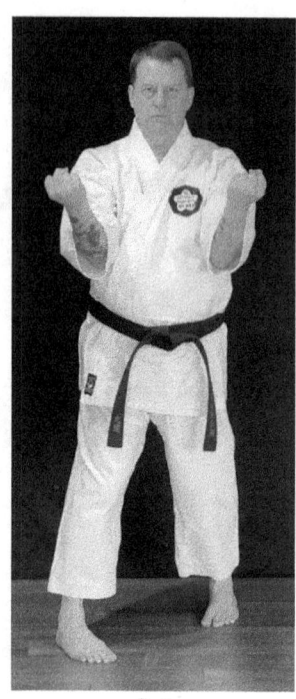 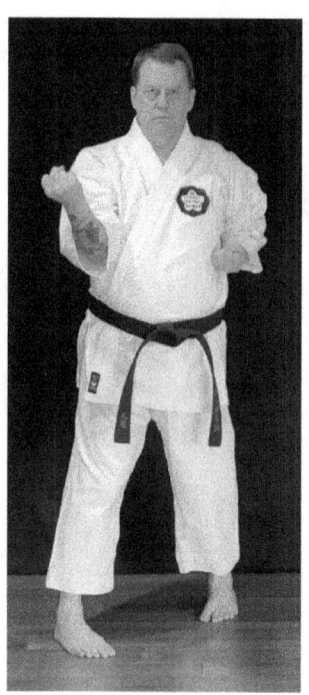

Set
Chamber Left Hand

Gekisai Ichi

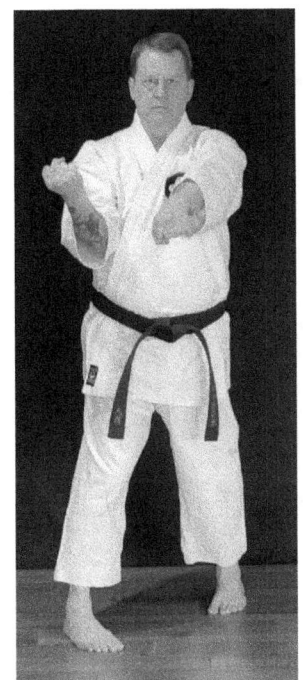
Complete Left Chudan Zuki

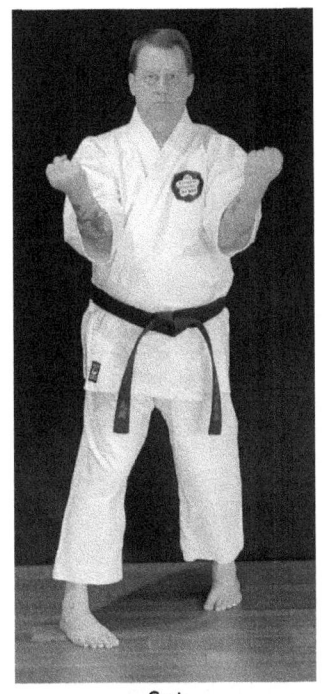
Set

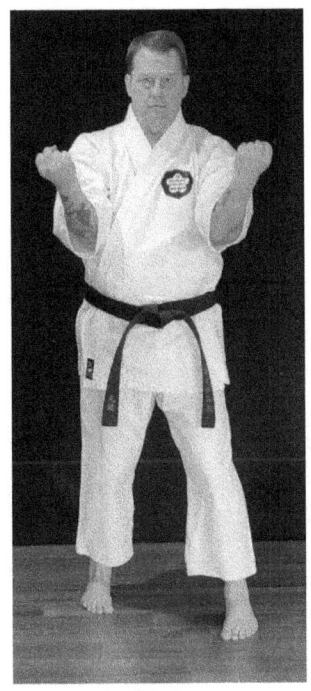
Step

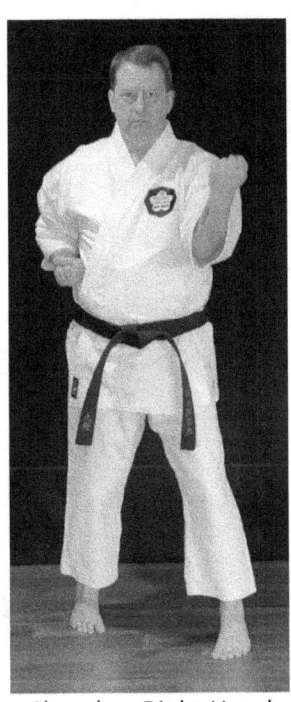
Chamber Right Hand

Gekisai Ichi

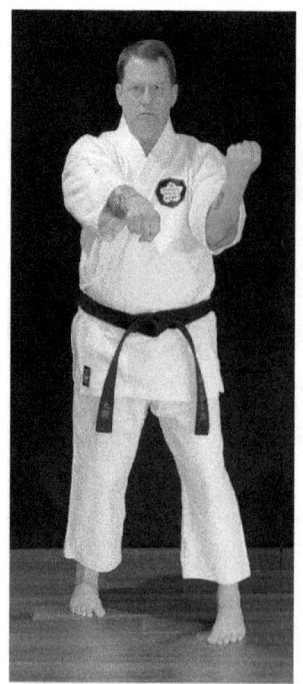
Complete Right Chudan Zuki

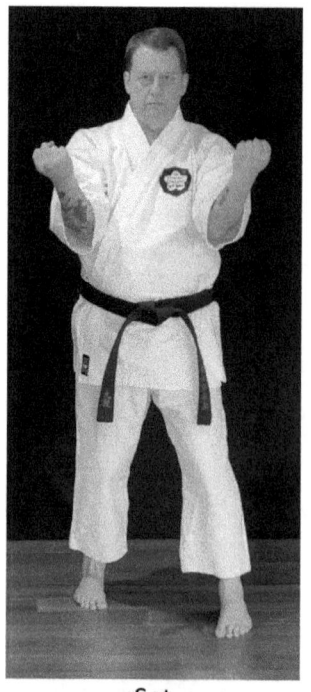
Set

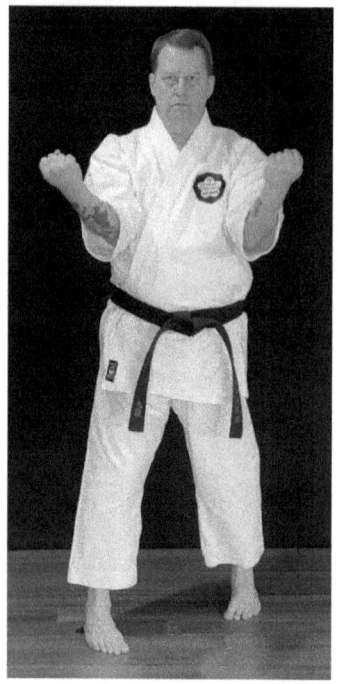
Step

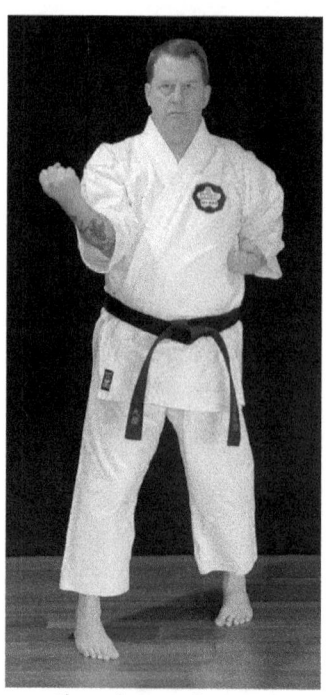
Chamber Left Hand

Gekisai Ichi

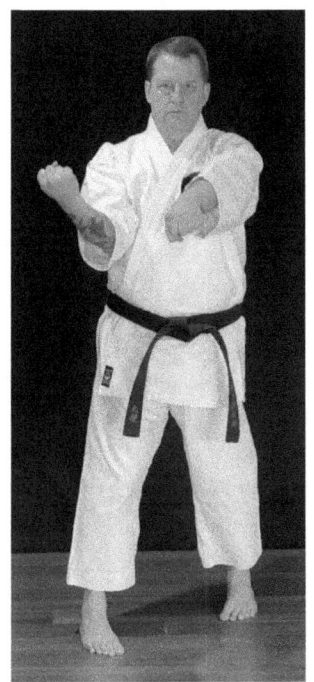
Complete Left Chudan Zuki

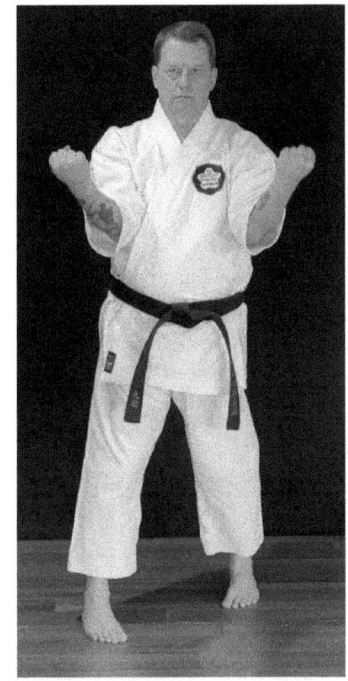
Set

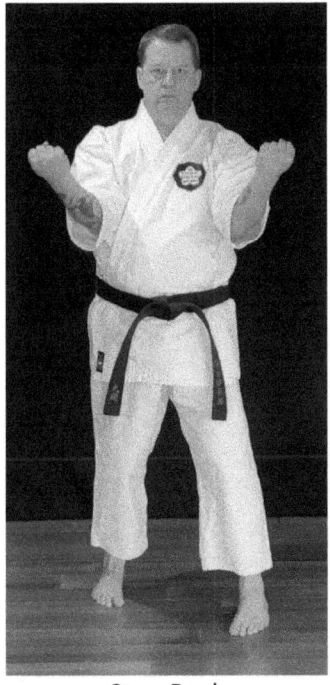
Step Back

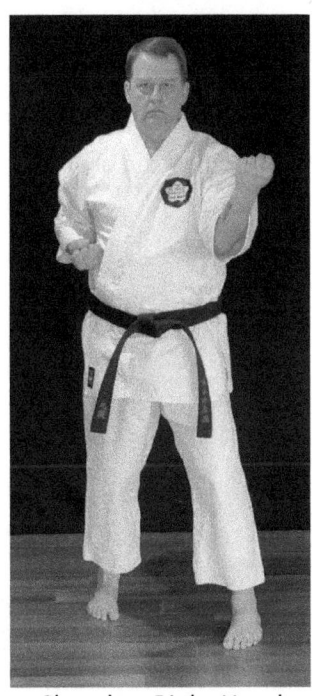
Chamber Right Hand

Gekisai Ichi

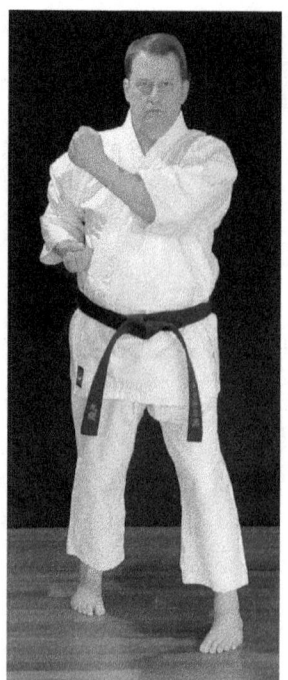 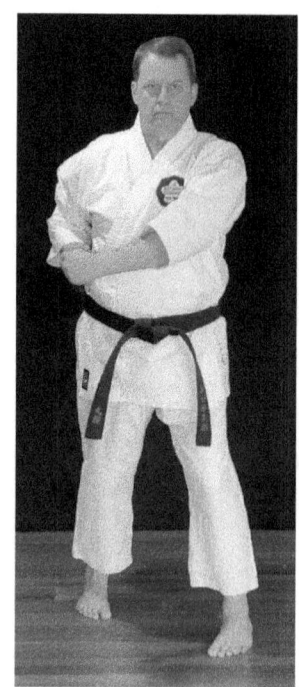

Complete Left Gedan Barai

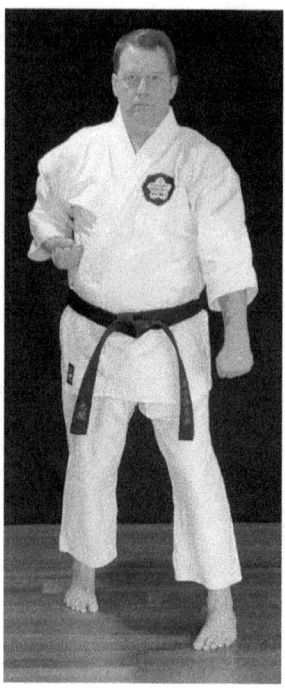 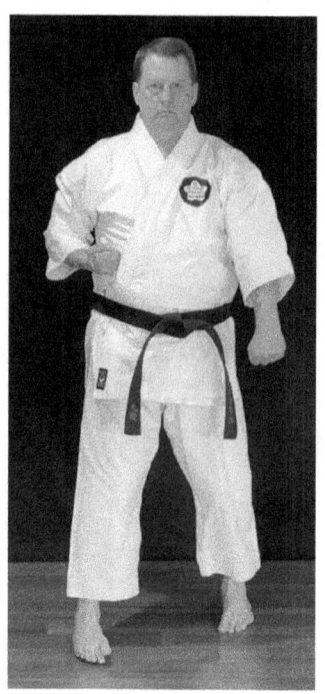

Gedan Barai (cont.)   Step Back

Gekisai Ichi

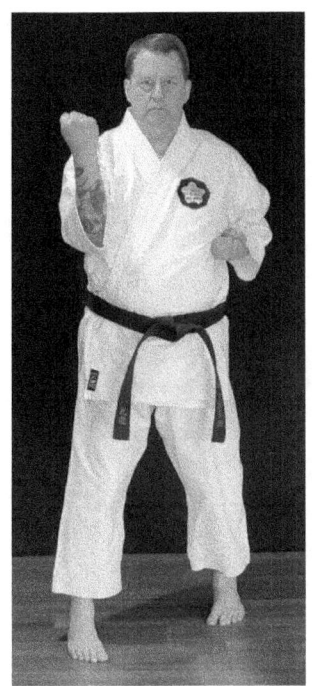 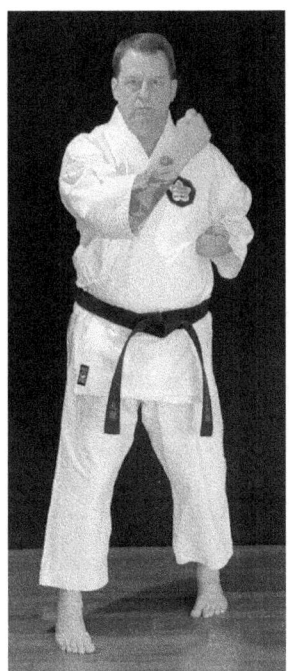

Complete Right Gedan Barai

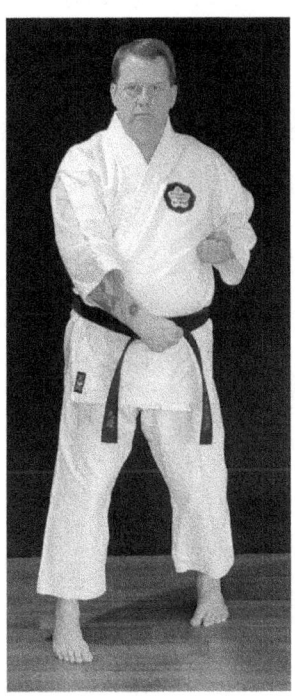 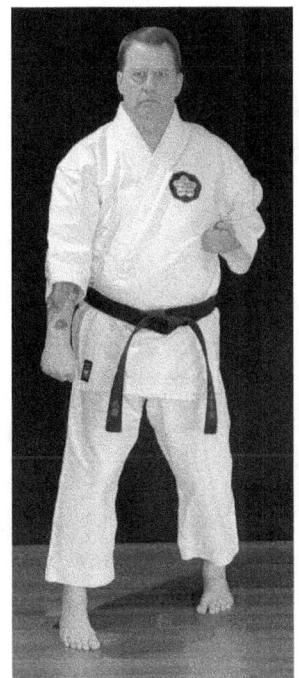

Gedan Barai (cont.)

Gekisai Ichi

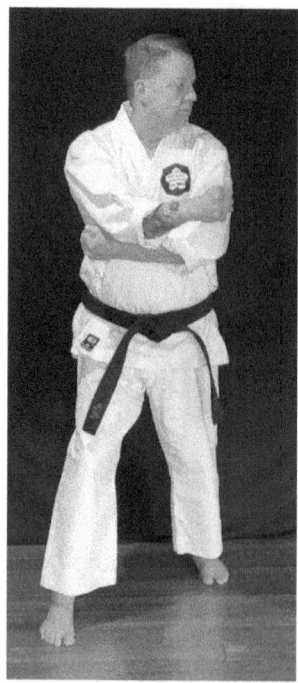

Look Left, then Begin Left Jodan Age Uke

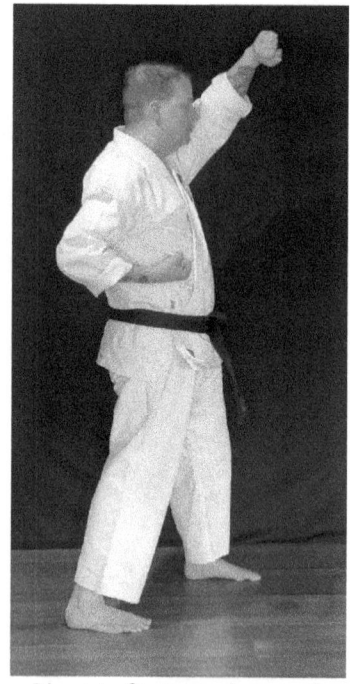

Pivot Left, Complete Left Jodan Age Uke

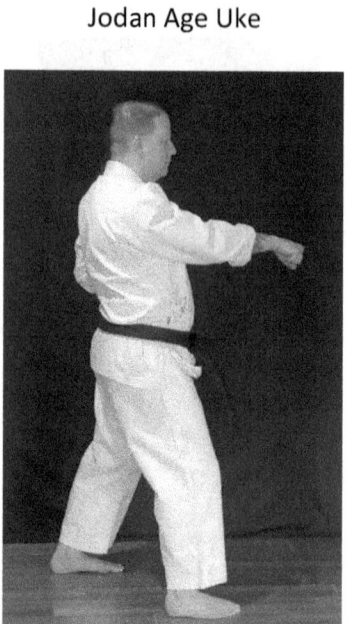

Step, then Complete Right Chudan Zuki

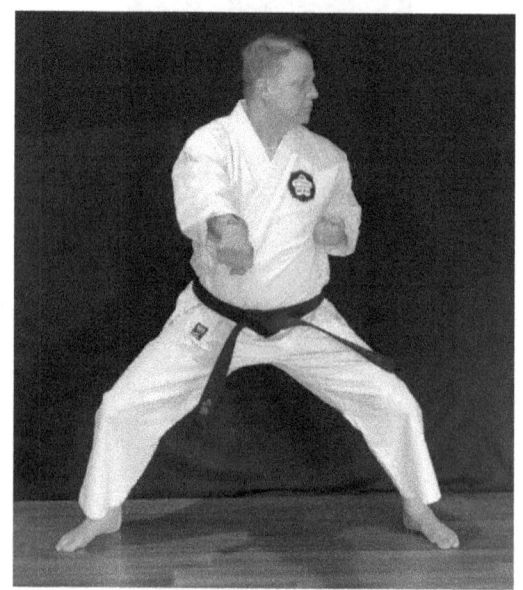

Right Foot Step Back into Shiko Dachi Facing Forward

Gekisai Ichi

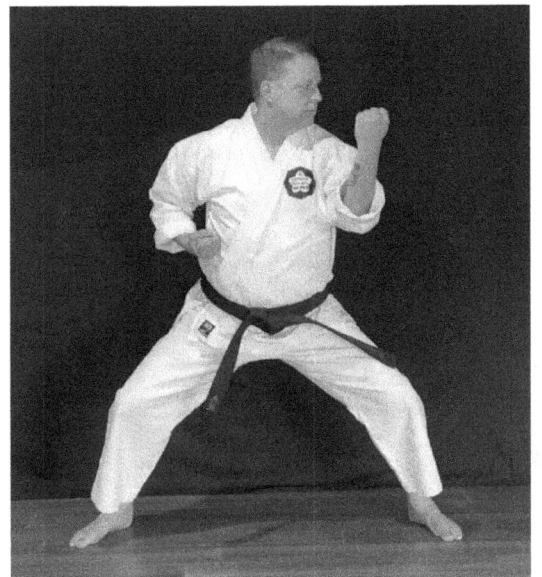
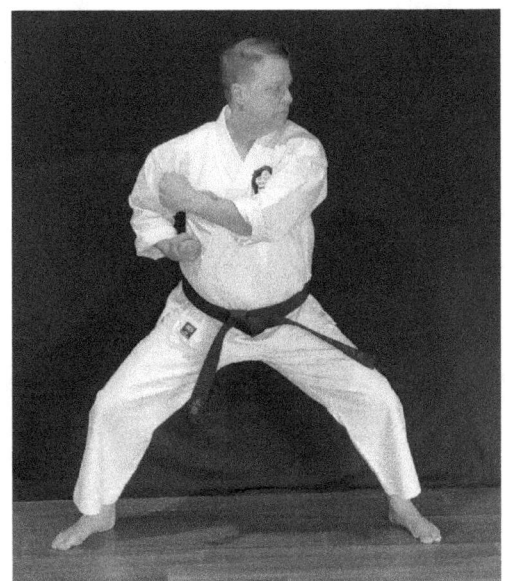

Complete Left Gedan Yoko Tettsui Uchi

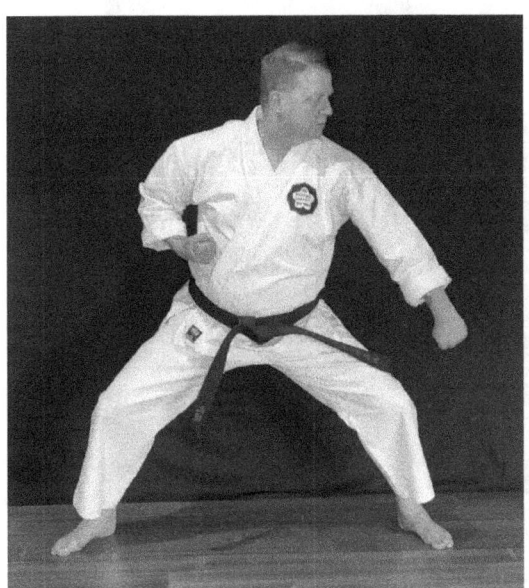
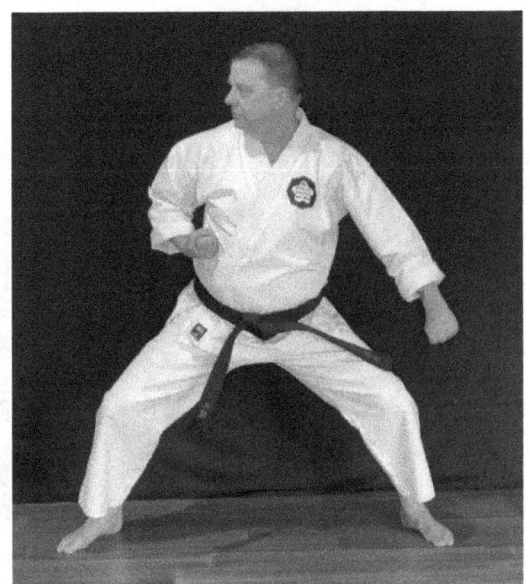

Gedan Tettsui Uchi (cont.)   Look Right

Gekisai Ichi

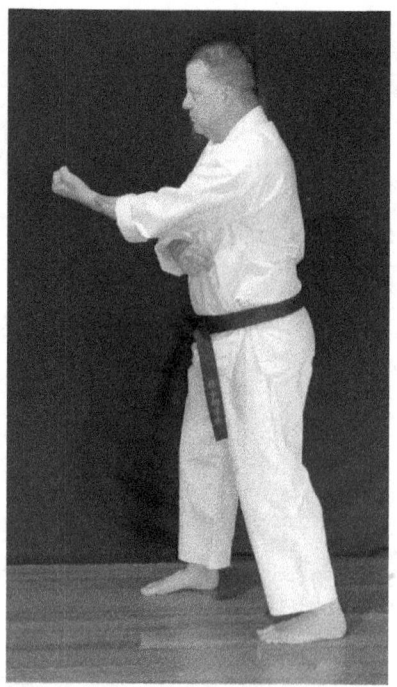 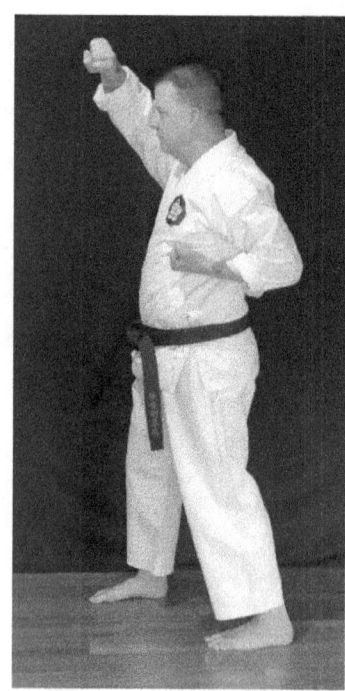

Pivot Right with Small Left Step, Complete Right Jodan Age Uke

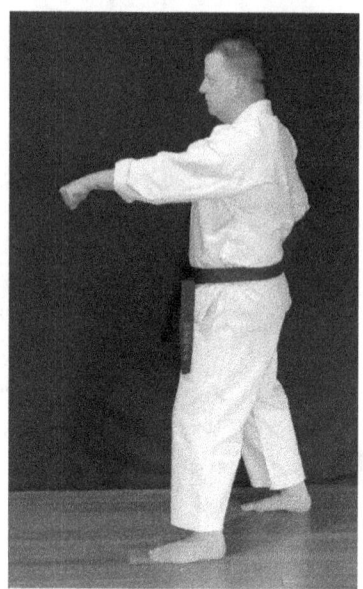 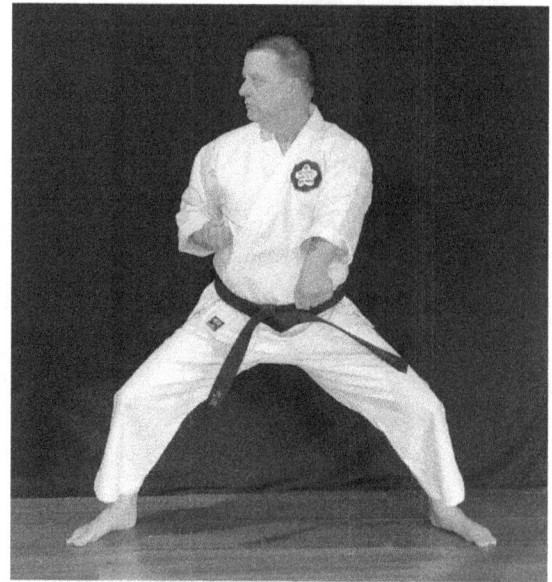

Step, Complete Left
Chudan Zuki

Left Foot Step Back into Shiko
Dachi Facing Forward

Gekisai Ichi

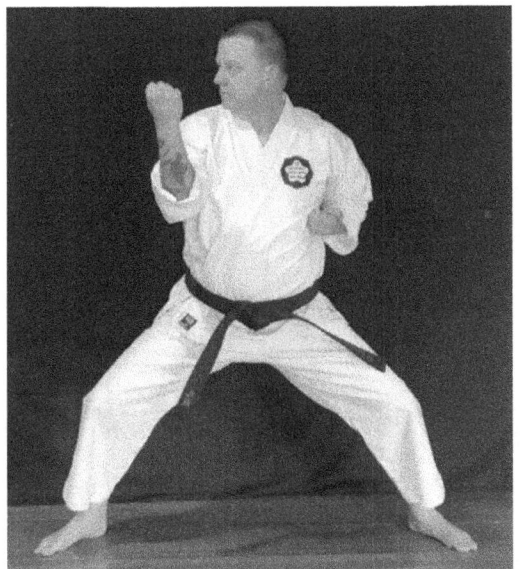
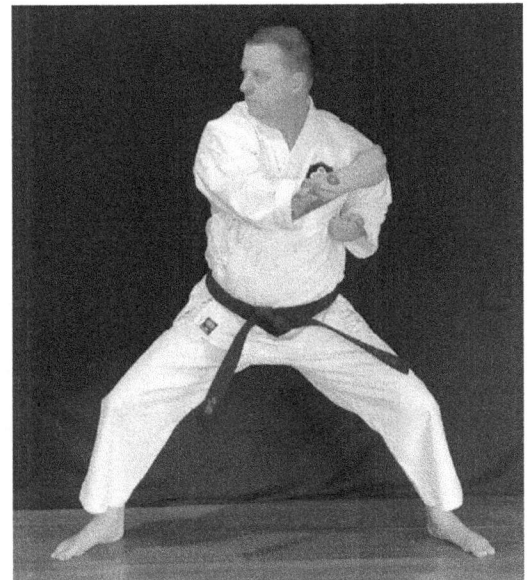

Complete Right Gedan Yoko Tettsui Uchi

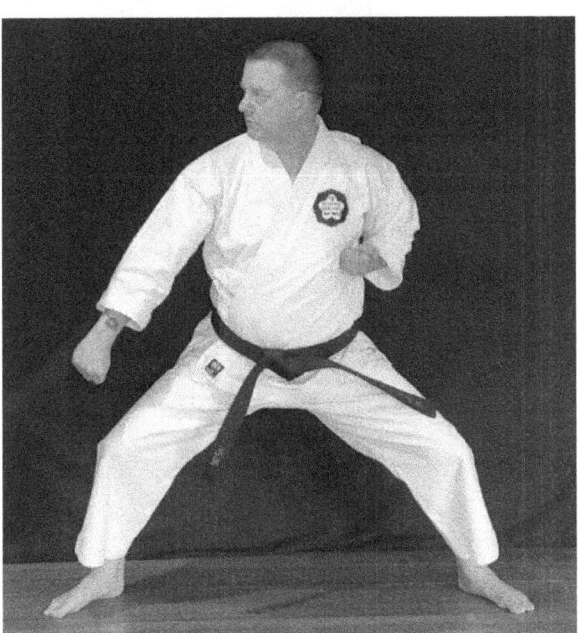

Gedan Yoko Tettsui Uchi (cont.)

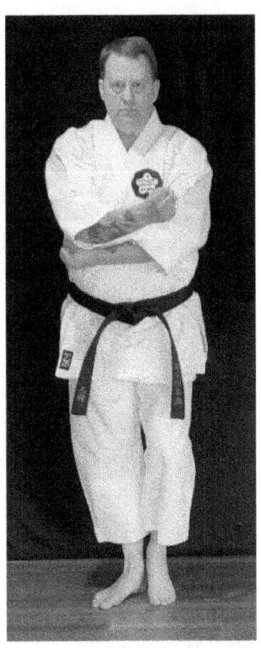

Step, Complete Slow Left Chudan Uke (inhale)

Gekisai Ichi

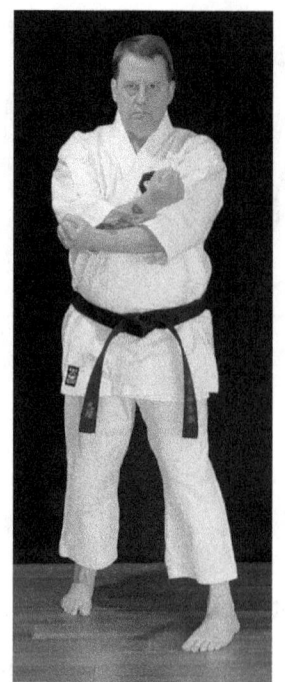 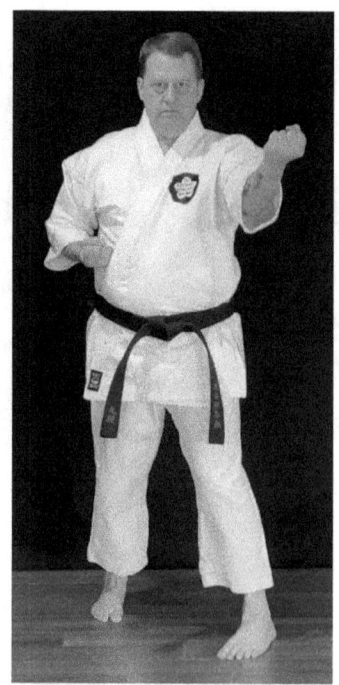

Chudan Uke (inhale) (cont.)

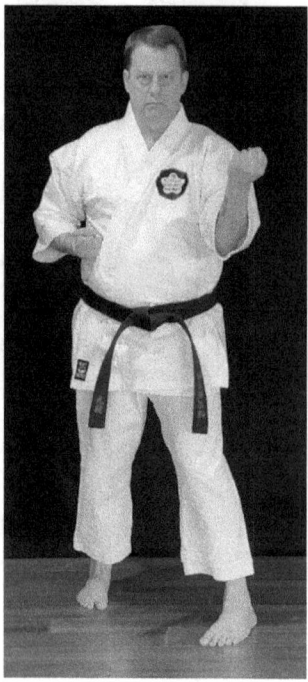 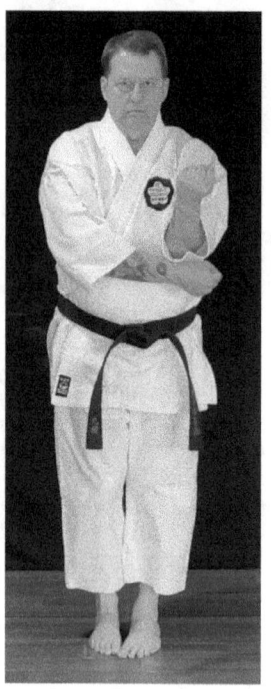

Set (exhale)   Step, Complete Slow Right Chudan Uke (inhale)

Gekisai Ichi

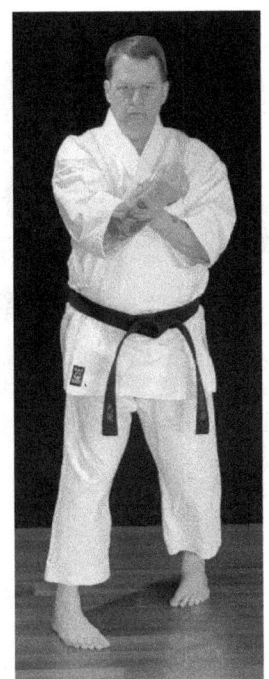
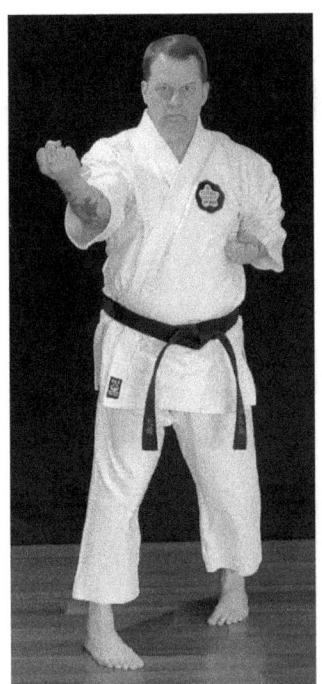

Chudan Uke (inhale) (cont.)

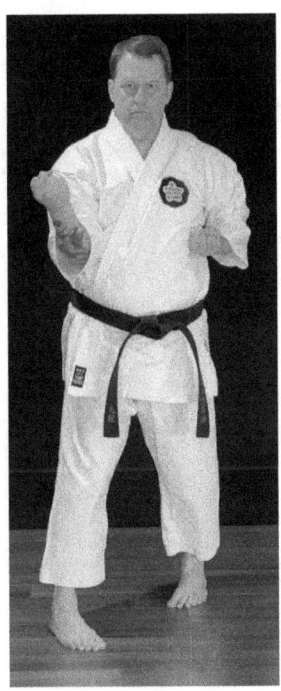
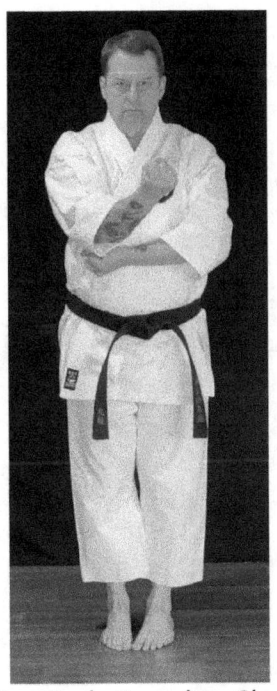

Set (exhale)

Step Back, Complete Slow
Left Chudan Uke (inhale)

Gekisai Ichi

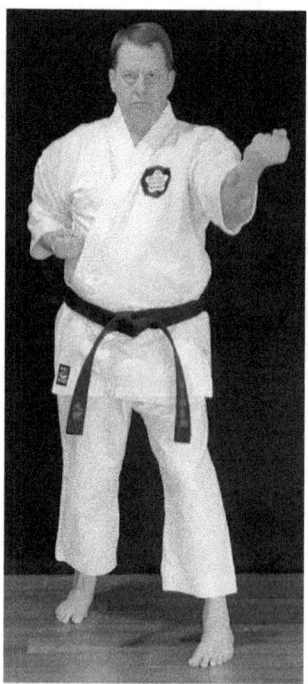

Slow Chudan Uke (inhale) (cont.)

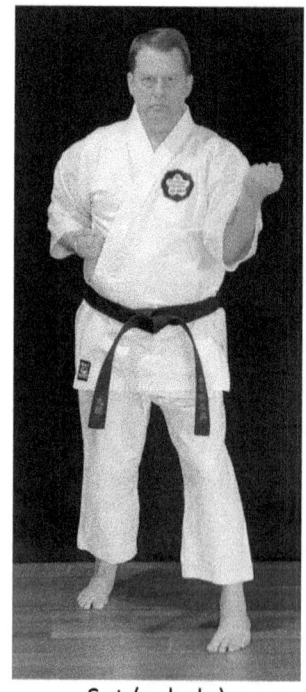

Set (exhale)

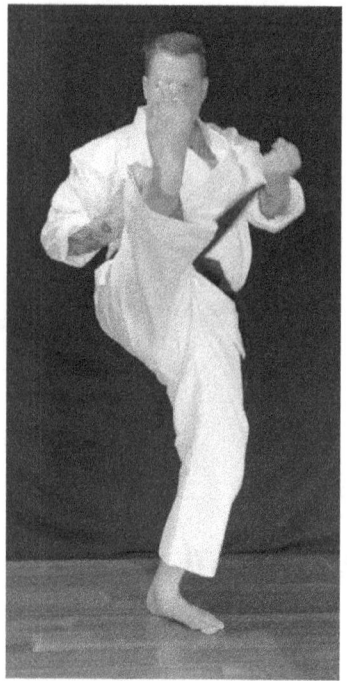

Complete Right Jodan
Mae Keage Geri (kiai)

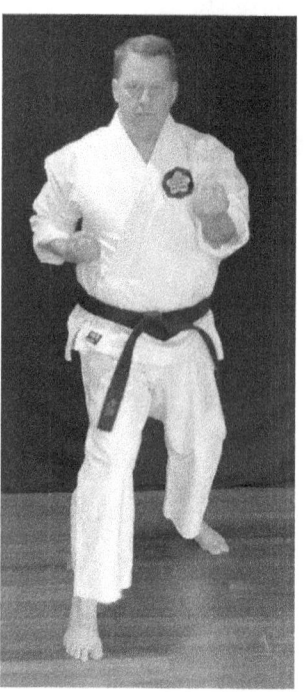

Set, Right Foot Forward
In Zenkutsu Dachi

Gekisai Ichi

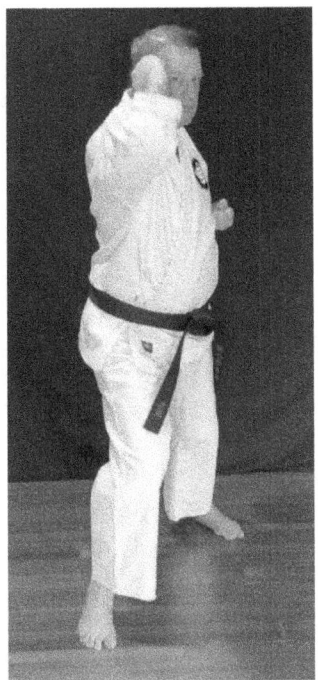
Complete Right Age Empi Uchi

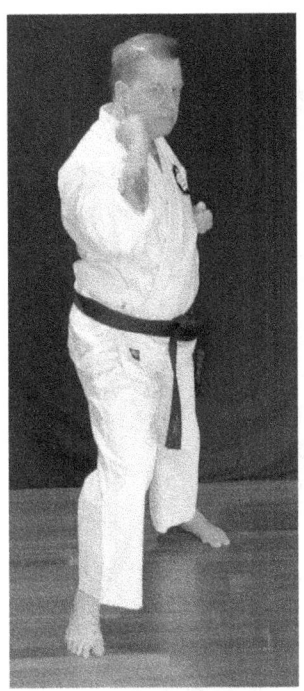
Bring Elbow Down

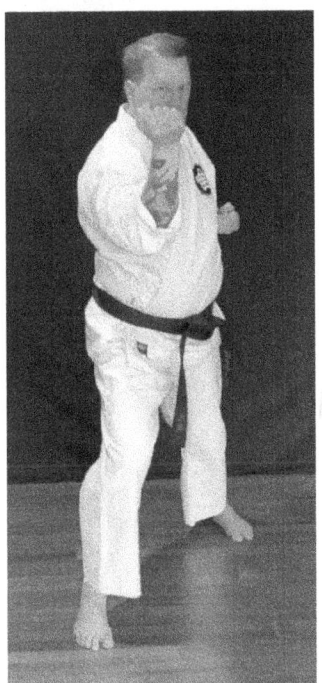
Complete Right Jodan Uraken Uchi

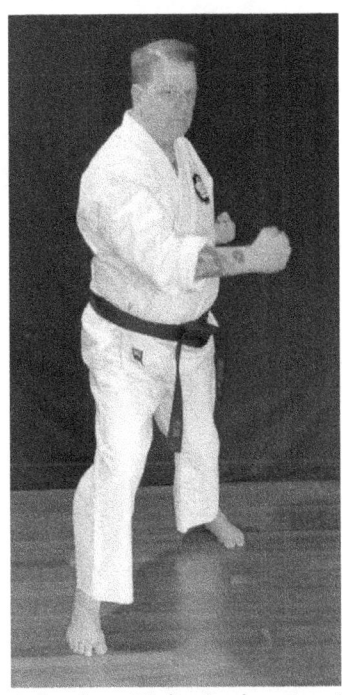
Complete Right Gedan Barai

Gekisai Ichi

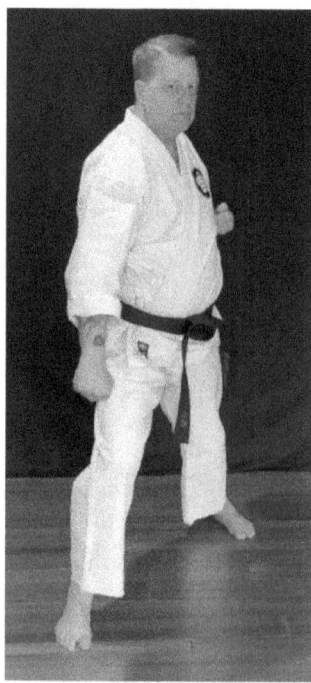

Gedan Barai (Cont.)

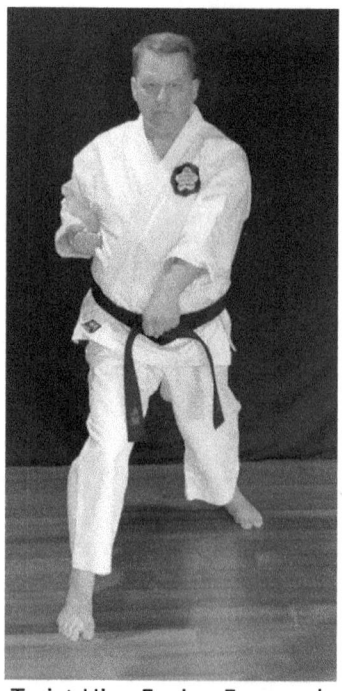

Twist Hips Facing Forward,
Complete Left Gedan Gyaku Zuki

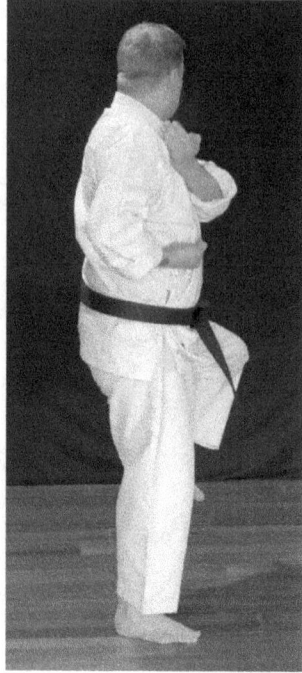

Bring Left Foot and Left Hand Up to
Chamber Looking Rear and Facing Left

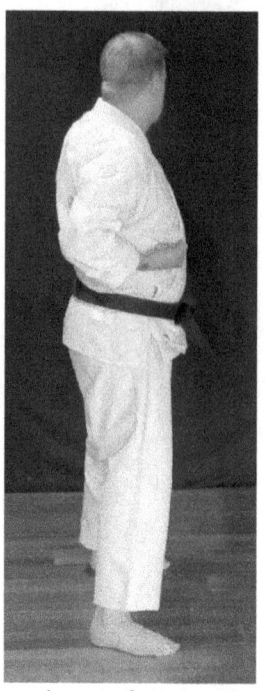

Complete Left Yoko Shuto
Uchi with Fumikomi Geri

Gekisai Ichi

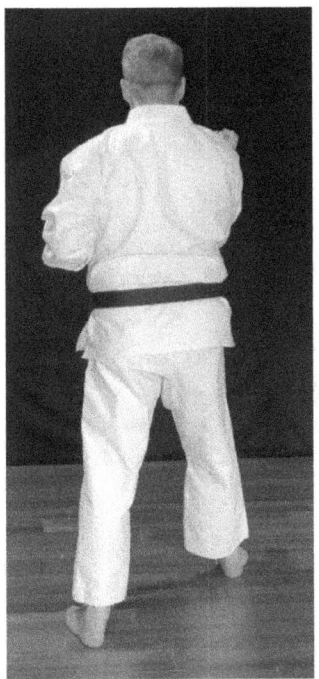

Step Towards Rear, Complete Slow Right Chudan Uke

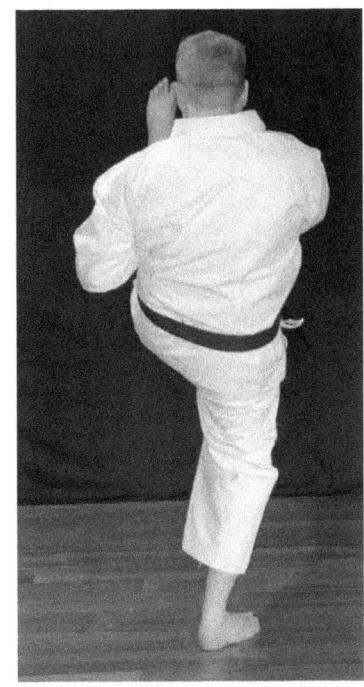

Complete Left Jodan Mae Keage Geri (kiai)

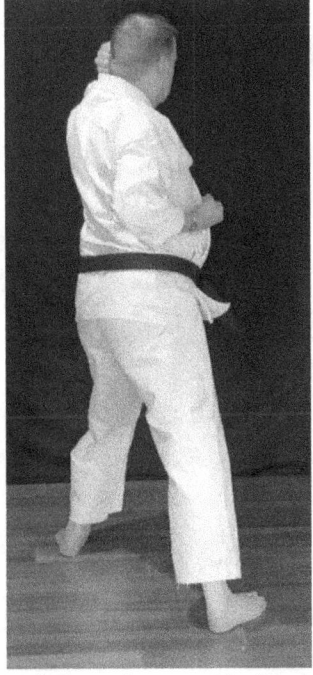

Set, Left Foot Forward in Zenkutsu Dachi, Complete Left Age Empi Uchi

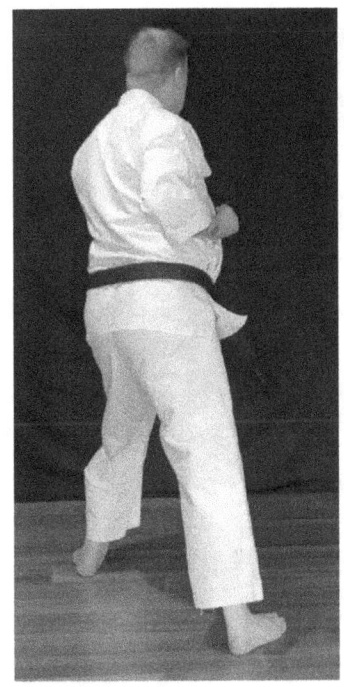

Bring Elbow Down

Gekisai Ichi

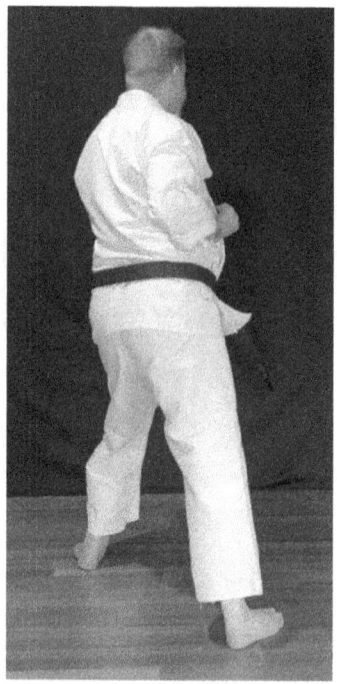

Complete Left Jodan
Uraken Uchi

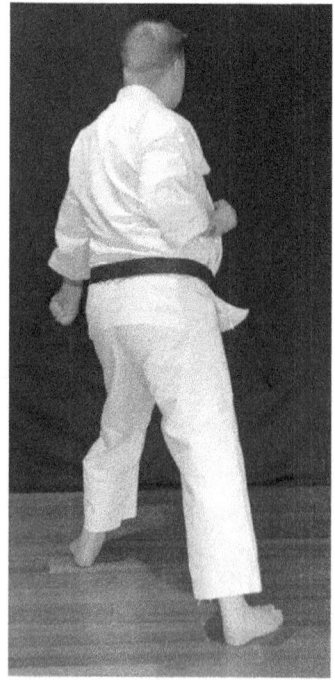

Complete Left Gedan Barai

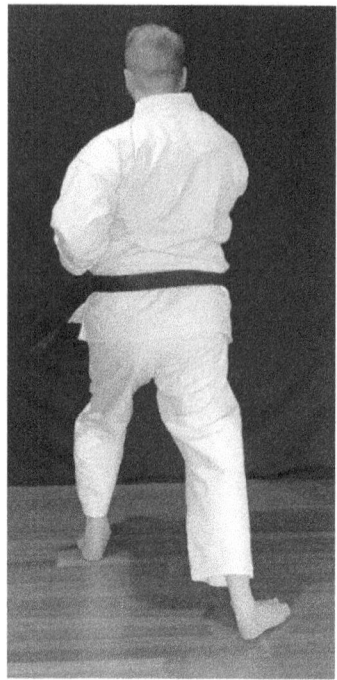

Twist Hips Facing Rear, Complete
Right Gedan Gyaku Zuki

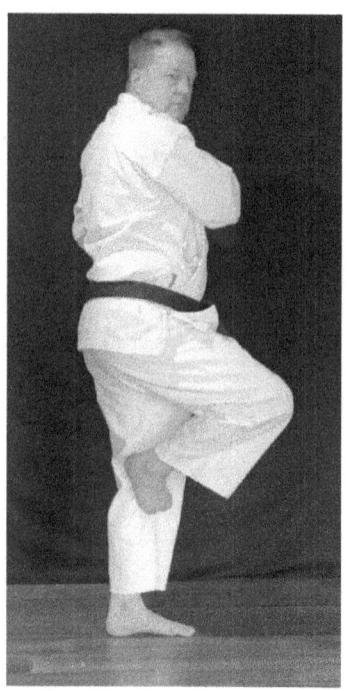

Bring Right Foot and Right Hand
Up to Chamber Looking Front
and Facing Right

Gekisai Ichi

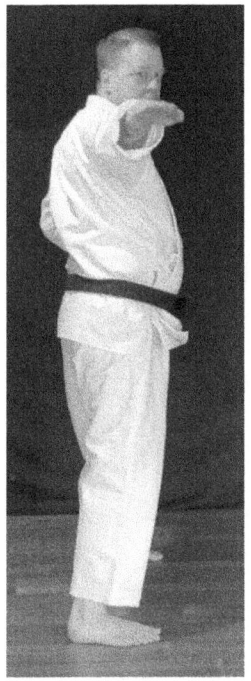

Complete Right Yoko Shuto Uchi with Fumikomi Geri

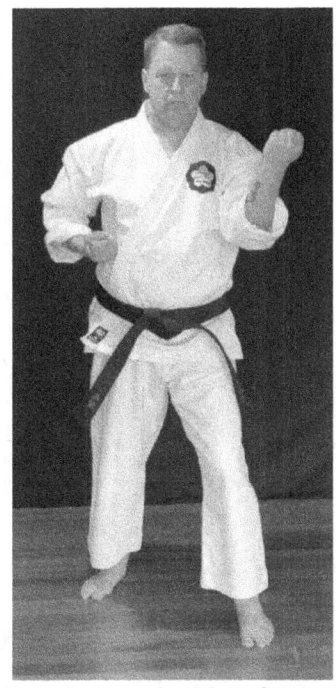

Step Forward with Left Foot, Complete Slow Left Chudan Uke

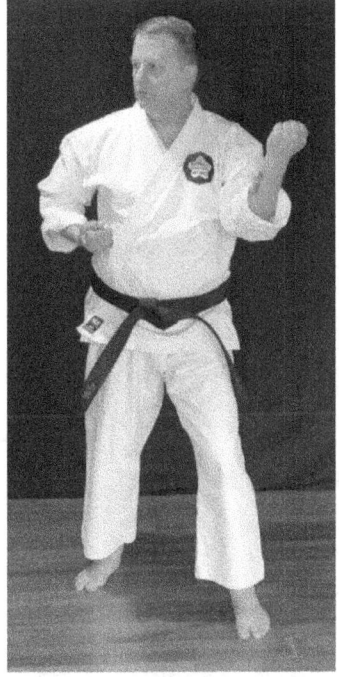

Look at Forward Right, 315° Angle

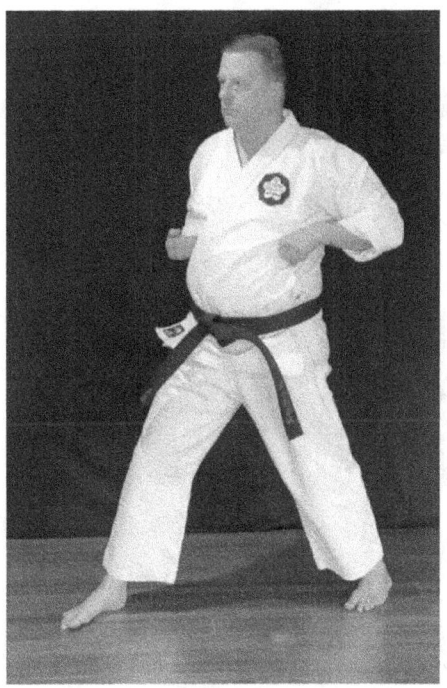

Step Back with Left Foot into Zenkutsu Dachi on 135° Angle while Chambering Left Hand, Palm Down

Gekisai Ichi

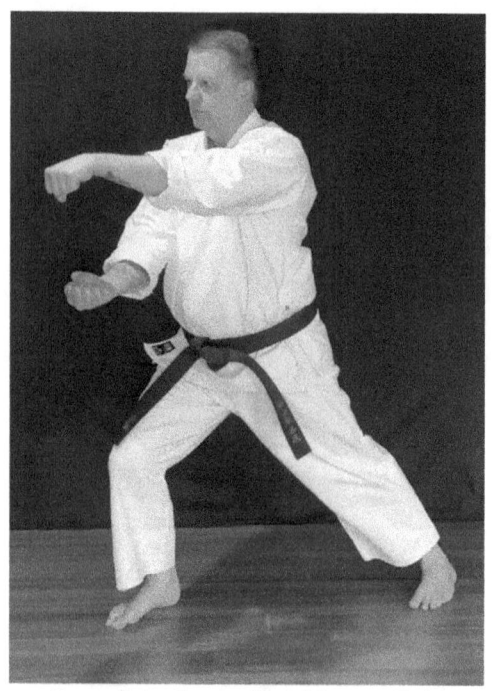

Complete Centerline Morote Zuki

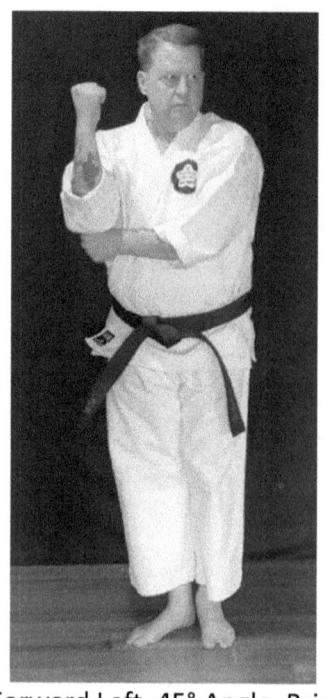

Look Forward Left, 45° Angle, Bring Left Foot to Right Foot, Chamber Left Hand Under Right Elbow

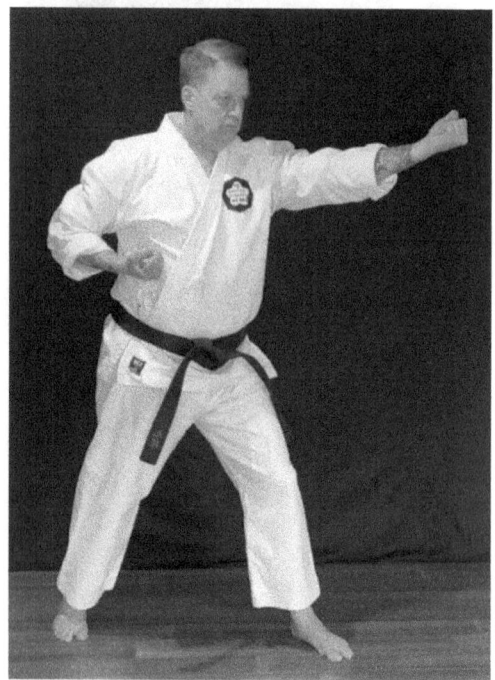

Complete Left Extended Chudan Uke while Stepping Back with Right Foot, 315° Angle

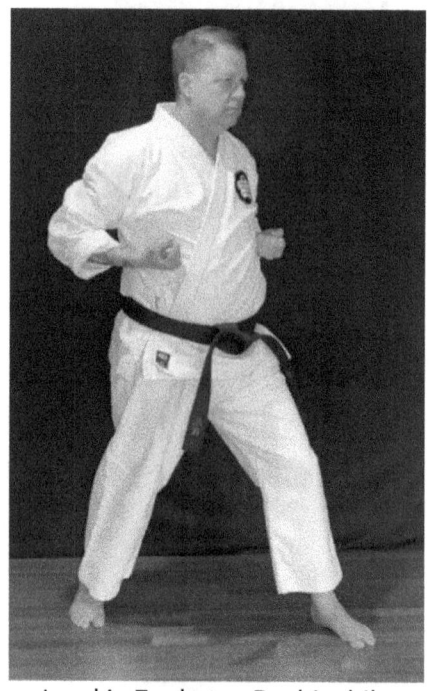

Land in Zenkutsu Dachi while Completing Left Chudan Uke, Both Palms Up

Gekisai Ichi

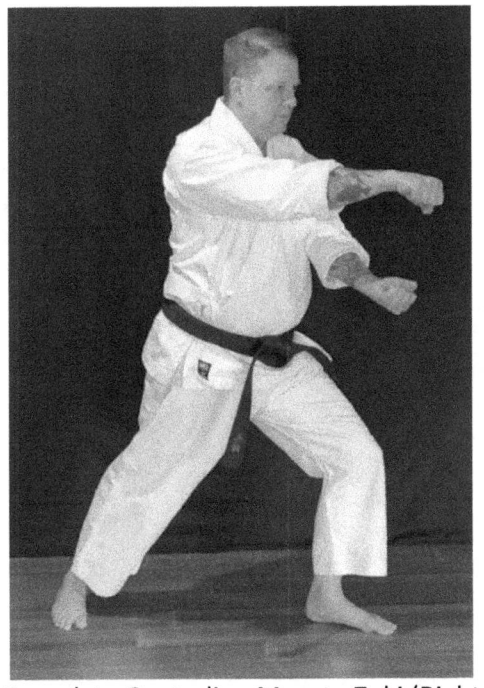

Complete Centerline Morote Zuki (Right Hand Twists to Palm Down with Strike)

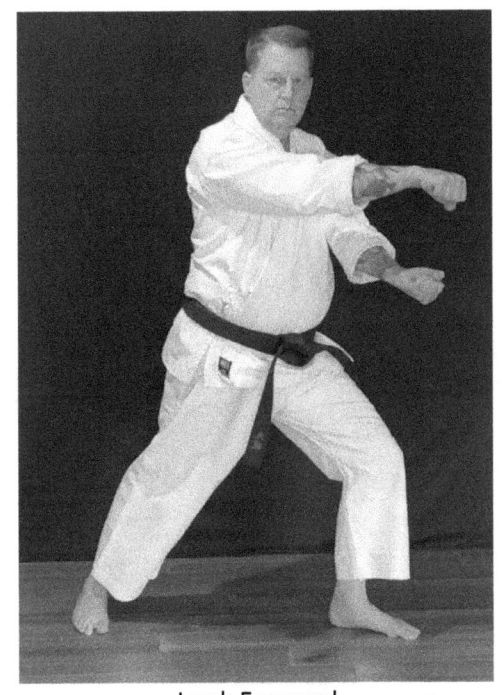

Look Forward

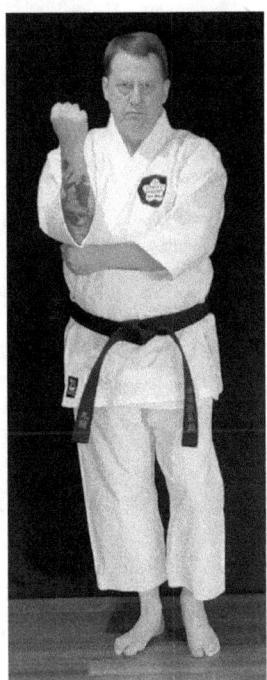

Bring Left Foot Inside While Chambering Left Hand Under Right Elbow

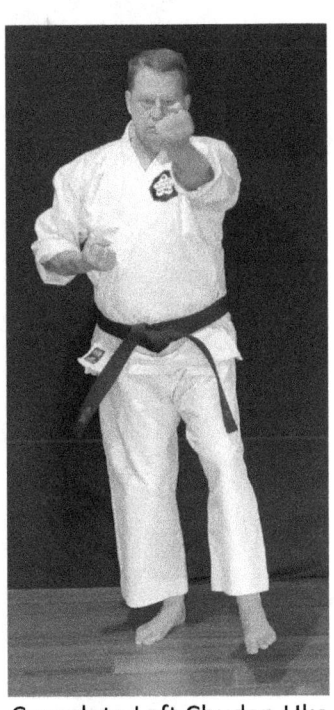

Complete Left Chudan Uke while Stepping Forward

Gekisai Ichi

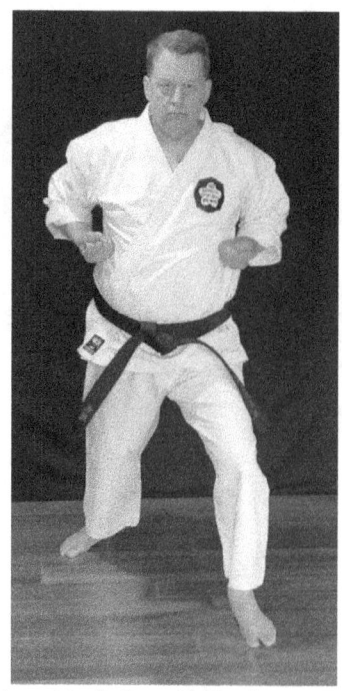 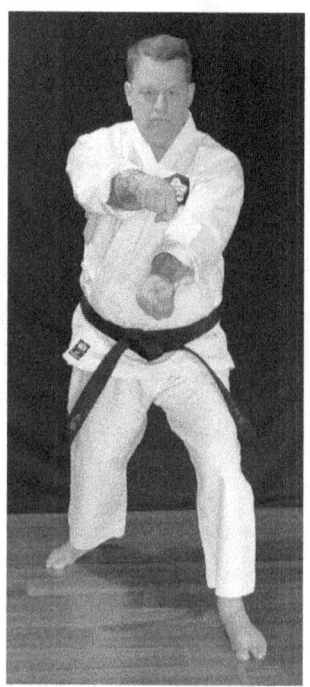

Land Left Foot in Zenkutsu Dachi while Completing Centerline Morote Zuki

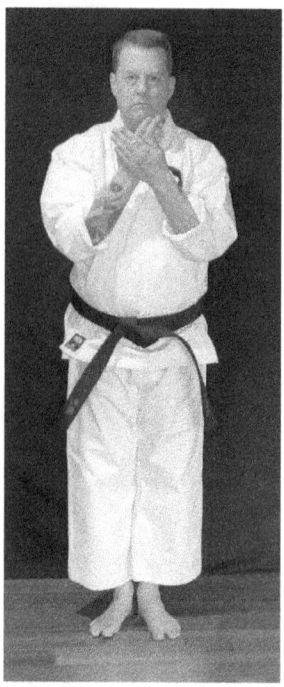

Step Back (Left Foot) to
Guard Throat

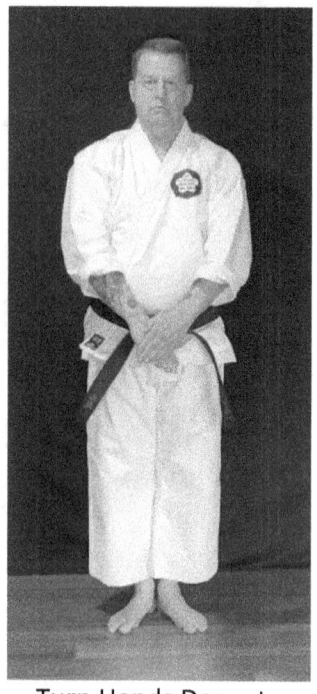

Turn Hands Down to
Guard Groin

Gekisai Ichi

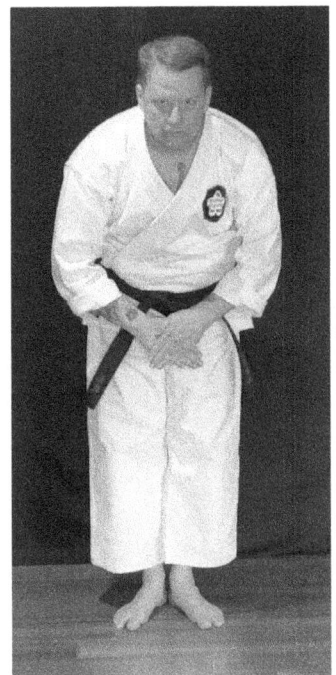

Rei

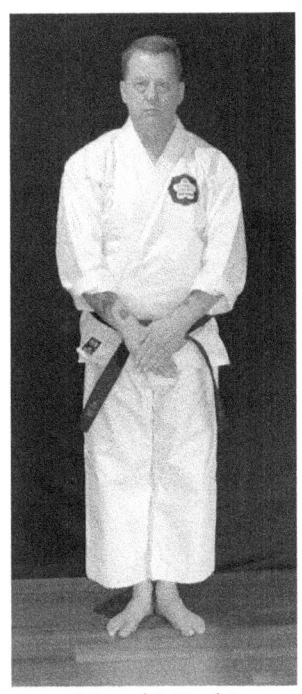

Musubi Dachi

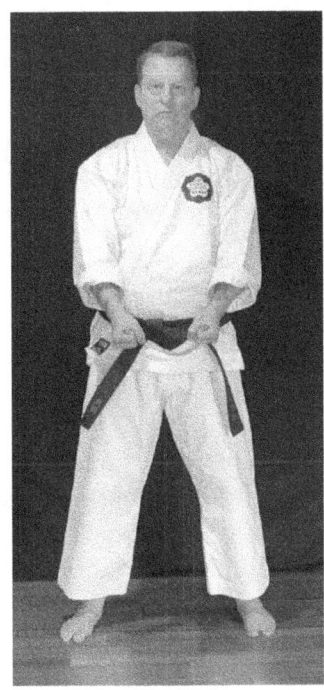

Heiko Dachi

Gekisai Ni

As originally designed, Gekisai Dai Ichi and Gekisai Dai Ni are nearly identical with just a few differences. Gekisai Dai Ichi uses closed hands while Ni introduces open handed techniques and new stances. It is in Gekisai Dai Ni that students are introduced to the neko ashi dachi stance and the wheel block (tora guchi), which is prevalent in Goju-Ryu katas. These are the first katas that Shodai made changes to, adding small elements of Seiunchin kata and Toguchi's Fukyu Ni kata, plus he brought the kick targets up to the chin instead of the groin. The Ketsugo Goju-Ryu system has kept Shodai's changes to honor his efforts to expand on the original system he was taught.

Below is the method by which Ketsugo Goju-Ryu performs Gekisai Ni kata. Complete details about each move are not included, as this is simply a demonstration. This demonstration is not meant to imply that it is the only way to do it, but it is the way at Ketsugo Goju-Ryu.

These are the Japanese terms used for this kata. Bear in mind, karate terms are not completely streamlined. There are terms that were used in the middle of the 20th Century that are no longer used today. Oftentimes there are more than one term that can be used for the same technique. The important thing is not what it is called, but the technique itself.

Age Empi Uchi – Rising Elbow Strike	**Neko Ashi Dachi** – Cat Leg Stance
Age Uke - Rising Block	**Oshi** – Push
Barai - Sweeping Block	**Otoshi** - Downward
Chudan - Middle	**Rei** – Bow (Respect)
Dachi – Stance	**Shiko Dachi** - Straddle Leg Stance
Fumikomi Geri – Stamping Kick	**Shotei** – Palm Heel
Gedan – Low	**Tettsui Uchi** - Hammer Fist Strike

Gekisai Ni

Hajime – Command to Begin	**Tora Guchi** – Wheel Block
Hari Uke – Open Hand Block (Palm Up)	**Tsukami Hiki** – Grab and Pull
Hiki Uke – Open Hand Block (Palm Down)/Pulling Block	**Tsuki/-Zuki** - Punch
Heiko Dachi - Parallel Stance	**Uchi** – Strike
Jodan - High	**Uke** – Block (Receive)
Mae Keage Geri – Front Snap Kick	**Ura Zuki** – Inverted Strike
Morote Chudan Uke – Double Chest Block	**Uraken Uchi** - Back Fist Strike
Morote Shotei Uchi – Double Palm Heel Strike	**Yoi** – Ready Command
	Yoko - Side
Morote Sukui Uke – Augmented Scooping Block	**Zenkutsu Dachi** - Forward Leaning Stance
Musubi Dachi - Attention Stance, Toes Out	

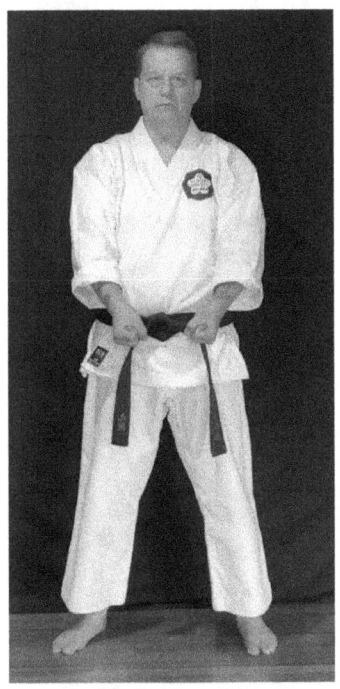

Heiko Dachi

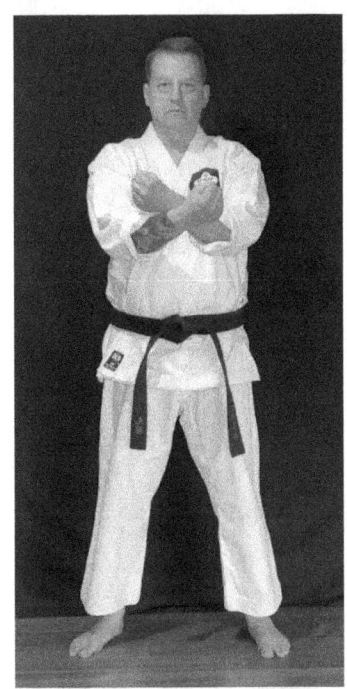

(Yoi) Brings Arms Up, Crossed at the Wrist

Gekisai Ni

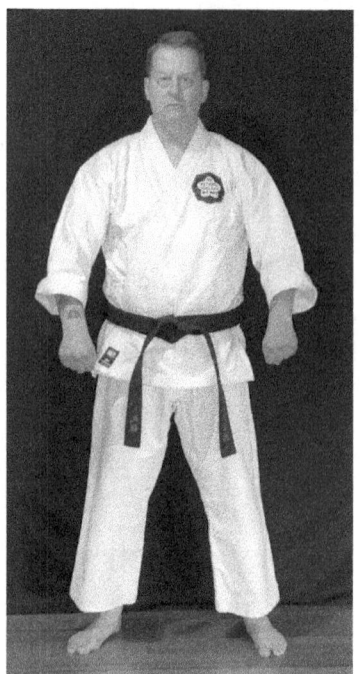
Bring Arms Down

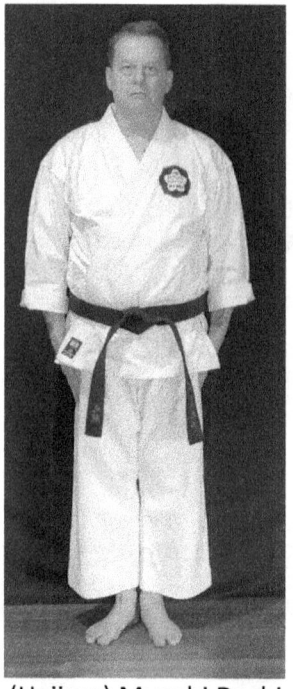
(Hajime) Musubi Dachi

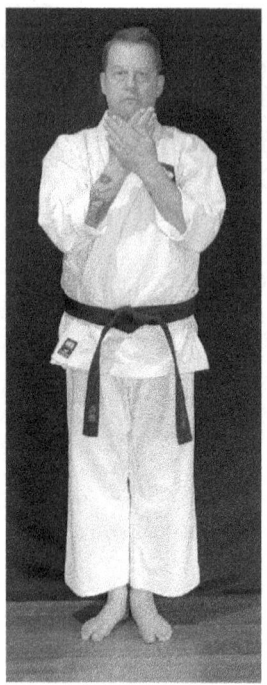
Guard Throat

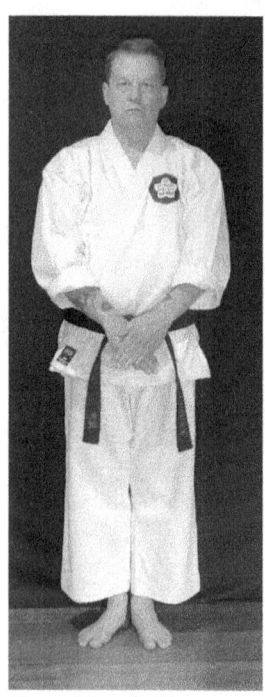
Turn Hands Down to Guard Groin

Gekisai Ni

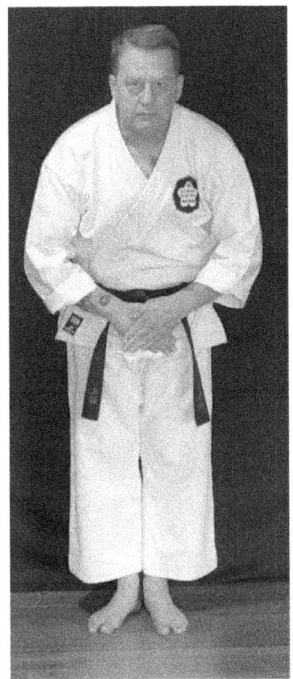

Rei

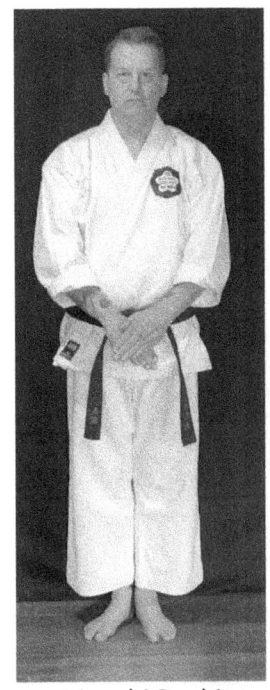

Musubi Dachi

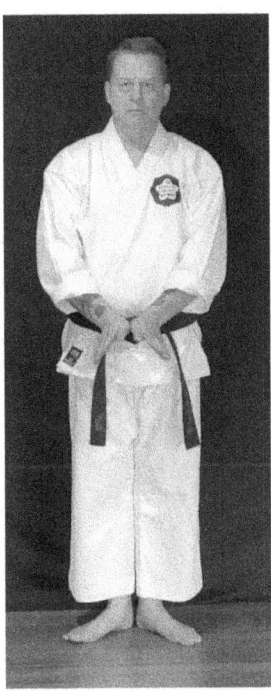

Open Hands at the Palm Heel
and Feet at the Heel

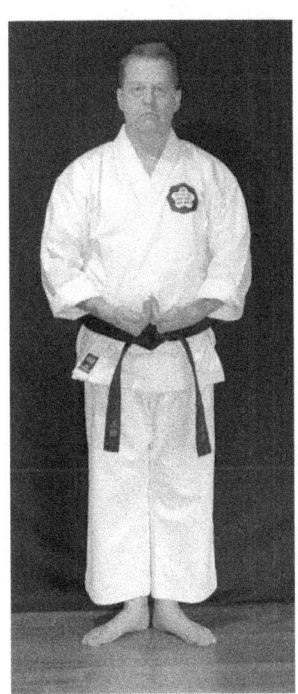

Complete Morote Sukui Uke,
Bring Hands Up Against the Body,
Keeping Back of Hands Together

Gekisai Ni

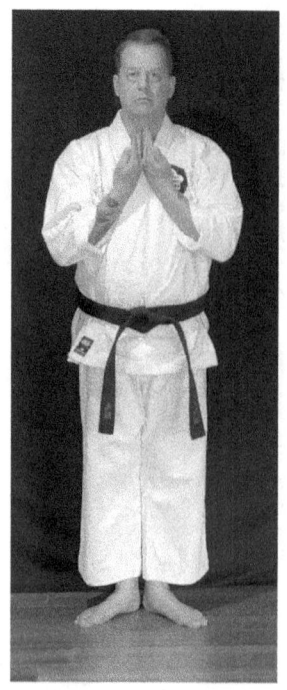 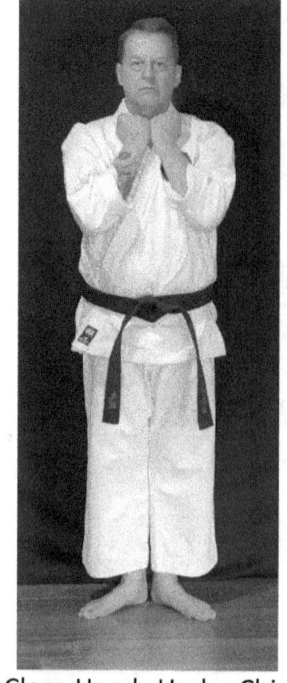

Close Hands Under Chin

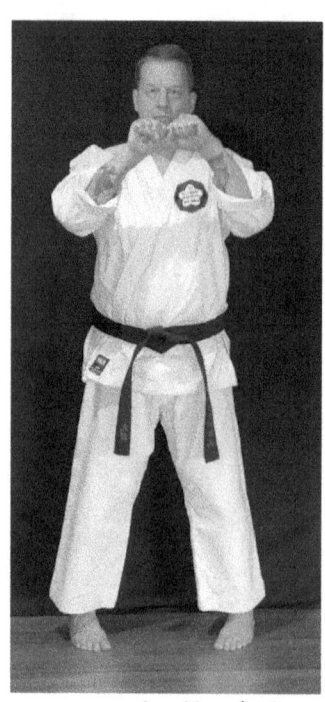 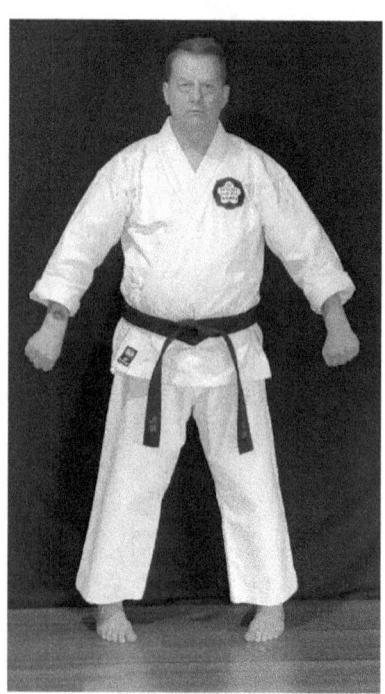

Arc Hands Out and Down While Moving Heels Out

Gekisai Ni

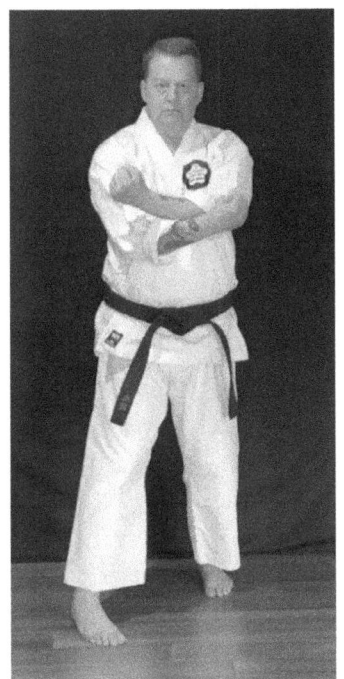
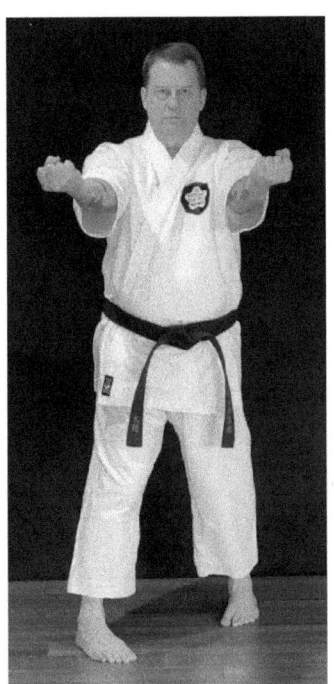

Complete Morote Chudan Uke

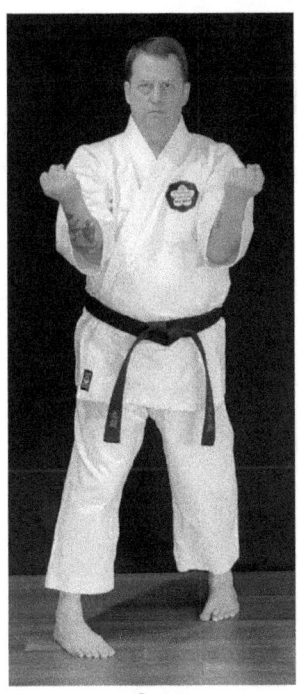
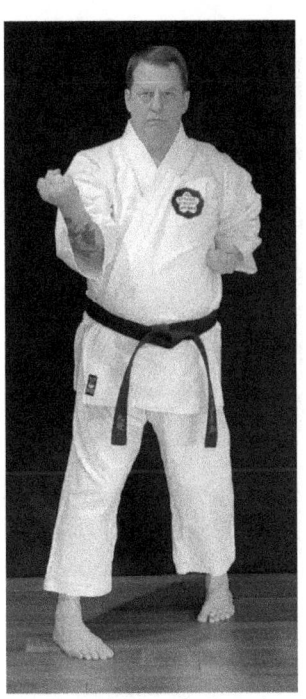

Set   Chamber Left Hand

Gekisai Ni

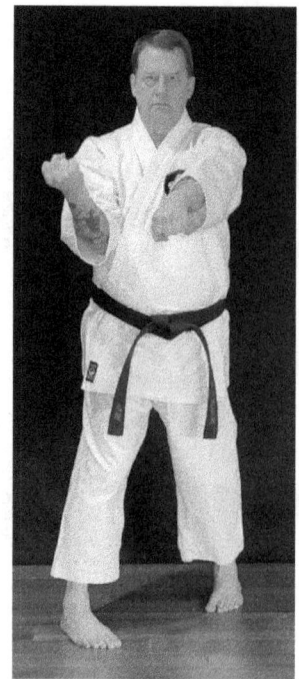
Complete Left Chudan Zuki

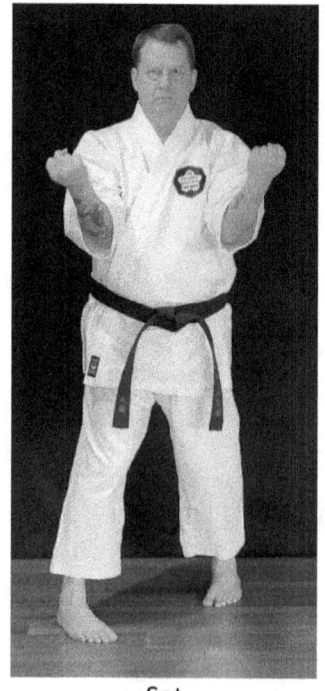
Set

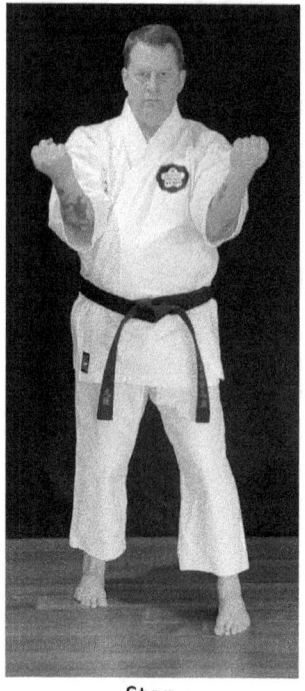
Step

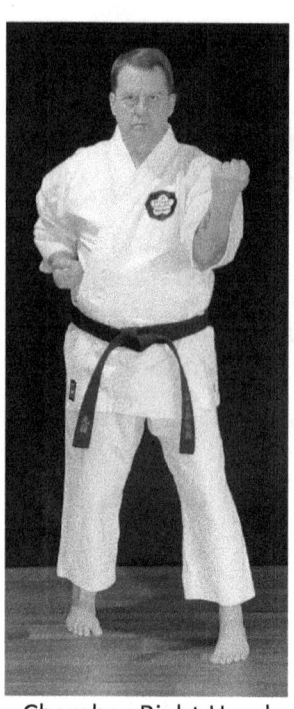
Chamber Right Hand

Gekisai Ni

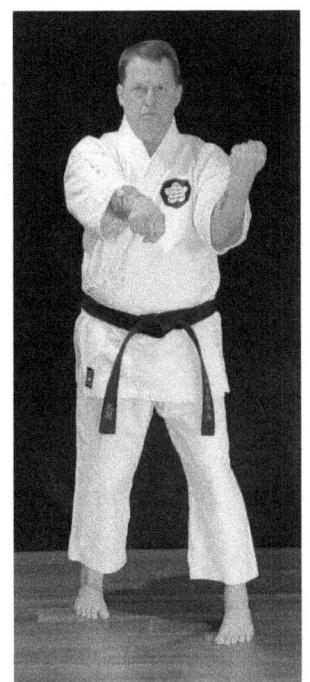
Complete Right Chudan Zuki

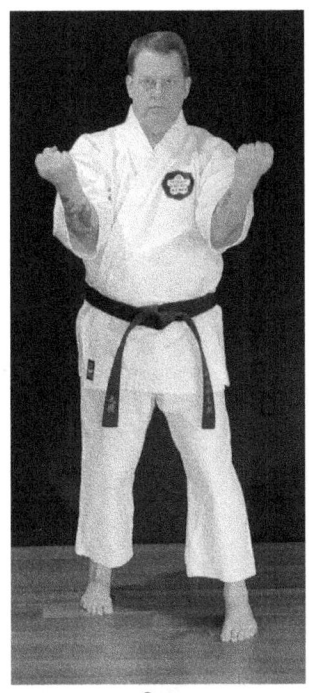
Set

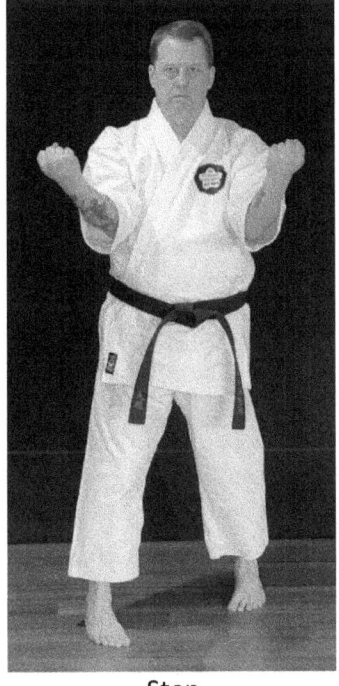
Step

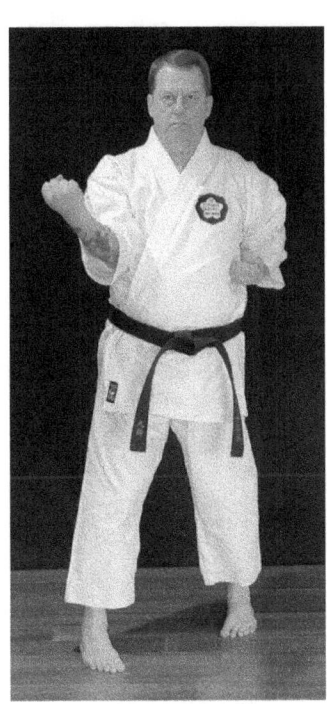
Chamber Left Hand

Gekisai Ni

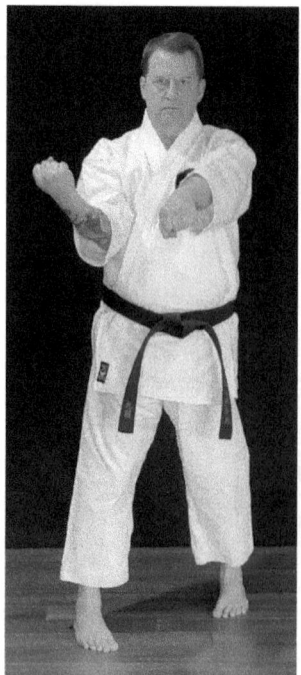
Complete Left Chudan Zuki

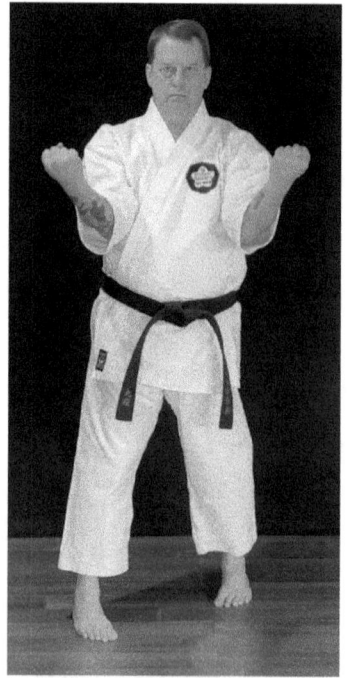
Set

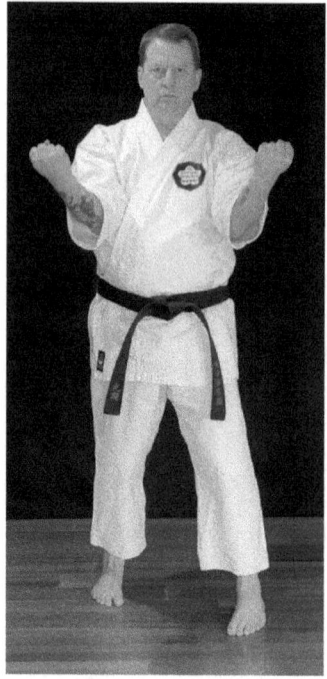
Step Back

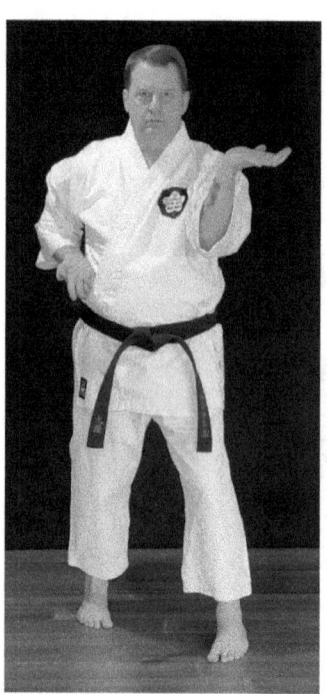
Complete Left Gedan Shotei Barai

Gekisai Ni

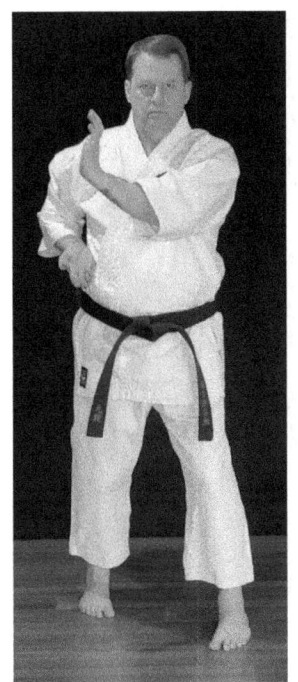 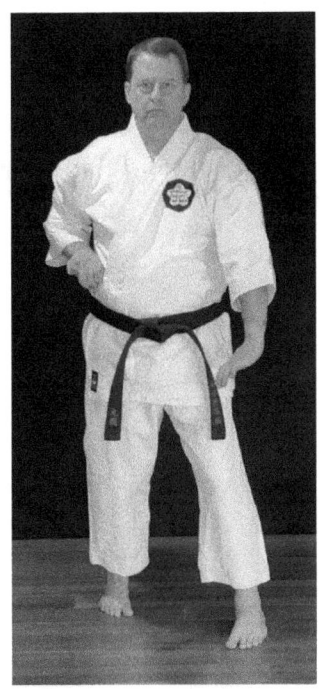

Gedan Shotei Barai (cont.)

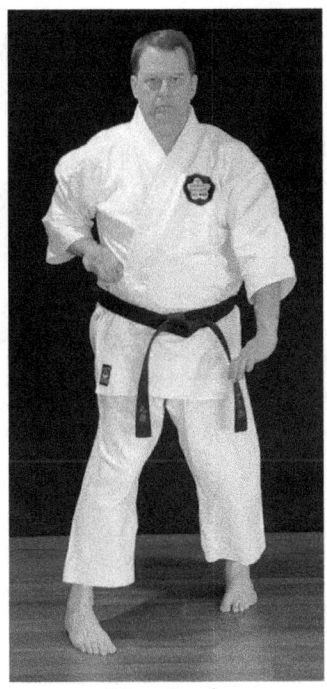 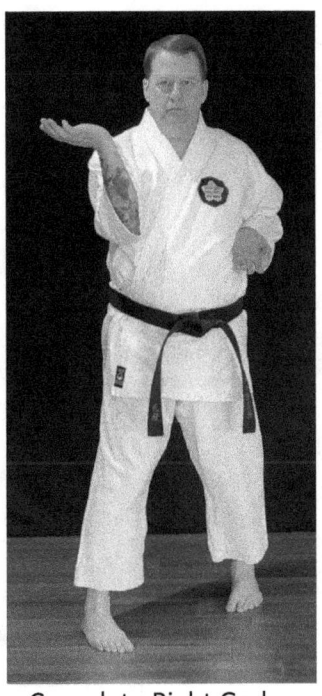

Step Back | Complete Right Gedan Shotei Barai

Gekisai Ni

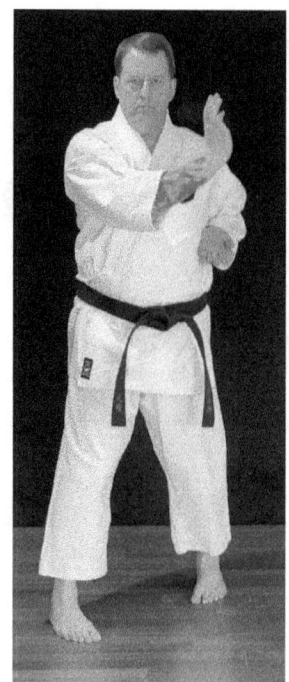
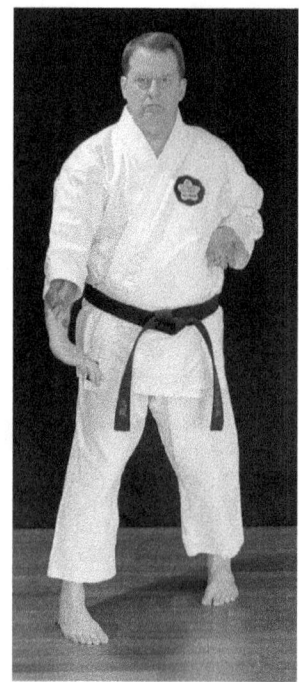

Gedan Shotei Barai (cont.)

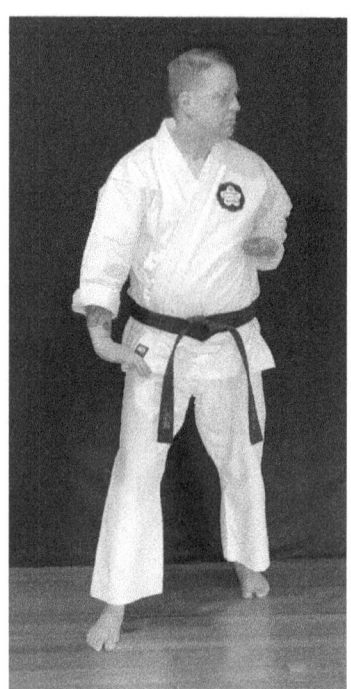

Look Left

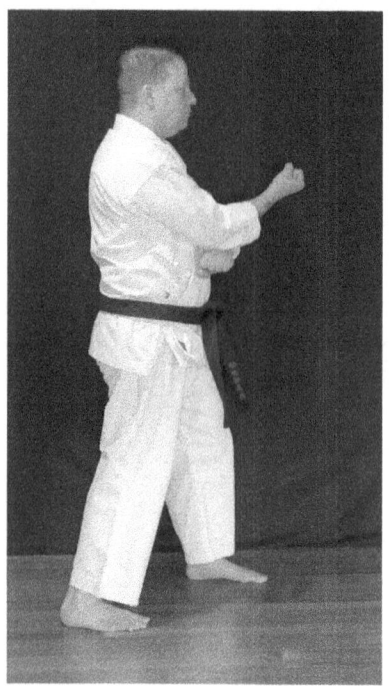

Pivot Left, Complete Left
Jodan Age Uke

Gekisai Ni

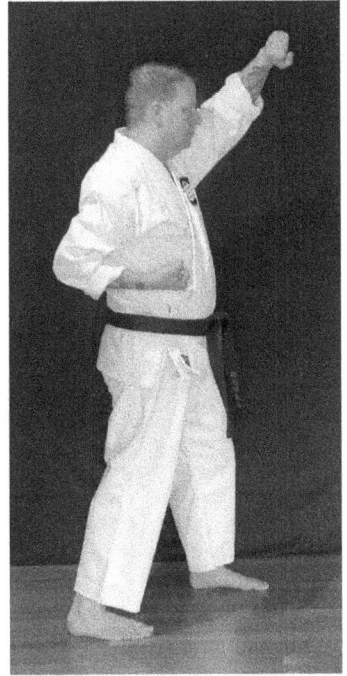
Jodan Uke (cont.)

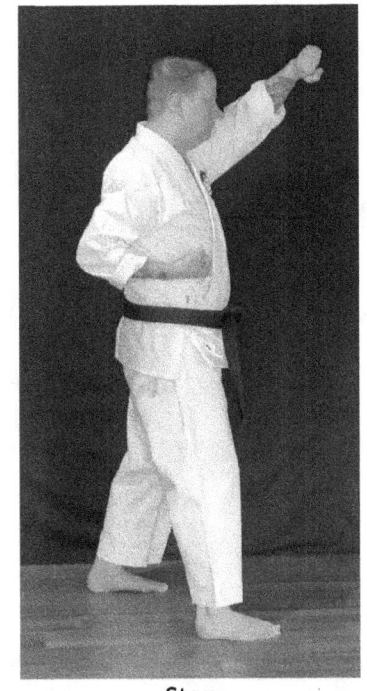
Step

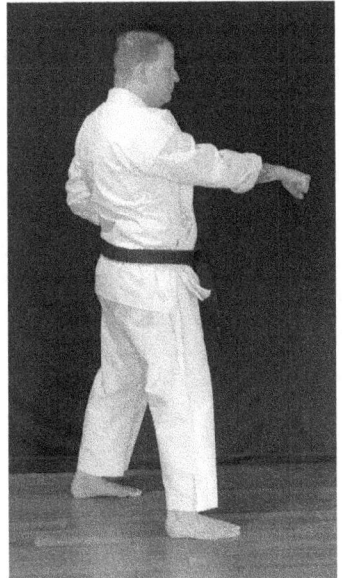
Complete Right Chudan Zuki

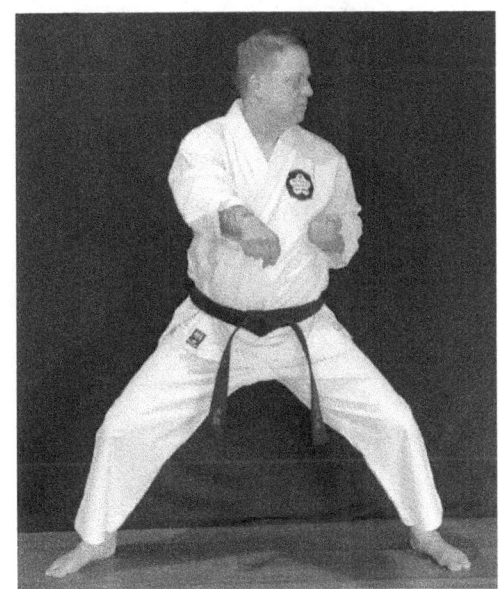
Right Foot Step Back into Shiko Dachi Facing Forward

Gekisai Ni

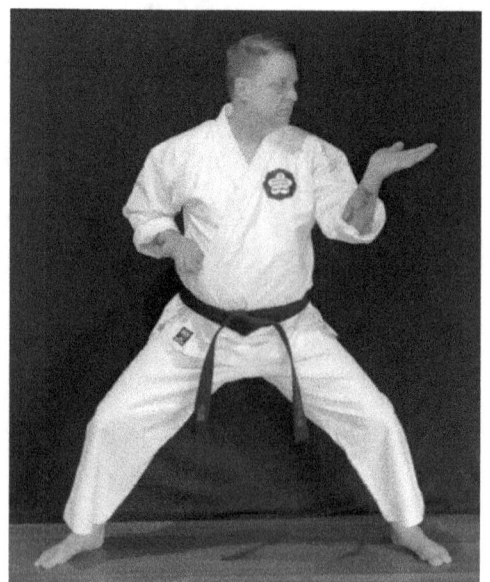 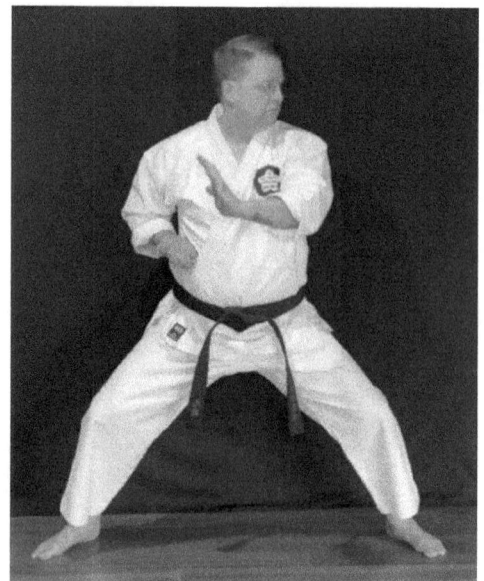

Complete Left Gedan Yoko Shotei Uchi

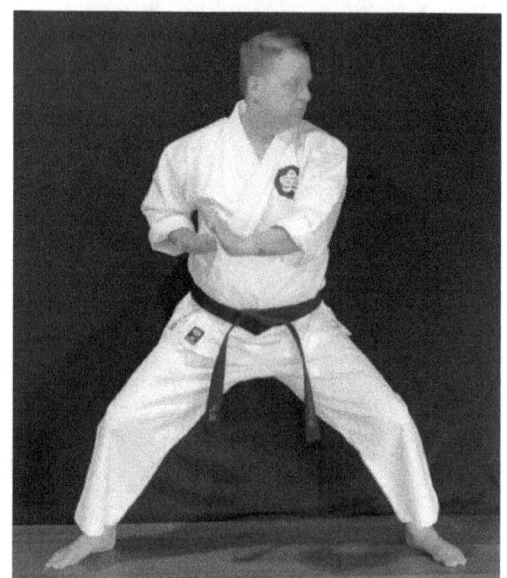 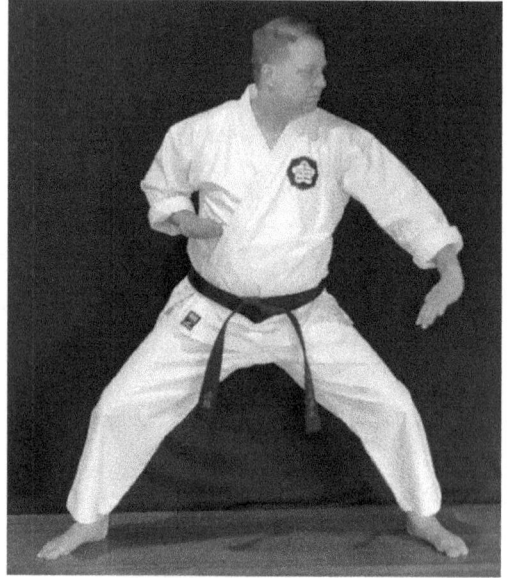

Left Gedan Yoko Shotei Uchi (cont.)

Gekisai Ni

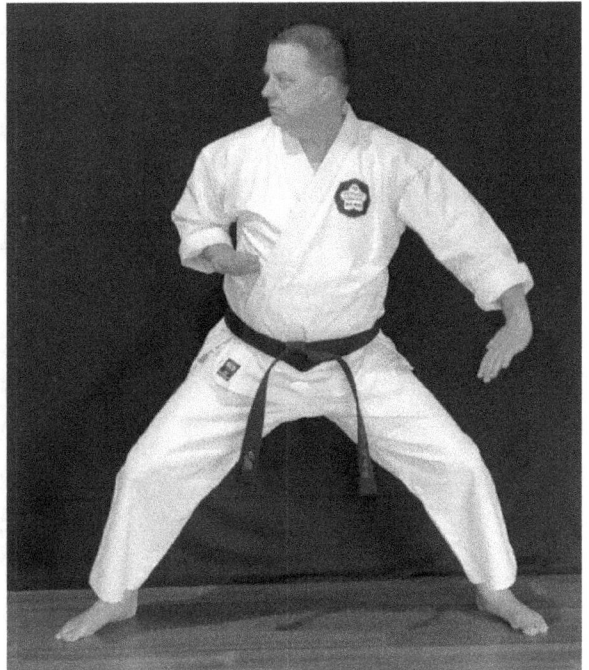
Look Right

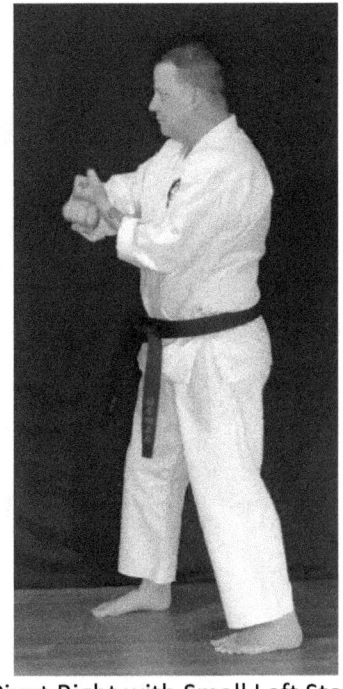
Pivot Right with Small Left Step, Complete Right Jodan Age Uke

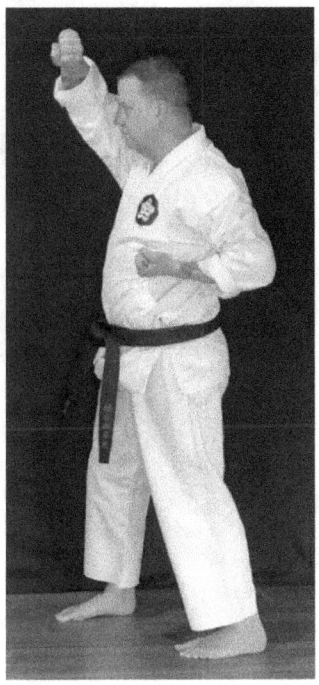
Jodan Age Uke (cont.)

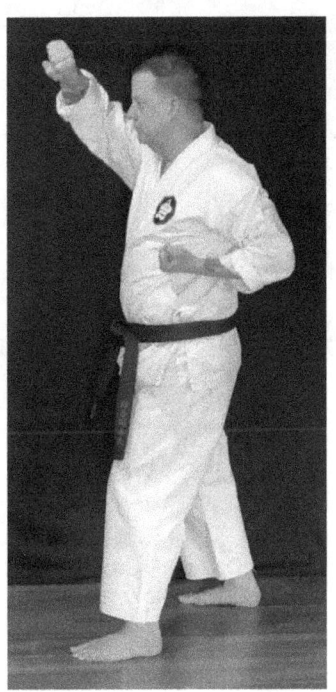
Step

Gekisai Ni

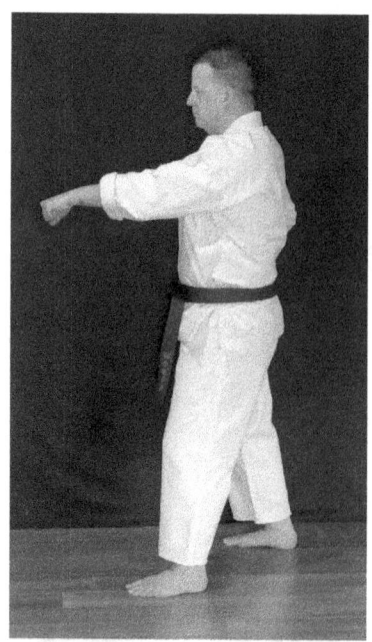

Complete Left Chudan Zuki

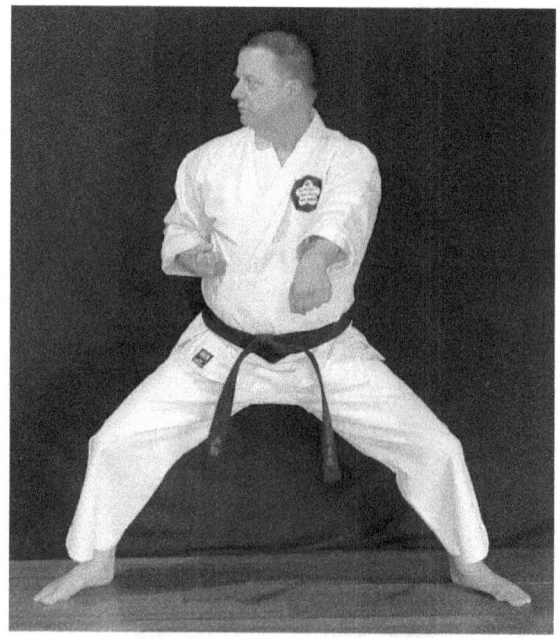

Left Foot Step Back into Shiko Dachi Facing Forward

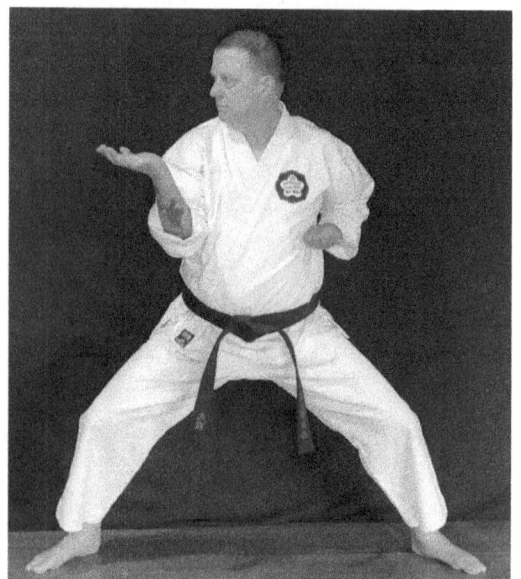

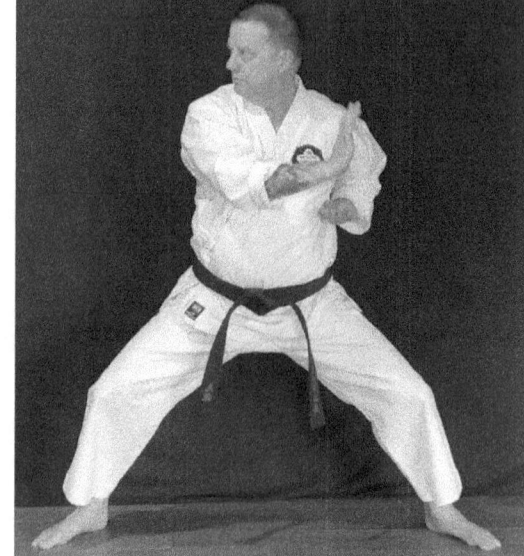

Complete Right Gedan Yoko Shotei Uchi

Gekisai Ni

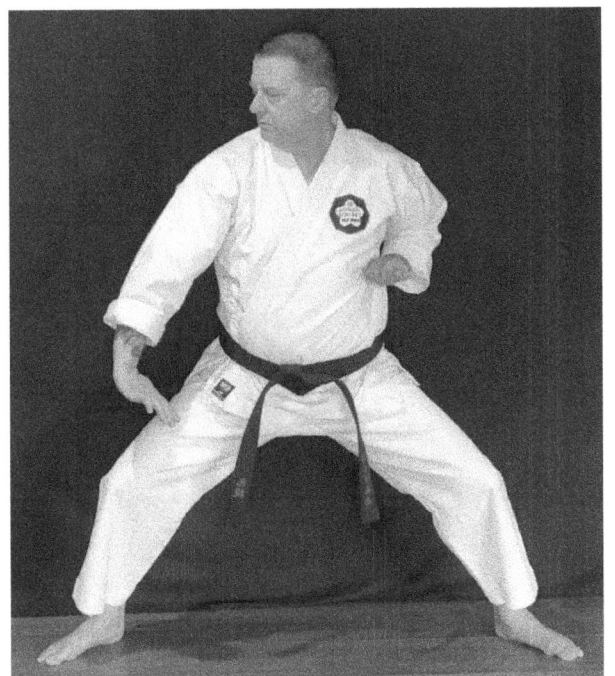

Gedan Yoko Shotei Uchi (cont.)

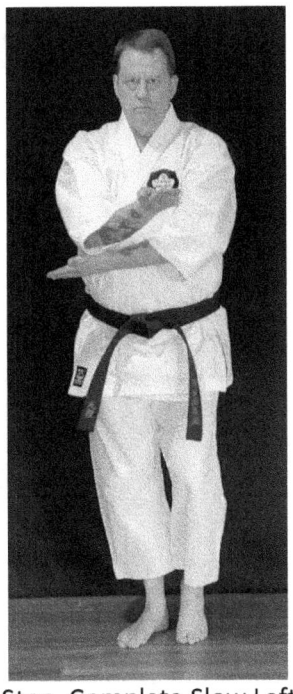

Step, Complete Slow Left Chudan Hari Uke (inhale)

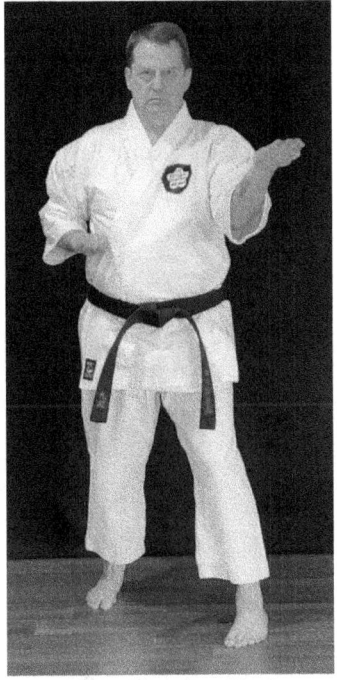

Slow Chudan Hari Uke (cont.) (inhale)

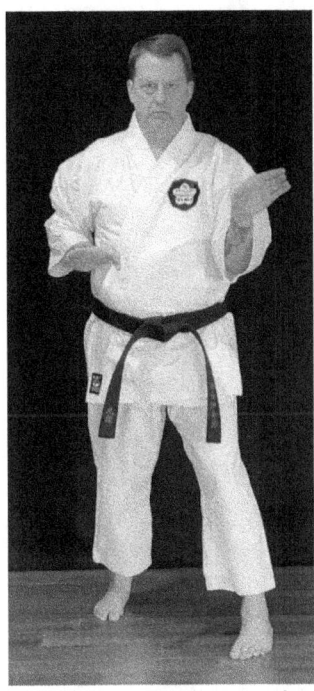

Turn Hands Over, Complete Slow Chudan Hiki Uke (exhale)

Gekisai Ni

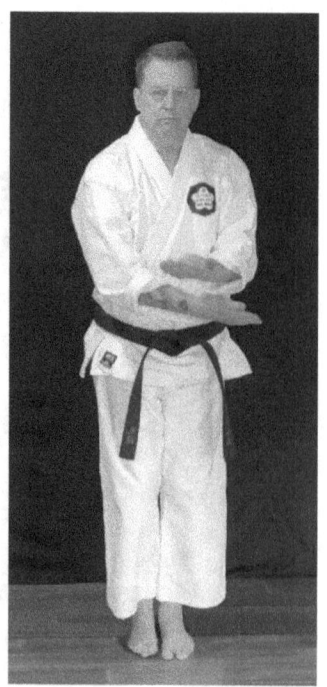 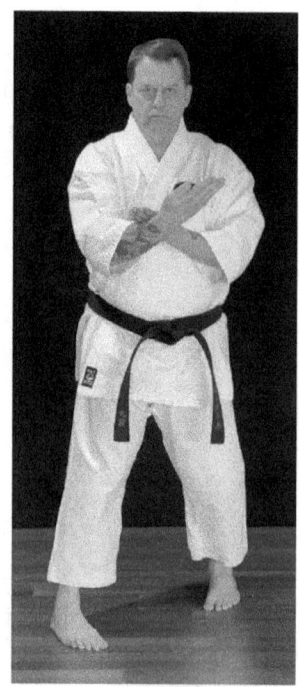

Step, Complete Slow Right Chudan Hari Uke (inhale)

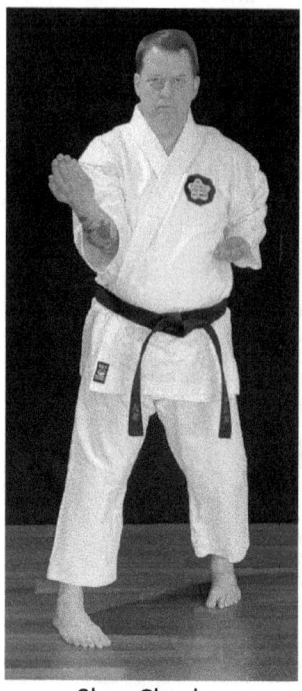 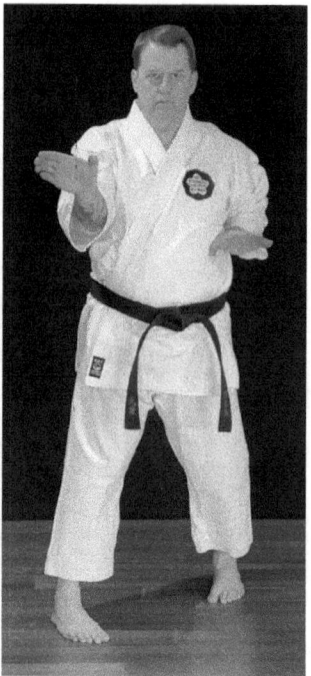

Slow Chudan Hari Uke (cont.) (inhale)

Turn Hands Over, Complete Slow Chudan Hiki Uke (exhale)

Gekisai Ni

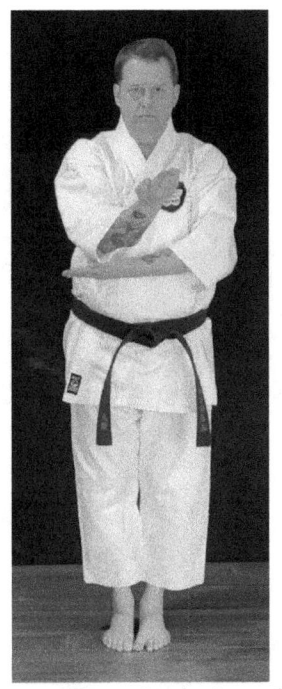
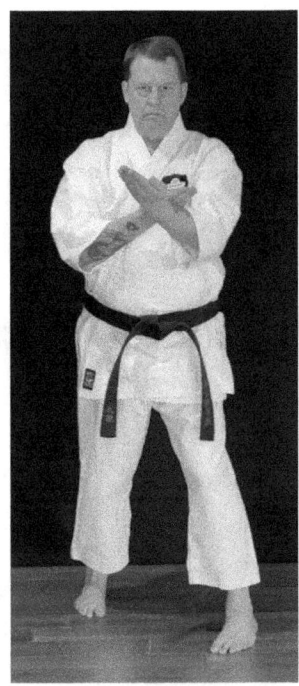

Step Back, Complete Slow Left Chudan Hari Uke (inhale)

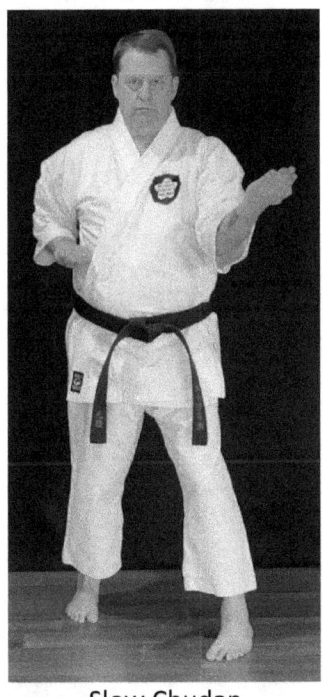
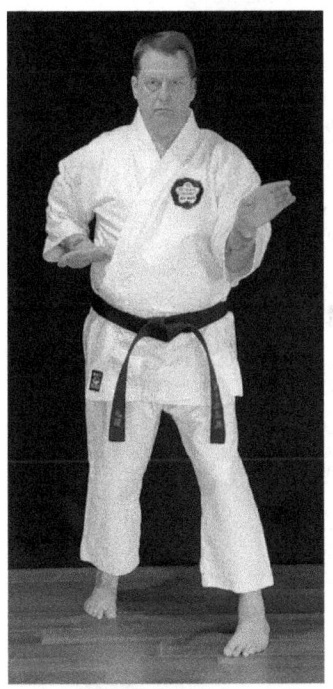

Slow Chudan
Hari Uke (inhale) (cont.)

Turn Hands Over, Complete
Slow Chudan Hiki Uke (exhale)

Gekisai Ni

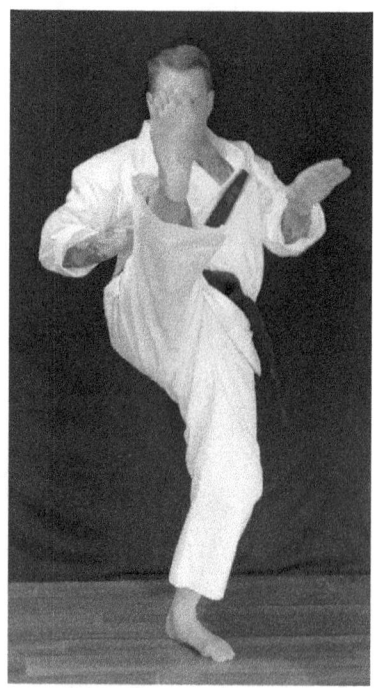

Complete Right Jodan
Mae Keage Geri (kiai)

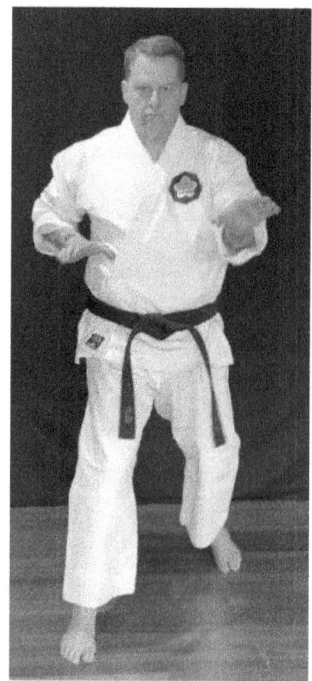

Set, Right Foot Forward
in Zenkutsu Dachi

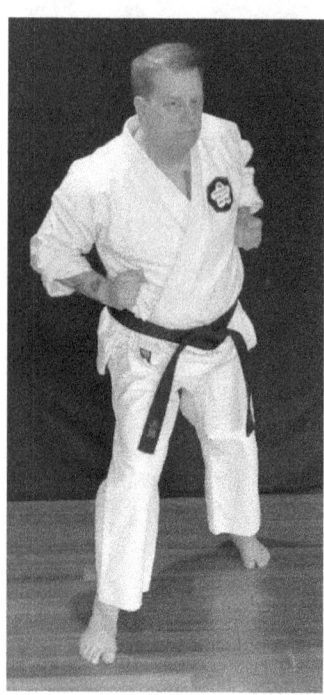

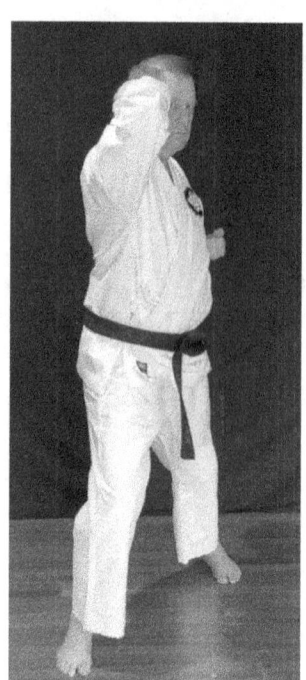

Complete Right Age Empi Uchi

Gekisai Ni

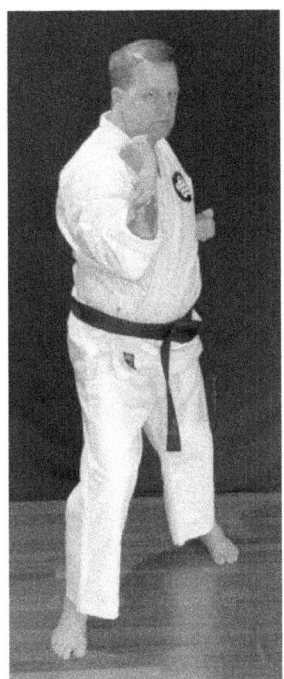

Bring Elbow Down

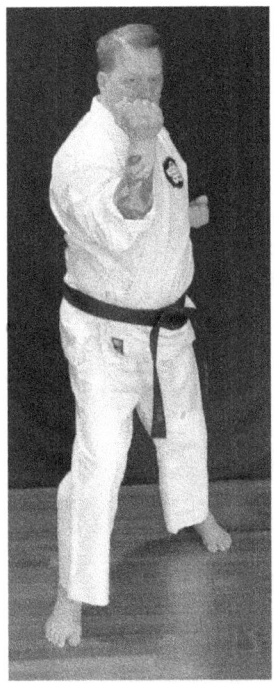

Complete Right Jodan Uraken Uchi

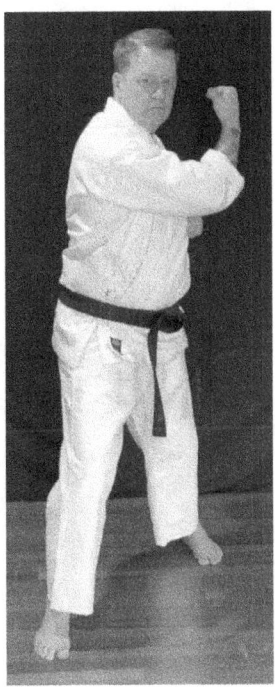

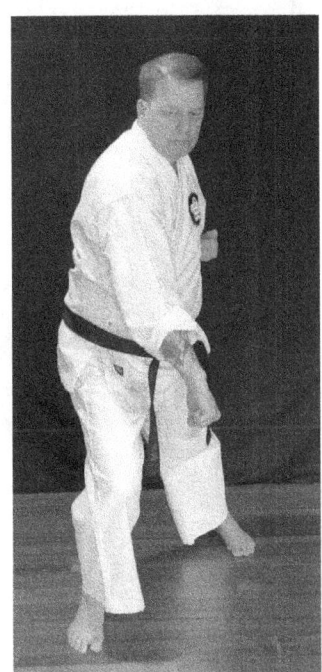

Complete Right Gedan Tettsui Uchi

Gekisai Ni

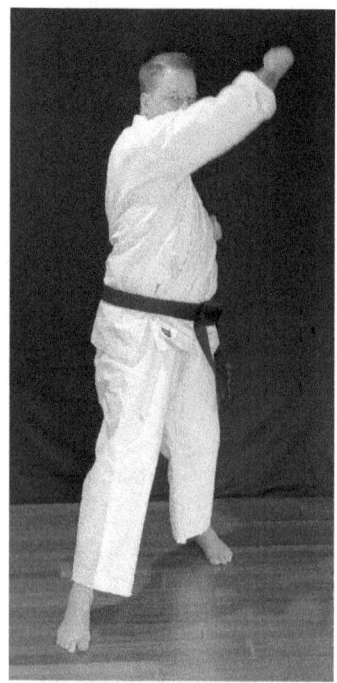 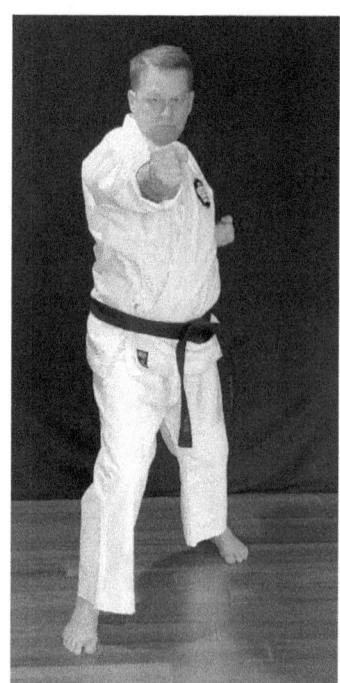

Same Hand Swing Around For Jodan Otoshi Tettsui Uchi

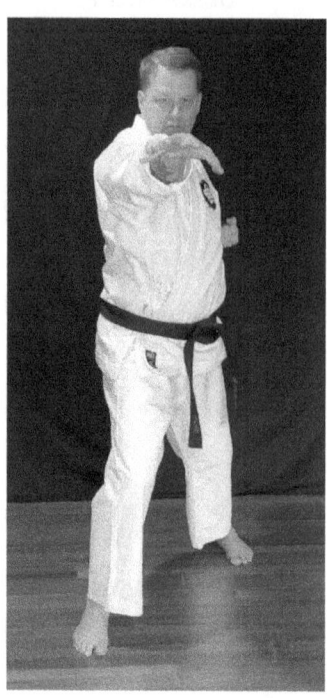 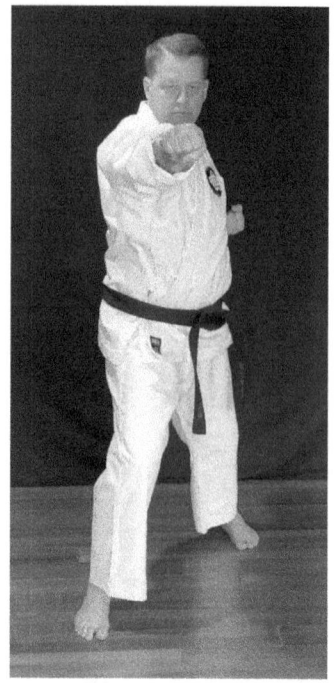

Complete Tsukami Hiki

Gekisai Ni

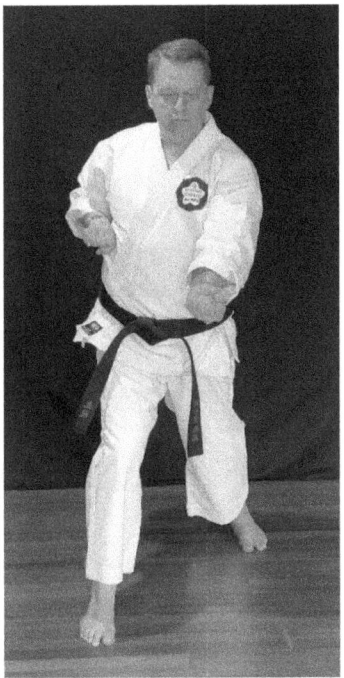

Twist Hips Facing Forward, Pull Back with Right Hand while Completing Left Ura Zuki

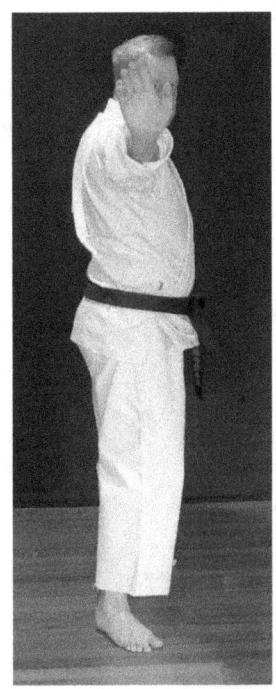

Bring Left Foot Back into Heiko Dachi, Oshi

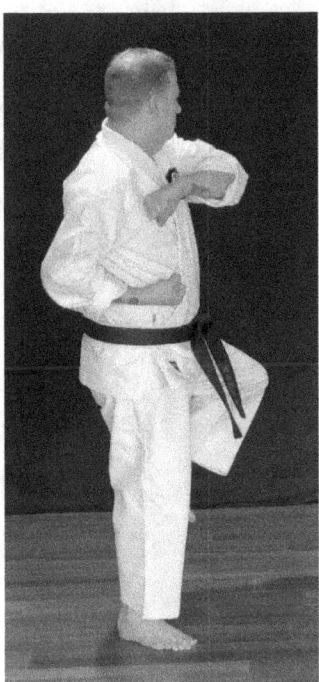

Bring Left Foot and Left Hand to Chamber Looking Rear and Facing Left

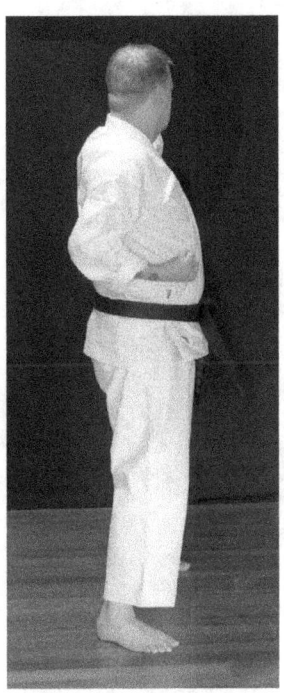

Complete Left Otoshi Tettsui Uchi with Fumikomi Geri

Gekisai Ni

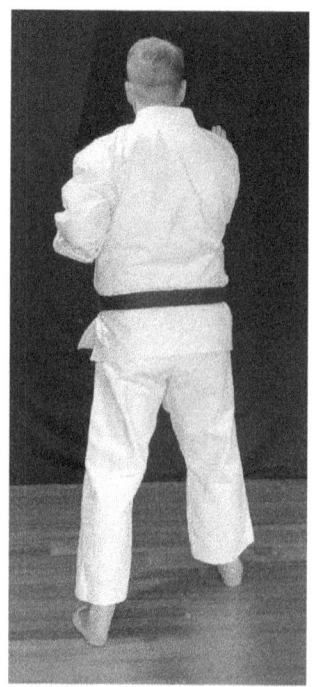

Step Toward Rear, Complete Slow Right Chudan Hari Uke

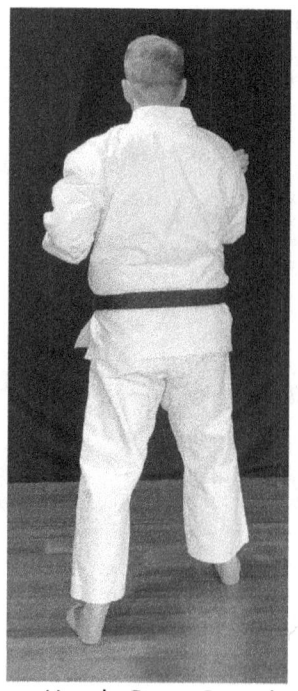

Turn Hands Over, Complete Slow Right Chudan Hiki Uke

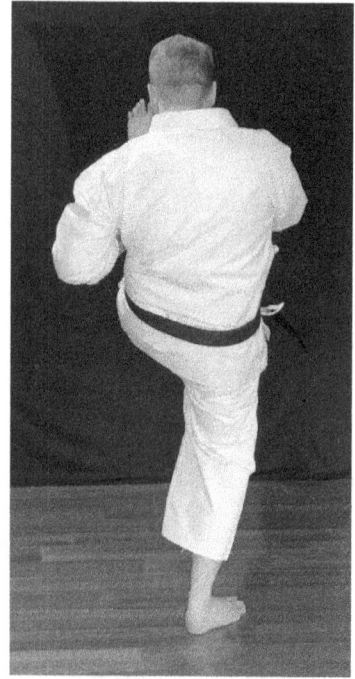

Complete Left Jodan Mae Keage Geri (kiai)

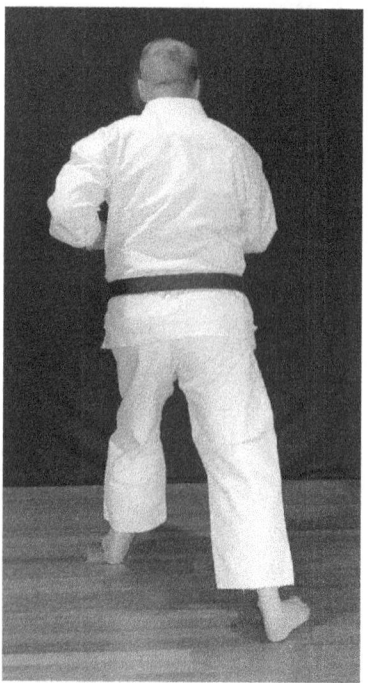

Set, Left Foot Forward in Zenkutsu Dachi

Gekisai Ni

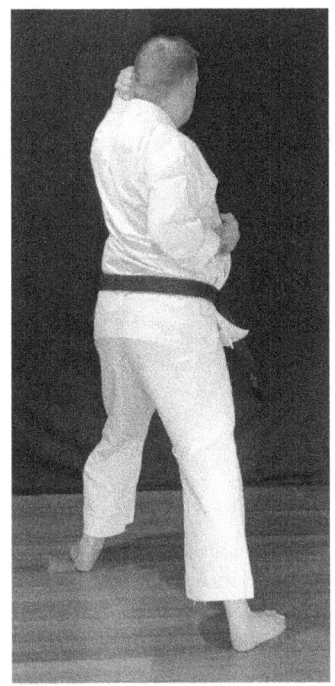

Complete Left Age Empi Uchi

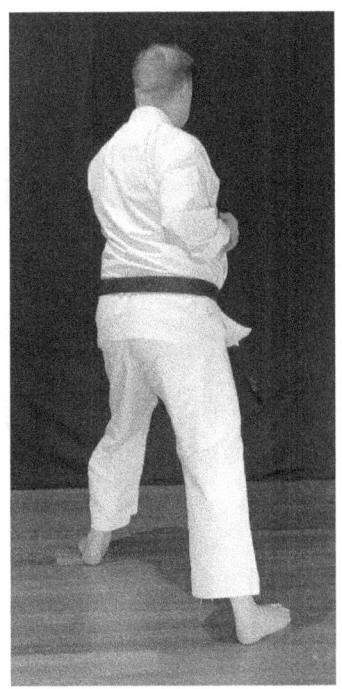

Bring Elbow Down

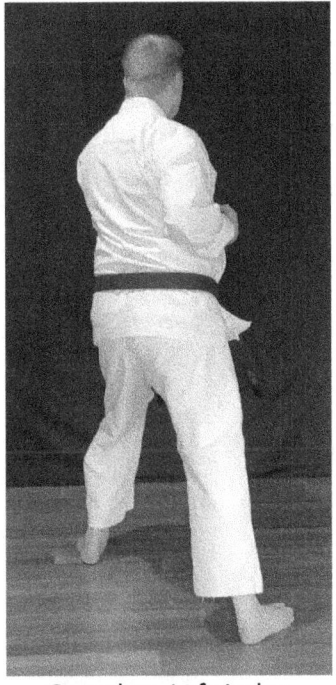

Complete Left Jodan
Uraken Uchi

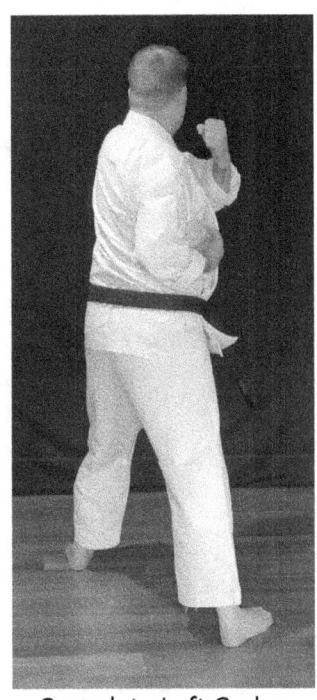

Complete Left Gedan
Tettsui Uchi

Gekisai Ni

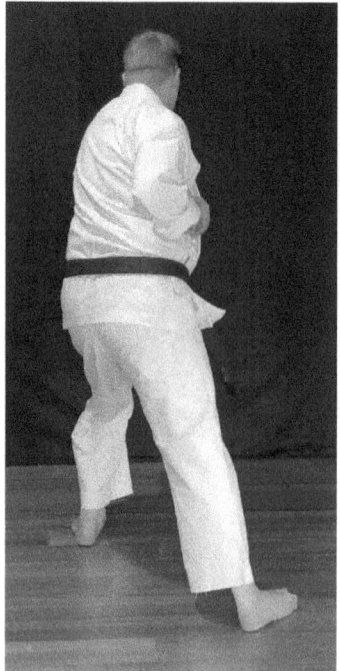
Gedan Tettsui Uchi (cont.)

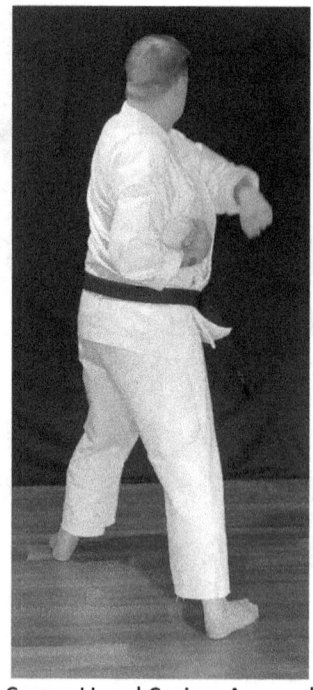
Same Hand Swing Around
For Jodan Otoshi Tettsui Uchi

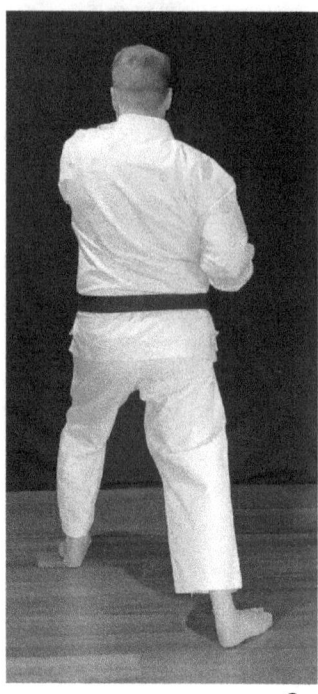

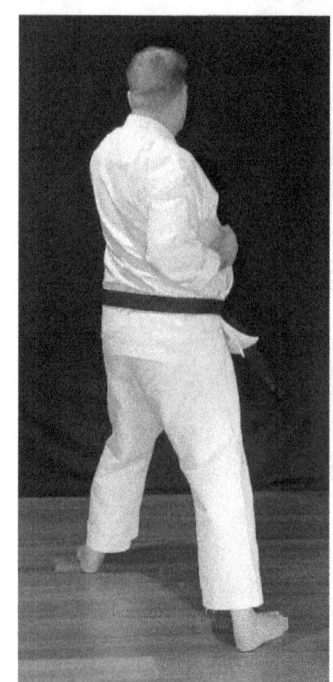

Complete Tsukami Hiki

Gekisai Ni

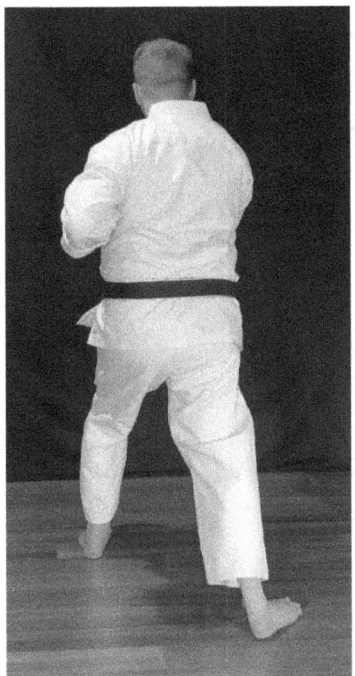

Twist Hips Facing Rear, Pull Back with Left Hand while Completing Right Ura Zuki

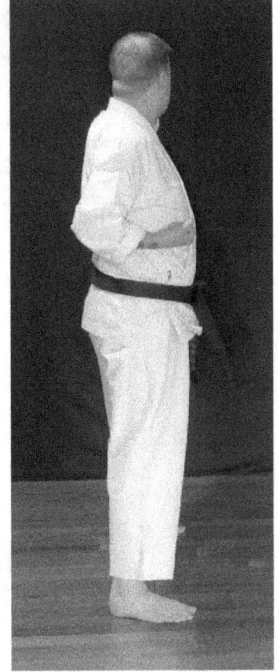

Bring Right Foot Back into Heiko Dachi, Oshi

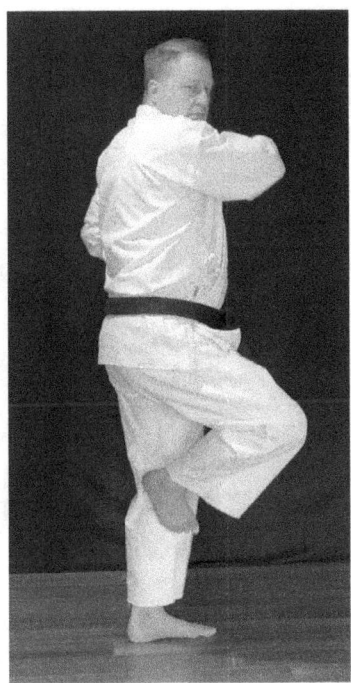

Bring Right Foot and Right Hand Up to Chamber Looking Front and Facing Left

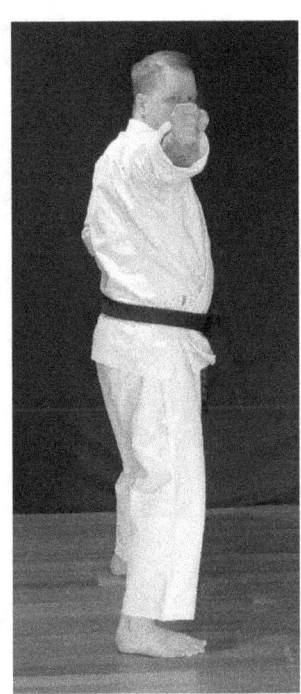

Complete Right Otoshi Tettsui Uchi with Fumikomi Geri

Gekisai Ni

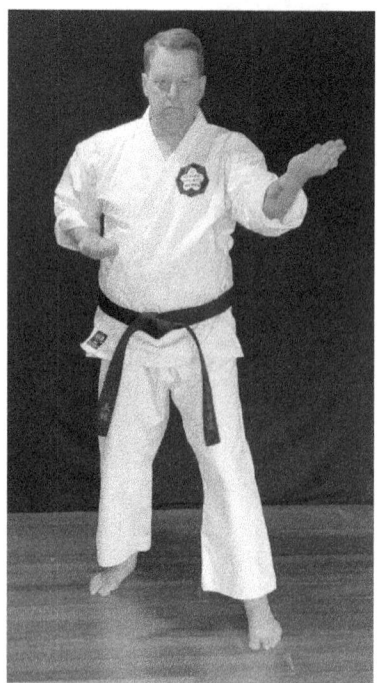

Step Forward with Left Foot, Complete Slow Left Chudan Hari Uke

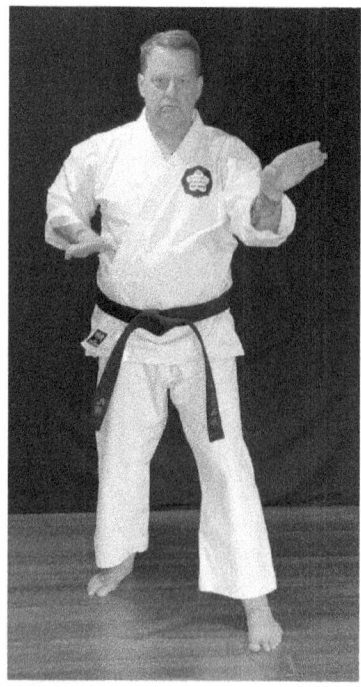

Turn Hands Over, Complete Slow Left Chudan Hiki Uke

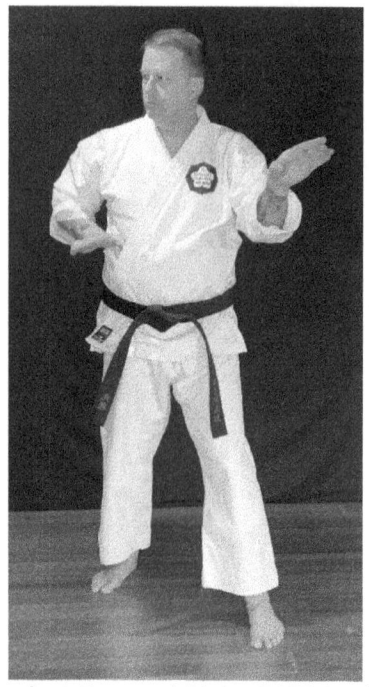

Look at Forward Right, 315° Angle

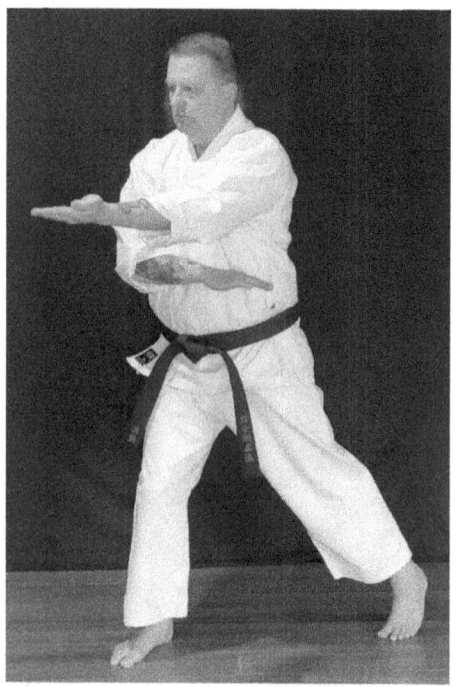

Step Back at 135° with Left Foot while Right Hand Positions Across Torso (palm down), Left Arm Reaches Out (palm up)

Gekisai Ni

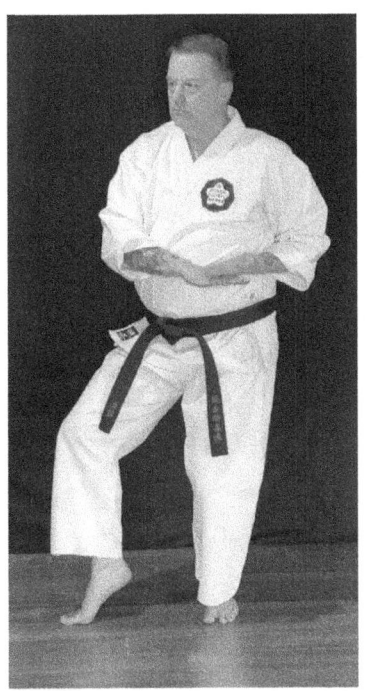

Land in Neko Ashi Dachi while Bringing Left Arm Straight Back

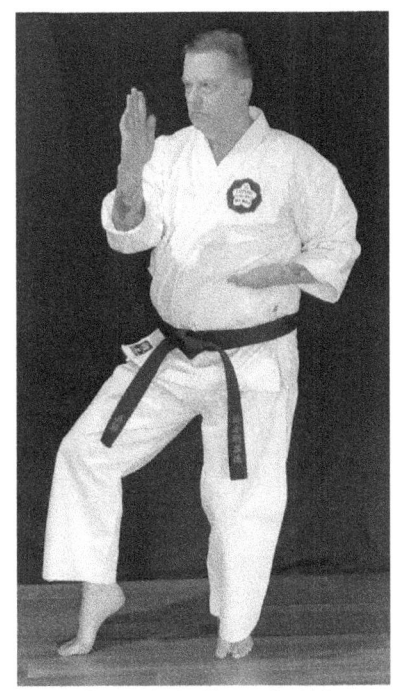

Complete Tora Guchi

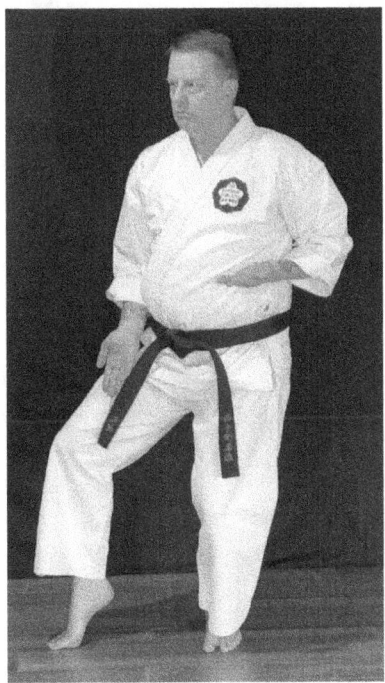

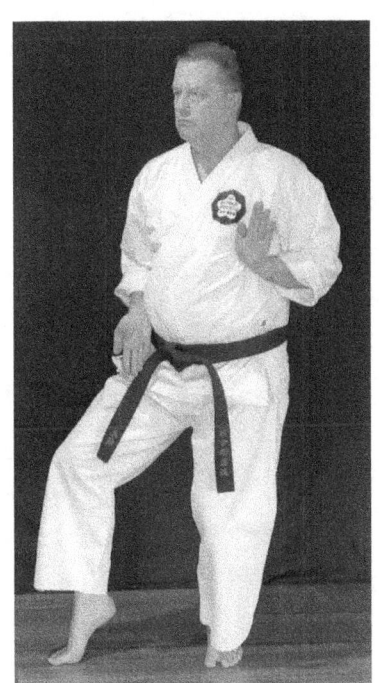

Tora Guchi (cont.)

Gekisai Ni

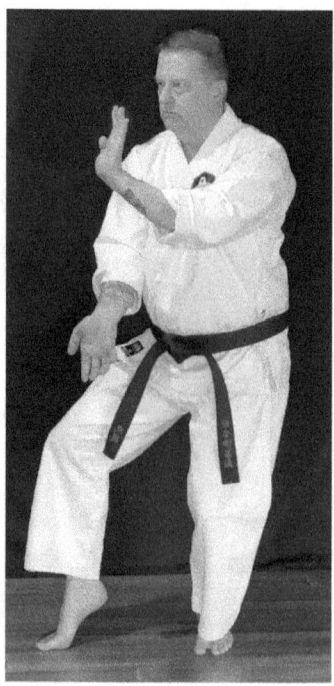

Complete Centerline
Morote Shotei Uchi

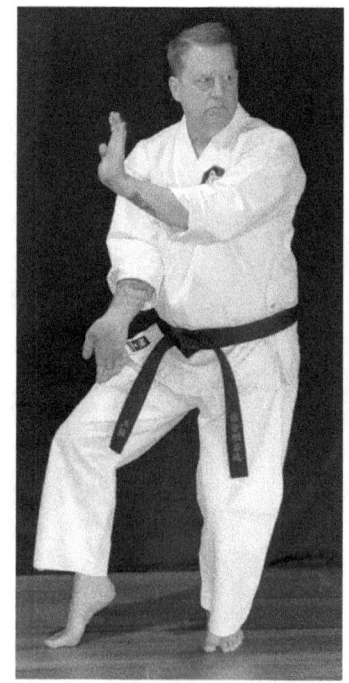

Look at Forward Left, 45° Angle

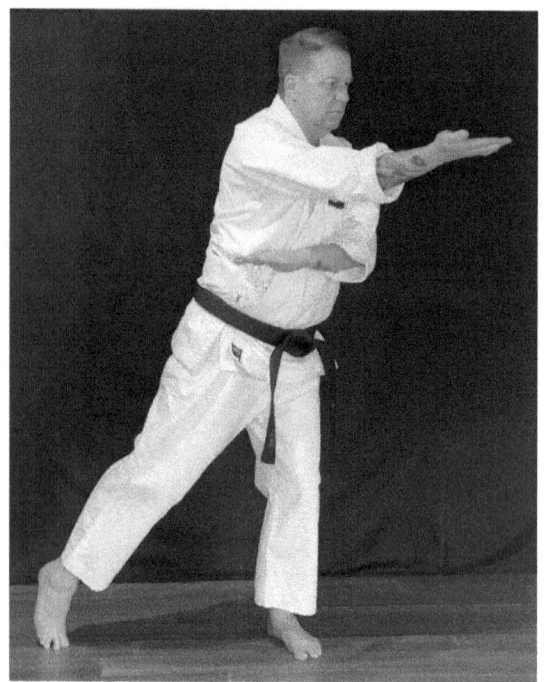

Step Back at 225° with Right Foot while Left
Hand Positions Across Torso (palm down),
Right Arm Reaches Out (palm up)

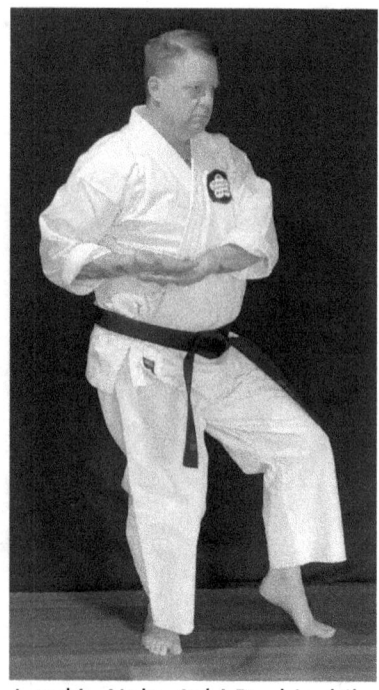

Land in Neko Ashi Dachi while
Bringing Right Arm Straight Back

Gekisai Ni

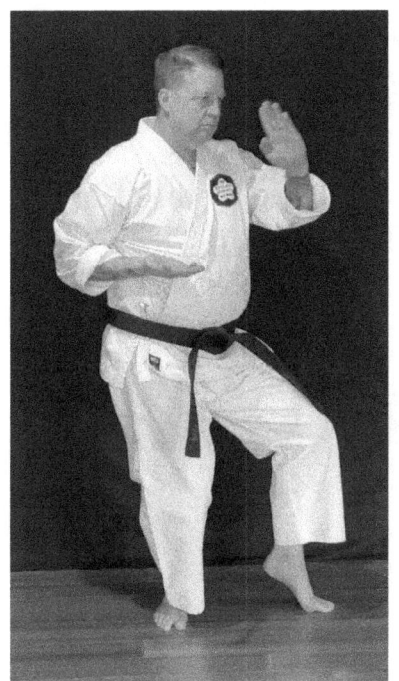
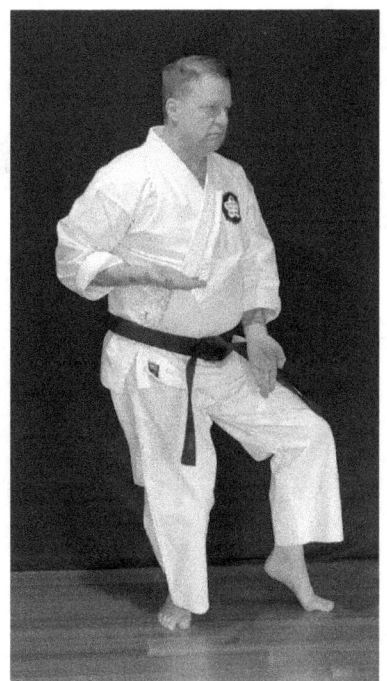

Complete Tora Guchi

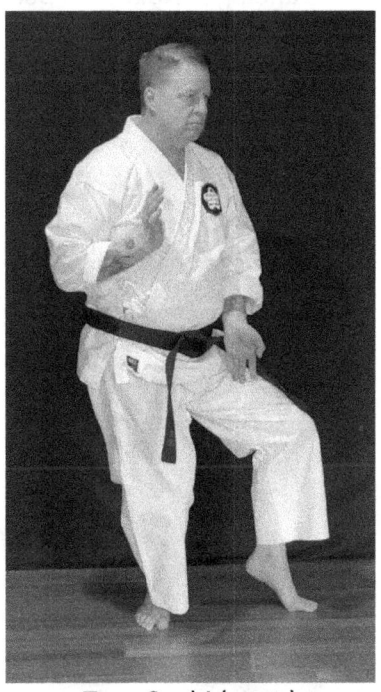
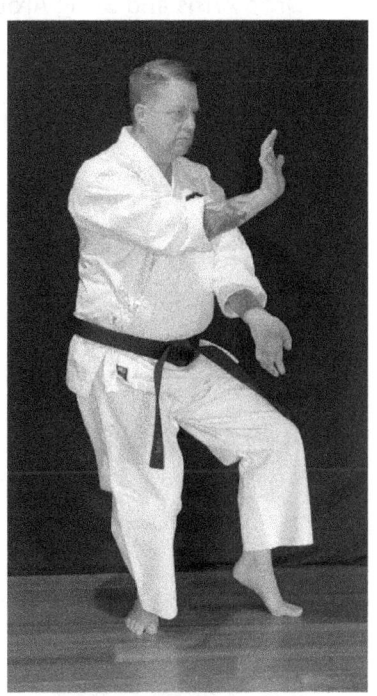

Tora Guchi (cont.)

Complete Centerline
Morote Shotei Uchi

Gekisai Ni

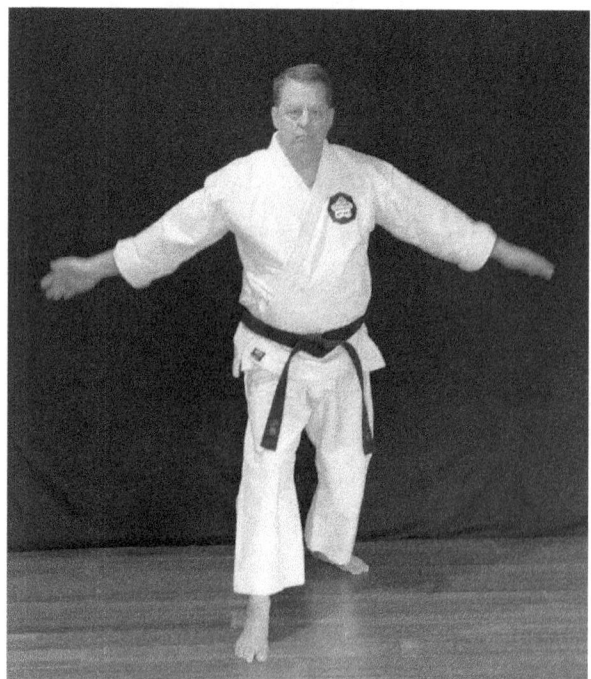

Left Step Back, Facing Forward, Drop Arms and Bring Around

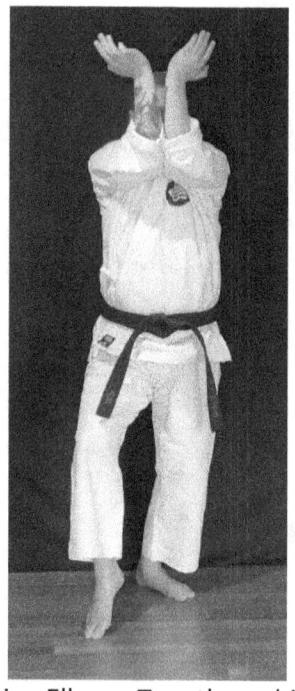

Bring Elbows Together while Landing in Neko Ashi Dachi

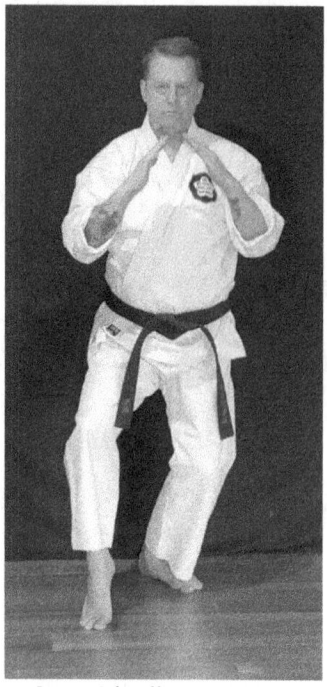

Set with Elbows Down and Hands Separated

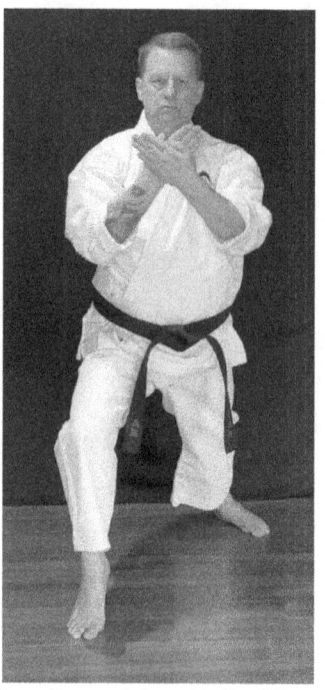

Step Forward on Ball of Foot while Guarding Throat

Gekisai Ni

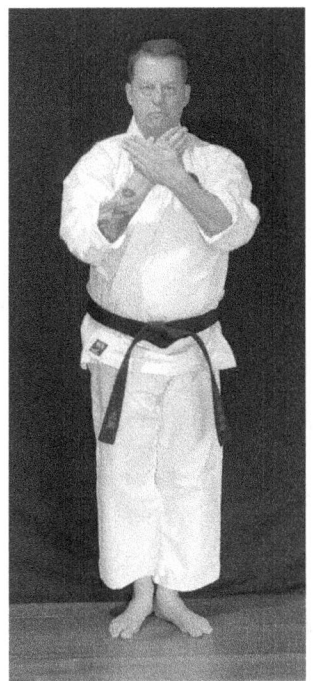

Step Back (Right Foot)
Keeping Throat Guarded

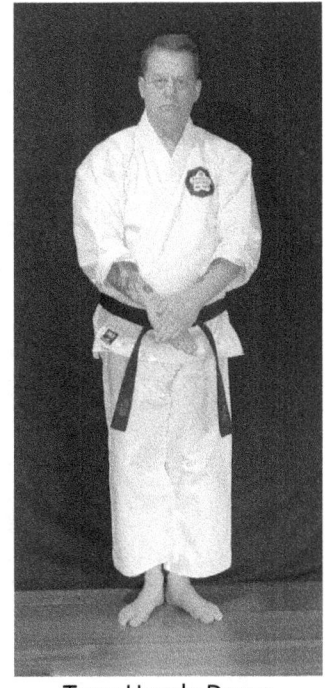

Turn Hands Down
to Guard Groin

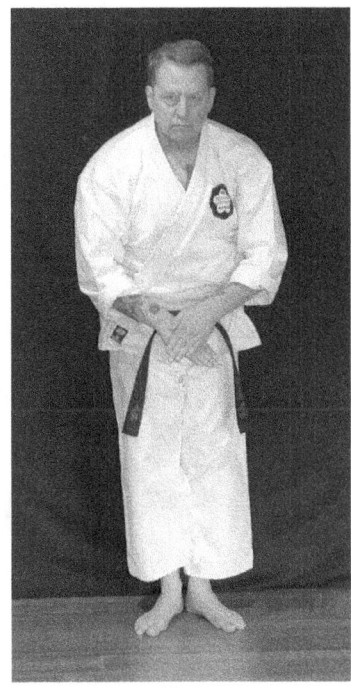

Rei

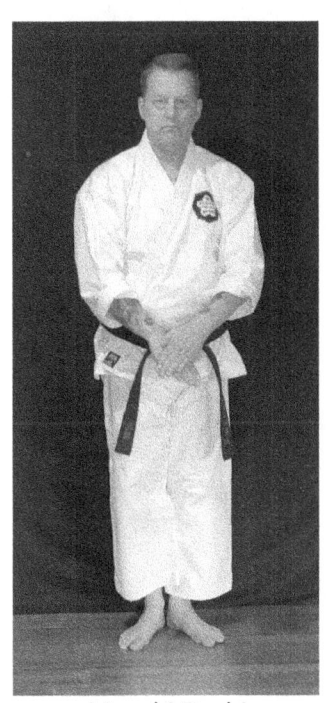

Musubi Dachi

Gekisai Ni

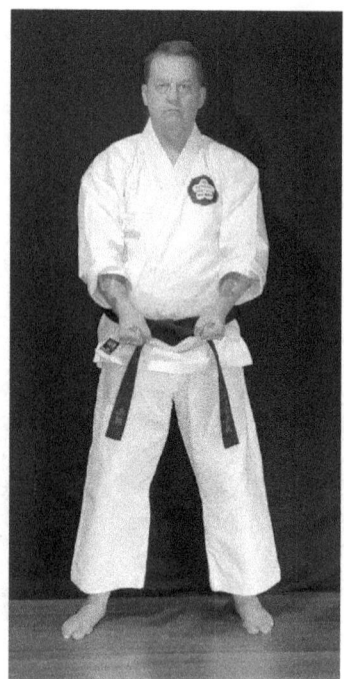

Heiko Dachi

Saifa

Saifa (砕破) can be translated as "destroy defeat[2]." Saifa has its origins in China and was said to be brought to Okinawa by Kanryo Higashionna[3]. It is one of the shortest katas in Goju-Ryu, containing approximately six attack sequences, repeated several times. The kata starts with a wrist grab defense turning into an elbow assisted takedown, leading into a rear hand shotei uke followed by a vertical uraken; this sequence is done three times. The second sequence includes a double hand block, hiza uchi, and gedan mae keage geri. This is followed by a defense against a ground attack, repeated from the rear, another short sequence involving an otoshi tettsui uchi, and the ending.

Below is the method by which Ketsugo Goju-Ryu performs Saifa kata. Complete details about each move are not included, as this is simply a demonstration. Saifa is a widespread kata, and many karate systems include it in their curriculum. This demonstration is not meant to imply that it is the only way to do it, but it is the way at Ketsugo Goju-Ryu.

These are the Japanese terms used for this kata. Bear in mind, karate terms are not completely streamlined. There are terms that were used in the middle of the 20th Century that are no longer used today. Oftentimes there are more than one term that can be used for the same technique. The important thing is not what it is called, but the technique itself.

Barai - Sweeping Block	**Oshi** – Push
Chudan - Middle	**Otoshi** - Downward
Dachi – Stance	**Rei** – Bow (Respect)
Fumikomi Geri – Stamping Kick	**Shiko Dachi** - Straddle Leg Stance
Gedan – Low	**Shotei** – Palm Heel

Saifa

Gyaku Zuki – Reverse Punch	**Sukui Uke** – Scooping Block
Haito Uchi – Ridge Hand Strike	**Tettsui Uchi** - Hammer Fist Strike
Hajime – Command to Begin	**Tora Guchi** – Wheel Block
Heiko Dachi - Parallel Stance	**Tsukami Hiki** – Grab and Pull
Hiki Uke – Open Hand Block (Palm Down)/Pulling Block	**Tsuki/-Zuki** - Punch
	Uchi – Strike
Hiza Uchi – Knee Strike	**Uke** – Block (Receive)
Jodan – High	**Uraken Uchi** – Back Fist Strike
Mae Keage Geri – Front Snap Kick	**Ura Zuki** – Inverted Strike
Morote Hiraken Zuki – Double Fore knuckle Punch	**Yoi** – Ready Command
	Yoko - Side
Morote Shotei Uchi – Double Palm Heel Strike	**Zenkutsu Dachi** - Forward Leaning Stance
Musubi Dachi - Attention Stance, Toes Out	
Neko Ashi Dachi – Cat Leg Stance	

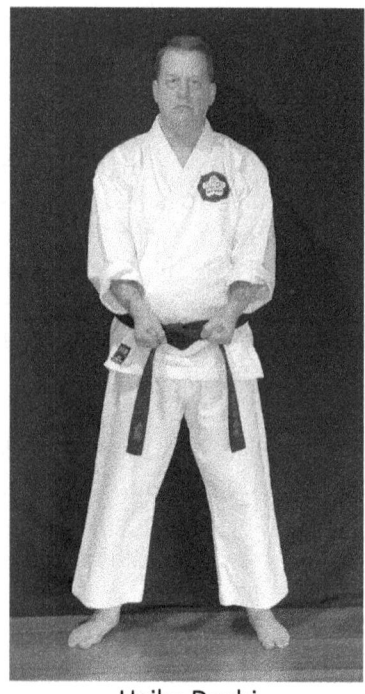

Heiko Dachi

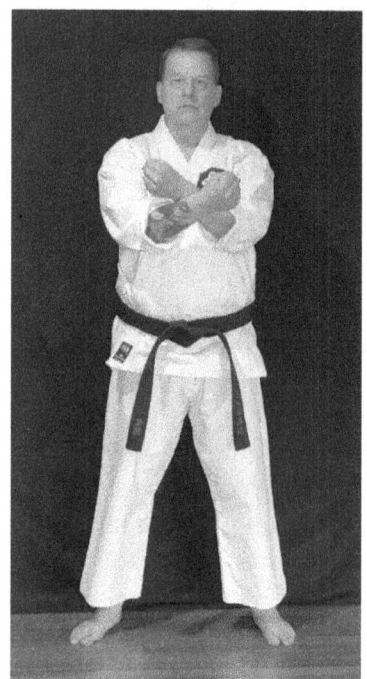

(Yoi) Brings Arms Up, Crossed at the Wrist

Saifa

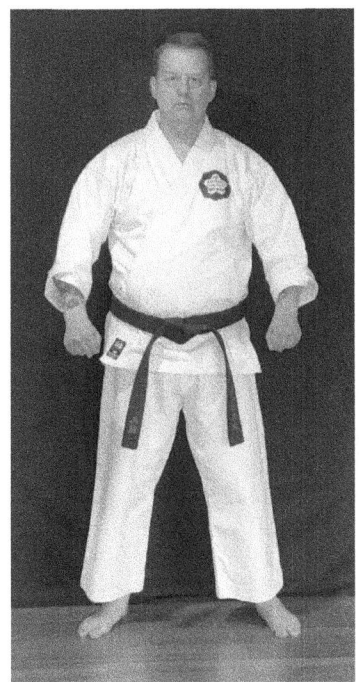

Bring Arms Down

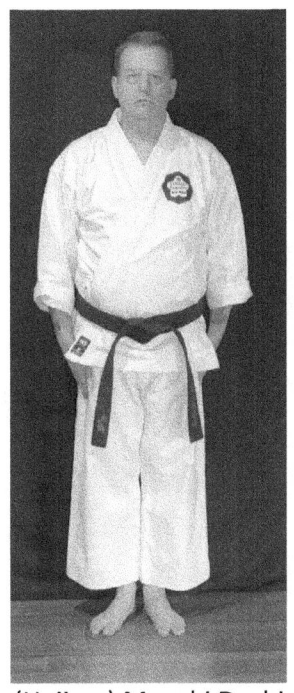

(Hajime) Musubi Dachi

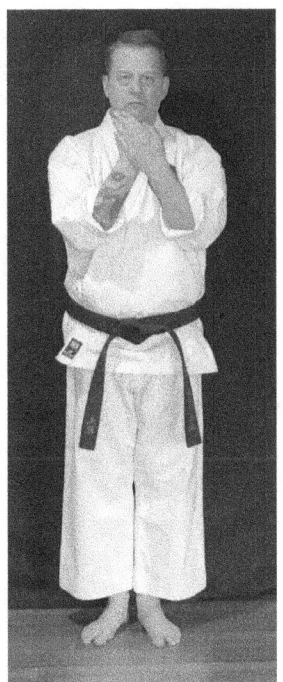

Guard Throat

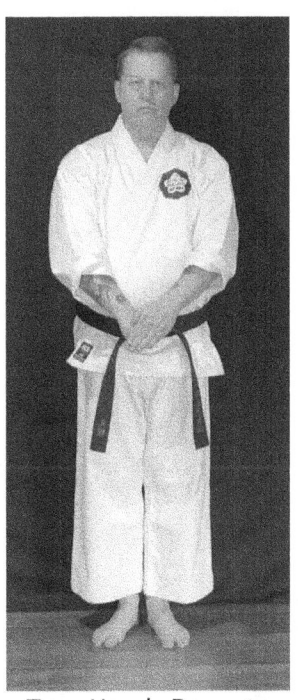

Turn Hands Down to
Guard Groin

Saifa

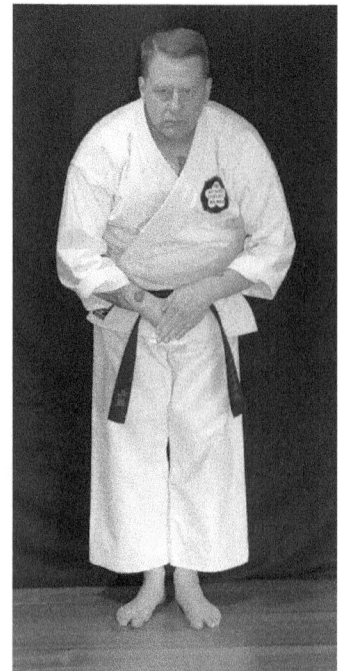
Rei

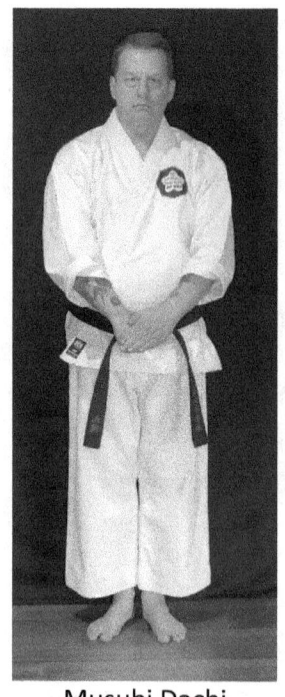
Musubi Dachi

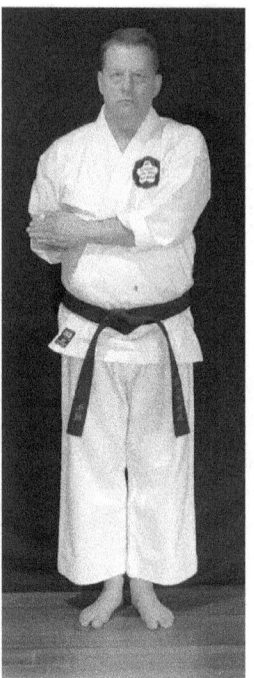
Cover Right Fist with Left Hand

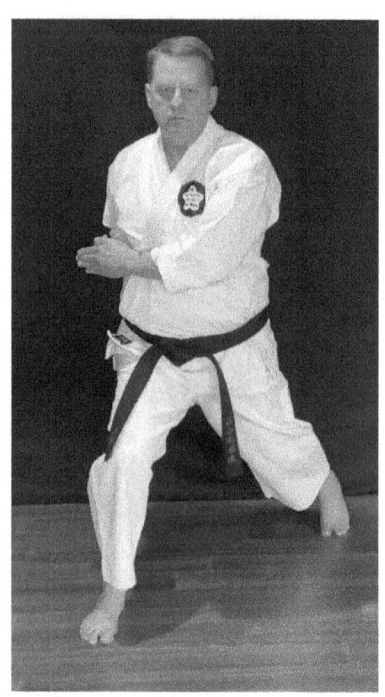
Keeping Hand Covered,
Right Step Forward, 315°

Saifa

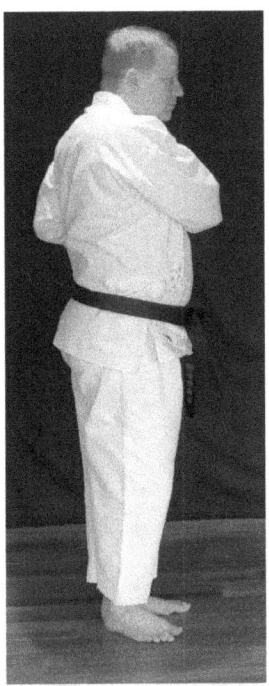

Turn Step 90° into Musubi Dachi, Facing the Side; Bring Right Elbow Across Torso to the Left Side

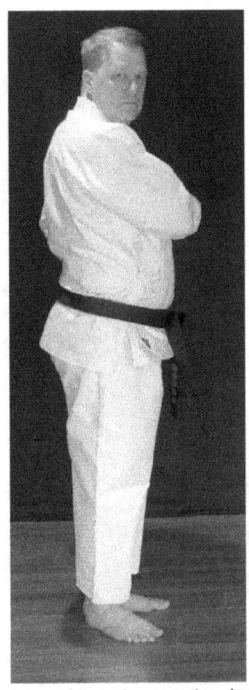

Turn Head to the Right (Front)

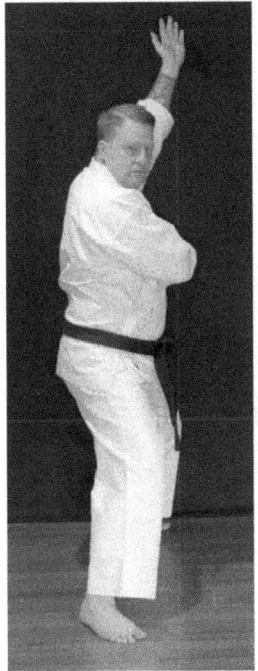

Bring Left Hand Back and Complete Shotei Otoshi Uke while Left Foot Step Back into Shiko Dachi

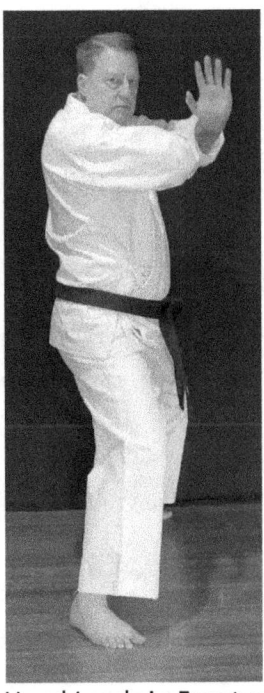

As Left Hand Lands in Front of Chest, Right Hand Begins Uraken Uchi

Saifa

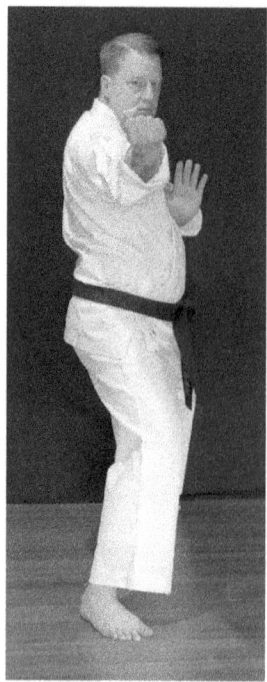

Complete Right Jodan Uraken Uchi

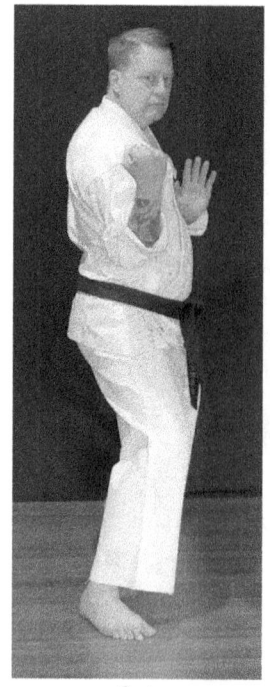

Set

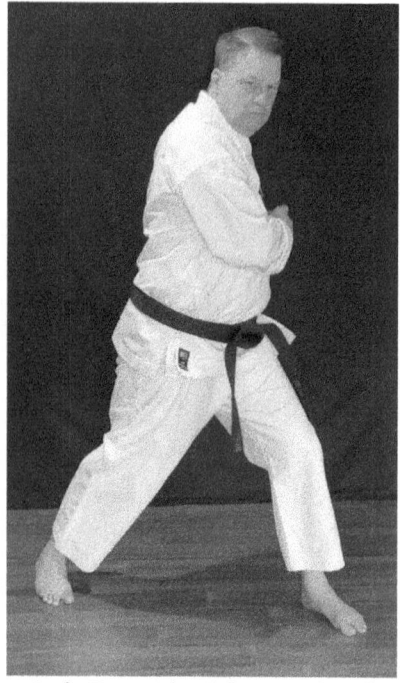

Close Left Fist with Right Hand, Left Step Forward, 45°

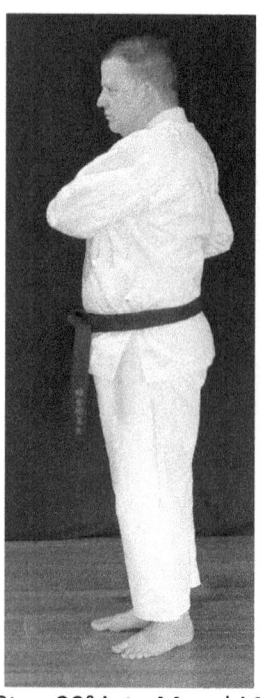

Turn Step 90° into Musubi Dachi, Facing the Side; Bring Left Elbow Across Torso to the Right

Saifa

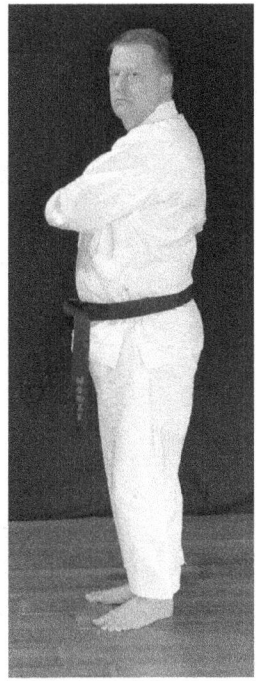

Turn Head to the Left (front)

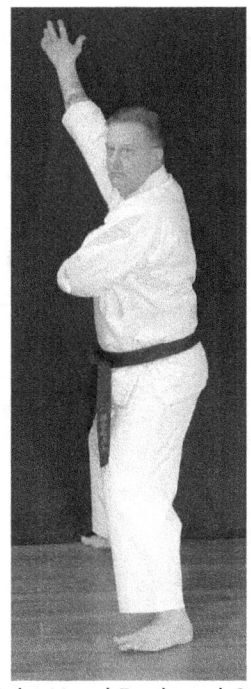

Bring Right Hand Back and Complete
Shotei Otoshi Uke while Right Foot
Step Back into Shiko Dachi

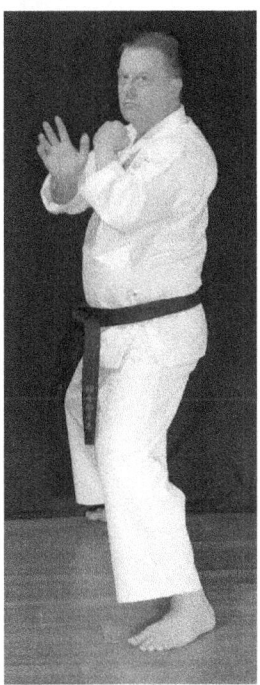

As Right Hand Lands in Front of
Chest, Left Hand Begins Uraken Uchi

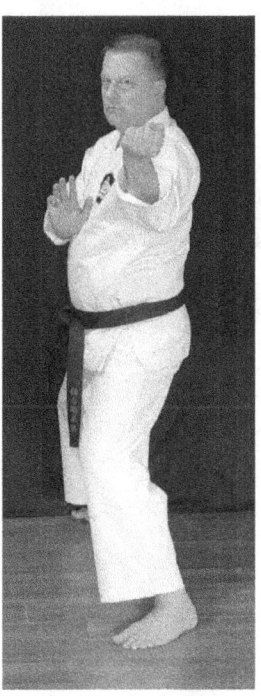

Complete Left Jodan
Uraken Uchi

Saifa

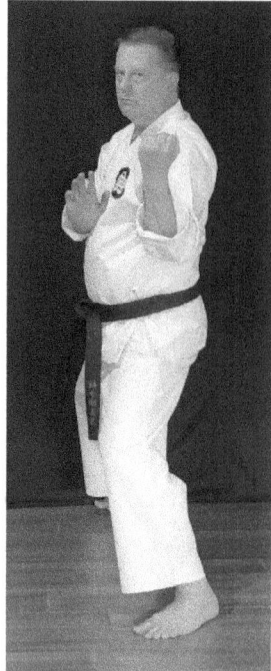

Set

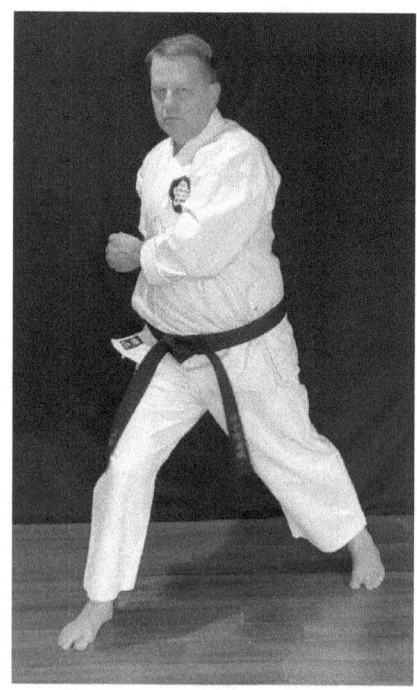

Right Step Forward, 315°

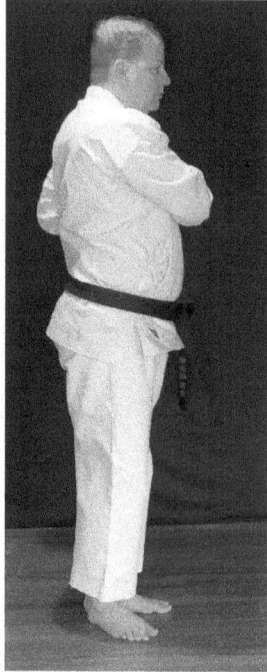

Turn Step 90° into Musubi Dachi, Facing the Side; Bring Right Elbow Across Torso to the Left

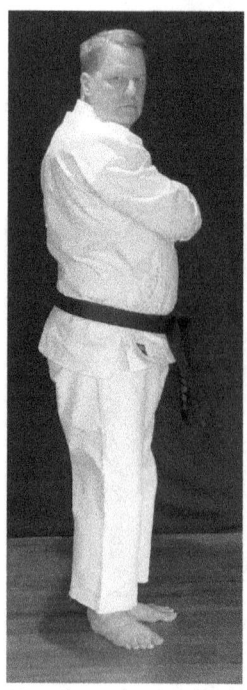

Turn Head to the Right (front)

Saifa

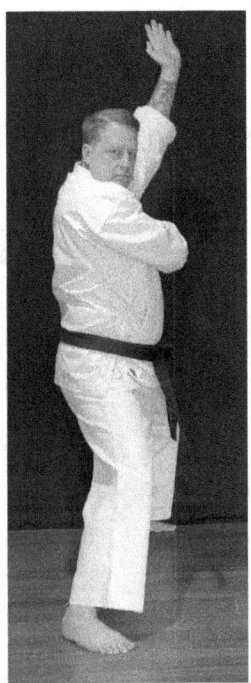

Bring Left Hand Back and Complete Shotei Otoshi Uke while Left Foot Steps into Shiko Dachi

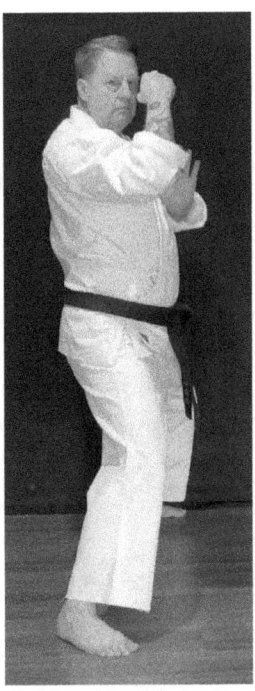

As Left Hand Lands in Front of Chest, Right Hand Begins Uraken Uchi

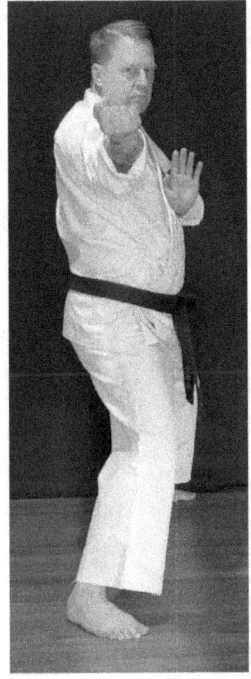

Complete Right Jodan Uraken Uchi

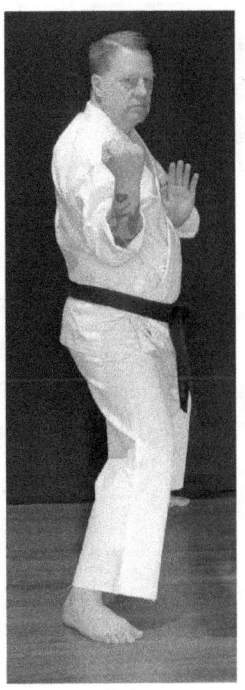

Set

Saifa

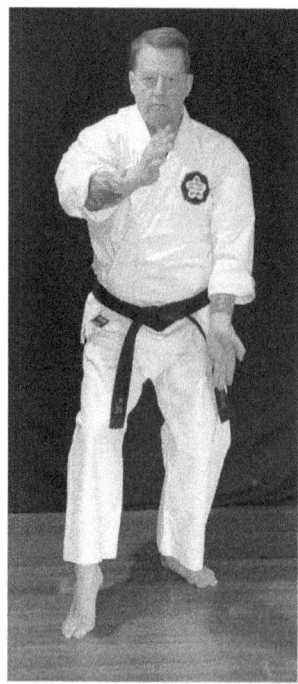

Step with Left Foot to Left Side, Drag Right Foot Across into Neko Ashi Dachi, while Dropping Left Hand Down, Right Hand Up

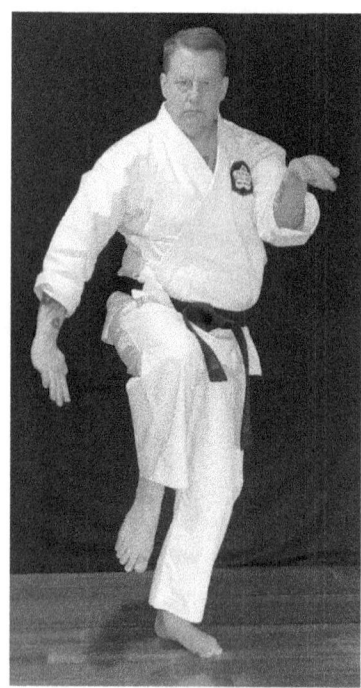

Right Hand Completes Gedan Shotei Barai while Left Hand Chudan Sukui Uke, while Completing Hiza Uchi

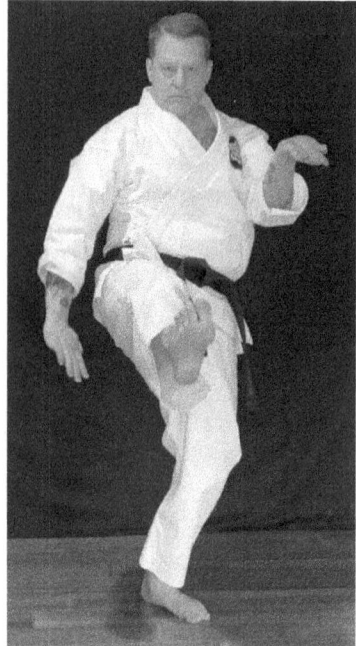

Complete Right Gedan Mae Keage Geri

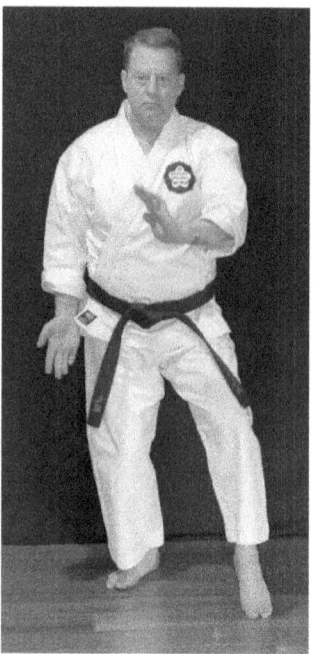

Step with Right Foot to Right Side, Drag Left Foot Across into Neko Ashi Dachi, while Turning Right Palm Up, Begin Left Gedan Shotei Barai

Saifa

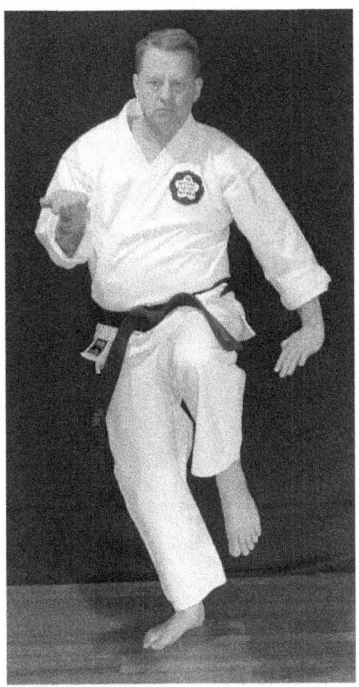

Left Hand Completes Gedan Shotei Barai while Right Hand Chudan Sukui Uke, while Completing Hiza Uchi

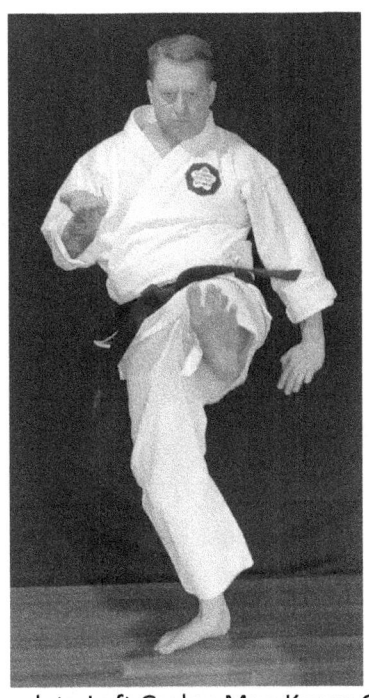

Complete Left Gedan Mae Keage Geri

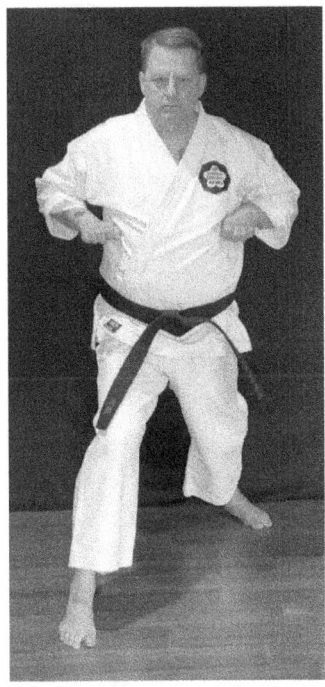

Left Step Back into Zenkutsu Dachi, Hiraken in Chamber

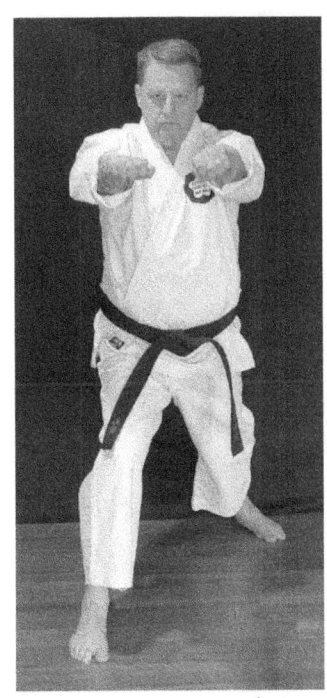

Complete Morote Hiraken Zuki

Saifa

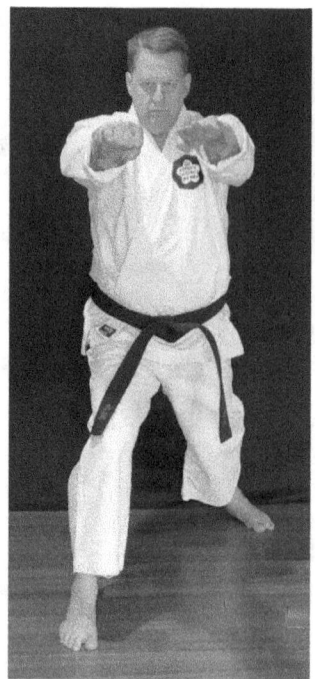
Close Right Hand, Open Left Hand

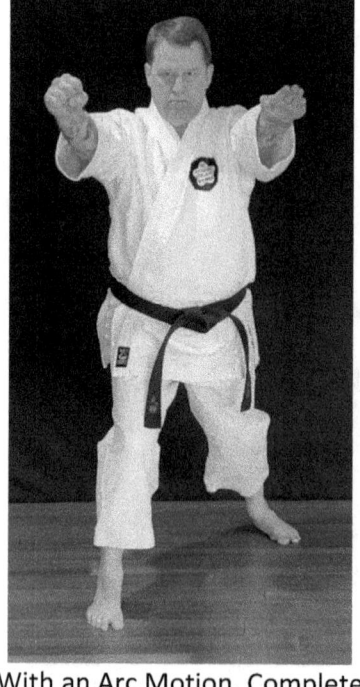
With an Arc Motion, Complete Tettsui Uchi with Right Hand into Open Left Hand

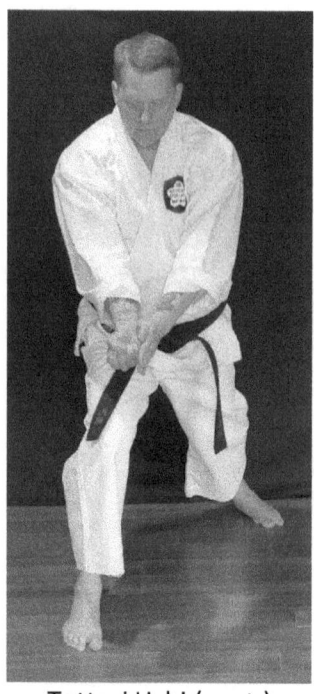
Tettsui Uchi (cont.)

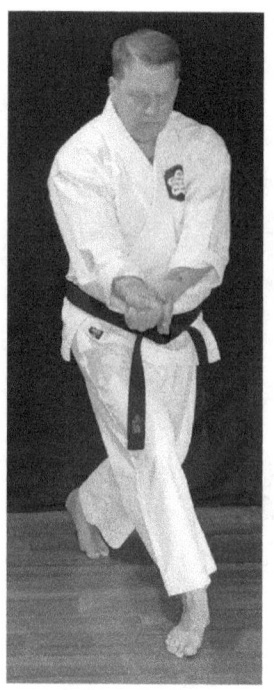
Step Left

Saifa

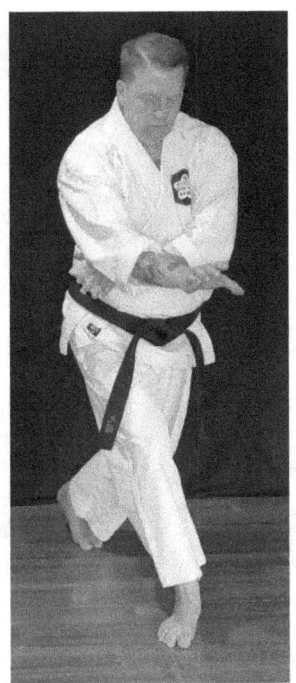

Open Hands, Prepare for Hiki Uke

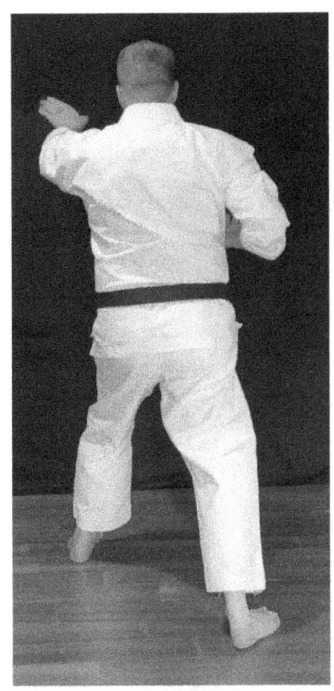

Spin Around 180°, Complete Left Chudan Hiki Uke

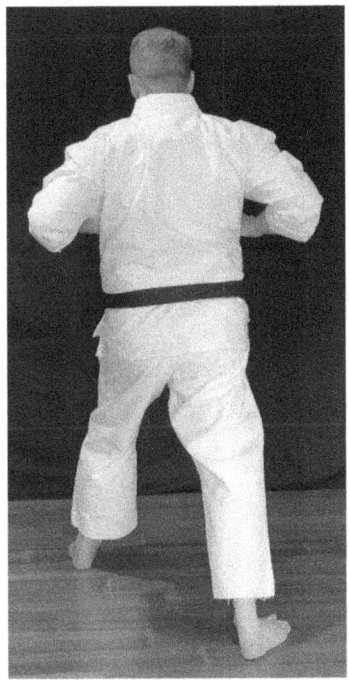

Chamber Hiraken

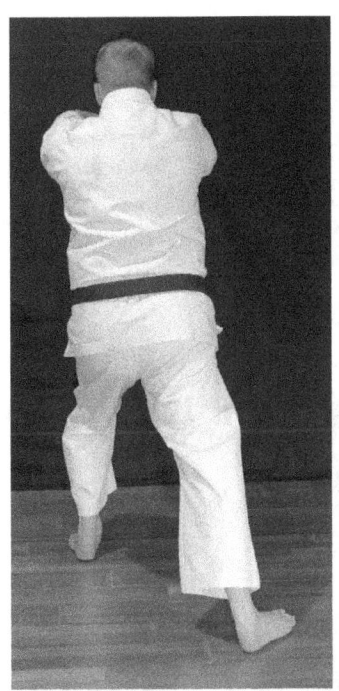

Complete Morote Hiraken Uchi

Saifa

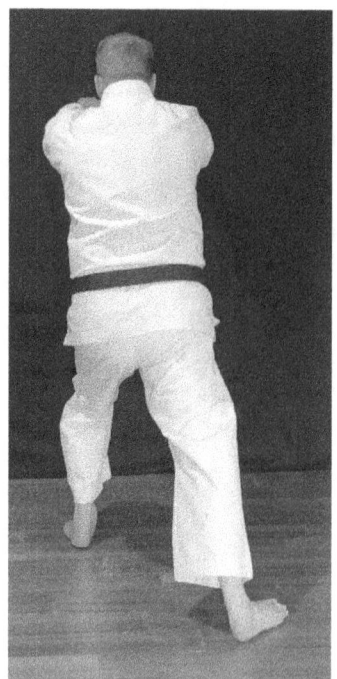

Close Left Hand, Open Right Hand

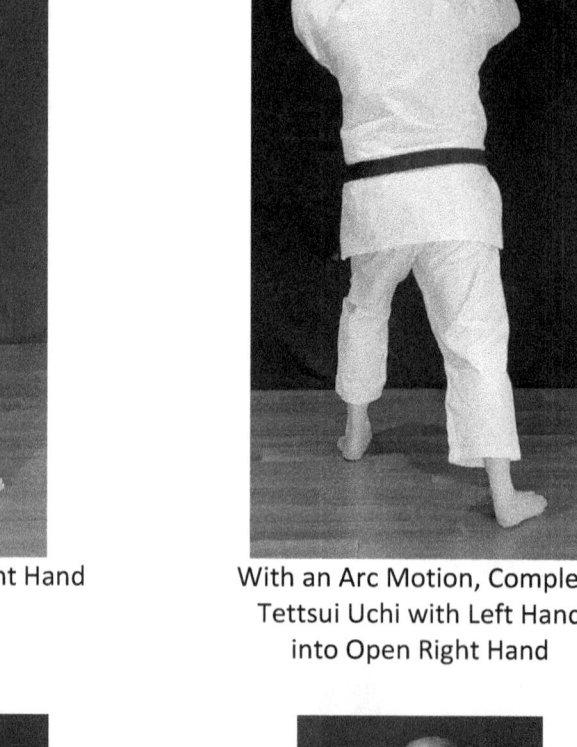

With an Arc Motion, Complete Tettsui Uchi with Left Hand into Open Right Hand

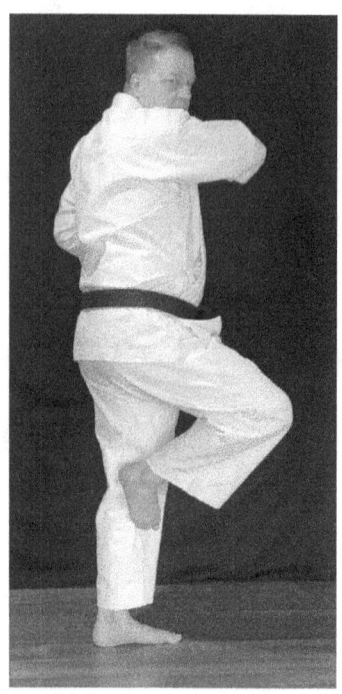

Bring Right Foot and Right Hand Up to Chamber Looking Front and Facing Left

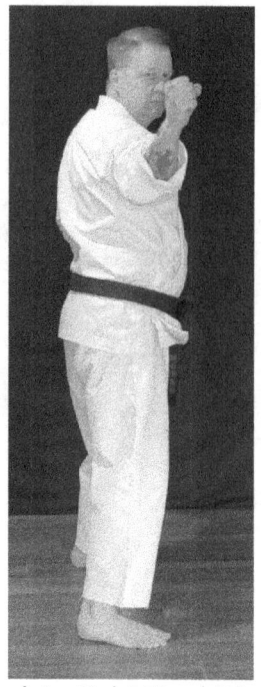

Complete Right Otoshi Tettsui Uchi with Fumikomi Geri (kiai)

Saifa

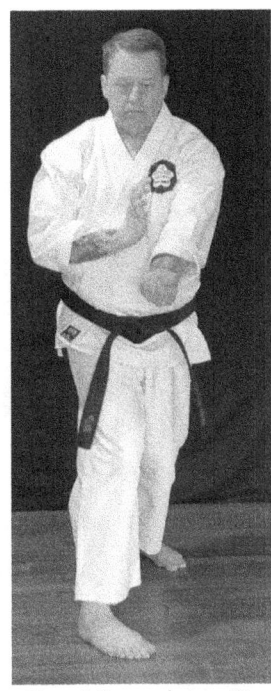

Right Hand Completes Tsukami Hiki while Left Hand Completes Yoko Ura Zuki

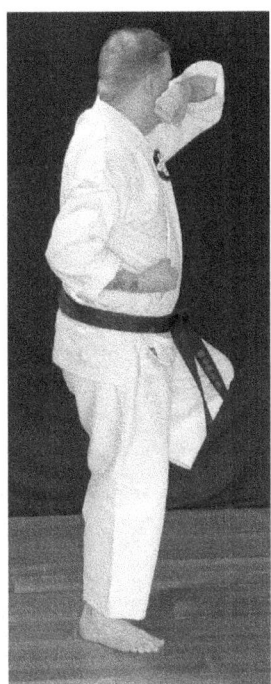

Bring Left Foot and Left Hand Up to Chamber Looking Rear and Facing Left

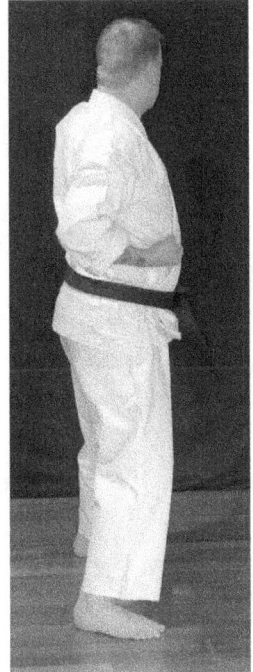

Complete Right Otoshi Tettsui Uchi with Fumikomi Geri (kiai)

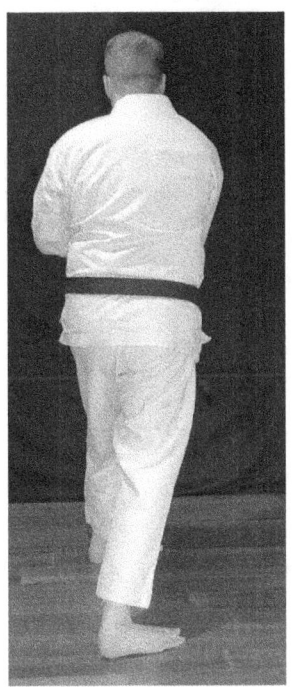

Left Hand Completes Tsukami Hiki while Right Hand Completes Yoko Ura Zuki

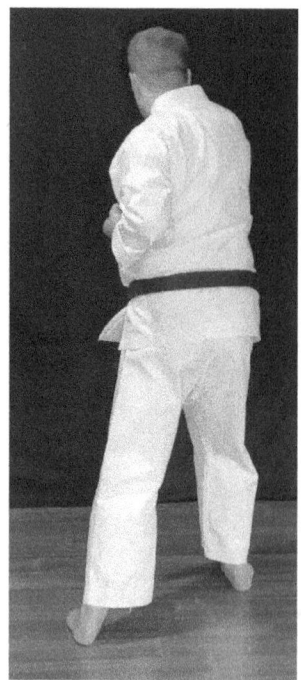 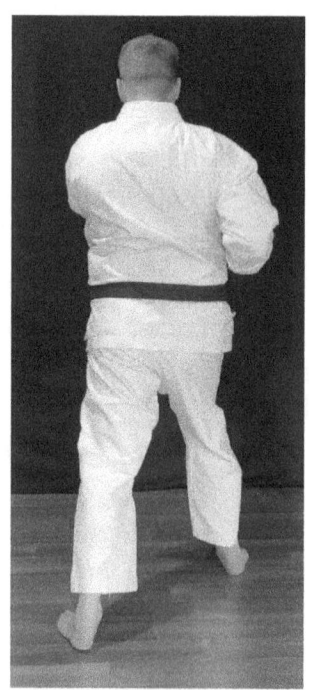

Right Step Towards Rear, Right Chudan Tsukami Hiki while Completing Left Gyaku Zuki

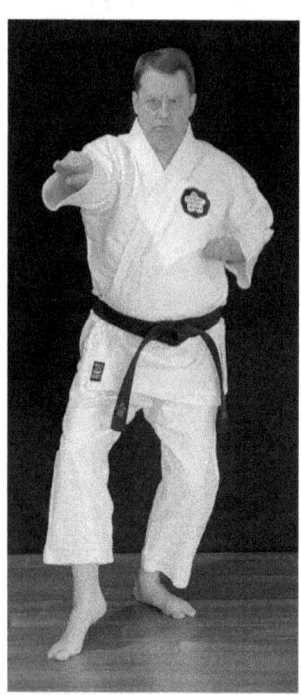 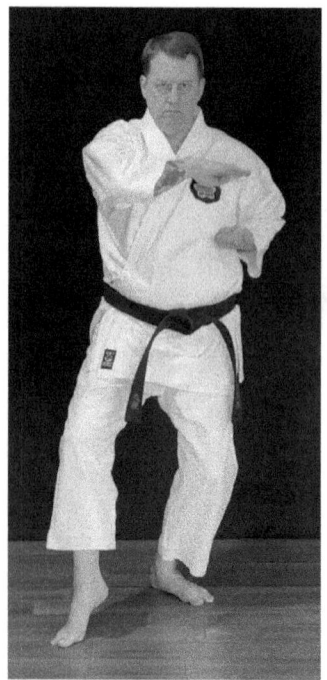

Step Around Facing Forward with Left Foot, Landing in Neko Ashi Dachi, while Swinging a Right Haito Uchi, Left Hand in Chamber

Saifa

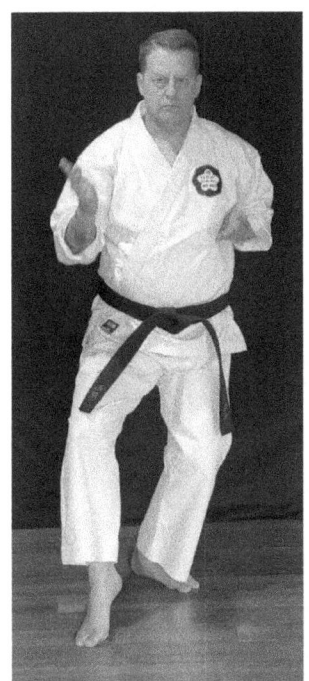 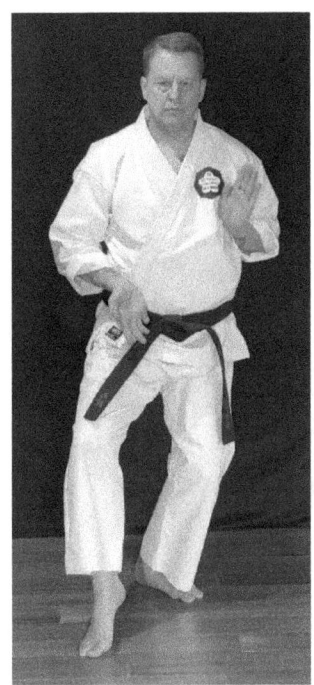

Complete Tora Guchi

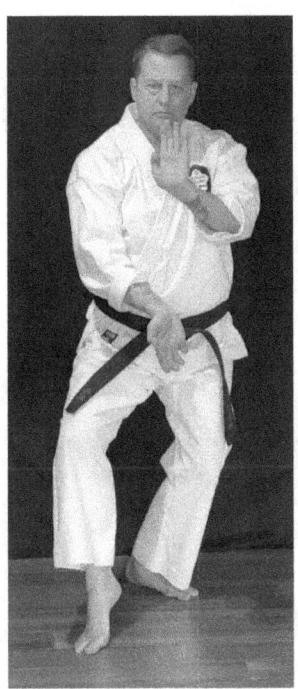 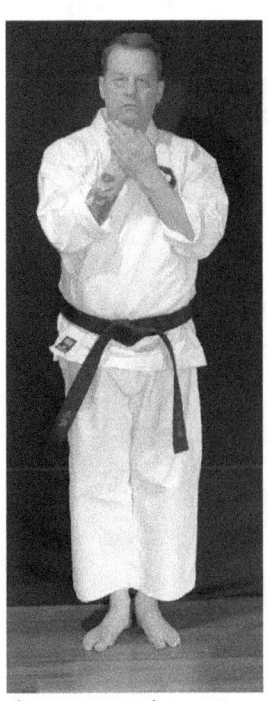

Complete Centerline
Morote Shotei Uchi

Right Step Back to Musubi
Dachi, Guarding Throat

Saifa

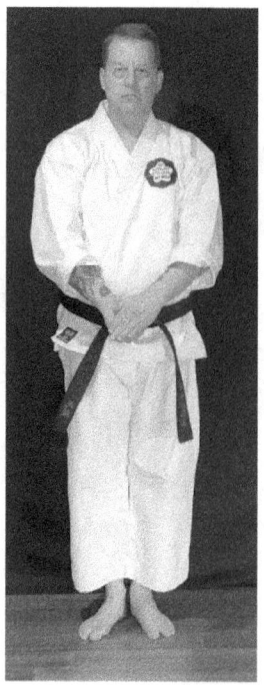

Turn Hands Down to Guard Groin

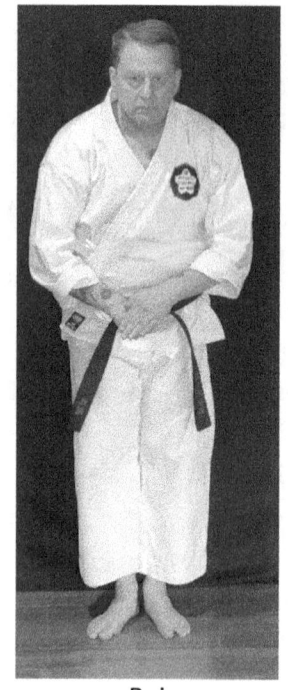

Rei

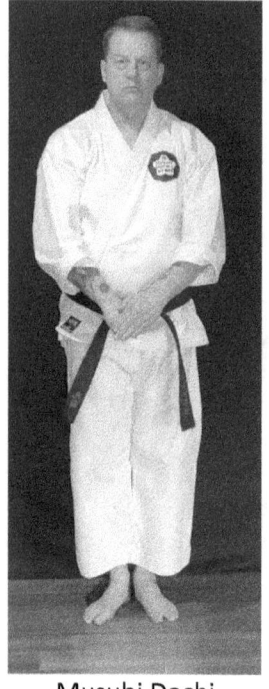

Musubi Dachi

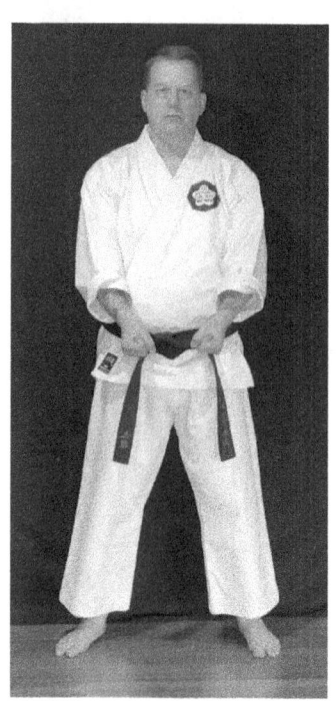

Heiko Dachi

Sanchin

Sanchin (三戦)means "three battles – body, mind and spirit." Sanchin was originally the first kata learned in the Goju-Ryu system and continues to be the cornerstone of any Goju-Ryu system. Its purpose is to harmonize the body, mind, and spirit (hence the name). The techniques are performed slowly, deliberately, and ibuki breathing moves perfectly with the strikes. The end of each breath stops at the same time as the strike or movement. This teaches the student to tighten the body upon exhalation in anticipation of a counterstrike.

Sanchin is practiced using a second person (typically the instructor), who gives strikes (shime) to various parts of the body of the person doing the kata. Shime is given to the stomach, groin, shoulders, lats, and outside of the knees. It is not a particularly difficult kata in movement, but the foundation of it is very important to master. In addition to the basic moves, the student must tense every muscle, gripping the floor with his feet, and tilting the pelvis upward after each step, which tucks the groin area. Of equal importance is the breathing, which is done in heavy ibuki style. The breathing matches the strikes, drawn in when the arm is drawn back and pushed out at the same pace as the strikes. Going through Sanchin with strikes can look difficult and intense, but students learn how to do it properly and practice accordingly.

There are many misconceptions about Sanchin. In Mark Bishop's book, Okinawan Karate[4], he warns against performing Sanchin because of harmful health impacts he claims he was told. He writes, "forceful closing of the anal sphincter...will result in hemorrhoids." Also, "blocking with the thumb side of the fist forced sideways causes pressure which will have an adverse effect on the lungs...which may result in TB and asthma." Finally, he claims that he was told that "punching and kicking the abdomen will have adverse effects on the intestines and may result in stomach cancer." To be fair, he does not list any sources for this information, and it is unknown how many people took his advice in 1989. But I will give the benefit of hindsight that sometimes information is given based on what one is told and occasionally time proves it incorrect.

According to a leaflet by the University Hospitals of Leicester[5], squeezing the anal sphincter muscles is a recommended exercise to prevent incontinence. To address his second and third points about the blocking fist and abdominal strikes, if while performing any exercises, a sharp pain is felt, the student may want to see a doctor about it, especially if the regular healing methods (rest, ice, compression, elevation) are not working. It is unclear if there are any links between blunt trauma to a specific part of the wrist and lung problems, and claims of getting cancer from blunt trauma are dubious at best. If that were the case, everyone who has ever trained with a medicine ball would be in danger of getting stomach cancer. The so-called danger in practicing Sanchin is the same danger as anything in martial arts or exercise. If a student has a previous condition, certain exercises may exacerbate the condition. This is why, if a student has a history of health problems, he or she should consult a physician prior to any kind of physical training. But speak to your instructor about the exercise itself too. Describing an exercise incorrectly will not help in communicating with a medical expert. And doing an exercise incorrectly is always a danger to the student. Technique first!

Below is the method by which Ketsugo Goju-Ryu performs Sanchin kata. Complete details about each move are not included, as this is simply a demonstration. Sanchin is a widespread kata, and many karate systems include it in their curriculum. This demonstration is not meant to imply that it is the only way to do it, but it is the way at Ketsugo Goju-Ryu.

These are the Japanese terms used for this kata. Bear in mind, karate terms are not completely streamlined. There are terms that were used in the middle of the 20th Century that are no longer used today. Oftentimes there are more than one term that can be used for the same technique. The important thing is not what it is called, but the technique itself.

Barai - Sweeping Block	**Musubi Dachi** - Attention Stance, Toes Out
Chudan - Middle	**Rei** – Bow (Respect)
Dachi – Stance	**Sanchin Dachi** – Hourglass Stance
Gedan – Low	**Shiko Dachi** - Straddle Leg Stance
Hajime – Command to Begin	**Shotei** – Palm Heel
Heiko Dachi - Parallel Stance	**Shuto Uchi** – Chop Strike
Jodan – High	**Tora Guchi** – Wheel Block
Kosa Dachi – Cross Leg Stance	**Tsuki/-Zuki** - Punch
Morote Chudan Uke – Double Arm Chest Block	**Uchi** – Strike
Morote Heiko Uchi – Double Parallel Strike	**Uke** – Block (Receive)
	Yoi – Ready Command
Morote Shotei Uchi – Double Palm Heel Strike	**Yoko** - Side

Sanchin

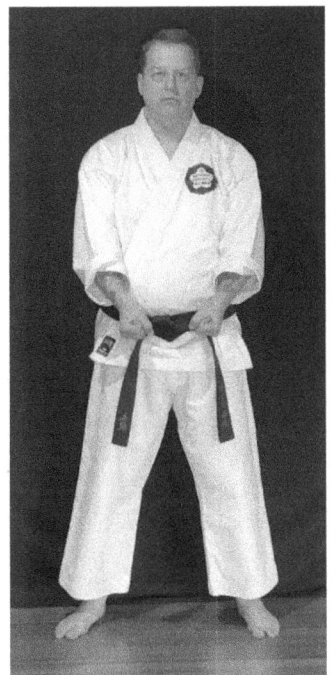

Heiko Dachi

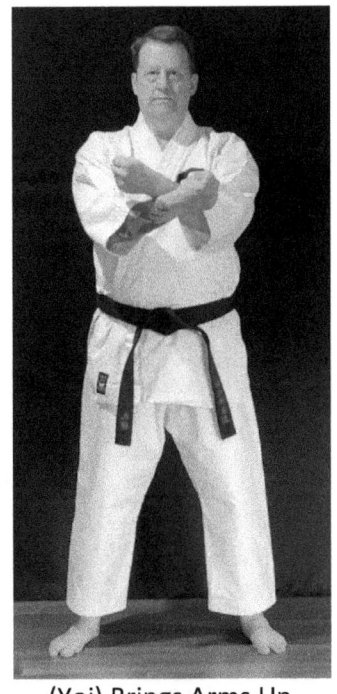

(Yoi) Brings Arms Up, Crossed at the Wrist

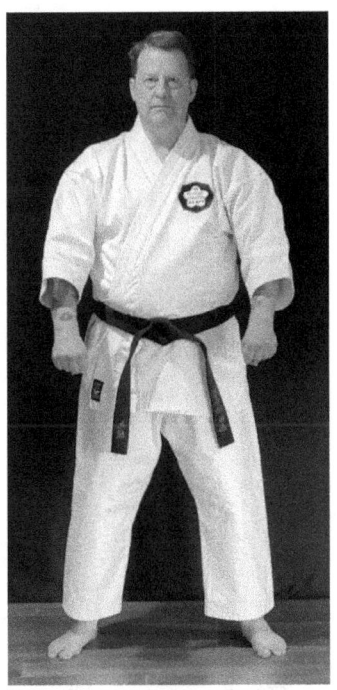

Bring Arms Down

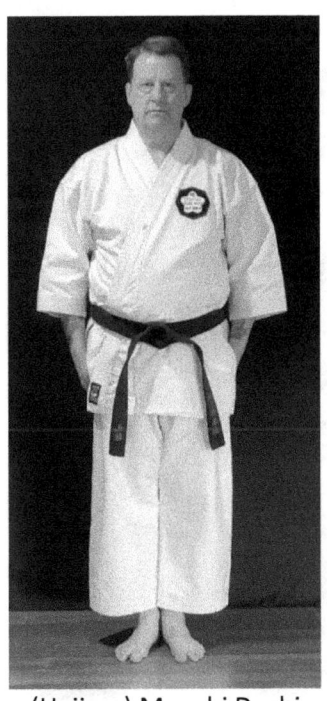

(Hajime) Musubi Dachi

Sanchin

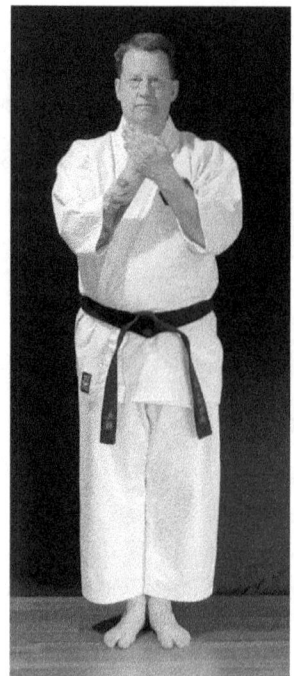

Guard Throat

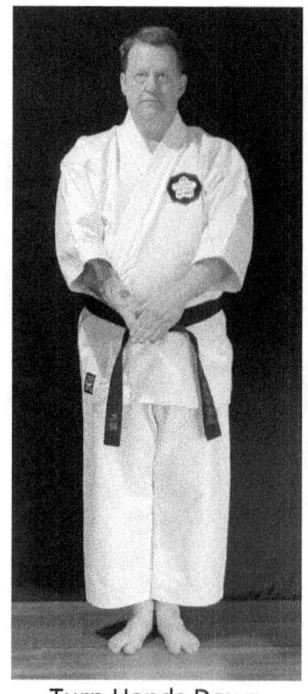

Turn Hands Down
to Guard Groin

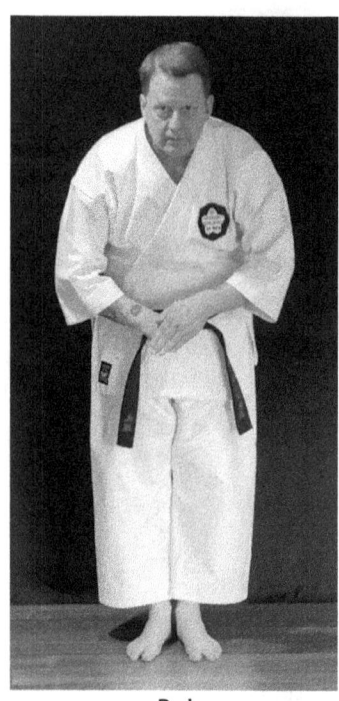

Rei

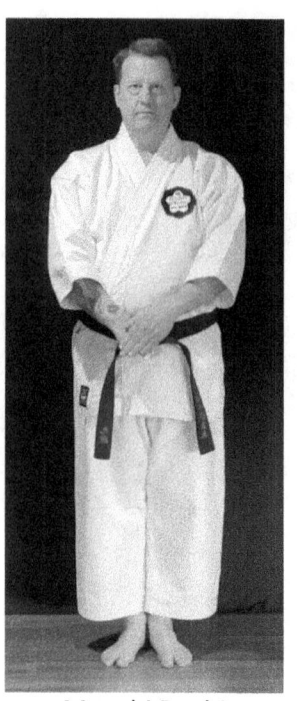

Musubi Dachi

Sanchin

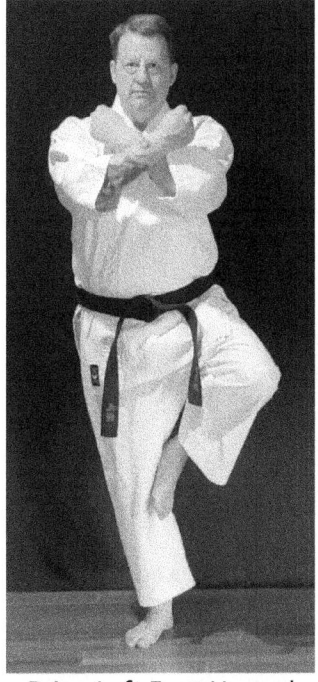

Bring Left Foot Up and Cross Arms (long inhale)

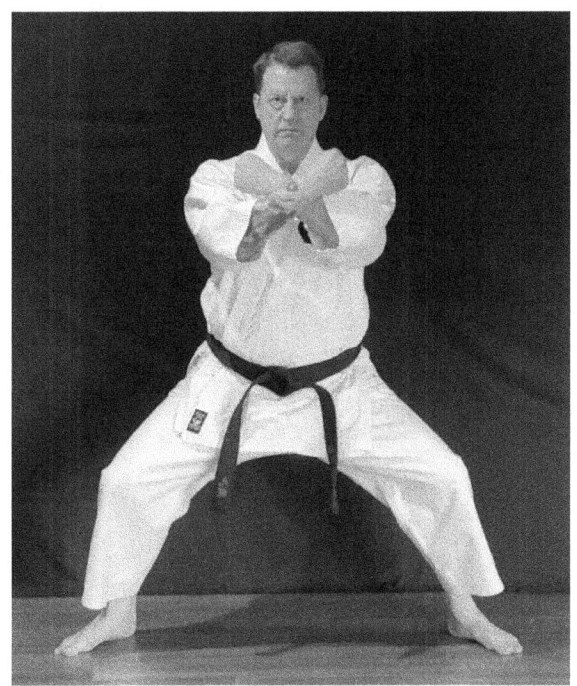

Come Down into Shiko Dachi

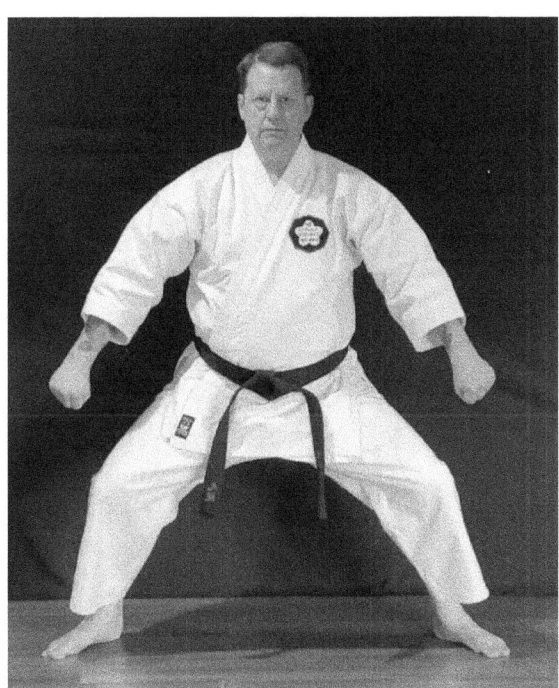

Complete Morote Gedan Barai Slowly (long exhale)

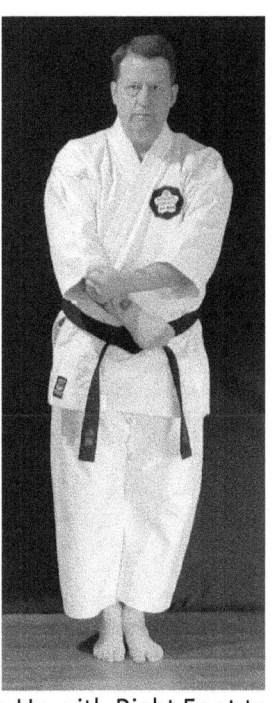

Come Up with Right Foot to Left, Step into Sanchin Dachi, Beginning Right Chudan Uke (long inhale)

Sanchin

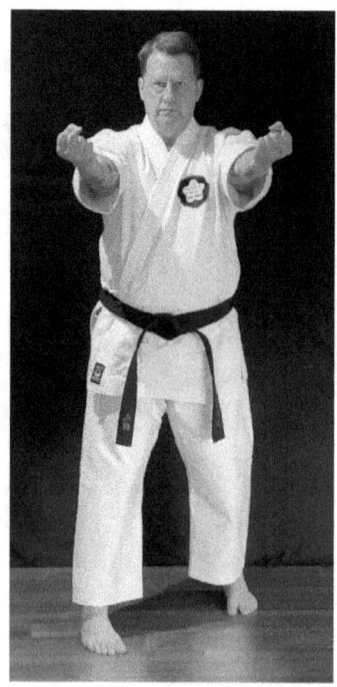

Complete Slow, Extended
Morote Chudan Uke (long inhale)

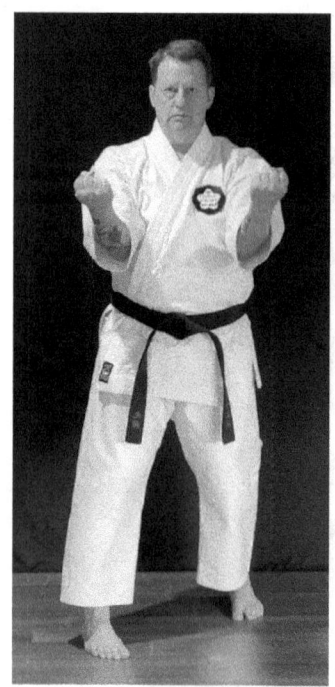

Set (long exhale)

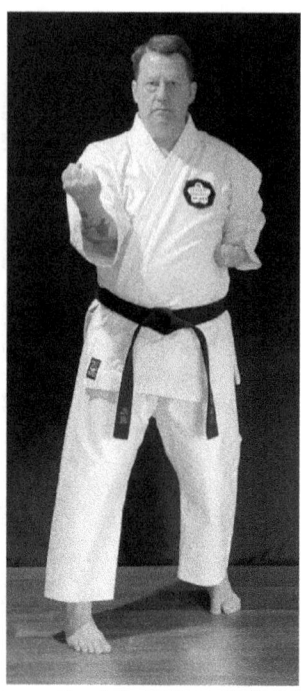

Draw Back Left Hand Slowly
into Chamber (long inhale)

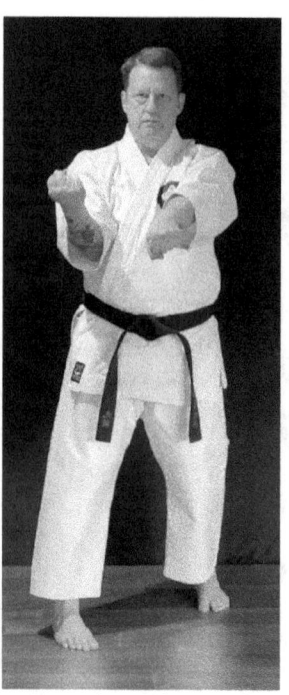

Complete Slow Left
Chudan Zuki (long exhale)

Sanchin

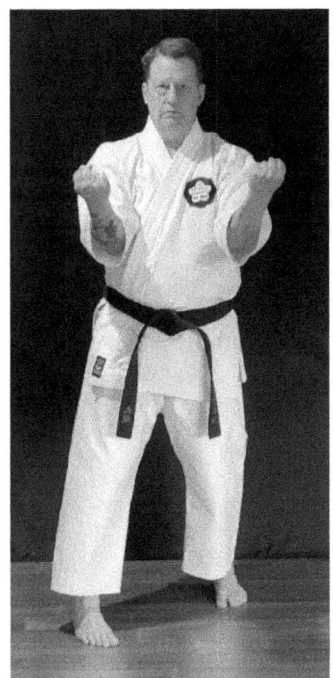
Set (short inhale/exhale)

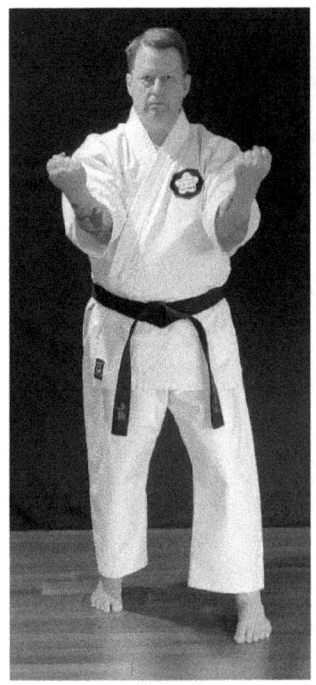
Step

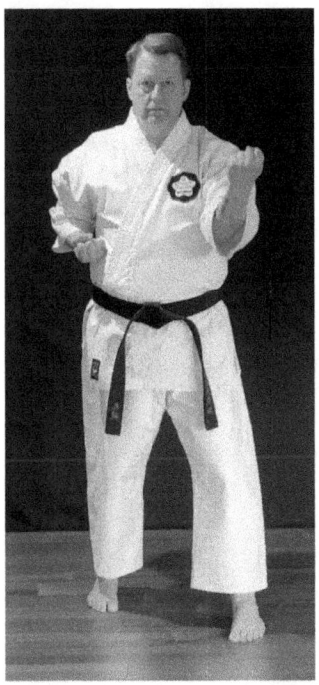
Draw Back Right Hand Slowly into Chamber (long inhale)

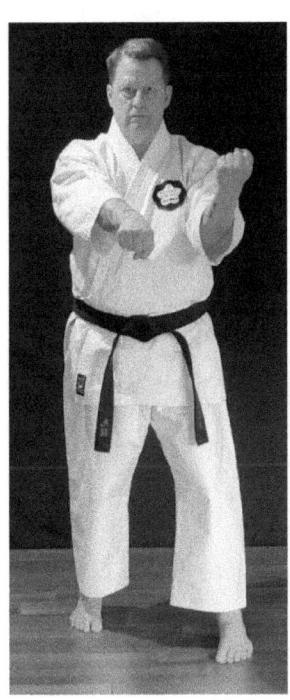
Complete Slow Right Chudan Zuki (long exhale)

Sanchin

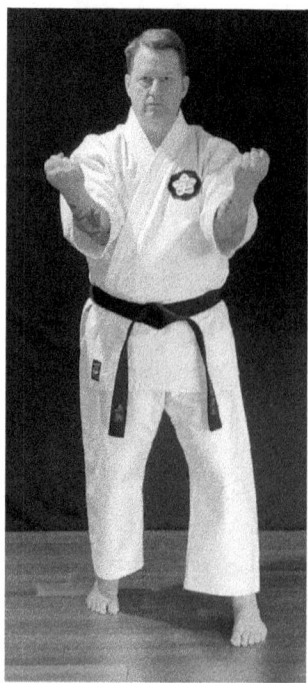
Set (short inhale/exhale)

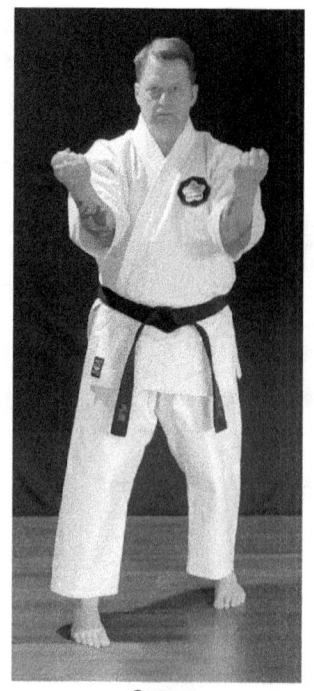
Step

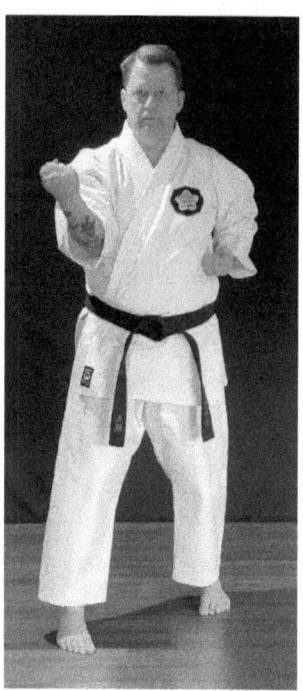
Draw Back Left Hand Slowly into Chamber (long inhale)

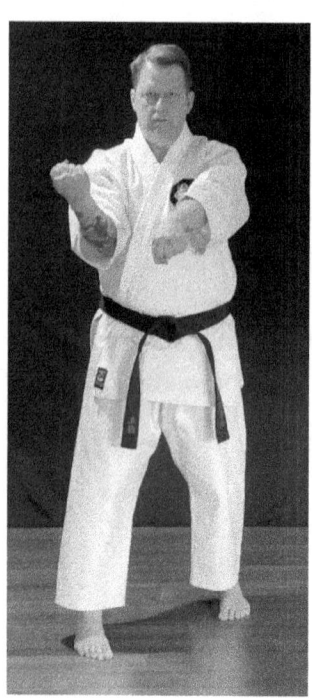
Complete Slow Left Chudan Zuki (long exhale)

Sanchin

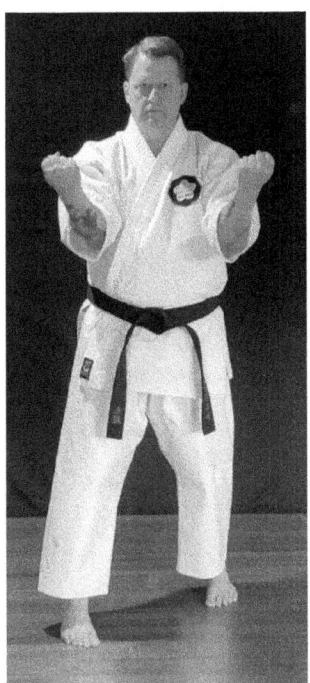

Set (short inhale/exhale)

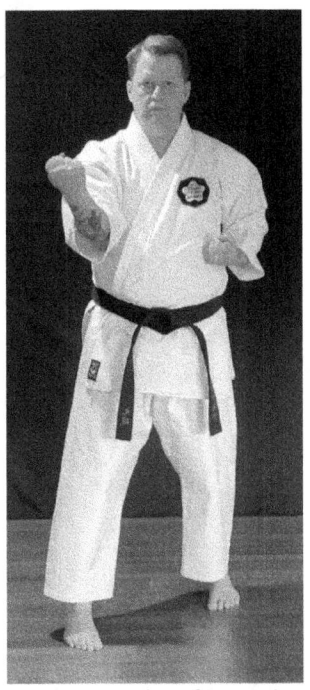

Draw Back Left Hand
Slowly into Chamber

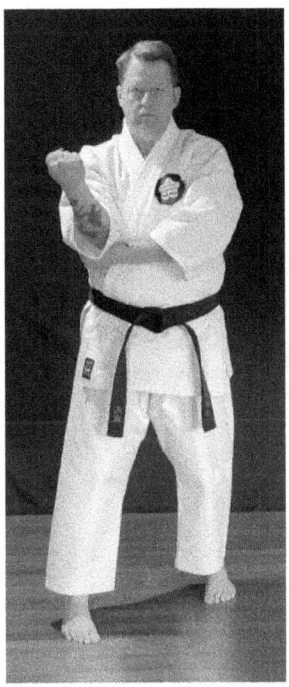

Chamber Left Hand
Under Right Elbow

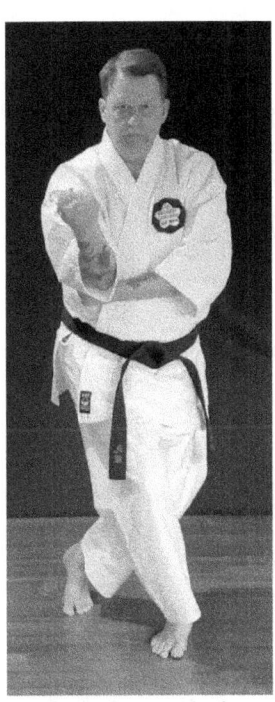

Step Across Left
into Kosa Dachi

Sanchin

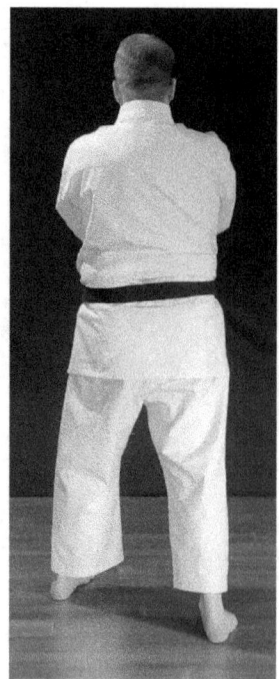

Spin Around 180°

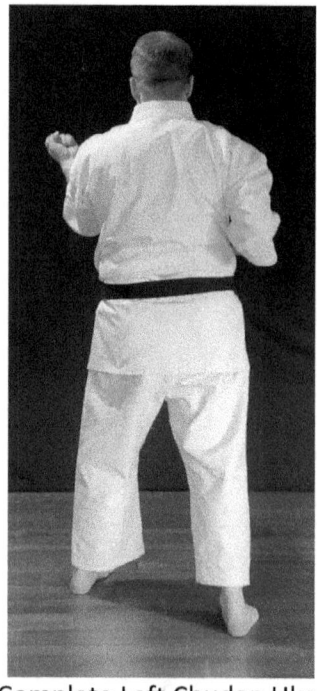

Complete Left Chudan Uke,
Drawing Right Hand into
Chamber (long inhale)

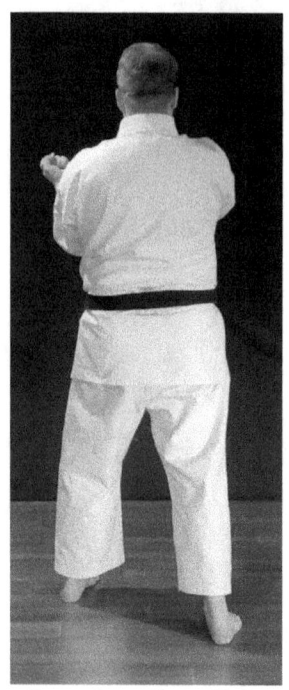

Complete Slow Right
Chudan Zuki (long exhale)

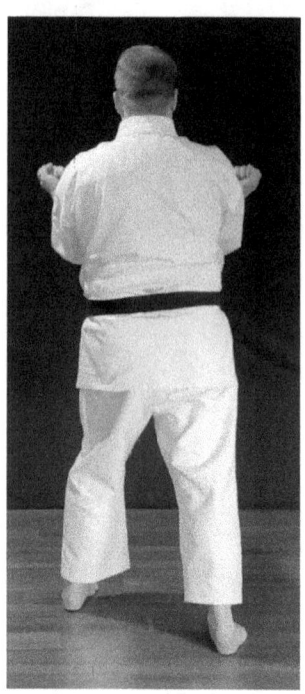

Set (short inhale/exhale)

Sanchin

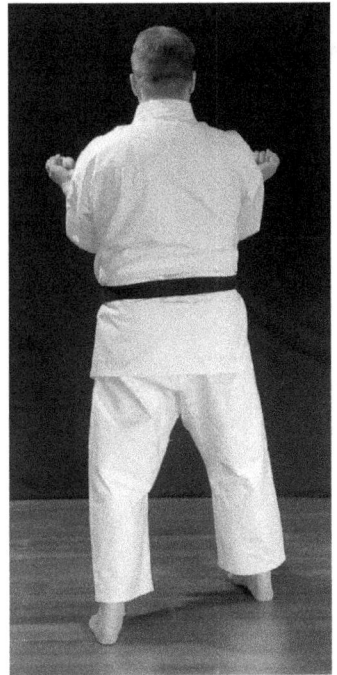

Step

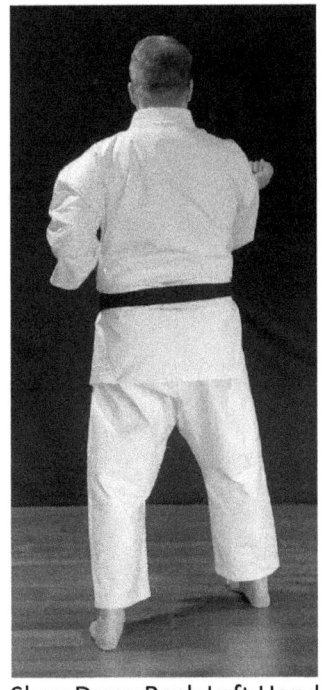

Slow Draw Back Left Hand into Chamber (long inhale)

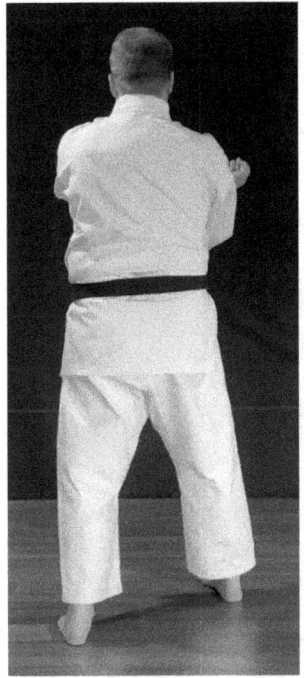

Complete Slow Left Chudan Zuki (long exhale)

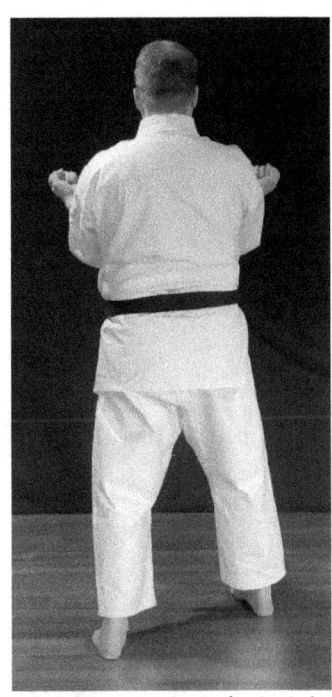

Set (short inhale/exhale)

Sanchin

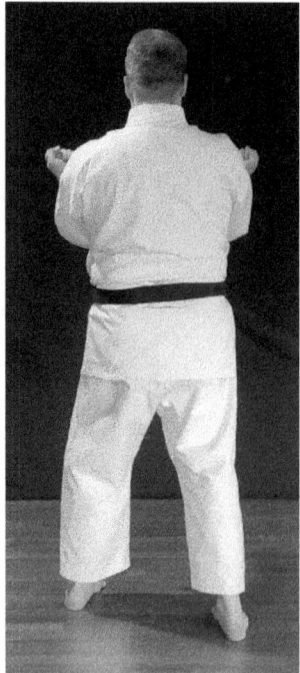

Step

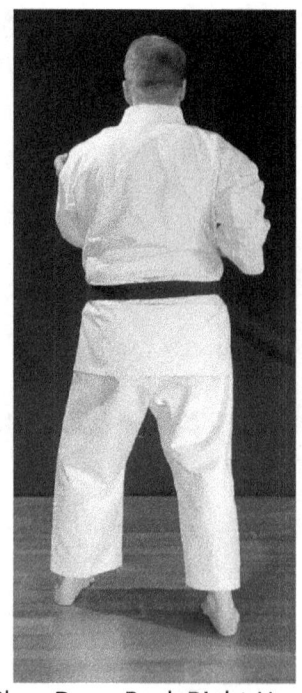

Slow Draw Back Right Hand into Chamber (long inhale)

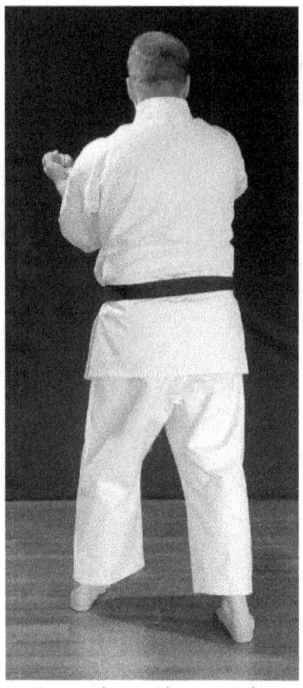

Complete Slow Right Chudan Zuki (long exhale)

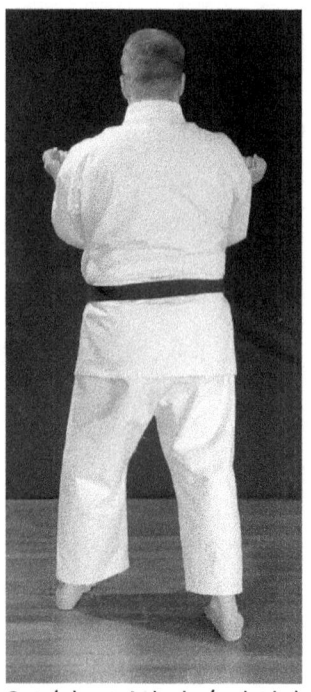

Set (short inhale/exhale)

Sanchin

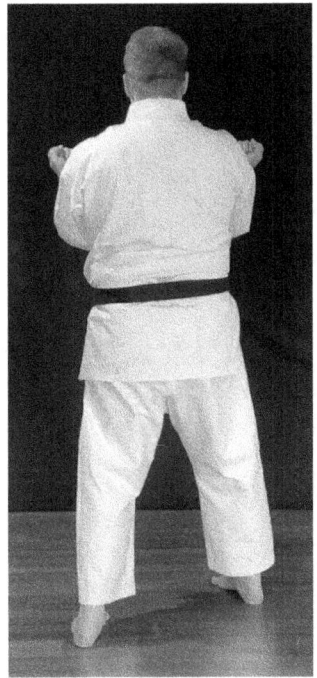

Step

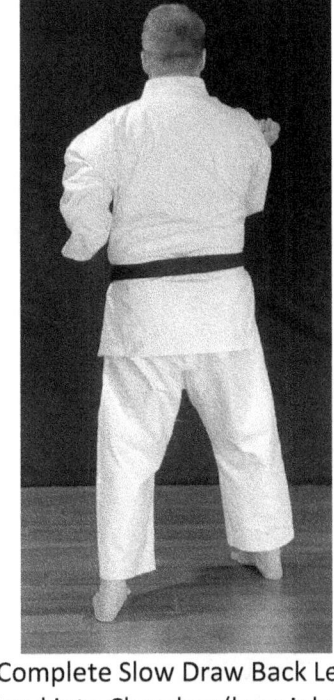

Complete Slow Draw Back Left
Hand into Chamber (long inhale)

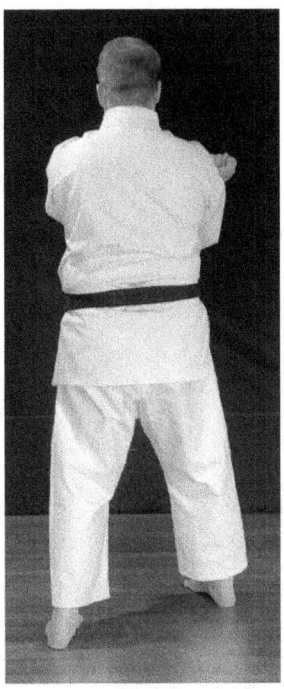

Complete Slow Left
Chudan Zuki (long exhale)

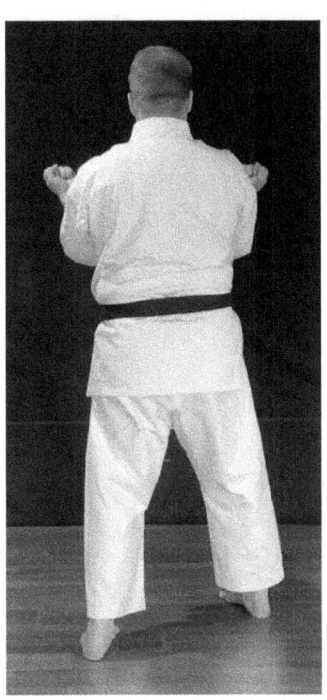

Set (short inhale/exhale)

Sanchin

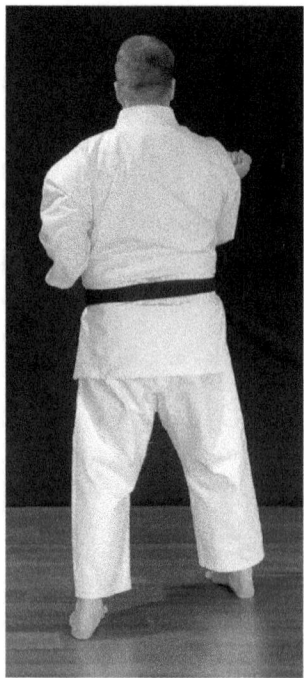

Draw Back Left Hand into Chamber

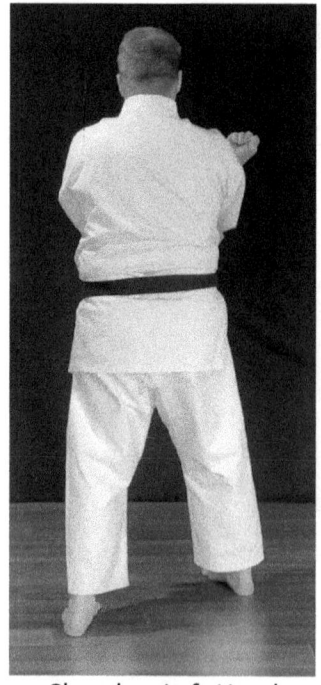

Chamber Left Hand Under Right Elbow

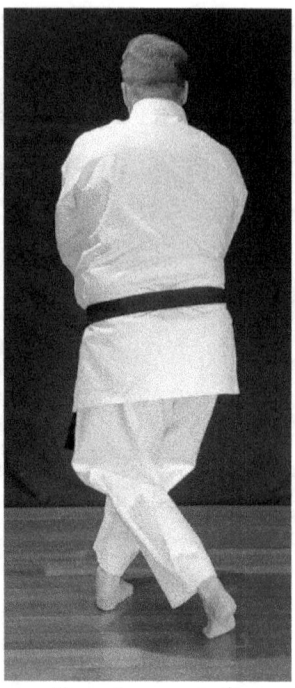

Step Across Left into Kosa Dachi

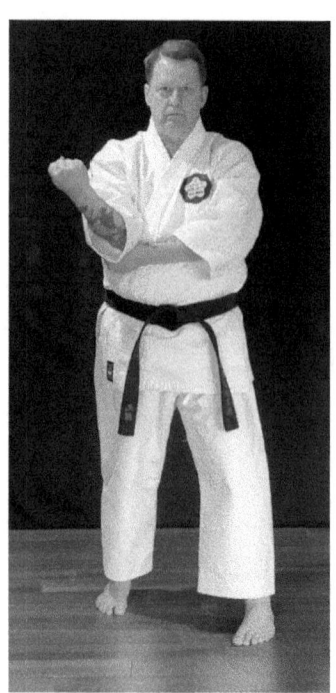

Spin Around Facing Forward

Sanchin

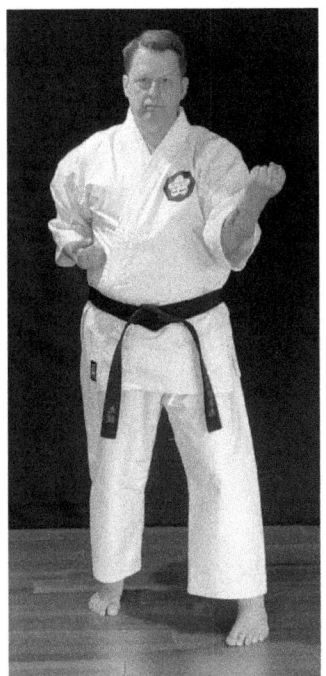

Complete Left Chudan Uke, Drawing Right Hand into Chamber (long inhale)

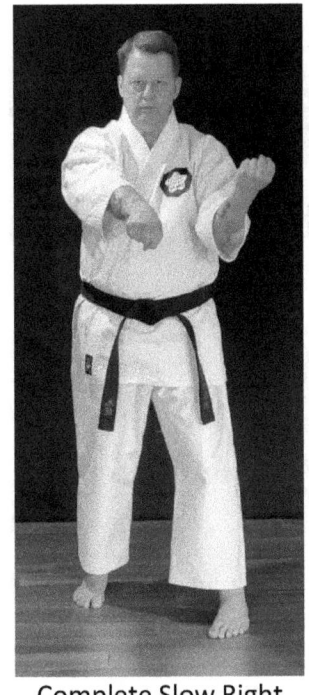

Complete Slow Right Chudan Zuki (long exhale)

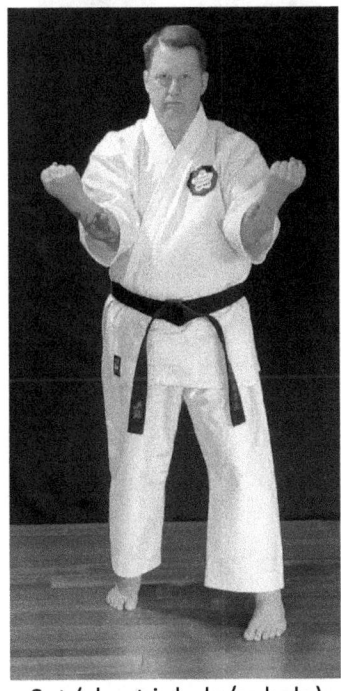

Set (short inhale/exhale)

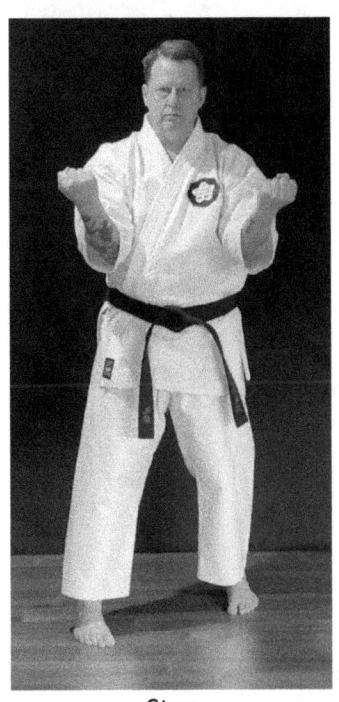

Step

Sanchin

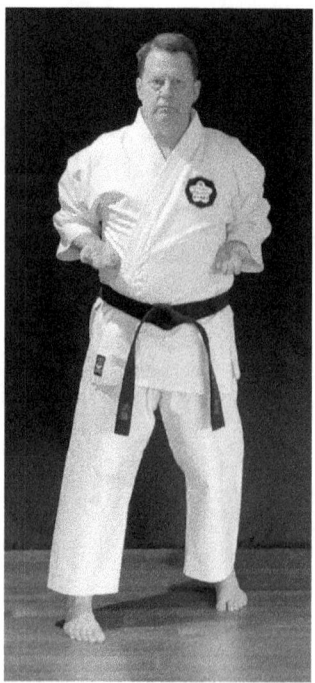

Bring Open Hands Back into
Chamber (long inhale)

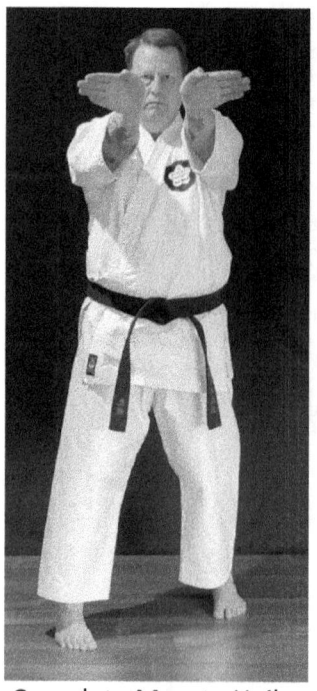

Complete Morote Heiko
Jodan Shotei Uchi (long exhale)

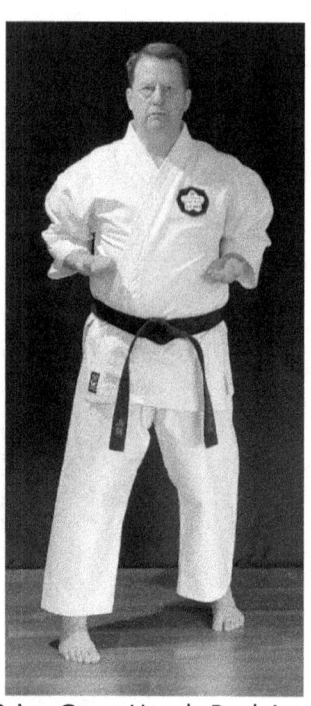

Bring Open Hands Back into
Chamber (long inhale)

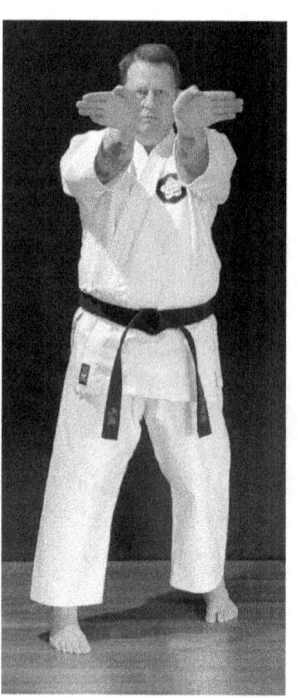

Complete Morote Heiko
Jodan Shotei Uchi (long exhale)

Sanchin

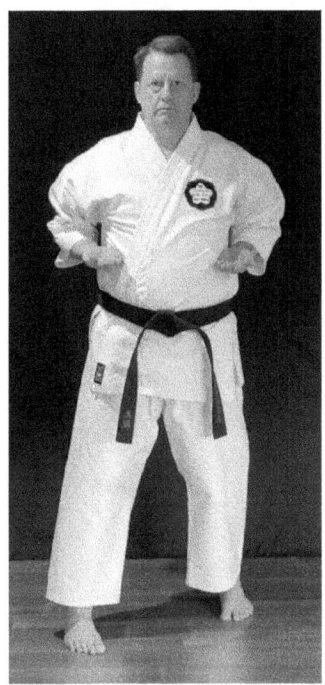

Bring Open Hands Back into
Chamber (long inhale)

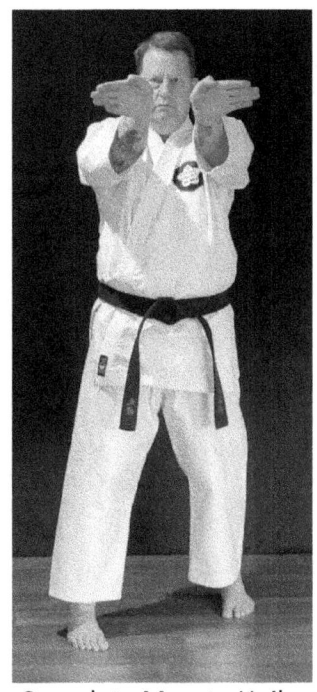

Complete Morote Heiko
Jodan Shotei Uchi (long exhale)

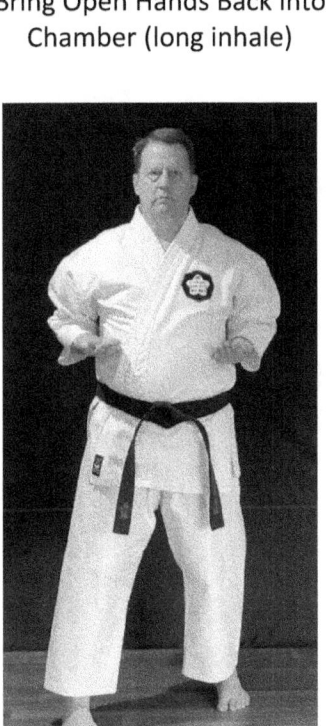

Bring Open Hands Back into
Chamber (long inhale)

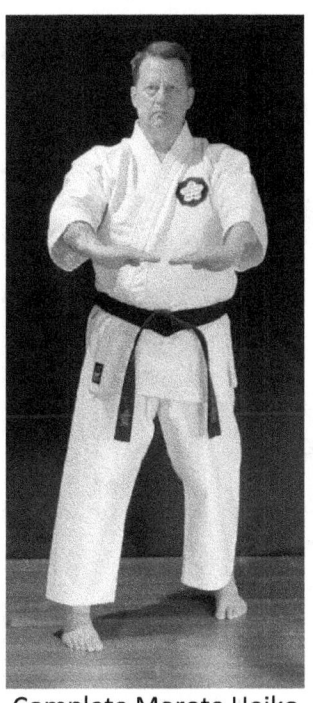

Complete Morote Heiko
Chudan Shuto Uchi (long exhale)

Sanchin

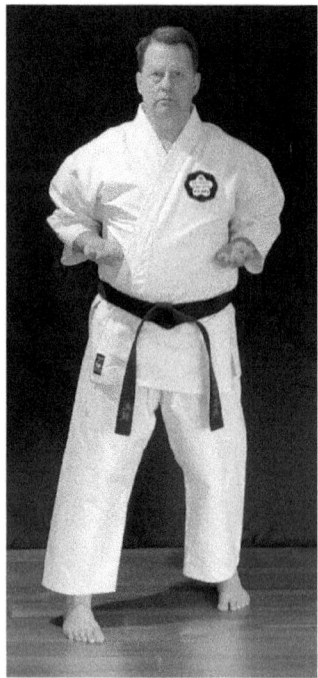

Bring Open Hands Back into Chamber (long inhale)

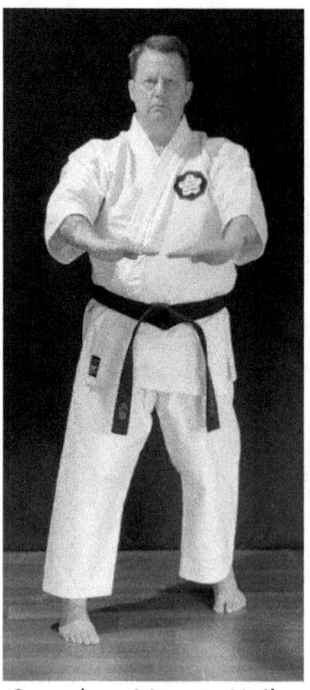

Complete Morote Heiko Chudan Shuto Uchi (long exhale)

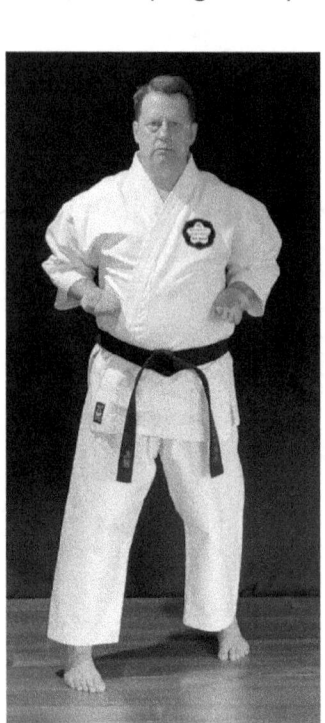

Bring Open Hands Back into Chamber (long inhale)

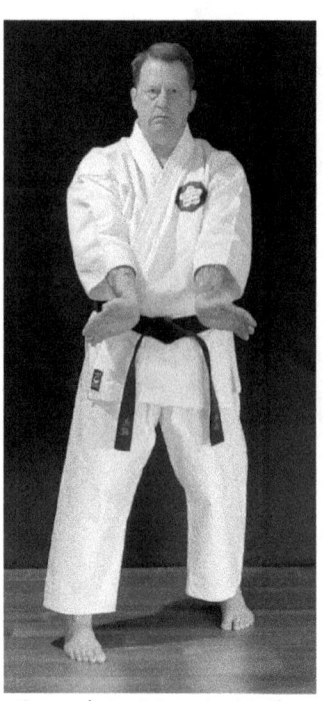

Complete Morote Heiko Gedan Shotei Uchi (long exhale)

Sanchin

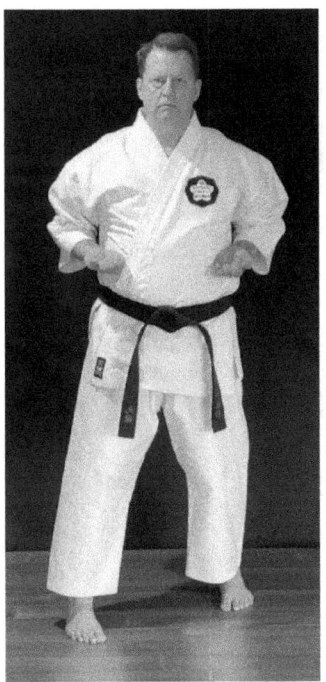

Bring Open Hands Back into Chamber (long inhale)

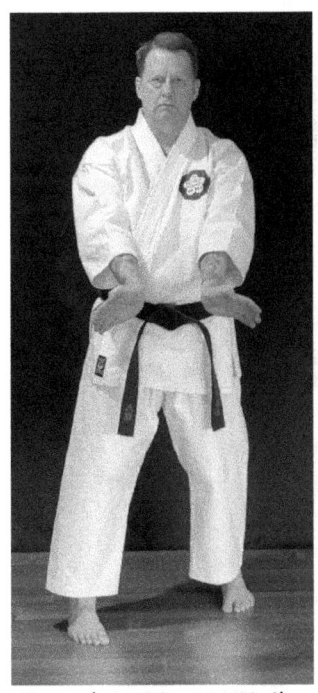

Complete Morote Heiko Gedan Shotei Uchi (long exhale)

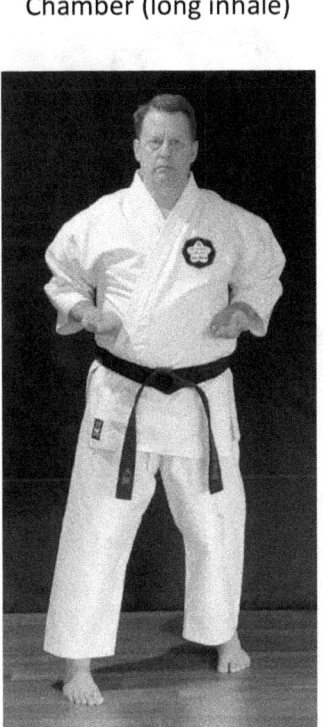

Bring Open Hands Back into Chamber (long inhale)

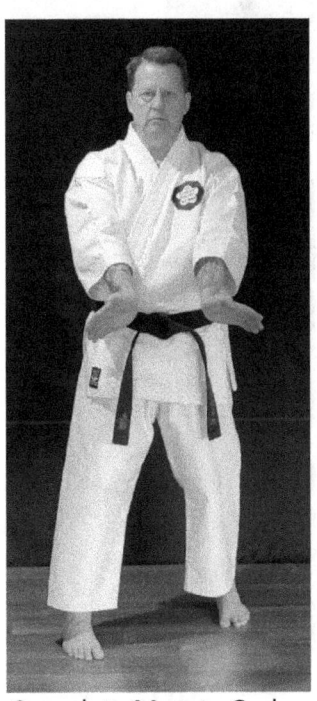

Complete Morote Gedan Shotei Uchi (long exhale)

Sanchin

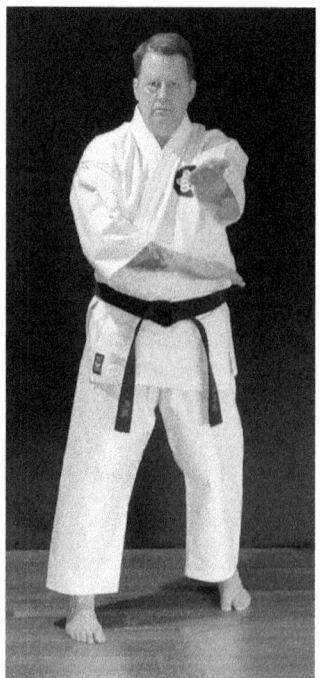
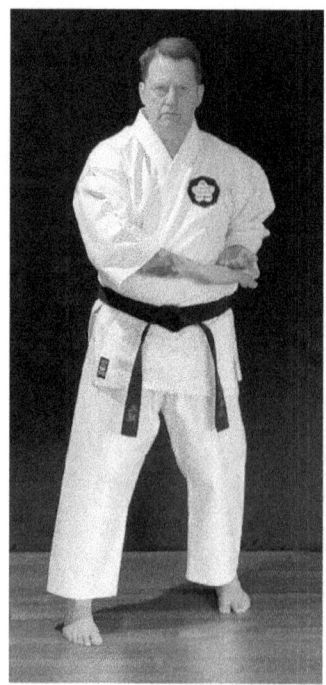

Complete Tora Guchi (long inhale)

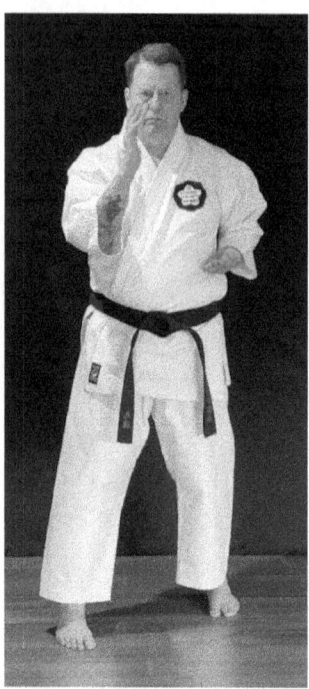
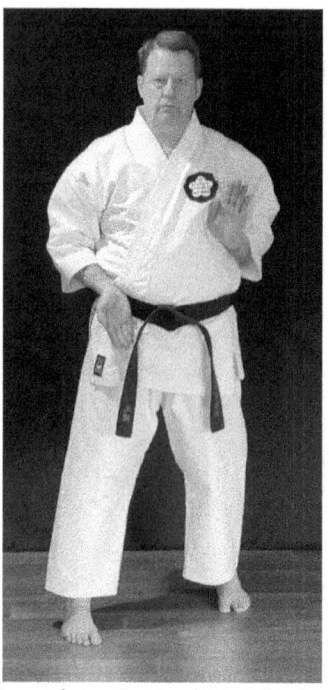

Tora Guchi (long inhale) (cont.)

Complete Centerline Morote Shotei Uchi (long exhale)

Sanchin

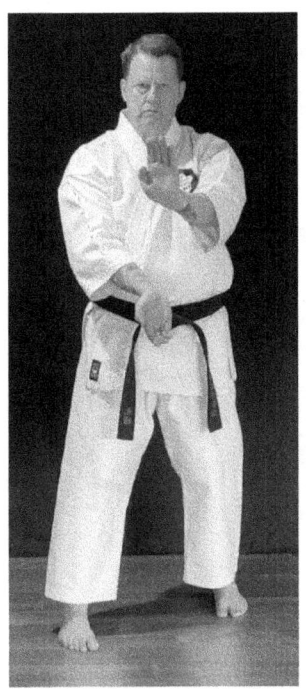

Centerline Morote Shotei Uchi (long exhale) (cont.)

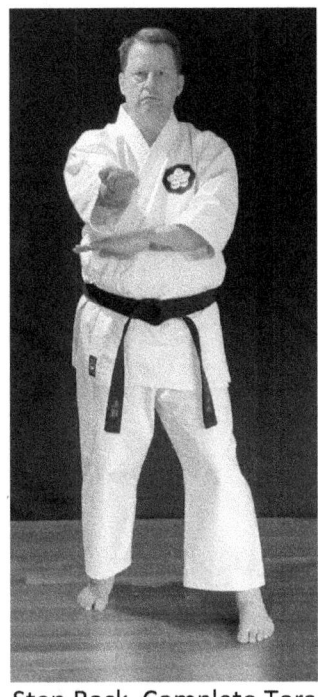

Step Back, Complete Tora Guchi (long inhale)

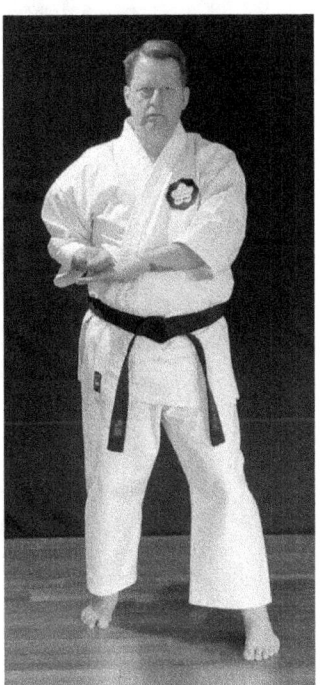

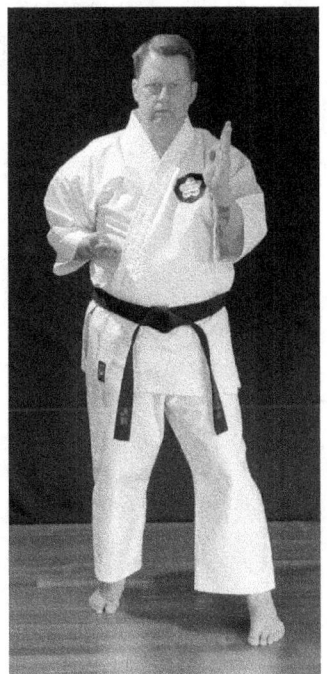

Tora Guchi (long inhale) (cont.)

Sanchin

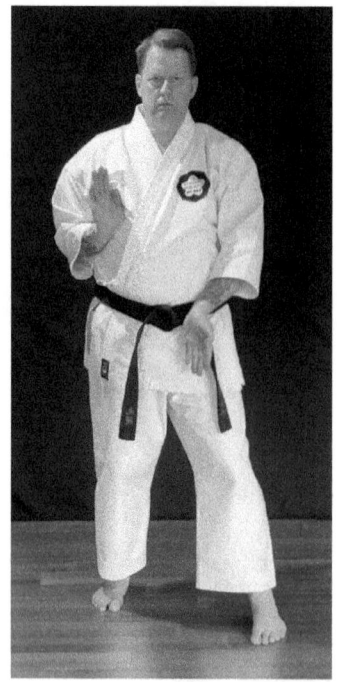 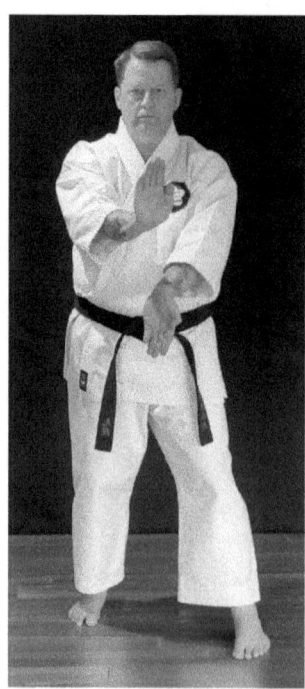

Complete Centerline Morote Shotei Uchi (long exhale)

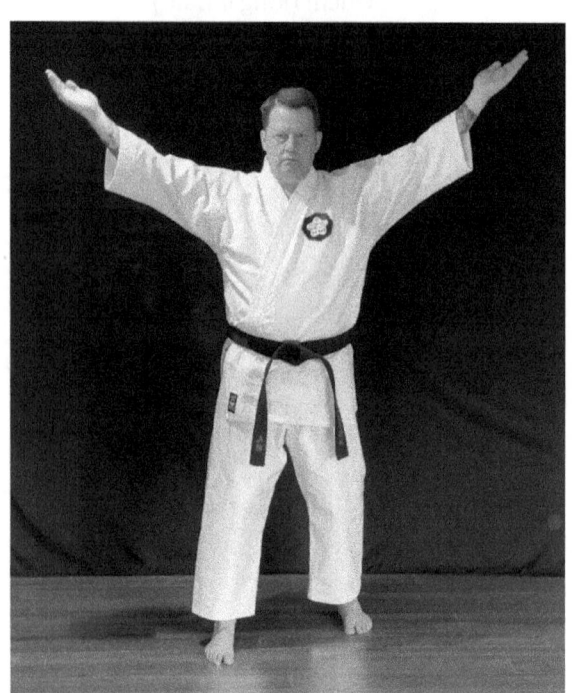 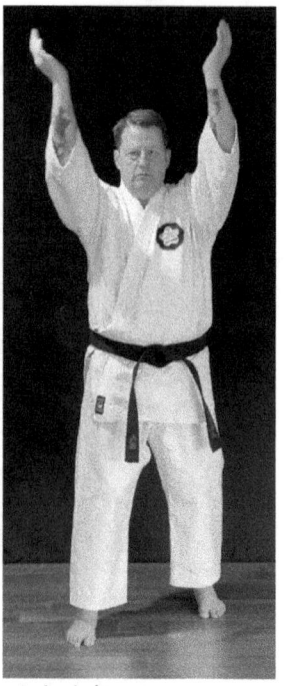

Step Back, Bring Arms Around (long inhale)

Sanchin

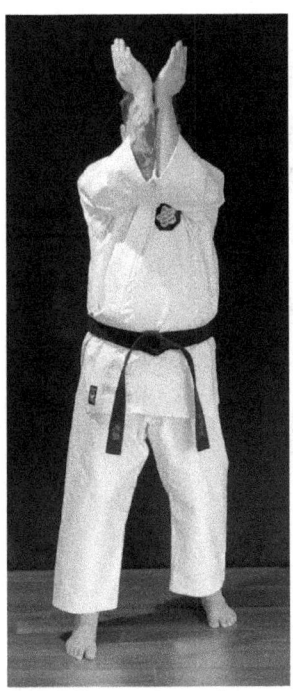

Bring Elbows Together and Down (long exhale)

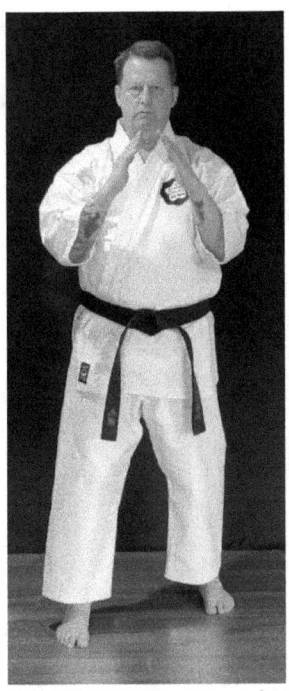

Set with Elbows Down and Hands Separated (long exhale cont.)

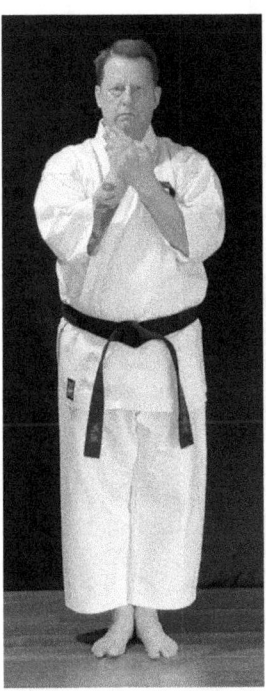

Step Back (Right Foot) Guard Throat (three short exhales)

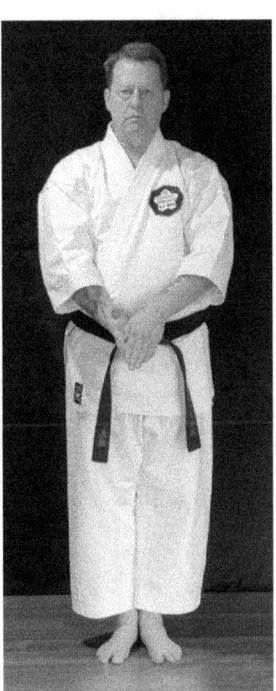

Turn Hands Down to Guard Groin

Sanchin

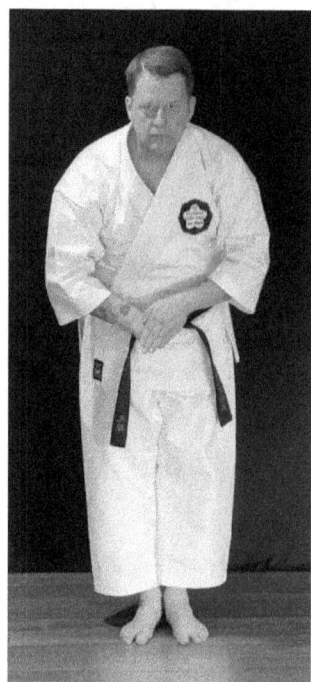

Rei

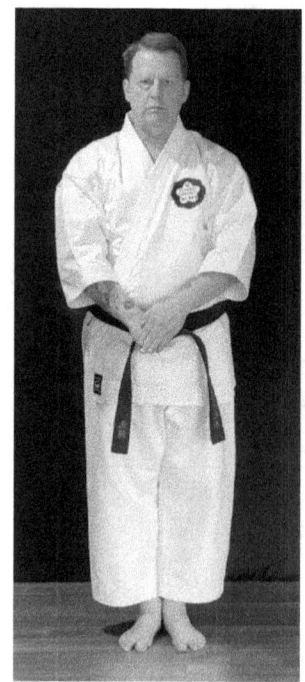

Musubi Dachi

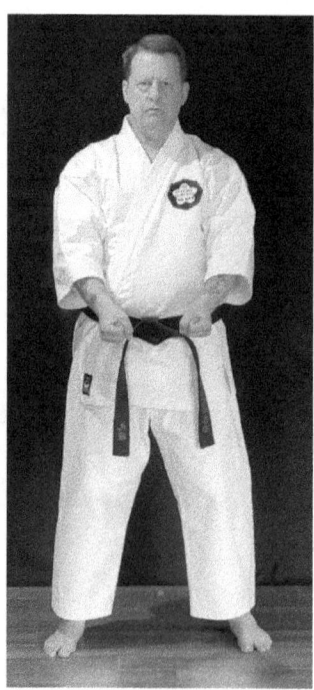

Heiko Dachi

Seiunchin

Seiunchin (征遠鎮) means "calmness conquers," which is a translation of the kanji[6]. Seiunchin kata is a low stance kata without kicks. For most of the kata, the student is in shiko dachi. The only modification Shodai made to this asterisk shaped kata was in the beginning, adding a stomp to the three shiko dachi steps, emphasizing the downward palm heels as a self-defense technique. This was Shodai's favorite kata.

Below is the method by which Ketsugo Goju-Ryu performs Seiunchin kata. Complete details about each move are not included, as this is simply a demonstration. Seiunchin is a widespread kata, and many karate systems include it in their curriculum. This demonstration is not meant to imply that it is the only way to do it, but it is the way at Ketsugo Goju-Ryu.

These are the Japanese terms used for this kata. Bear in mind, karate terms are not completely streamlined. There are terms that were used in the middle of the 20th Century that are no longer used today. Oftentimes there are more than one term that can be used for the same technique. The important thing is not what it is called, but the technique itself.

Age Hiji Ate – Rising Elbow Strike	**Morote Sukui Uke** – Double Scooping Block
Age - Rising	
Barai - Sweeping Block	**Musubi Dachi** - Attention Stance, Toes Out
Chudan - Middle	
Dachi – Stance	**Neko Ashi Dachi** – Cat Leg Stance
Gedan – Low	**Otoshi Tettsui Uchi** – Down Hammer Fist Strike
Hajime – Command to Begin	
Hari Uke - Open Hand Block (Palm Up)	**Rei** – Bow (Respect)
Heiko Dachi - Parallel Stance	**Shiko Dachi** - Straddle Leg Stance
Hiki Uke - Open Hand Block (Palm Down)/Pulling Block	**Shotei** – Palm Heel
	Soto Uke – Outside Forearm Block

Seiunchin

Hojo Osae Uke – Augmented Pressing Block	**Tsuki/-Zuki** - Punch
Hojo Oshi – Augmented Push	**Uchi** – Strike
Hojo Uke – Augmented Block	**Uchi Uke** – Inside Block (Pinky Side of Arm)
Jodan – High	**Uke** – Block (Receive)
Kagi Zuki – Hook Punch	**Uraken Uchi** – Back Fist Strike
Morote Gedan Barai – Double Down Block	**Ushiro Empi Uchi** – Rear Elbow Strike
Morote Otoshi Shotei Uchi – Double Palm Strike	**Yoi** – Ready Command

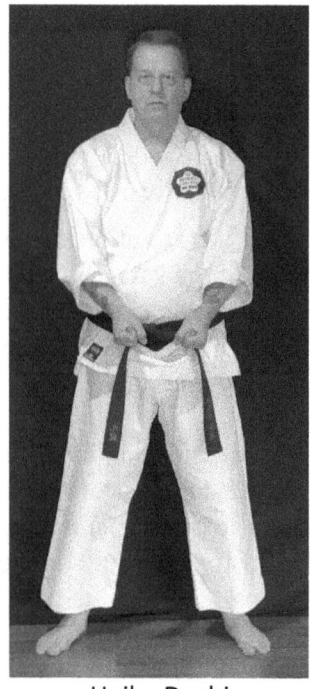

Heiko Dachi

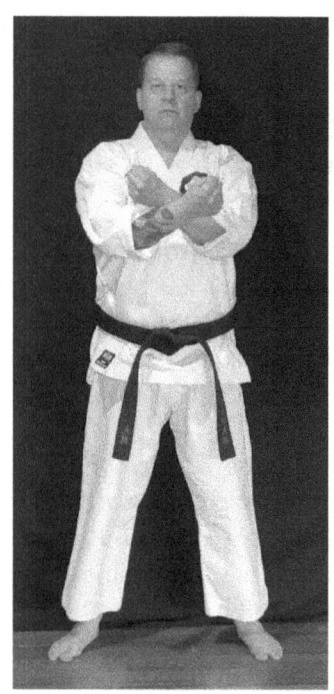

(Yoi) Brings Arms Up, Crossed at the Wrist

Seiunchin

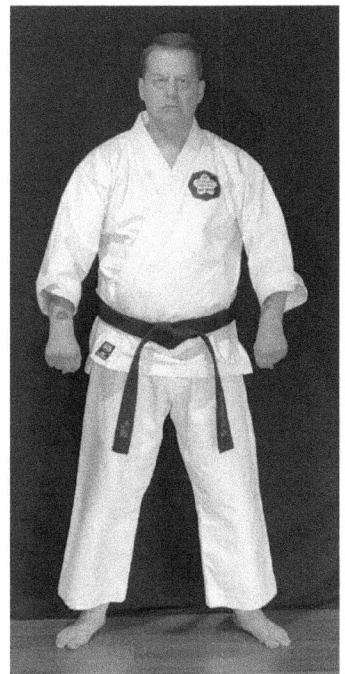

Bring Arms Down

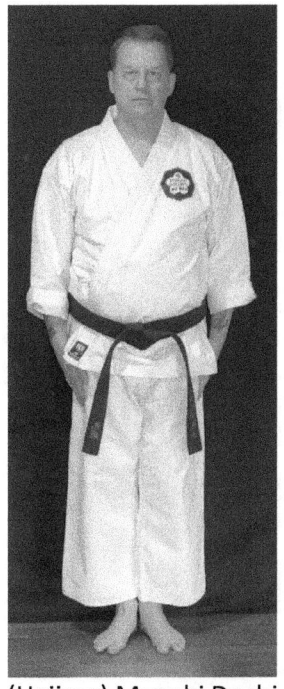

(Hajime) Musubi Dachi

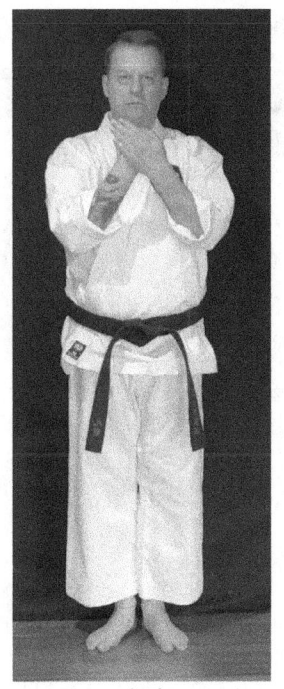

Guard Throat

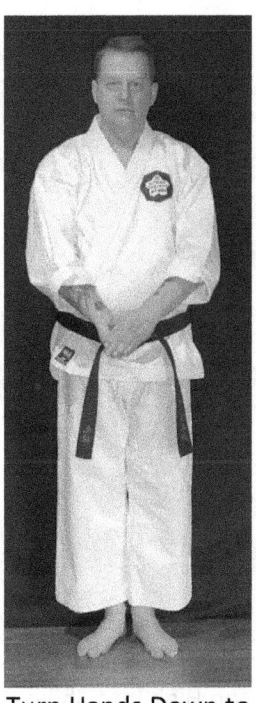

Turn Hands Down to Guard Groin

Seiunchin

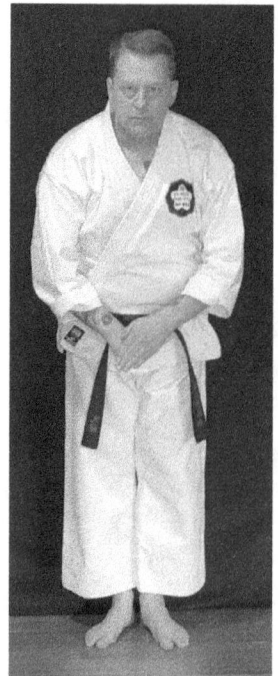

Rei

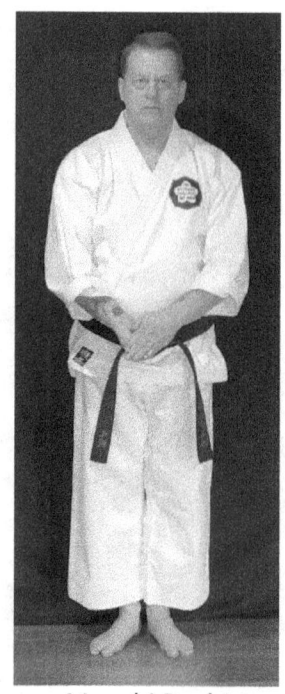

Musubi Dachi

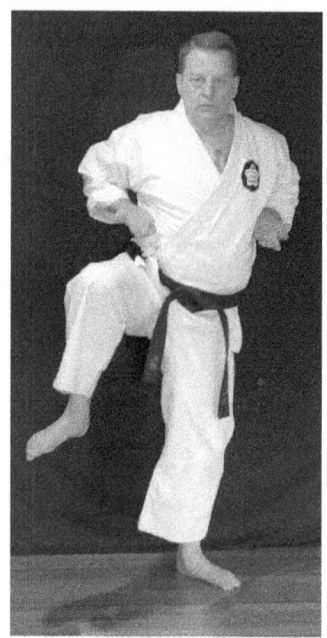

Bring Open Hands to Chamber
and Step High into Shiko Dachi
at 315° Angle

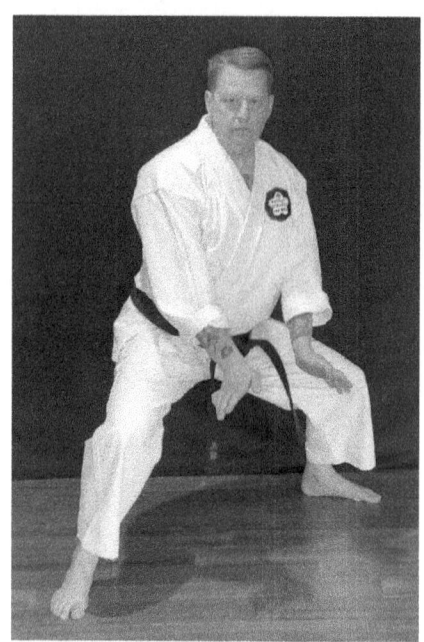

Land Hard while Completing
Morote Otoshi Shotei Uchi

Seiunchin

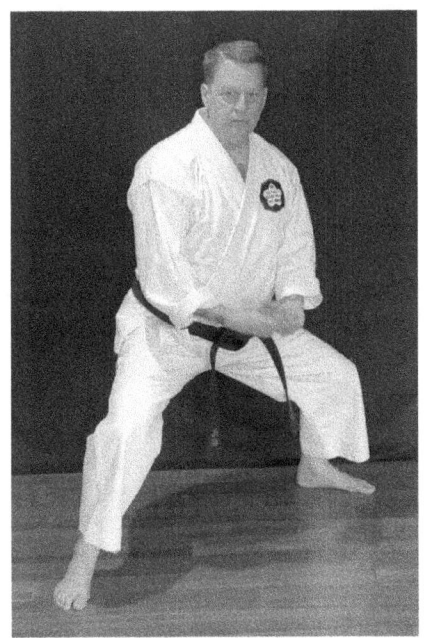

Land Hard while Completing Morote Otoshi Shotei Uchi

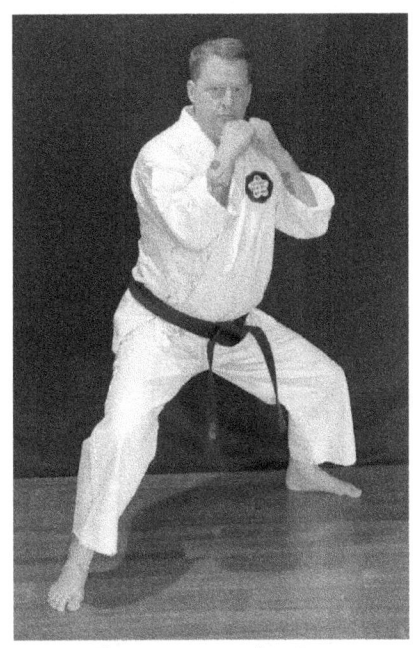

Close Fists at the Top

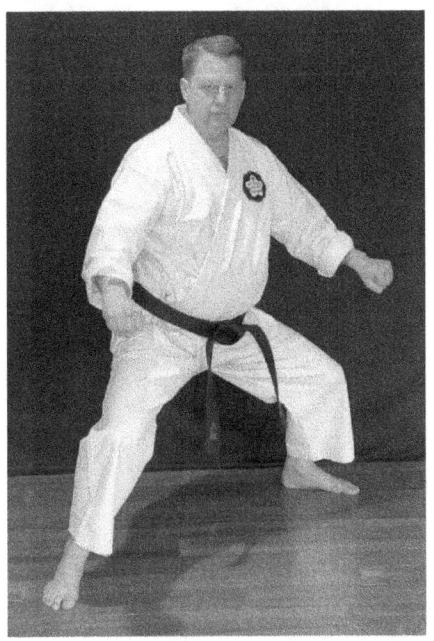

Complete Morote Gedan Barai

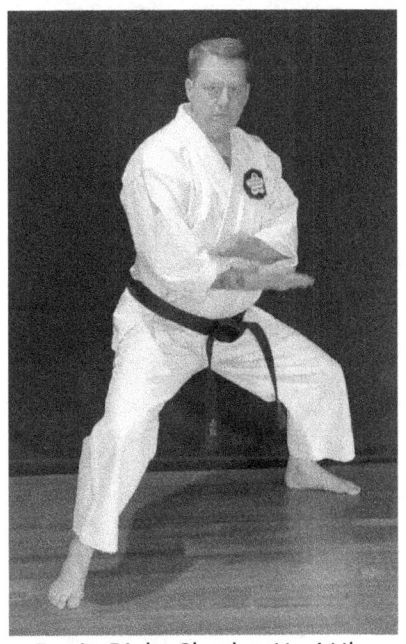

Begin Right Chudan Hari Uke

Seiunchin

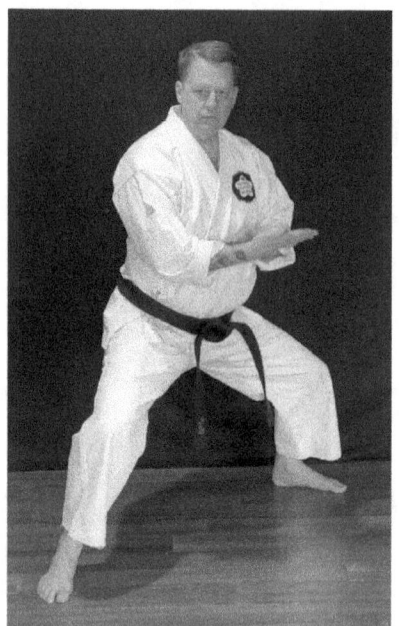
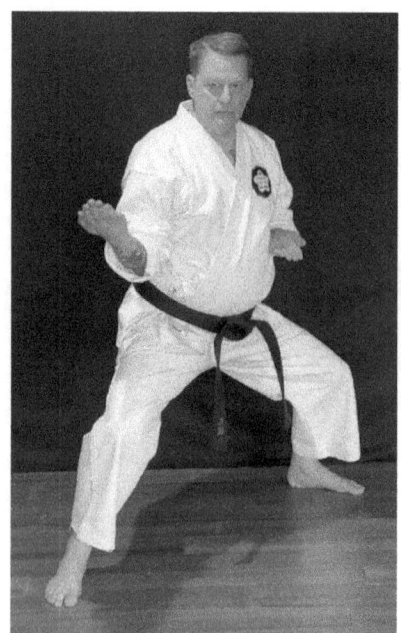

Complete Chudan Hari Uke

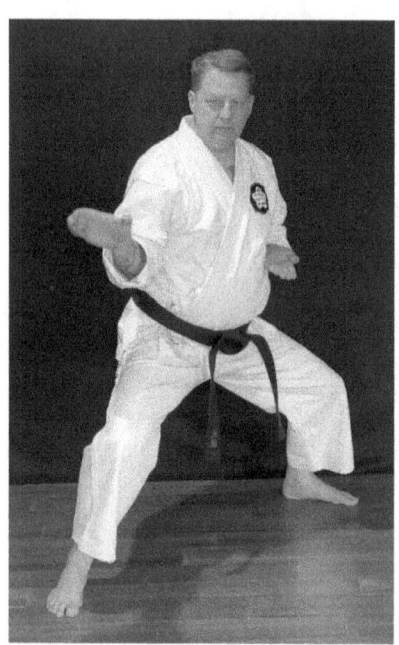

Reach Lead Hand Around Opponent's Wrist

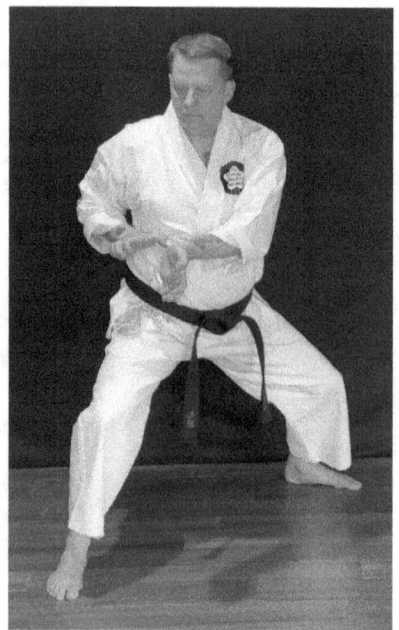

Complete Right Hiki Uke while Rear Hand Completes Shotei Uchi to Opponent's Arm/Elbow

Seiunchin

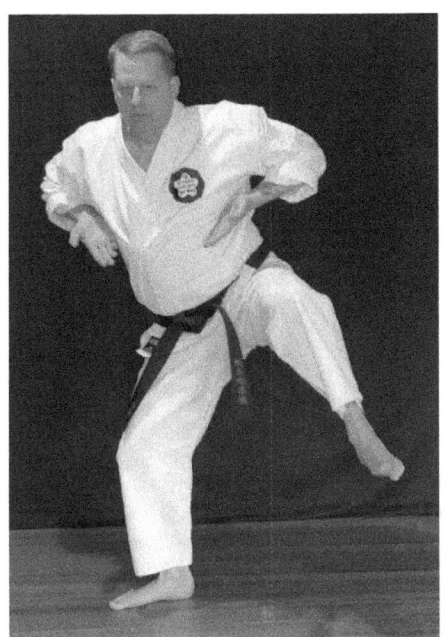

Bring Open Hands to Chamber and Step High into Shiko Dachi at 45° Angle

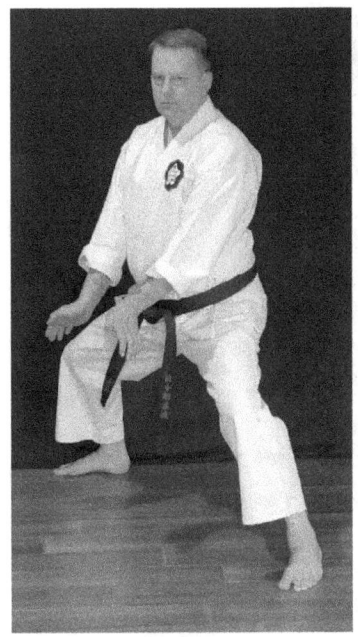

Land Hard while Completing Morote Otoshi Shotei Uchi

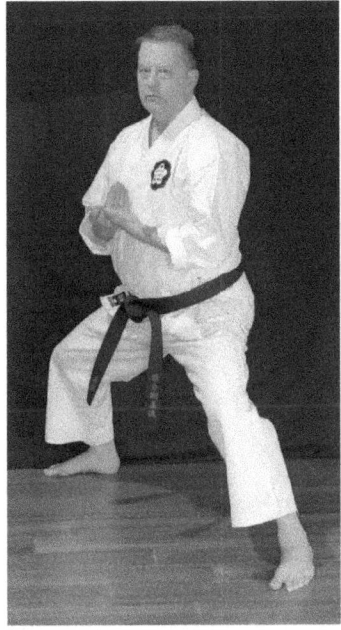

Complete Morote Sukui Uke, Bring Hands Up, Keeping Back of Hands Together

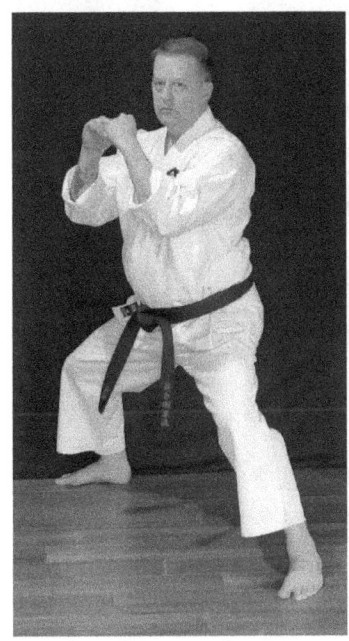

Close Fists at the Top

Seiunchin

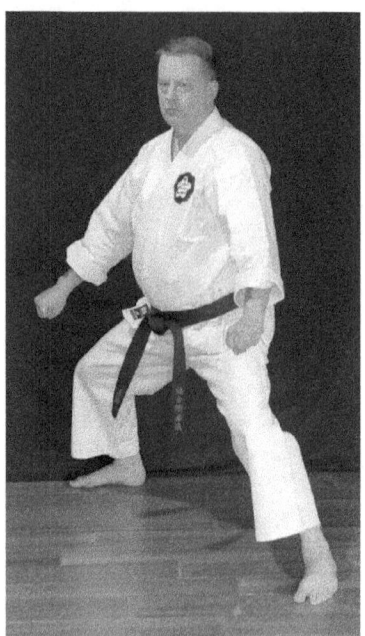

Complete Morote Gedan Barai

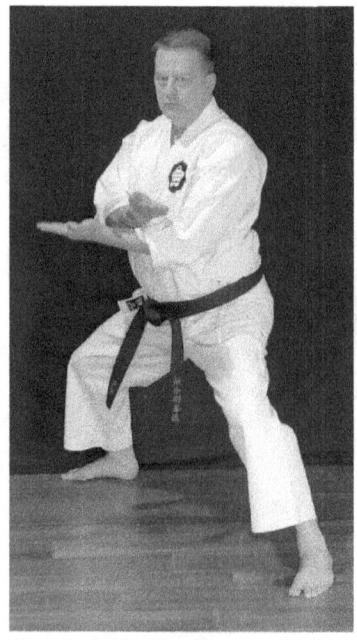

Begin Left Chudan Hari Uke

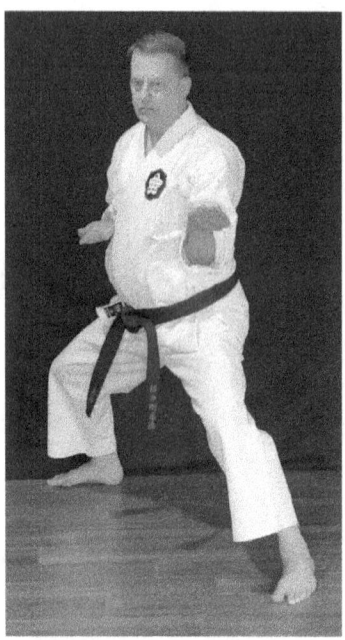

Complete Chudan Hari Uke

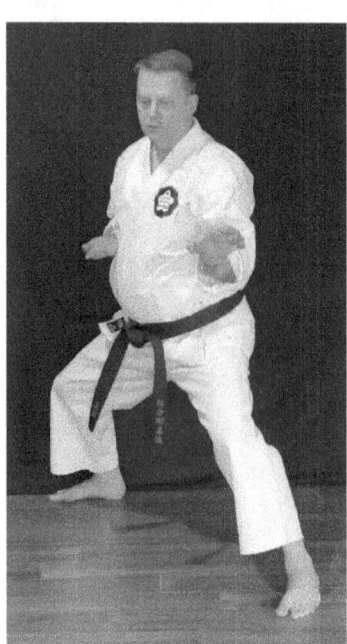

Reach Lead Hand Around Opponent's Wrist

Seiunchin

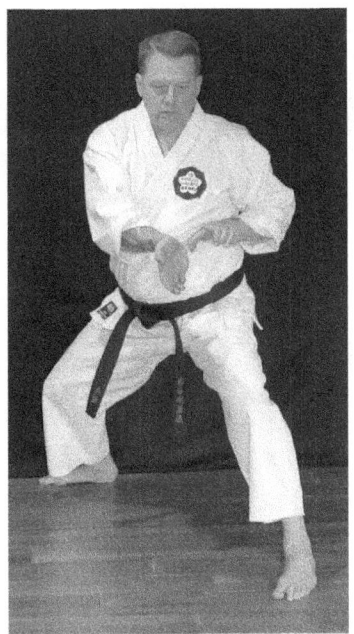

Complete Left Hiki Uke while Rear Hand Completes Shotei Uchi to Opponent's Arm/Elbow

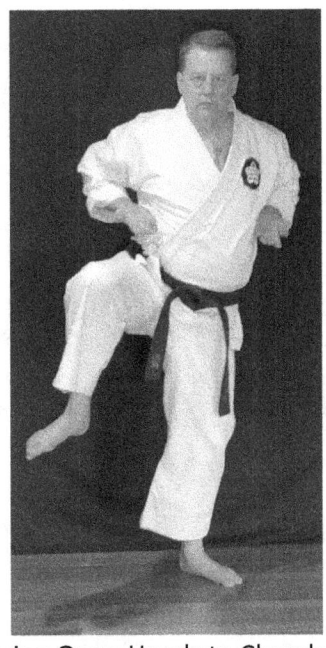

Bring Open Hands to Chamber and Step High into Shiko Dachi at 315° Angle

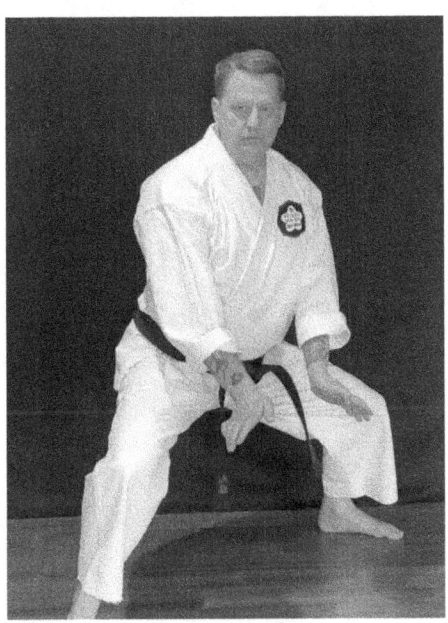

Land Hard while Completing Morote Otoshi Shotei Uchi

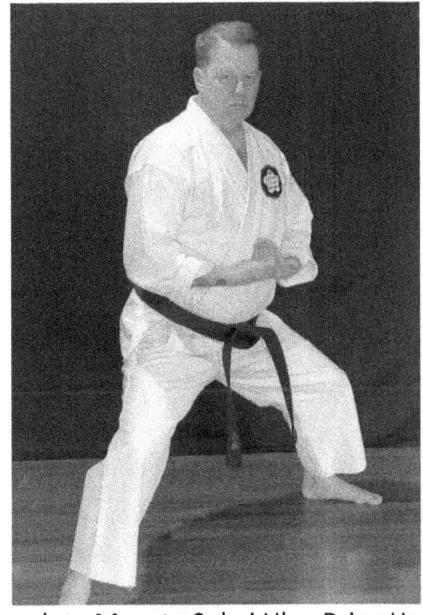

Complete Morote Sukui Uke, Bring Hands Up, Keeping Back of Hands Together

Seiunchin

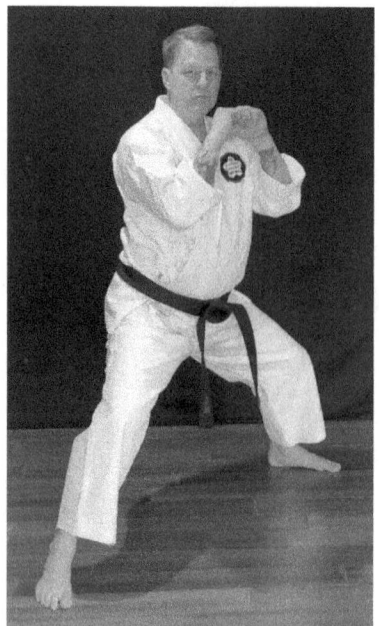
Close Fists at the Top

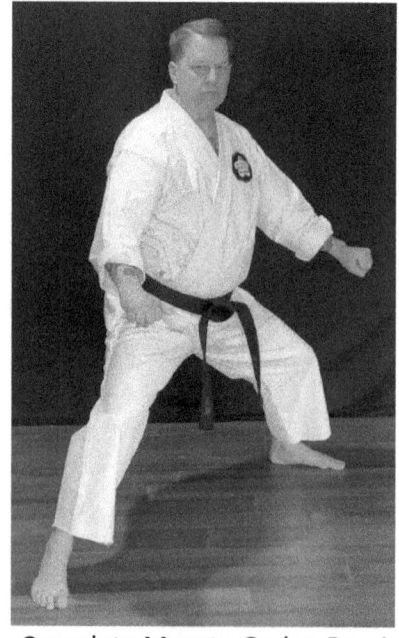
Complete Morote Gedan Barai

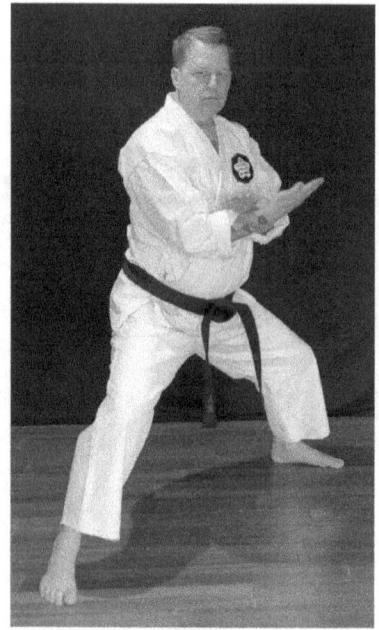
Begin Right Chudan Hari Uke

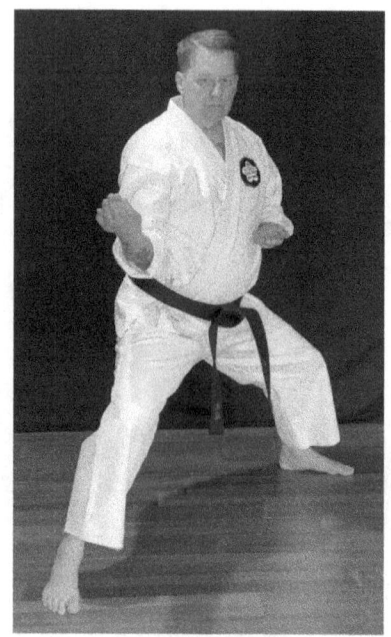
Complete Chudan Hari Uke

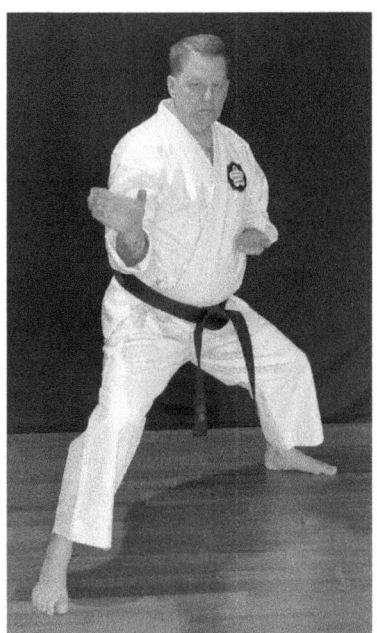

Reach Lead Hand Around Opponent's Wrist

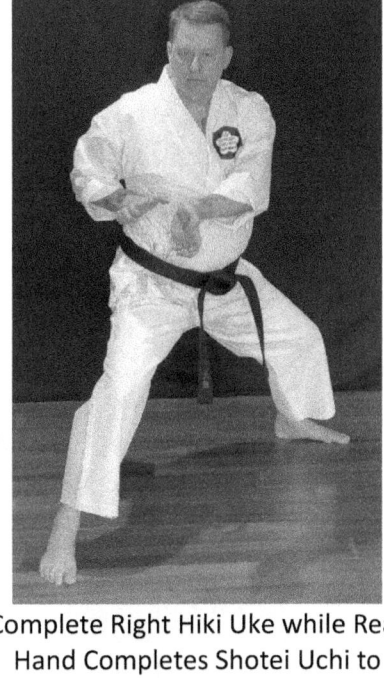

Complete Right Hiki Uke while Rear Hand Completes Shotei Uchi to Opponent's Arm/Elbow

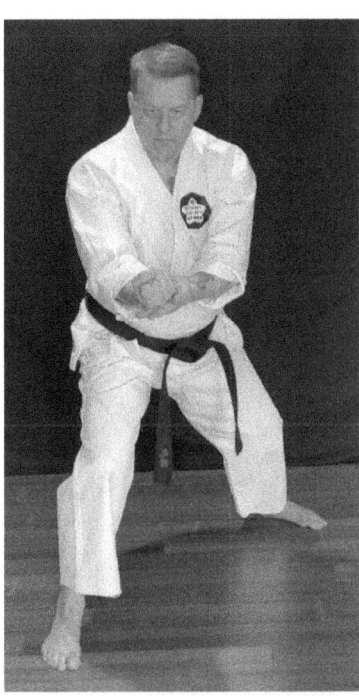

Facing Forward, Close Right Hand in Front, Open Left Hand Under Right Fist

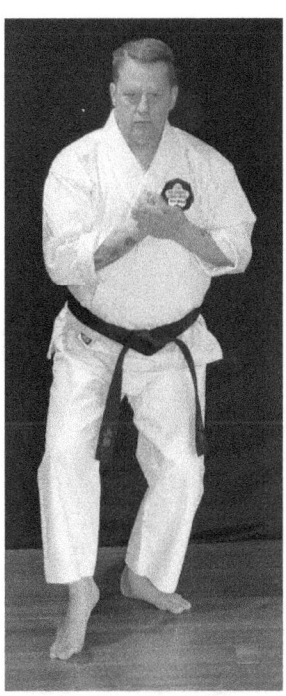

Slide Right Foot Back into Neko Ashi Dachi, while Bringing Hand Back to Chest

Seiunchin

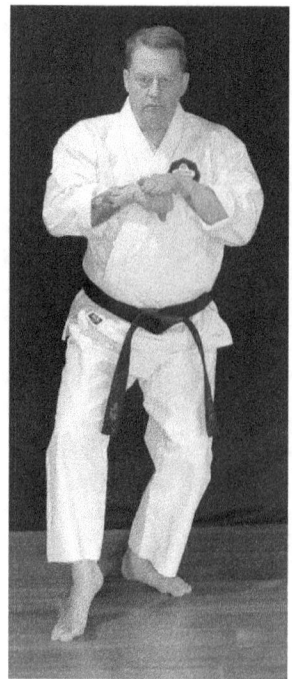

Turn Right Fist Over, Leaving Open Hand on Fist

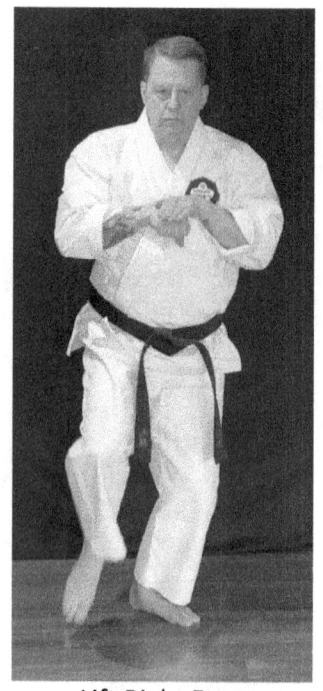

Lift Right Foot

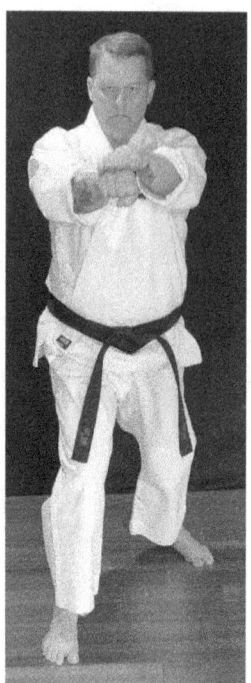

Slide Right Foot Forward while Completing Hojo Oshi

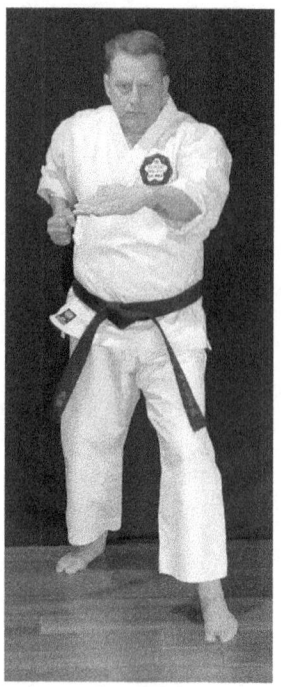

Step Back while Bringing Right Elbow Back, Leaving Left Arm Across

Seiunchin

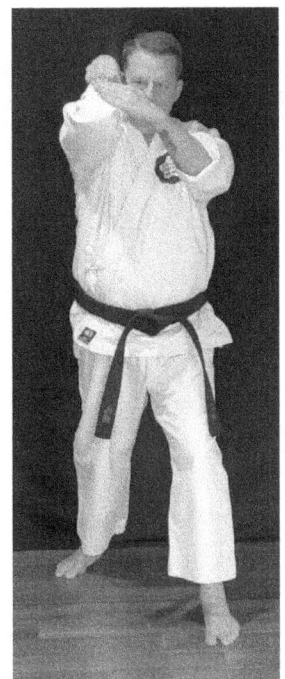

Complete Right Empi Uchi into Left Palm

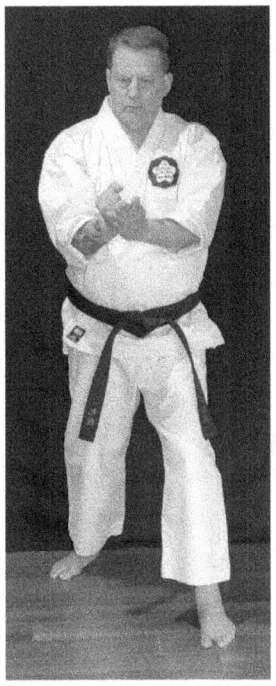

Slide Arm Down, Right Fist into Left Palm

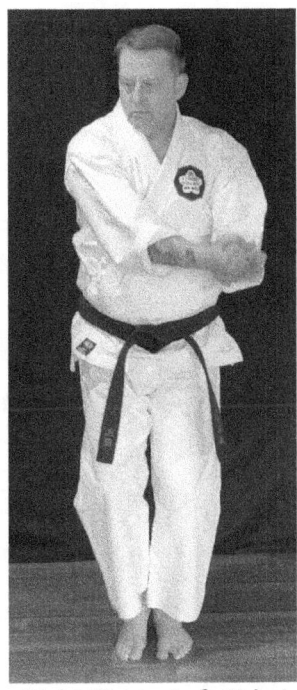

Bring Right Fist to Left Side in Left Hand while Bringing Right Foot to the Left

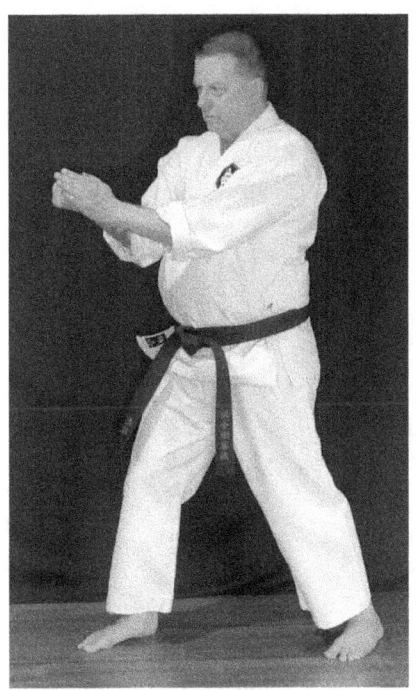

Complete Hojo Uke while Stepping into 315° Angle

Seiunchin

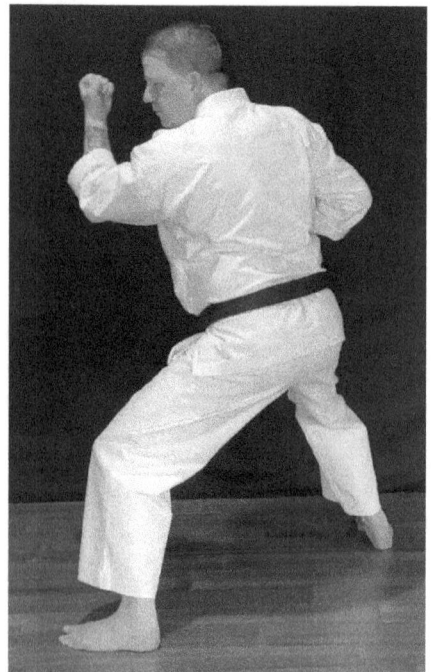 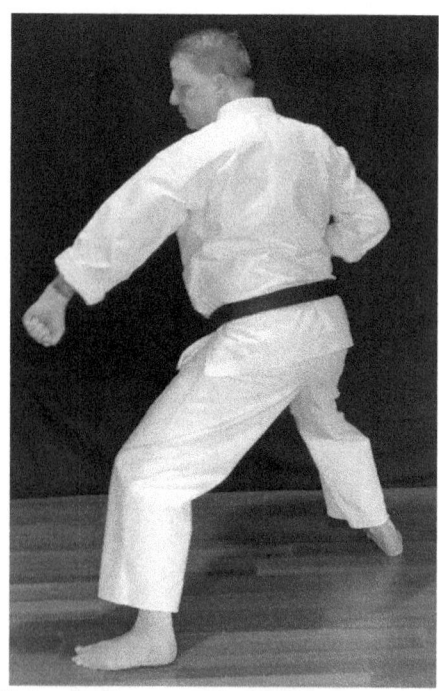

Keeping on the Same Angle, Step Around into Shiko Dachi, Complete Left Gedan Barai

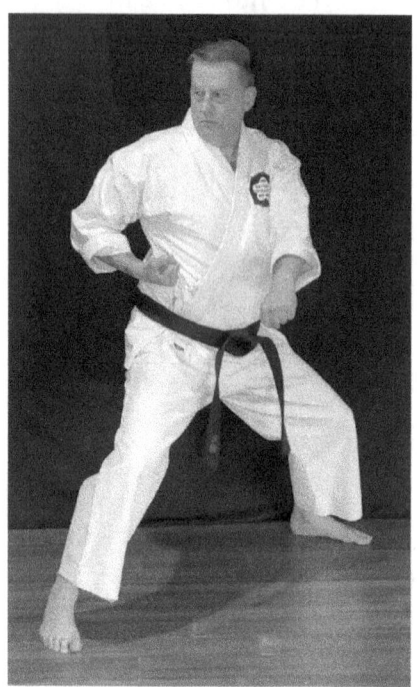 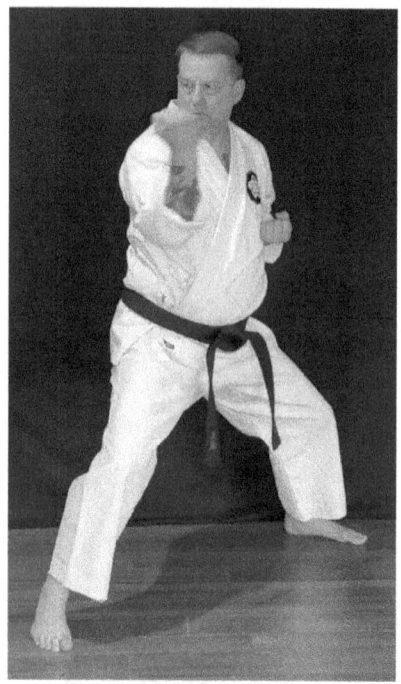

Step Back on Same Angle in Shiko Dachi

Complete Right Gedan Barai

Seiunchin

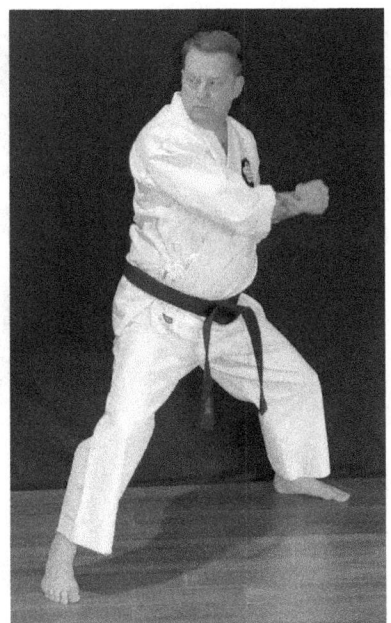
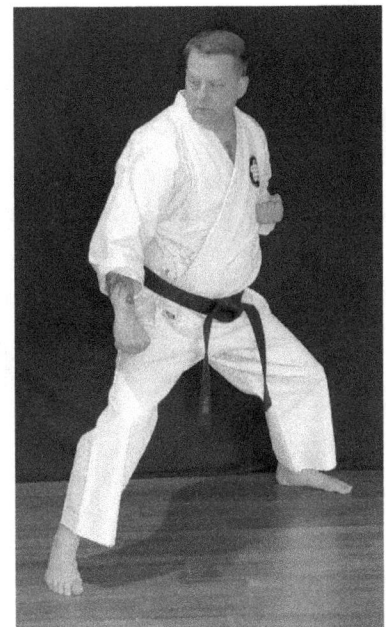

Gedan Barai (cont.)

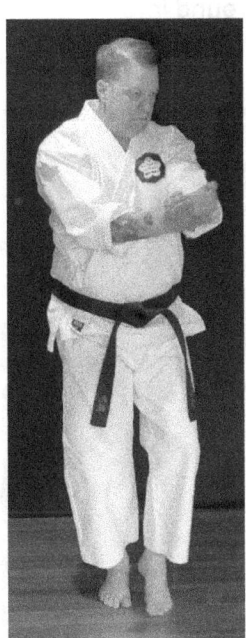

Bring Left Fist to Right Side in Right Hand
while Bringing Left Foot to the Right

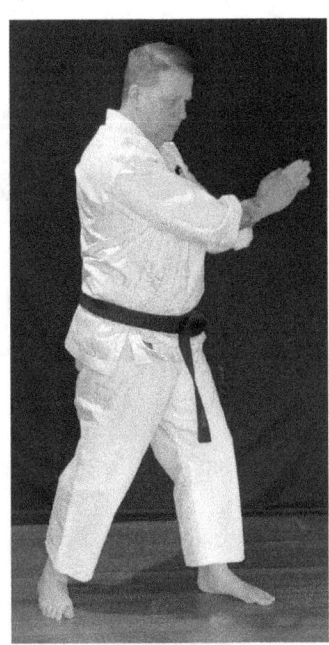

Complete Hojo Uke while
Stepping into 45° Angle

Seiunchin

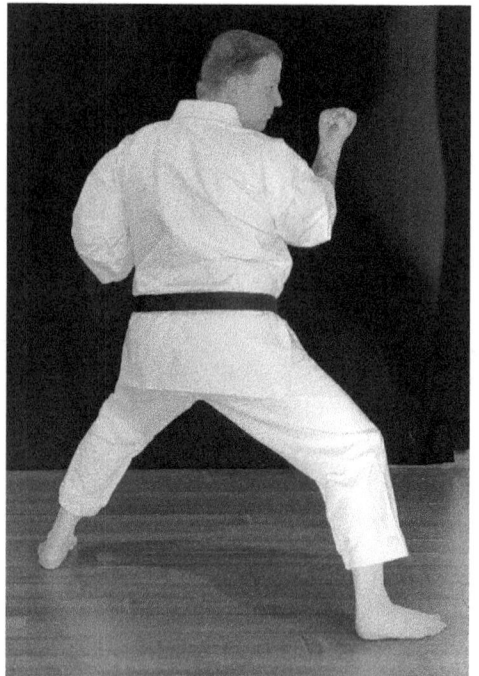
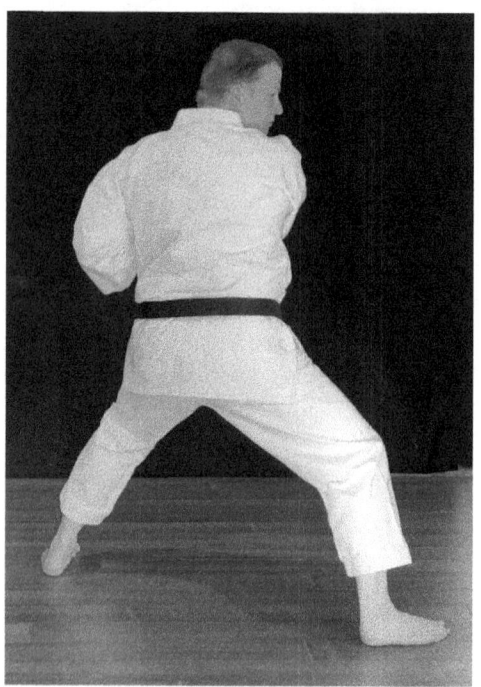

Keeping on the Same Angle, Step Around into
Shiko Dachi, Complete Right Gedan Barai

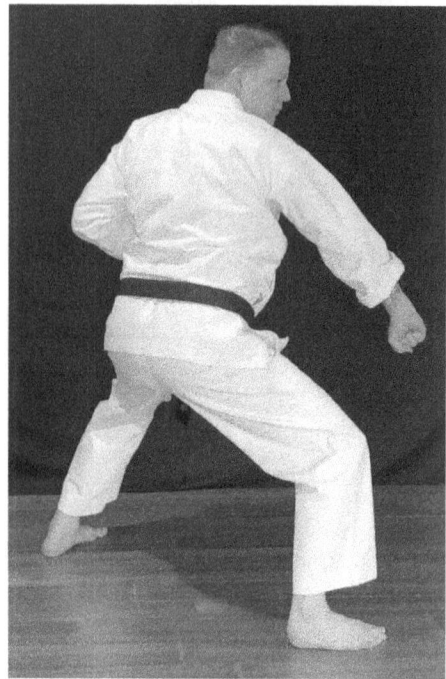

Gedan Barai (cont.)

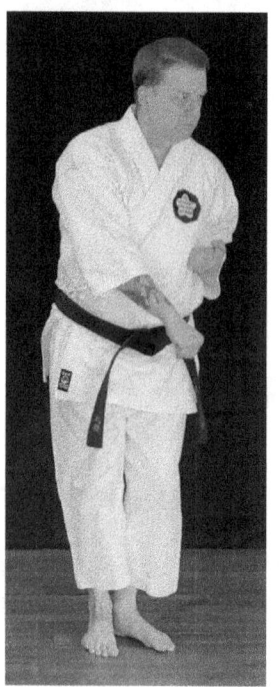

Step Back on Same Angle

Seiunchin

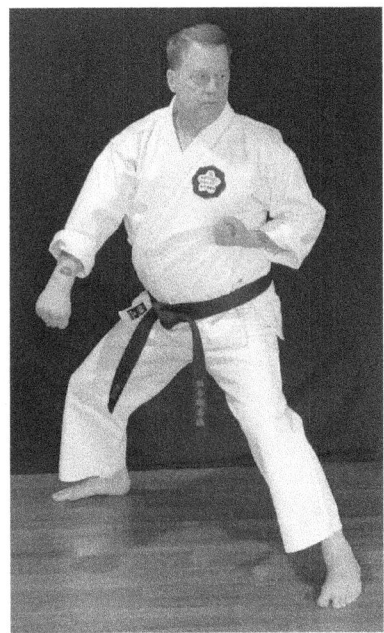
Land in Shiko Dachi

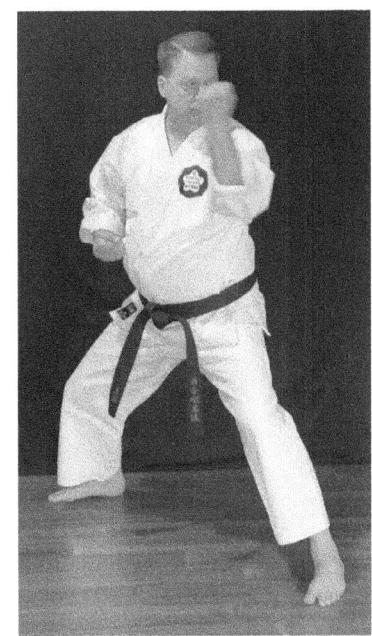
Complete Left Gedan Barai

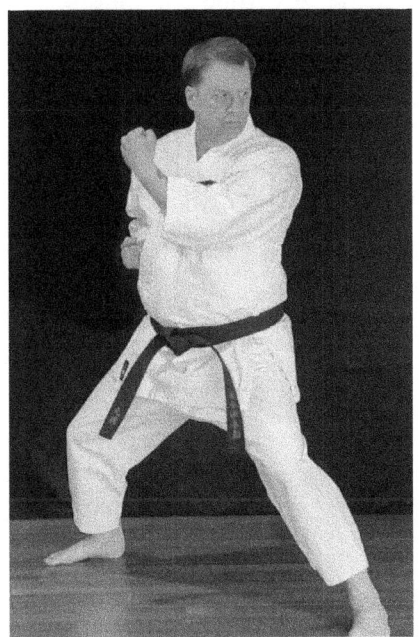

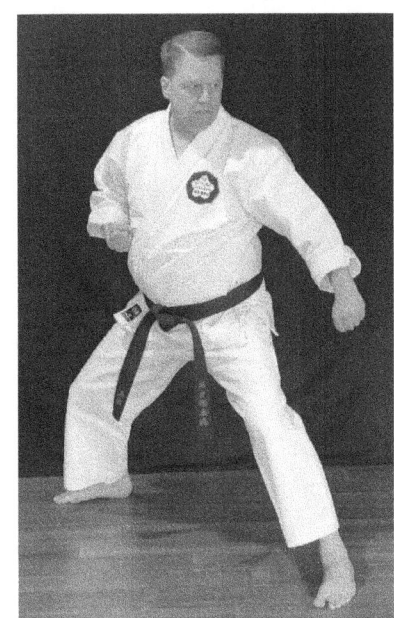
Gedan Barai (cont.)

Seiunchin

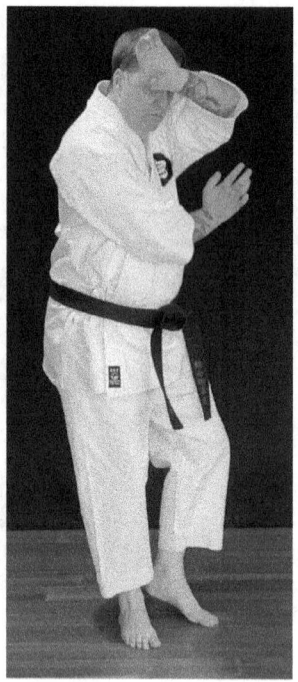 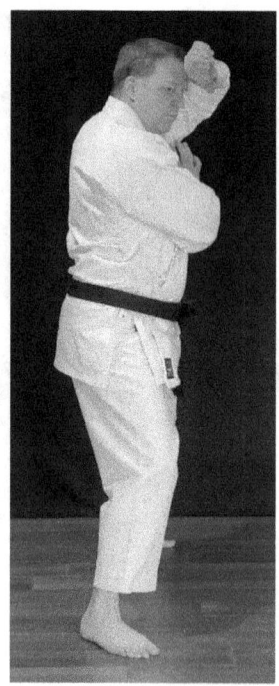

Step Back with Left Foot into Shiko Dachi Facing Left while Completing Right Gedan Shotei Barai and Left Jodan Age Uke

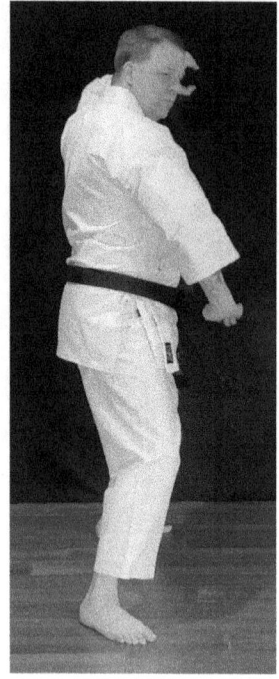 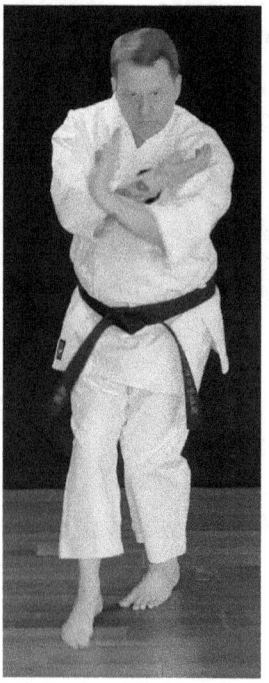

Step Back with Right Foot into Shiko Dachi Facing Right

Seiunchin

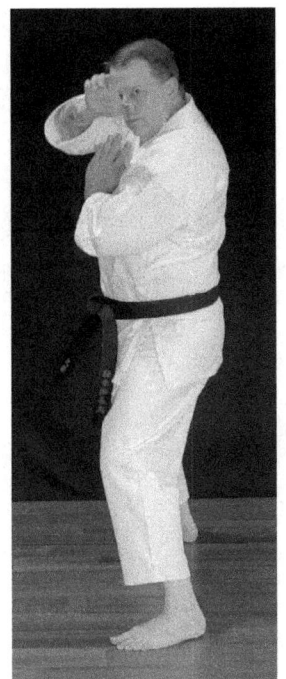
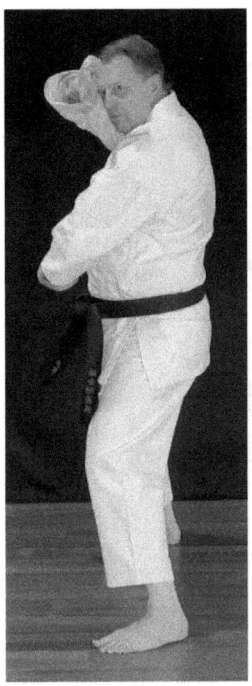

Complete Right Gedan Shotei Barai and Left Jodan Age Uke

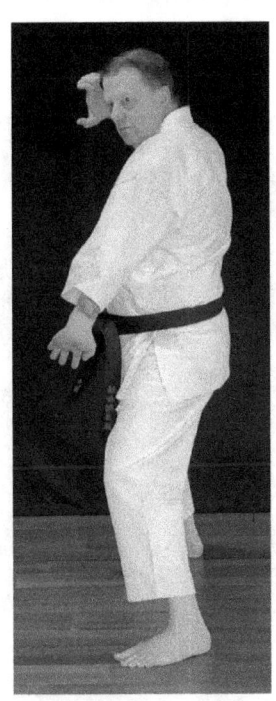
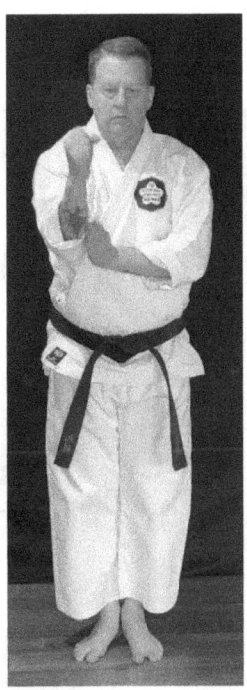

Step Around Facing Forward with Right Foot while Completing Soto Uke into Left Palm

Seiunchin

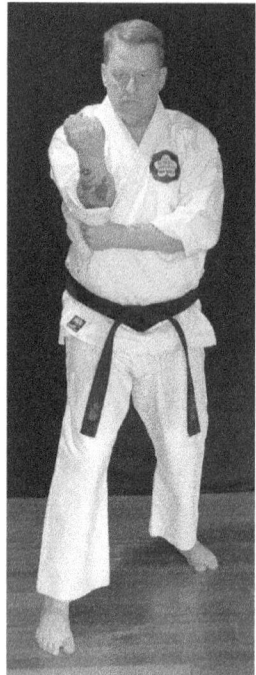

Step, Complete Right Uraken Uchi

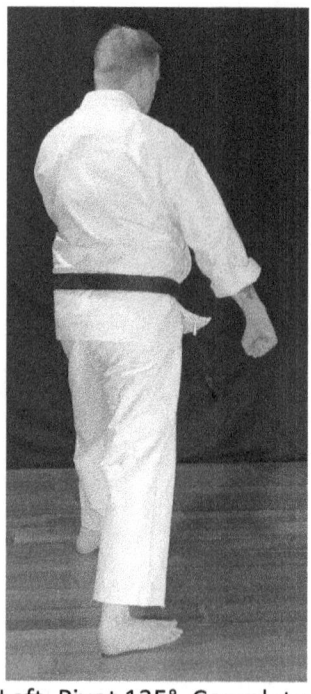

Step Left, Pivot 135°, Complete Right Gedan Barai and Left Chudan Uke Simultaneously

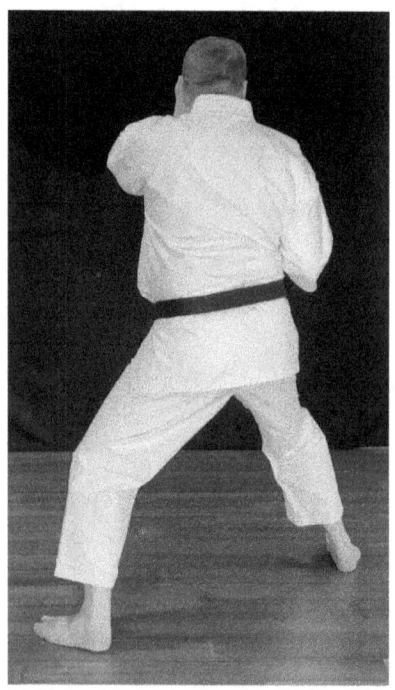

Right Step in on Same Angle into Shiko Dachi

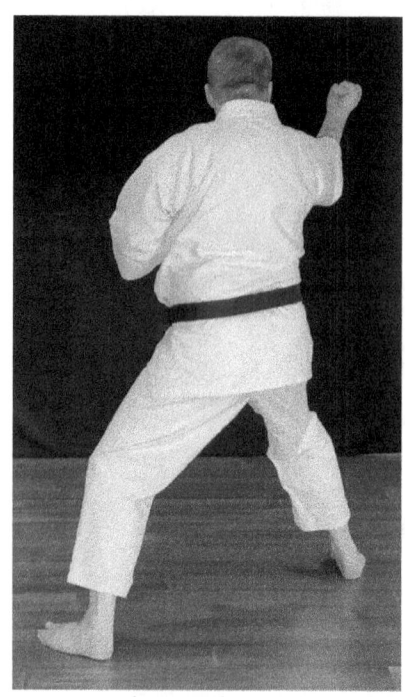

Complete Right Age Zuki

Seiunchin

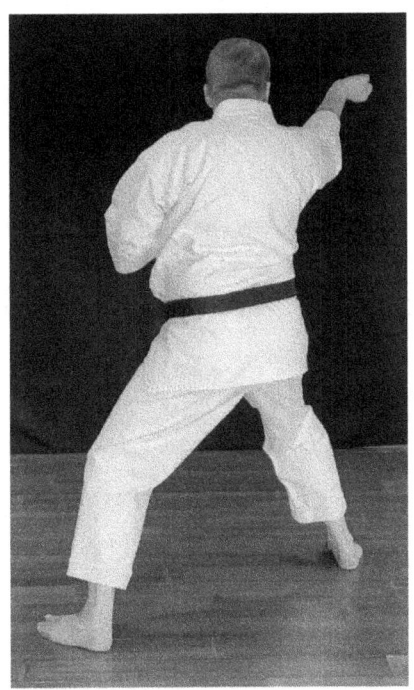
Complete Right Uraken Uchi

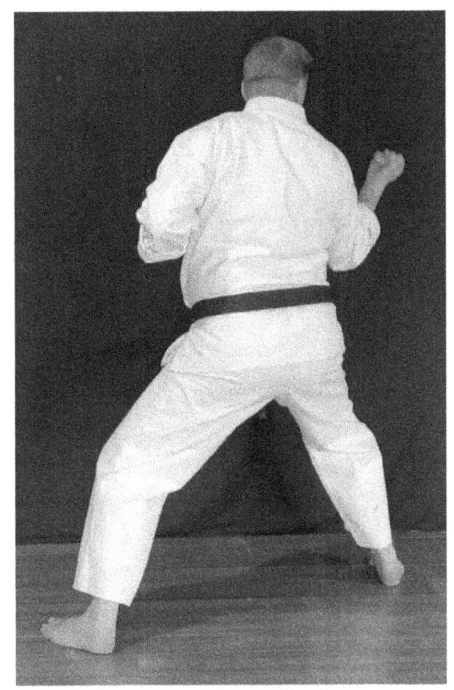
Bring Elbow Back

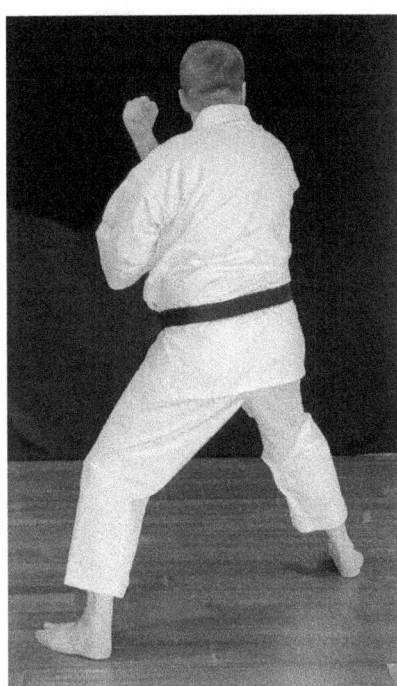

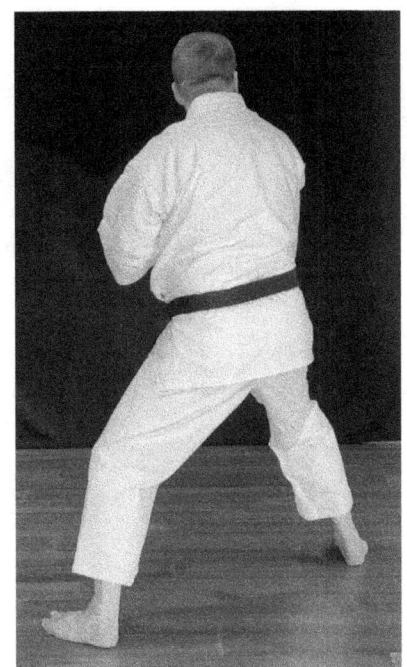
Complete Right Gedan Barai

Seiunchin

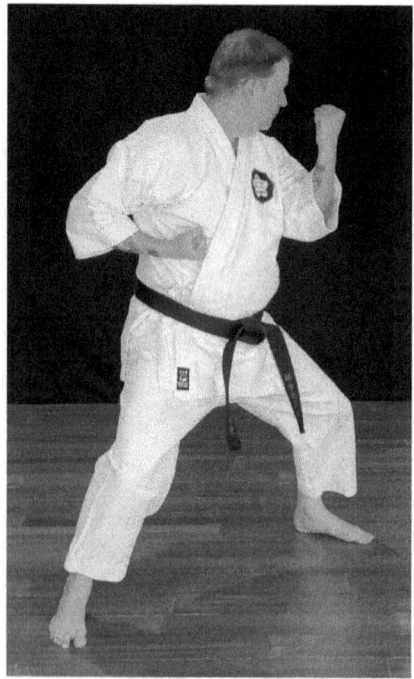
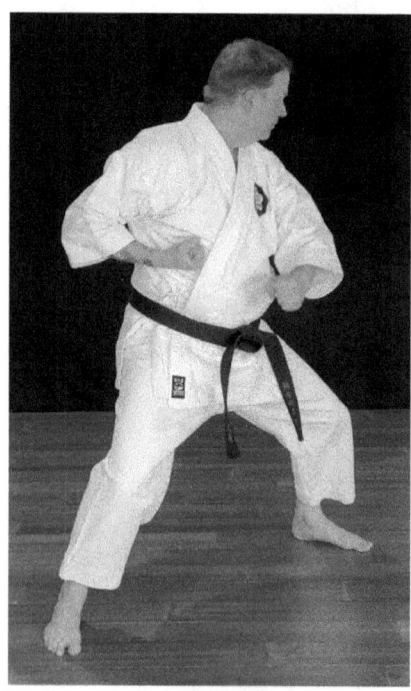

Step Back into Shiko Dachi on Same Angle, Complete Left Gedan Barai

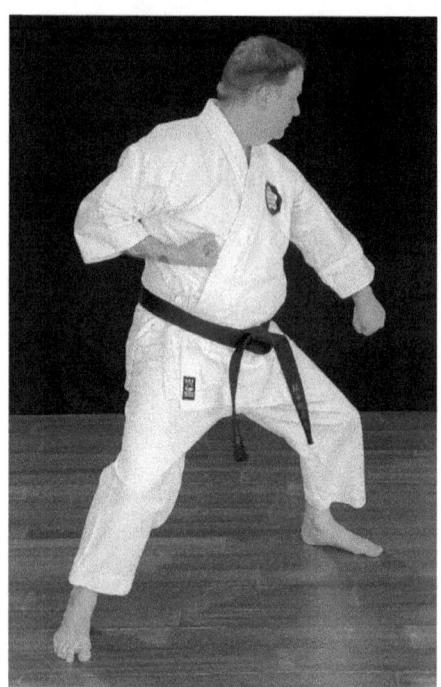

Gedan Barai (cont.)

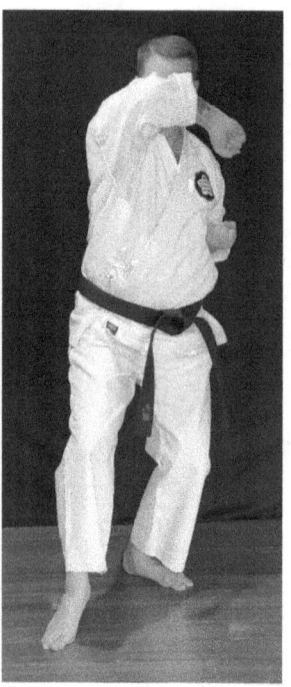

Realign Forward, Bring Right Foot Back into Neko Ashi Dachi, Complete Right Age Hiji Ate and Left Ushiro Empi Uchi

Seiunchin

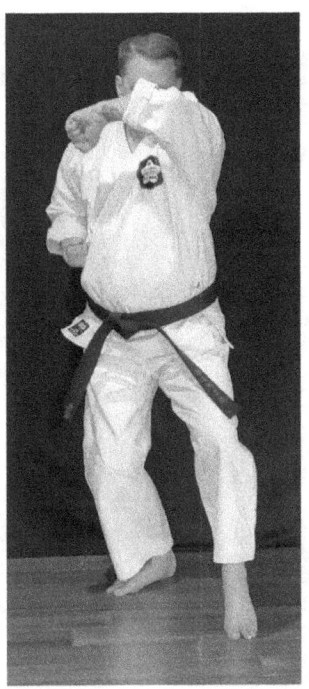

Right Step Back into Neko Ashi Dachi, Complete Left Age Hiji Ate and Right Ushiro Empi Uchi Simultaneously

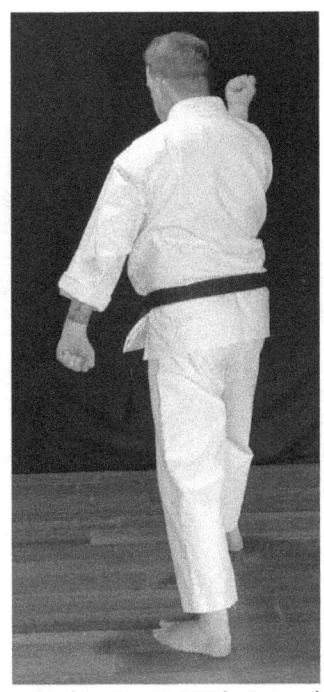

Step Right, Pivot 225°, Complete Left Gedan Barai and Right Chudan Uke Simultaneously

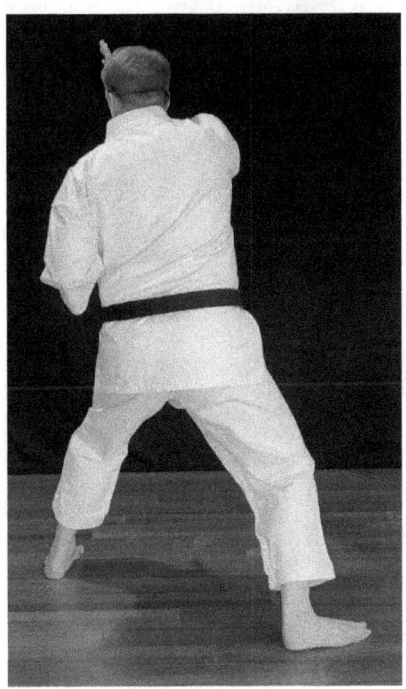

Left Step in on Same Angle into Shiko Dachi, Bring Right Open Hand to Chest

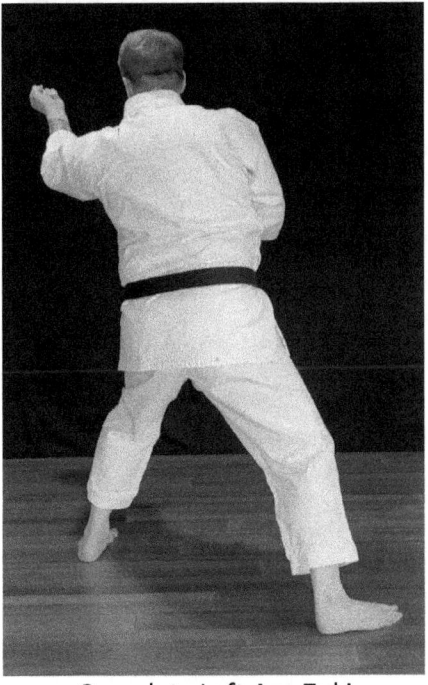

Complete Left Age Zuki

Seiunchin

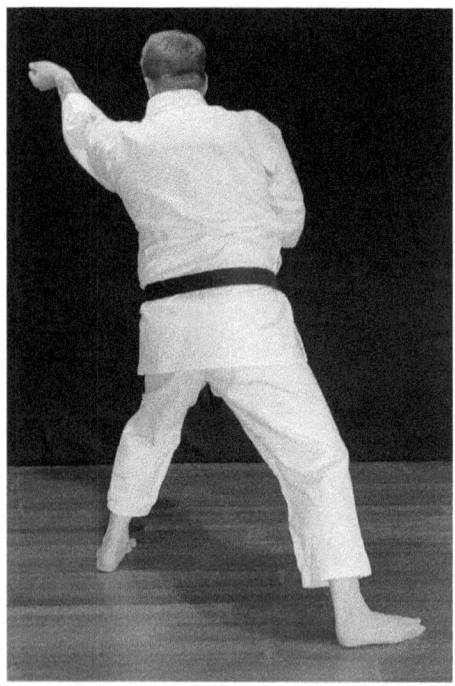
Complete Left Uraken Uchi

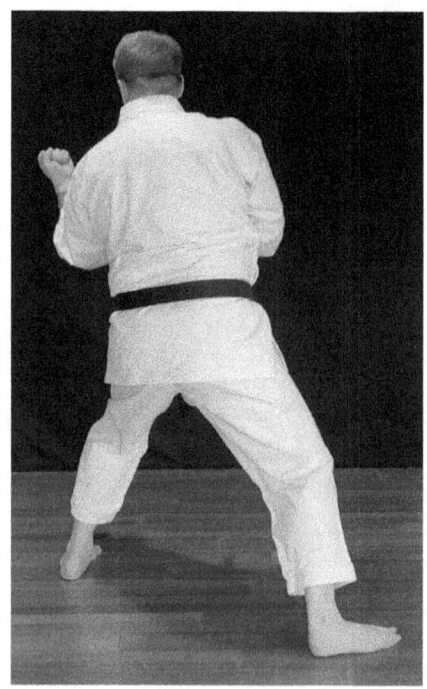
Bring Elbow Back

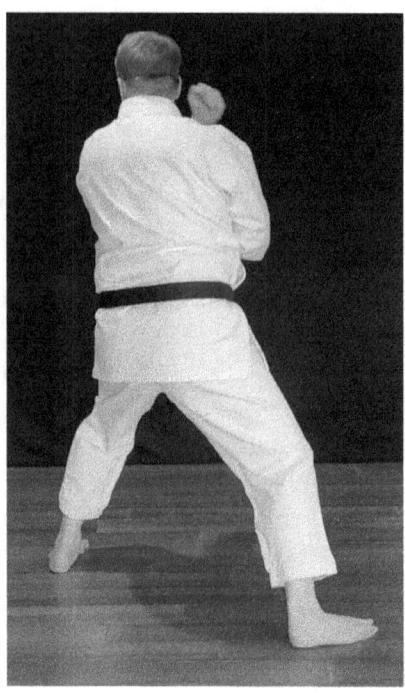
Complete Left Gedan Barai

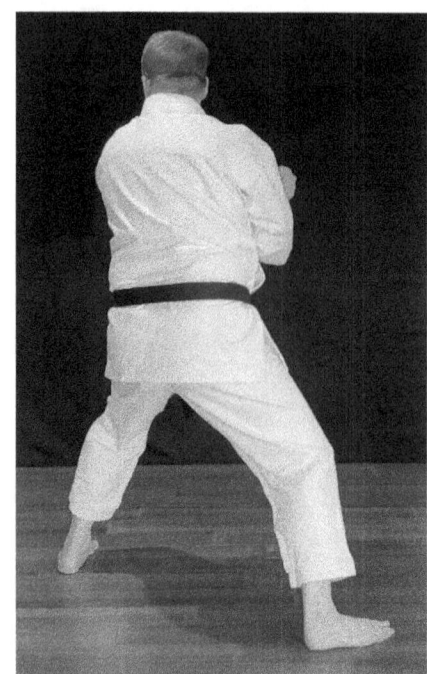

Seiunchin

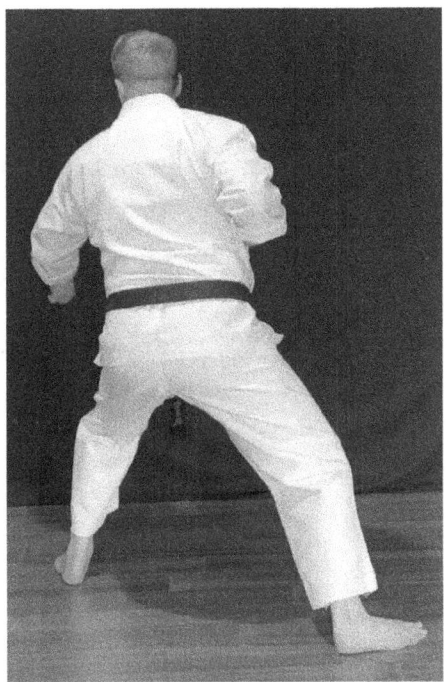
Gedan Barai (cont.)

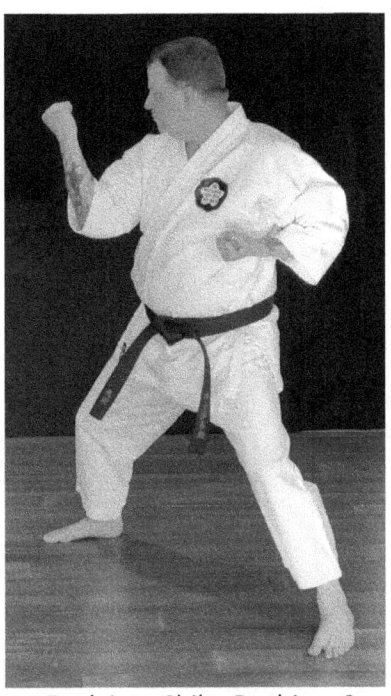
Step Back into Shiko Dachi on Same Angle, Complete Right Gedan Barai

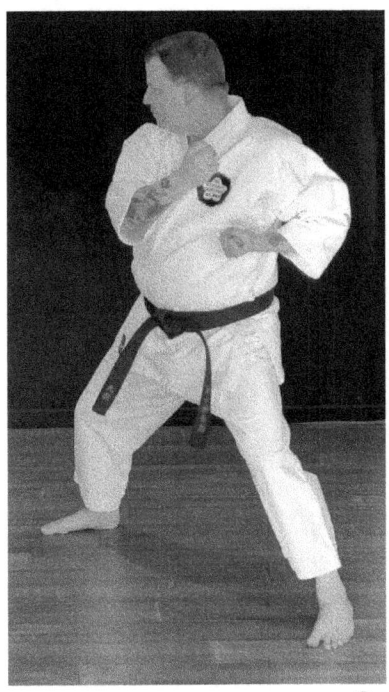

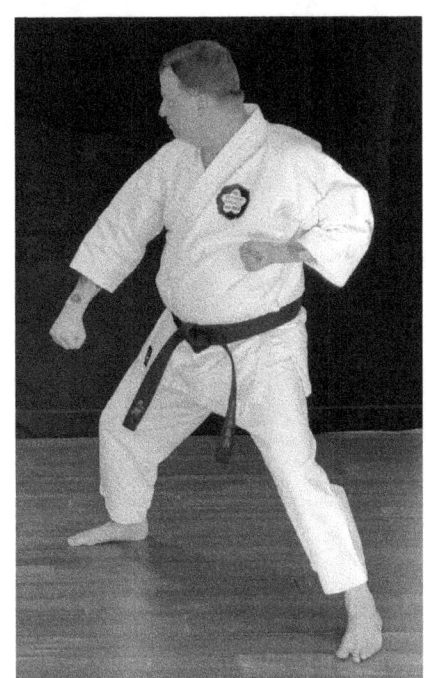

Gedan Barai (cont.)

Seiunchin

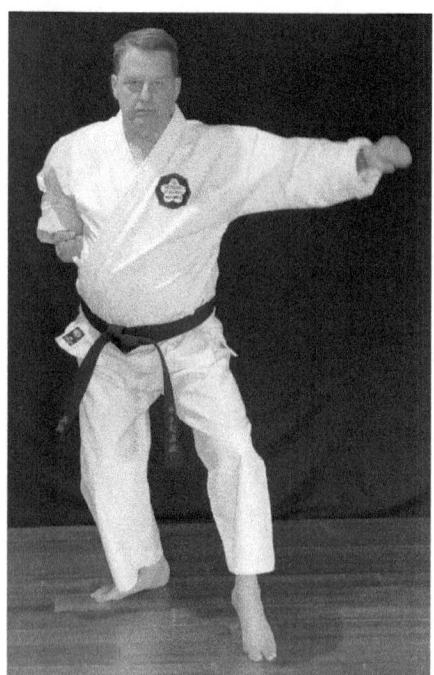
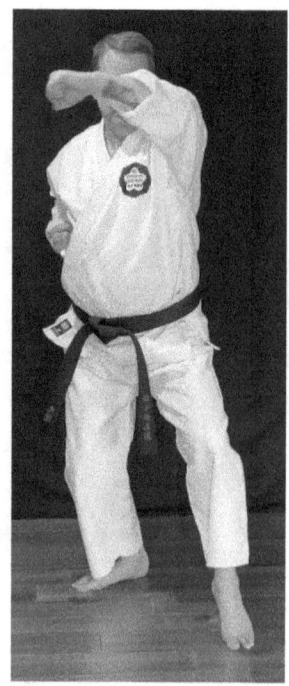

Realign Forward, Bring Back Left Foot into
Neko Ashi Dachi, Complete Left Kagi Zuki

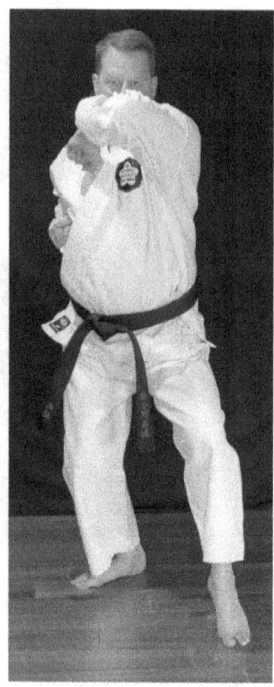
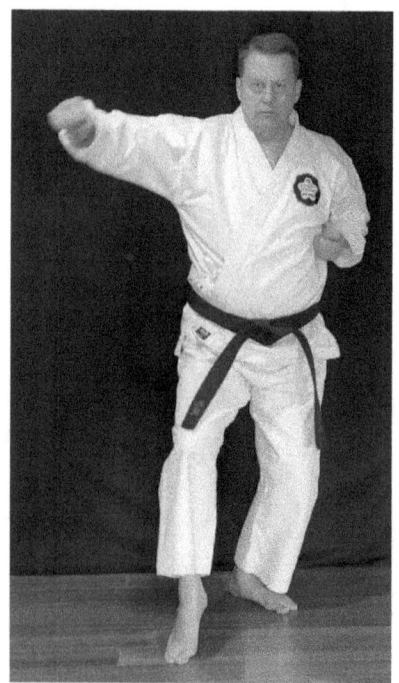

Kagi Zuki (cont.)

Left Step Back, Complete
Right Kagi Zuki

Seiunchin

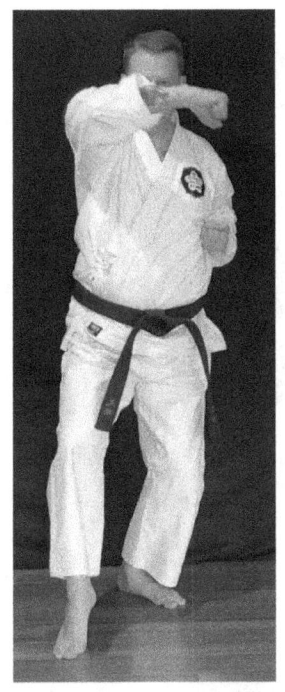 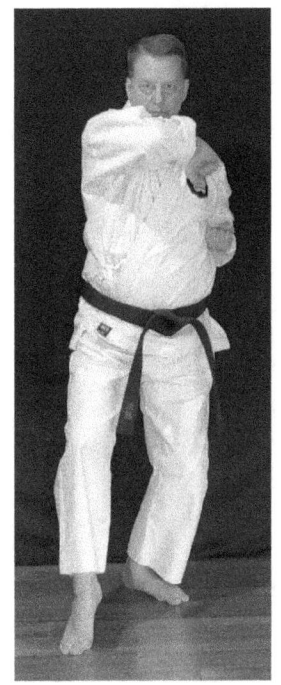

Kagi Zuki (cont.)

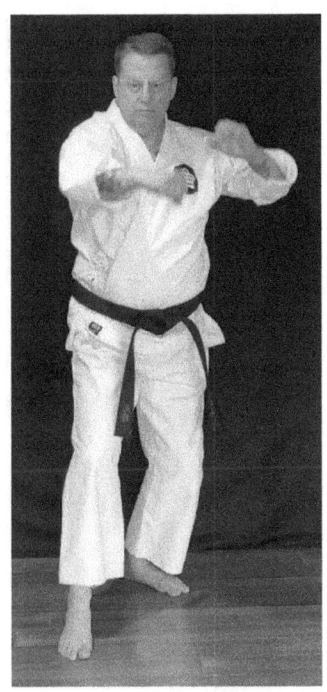 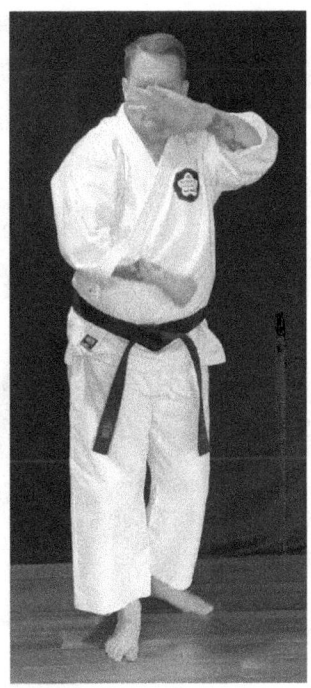

Step Forward and Complete Right Otoshi Tettsui
Uchi with Left Arm Across Torso

Seiunchin

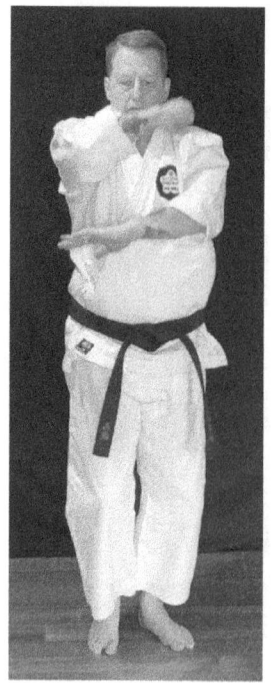 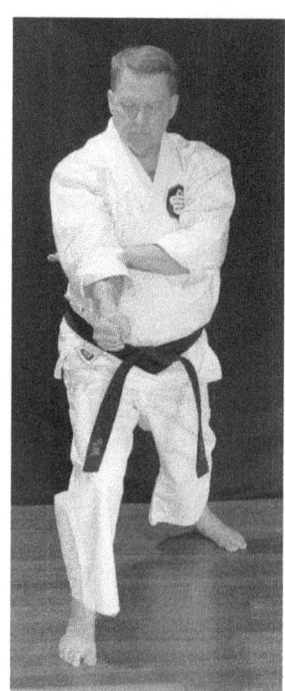

Complete Otoshi Tettsui Uchi (kiai)

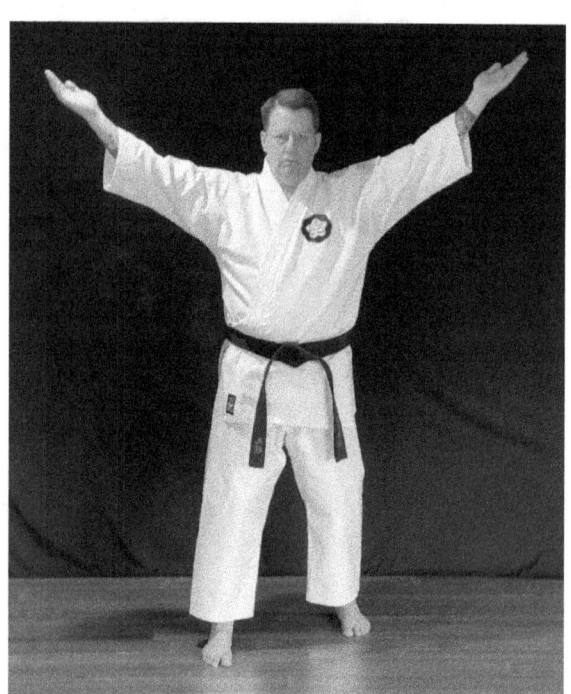 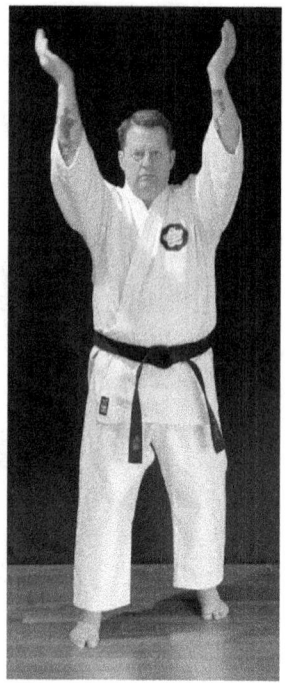

Step Back, Bring Arms Around

Seiunchin

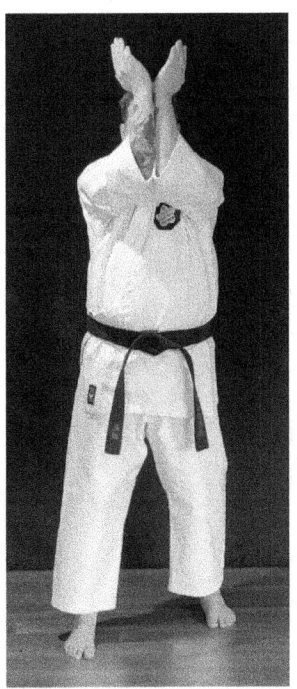

Bring Elbows Together and Down

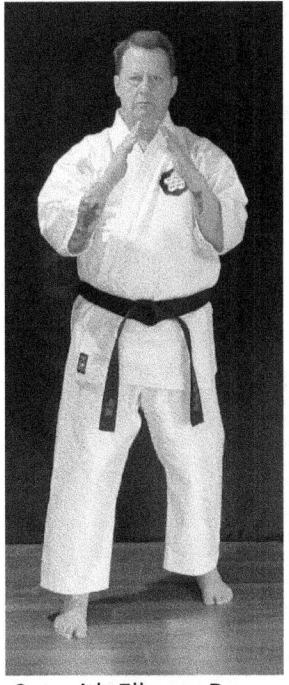

Set with Elbows Down and Hands Separated

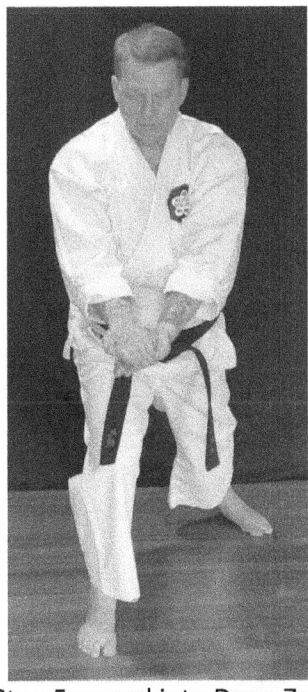

Right Step Forward into Deep Zenkutsu Dachi with Open Left Hand and Open Right Hand

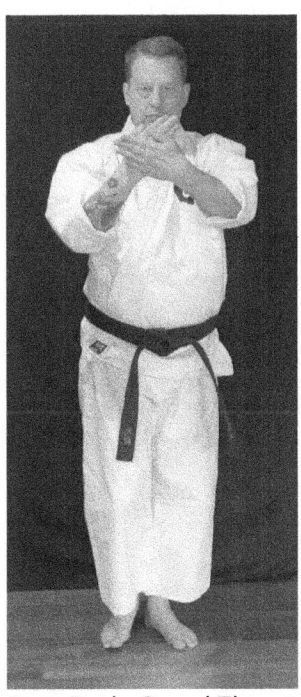

Step Back, Guard Throat

Seiunchin

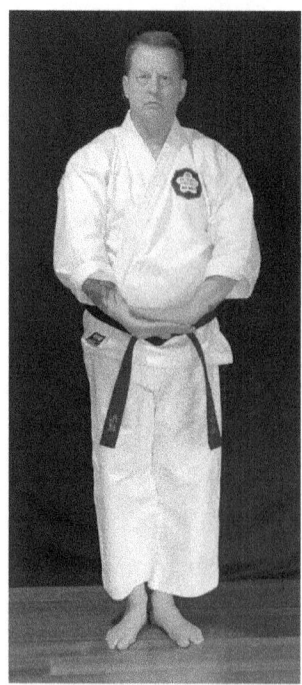

Turn Hands Down,
Complete Hojo Osae Uke

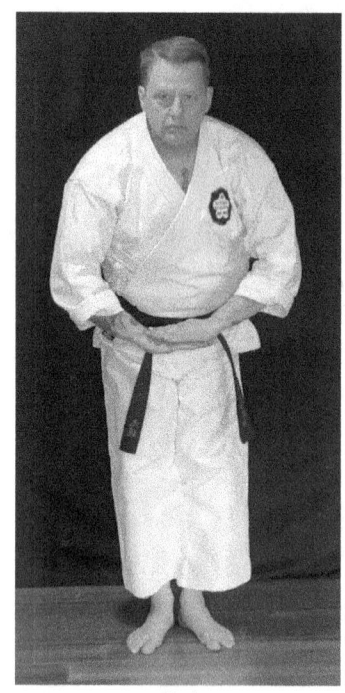

Rei

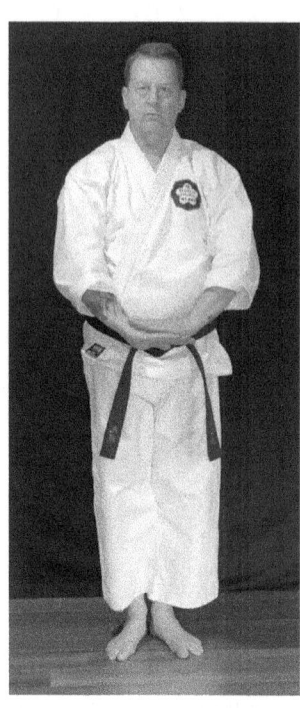

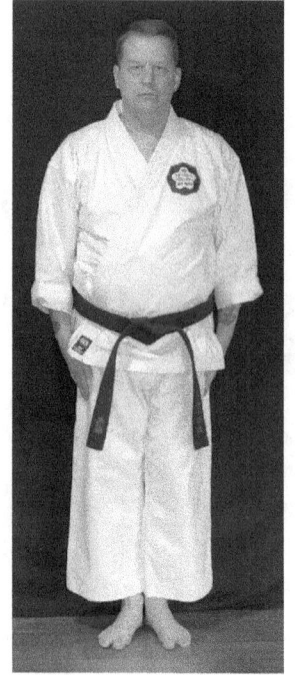

Musubi Dachi

Seiunchin

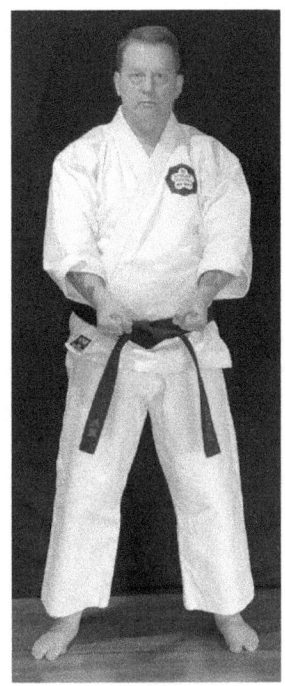

Heiko Dachi

Sepai

Sepai means eighteen, which is a translation of the kanji (十八). There is considerable discussion on what 18 refers to. It could mean number of techniques, or part of Buddhist numeral symbolism.[7] Regardless of the origin, the kata itself is one of the more unique katas in the Goju-Ryu curriculum. It contains the double strike furi zuki, an arm bar, and several takedown techniques.

Below is the method by which Ketsugo Goju-Ryu performs Sepai kata. Complete details about each move are not included, as this is simply a demonstration. Sepai is a widespread kata, and many karate systems include it in their curriculum. This demonstration is not meant to imply that it is the only way to do it, but it is the way at Ketsugo Goju-Ryu.

These are the Japanese terms used for this kata. Bear in mind, karate terms are not completely streamlined. There are terms that were used in the middle of the 20th Century that are no longer used today. Oftentimes there are more than one term that can be used for the same technique. The important thing is not what it is called, but the technique itself.

Age Empi Uchi – Rising Elbow Strike	**Oshi** – Push
Age Uke - Rising Block	**Otoshi** - Downward
Barai - Sweeping Block	**Rei** – Bow (Respect)
Chudan - Middle	**Shiko Dachi** - Straddle Leg Stance
Dachi – Stance	
Furi Uchi - Swinging or Hook Punch	**Shotei** – Palm Heel
Gedan – Low	**Suihei Osae** – Horizontal Pressing
Hajime – Command to Begin	
Hari Uke – Open Hand Block (Palm Up)	

Sepai

Hiki Uke – Open Hand Block (Palm Down)/Pulling Block **Heiko Dachi** - Parallel Stance **Jodan** - High **Mae Keage Geri** – Front Snap Kick **Morote Nakadakaken Uchi** – Double Middle Knuckle Fist Strike **Morote Shotei Uchi** – Double Palm Heel Strike **Morote Sukui Uke** – Augmented Scooping Block **Musubi Dachi** - Attention Stance, Toes Out **Neko Ashi Dachi** – Cat Leg Stance	**Tenchi no Kamae** – Position with One Palm Up and One Palm Down **Tettsui Uchi** - Hammer Fist Strike **Tsuki/-Zuki** - Punch **Uchi** – Strike **Uke** – Block (Receive) **Ura Zuki** – Inverted Strike **Uraken Uchi** - Back Fist Strike **Ushiro Empi Uchi** – Rear Elbow Strike **Yoi** – Ready Command **Yoko** - Side

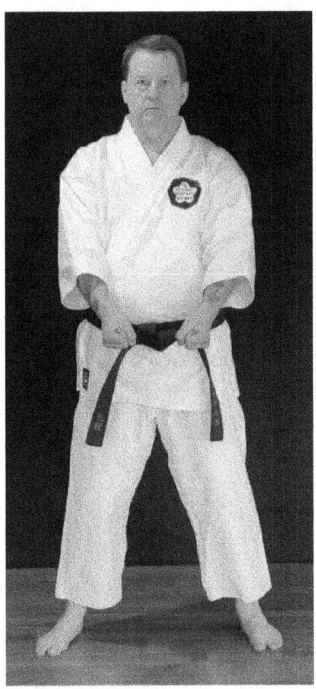

Heiko Dachi

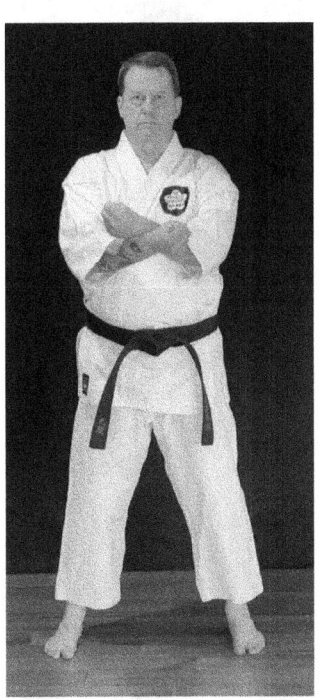

(Yoi) Brings Arms Up, Crossed at the Wrist

Sepai

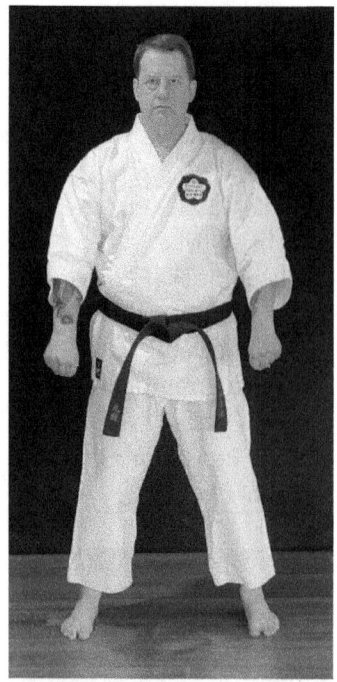
Bring Arms Down

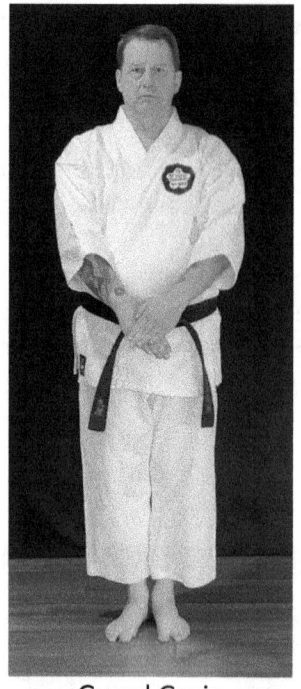
Guard Groin

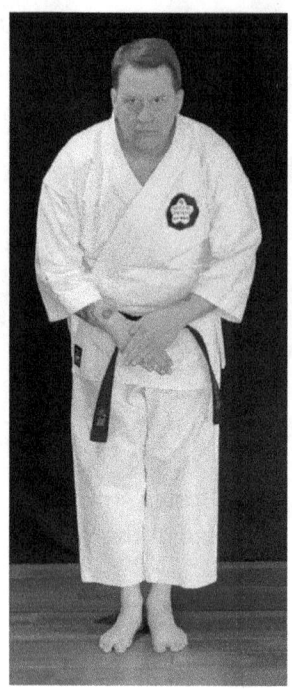
Rei

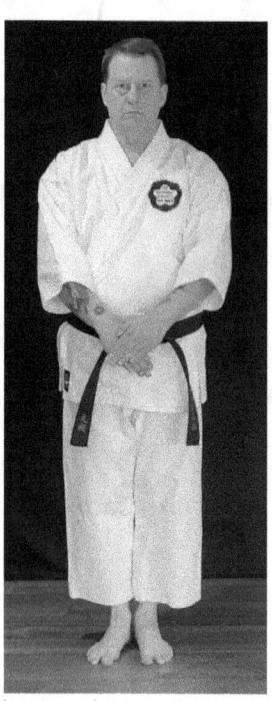
(Hajime) Musubi Dachi

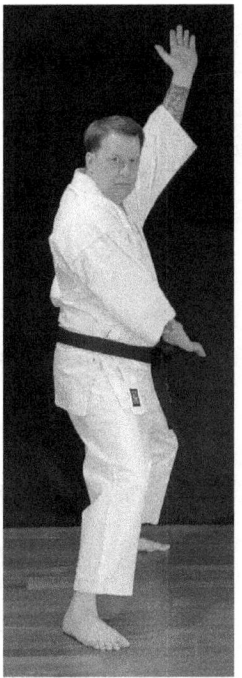 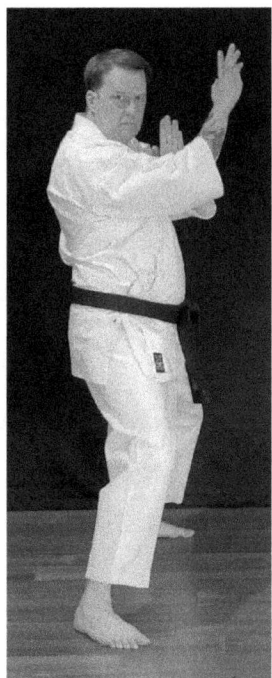

Left Foot Steps Back into Shiko Dachi while Left Hand Drops Back Completing Shotei Otoshi Uke and Right Hand Makes an Arc

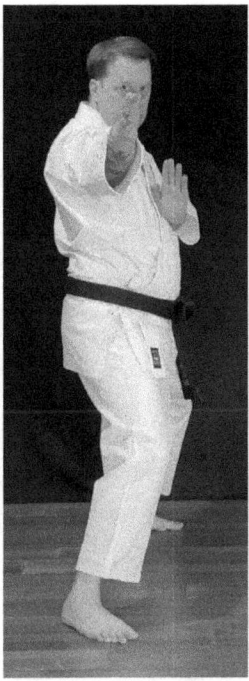 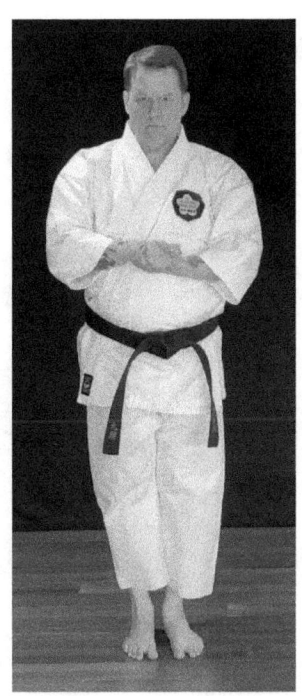

Right Hand Lands in Front, Arm Outstretched at Face Level

Back Foot Steps Up While Back Hand Clasps with Front Hand at Chest

Sepai

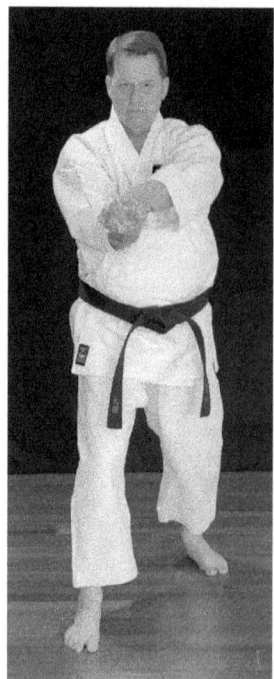

Right Step while Turning Hands
Over and Delivering a Strike

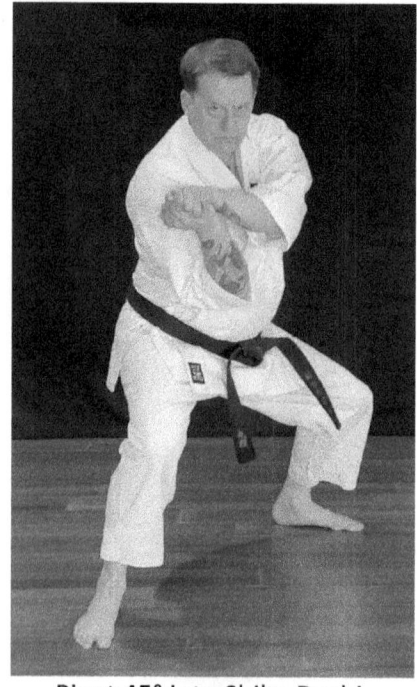

Pivot 45° into Shiko Dachi,
Holding Down Clasped Hands

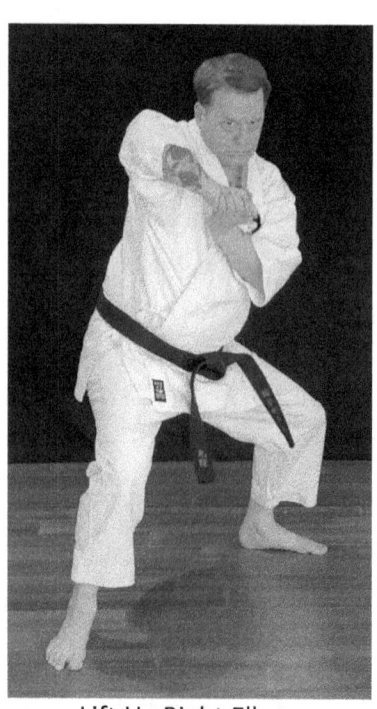

Lift Up Right Elbow
into Age Hiji Ate

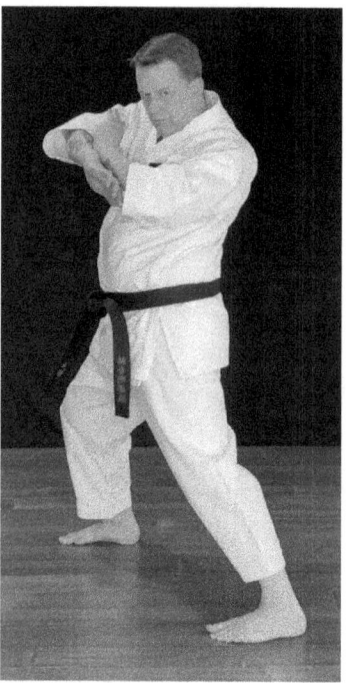

Left Step into Kokutsu Dachi,
Lift the Left Hand Over Right Forearm

Sepai

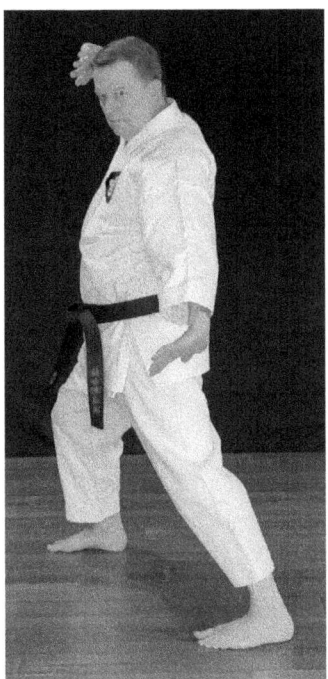

Right Hand Pulls Back to Head
While Left Hand Completes Shotei
Barai, then Left Kake Uke

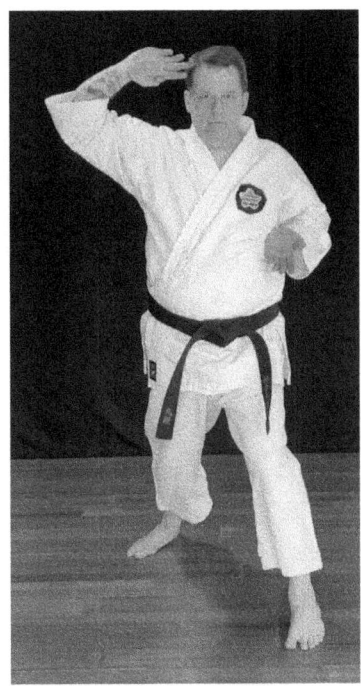

Pivot Facing Forward,
Chamber Hands for
Shuto Uchi

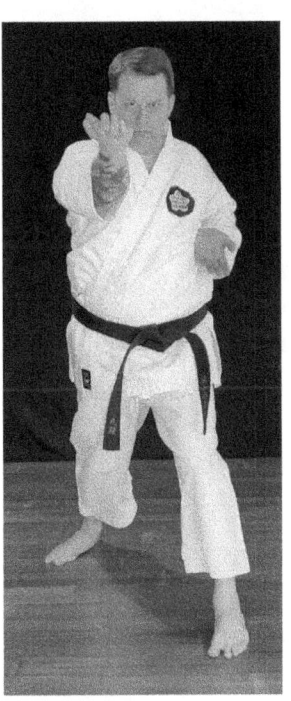

Complete Right Jodan
Shuto Uchi

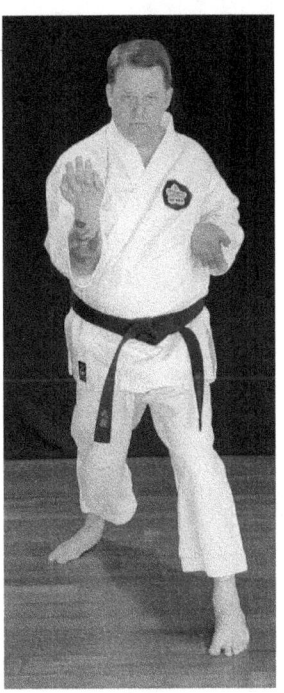

Set

Sepai

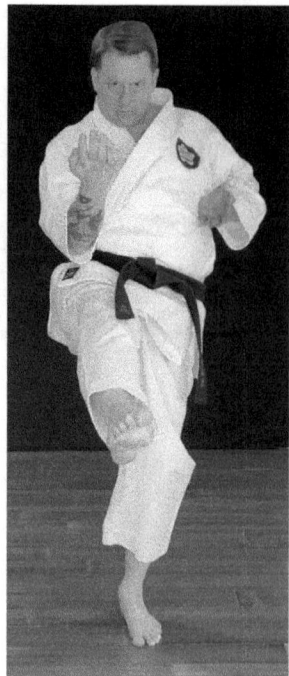

Complete Right Gedan Mae Keage Geri

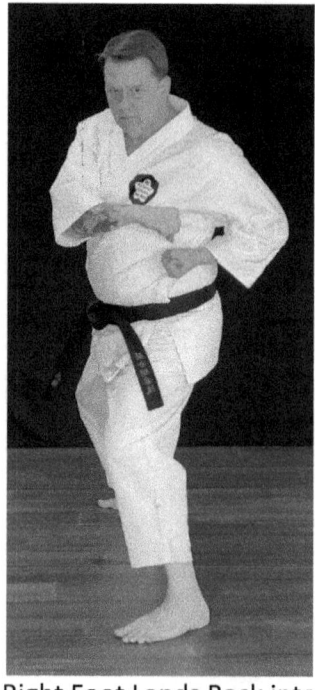

Right Foot Lands Back into Shiko Dachi Facing Right

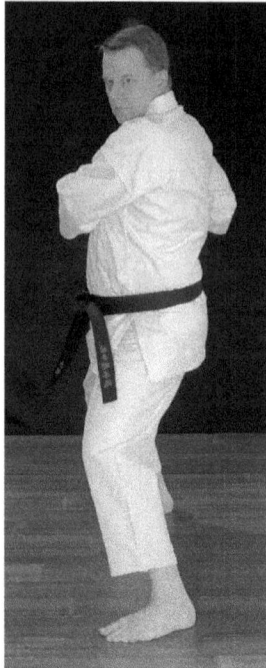

Left Elbow Completes Hiji Ate while Completing Right Ushiro Empi Uchi Simultaneously

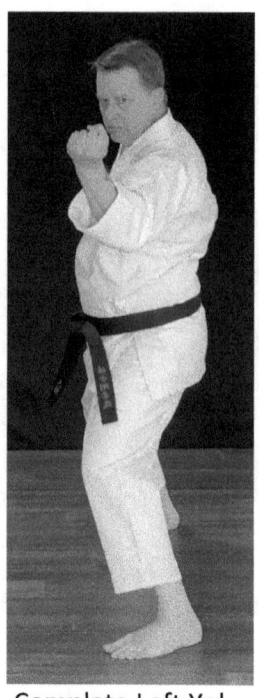

Complete Left Yoko Uraken Uchi

Sepai

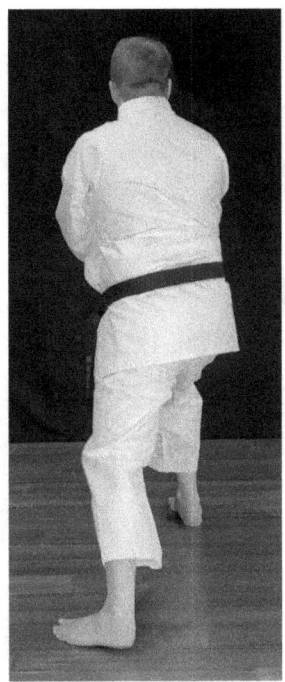

Pivot 180° Right
(Facing Rear)

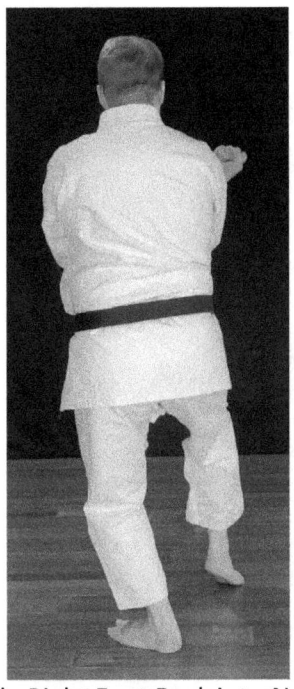

Slide Right Foot Back into Neko
Ashi Dachi while Lifting Right Arm
Up and Left Fist Under Right Elbow

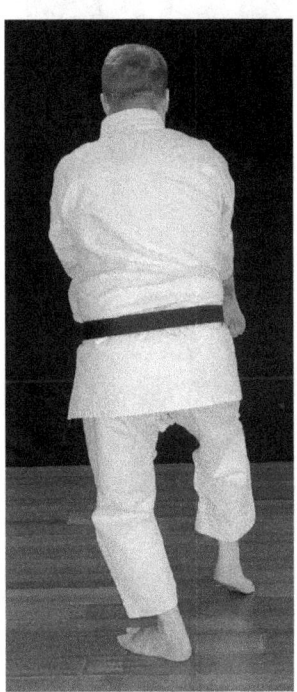

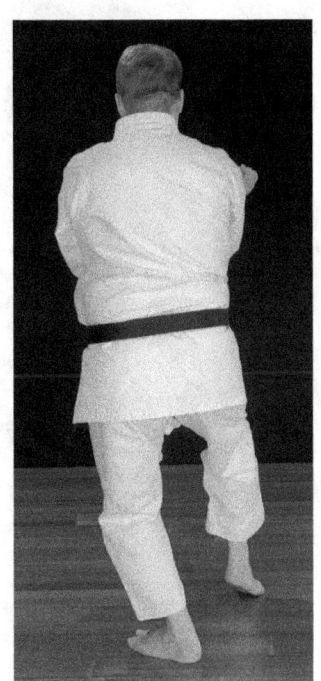

Complete Right Gedan Barai, then an Immediate Right Chudan Uke

Sepai

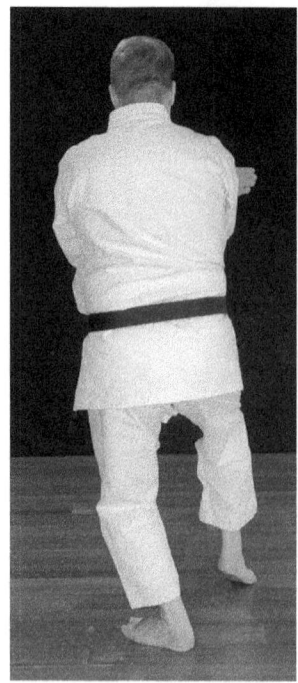

Turn Right Hand into Chudan Hiki Uke

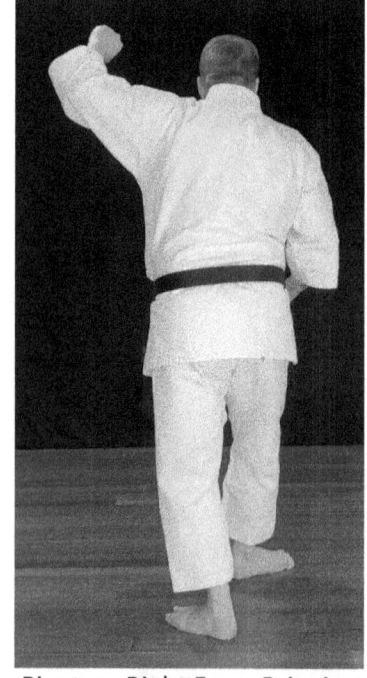

Pivot on Right Foot, Bringing Left Arm Up while Left Fist Drops

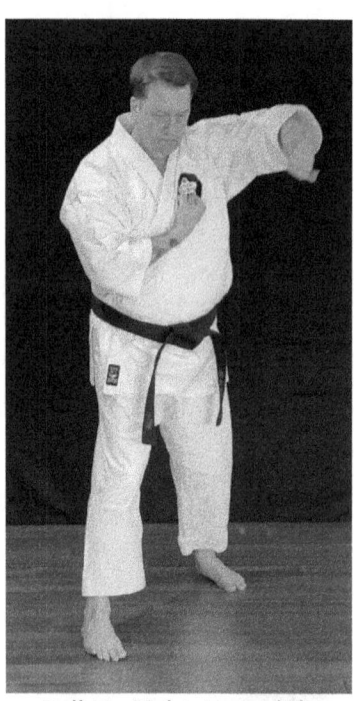

Pull Up Right Arm while Left Arm Circles Down

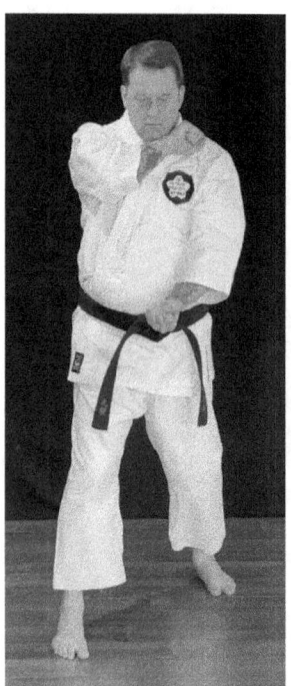

Turn Right Hand Over

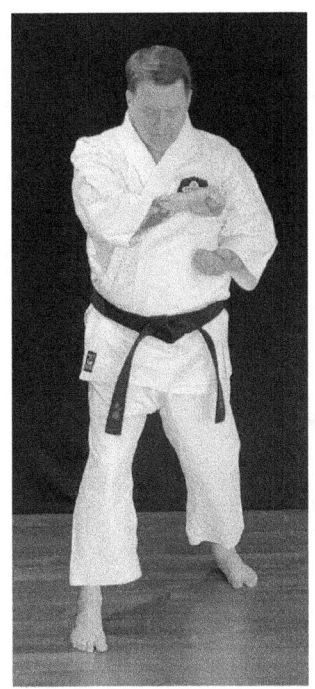

Bring Left Fist Up and Right Fist Down (Suihei Osae)

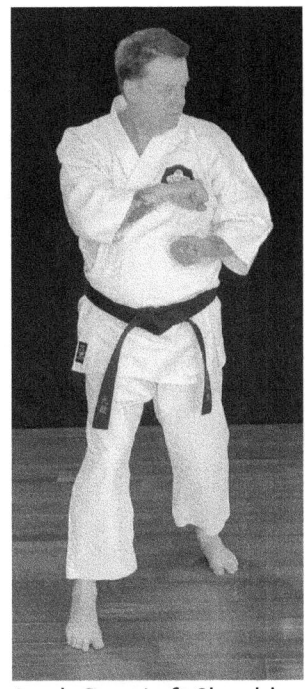

Look Over Left Shoulder

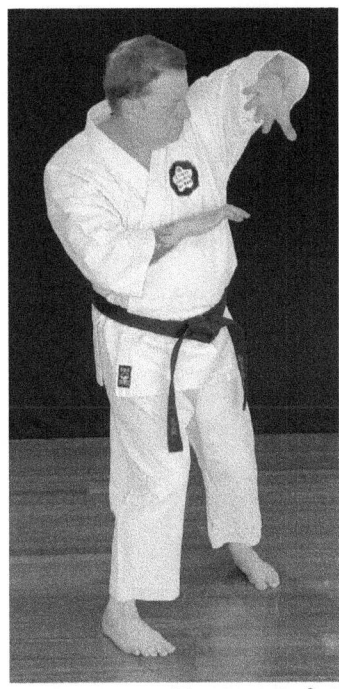
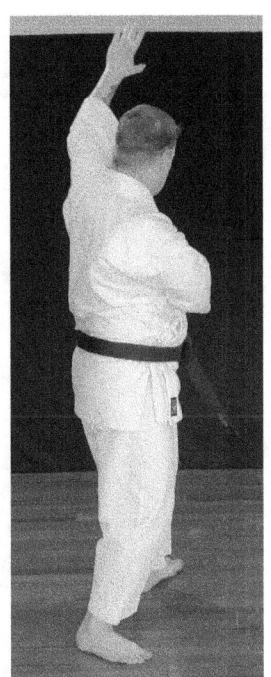

Pivot on Left Foot while Lifting Left Arm in Arc

Sepai

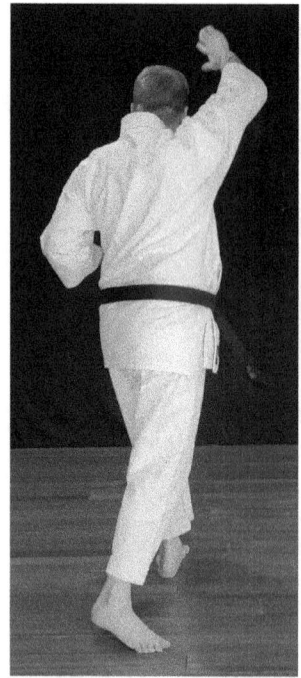

Bring Left Hand to Chamber while Right Hand Begins Arc

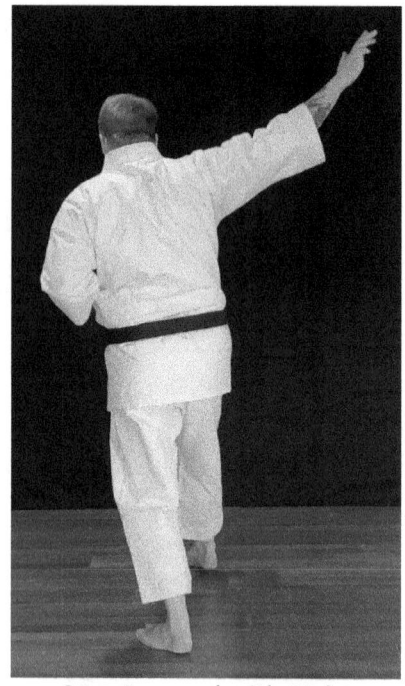

Step Forward with Right Foot in 225° Angle

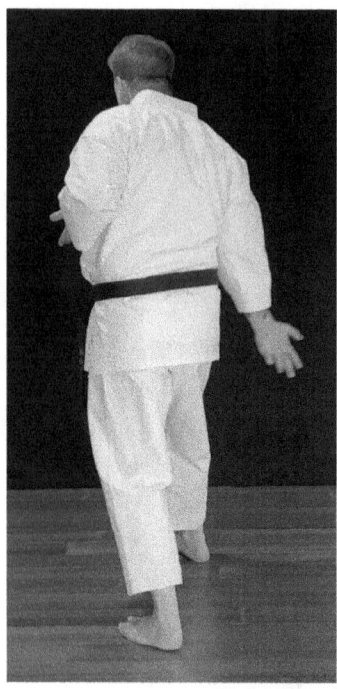

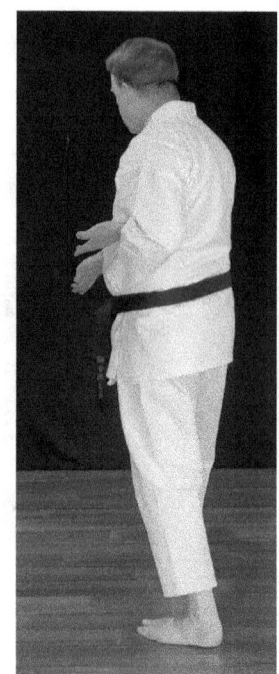

Right Hand Completes Gedan Furi Uchi

Sepai

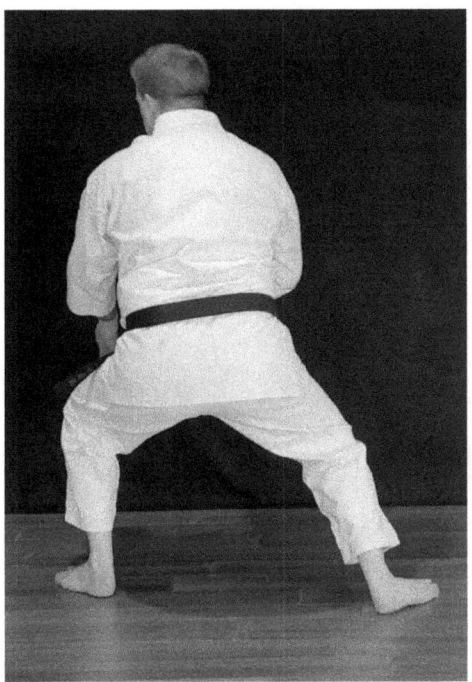

Slide Left Foot Followed By Right Foot

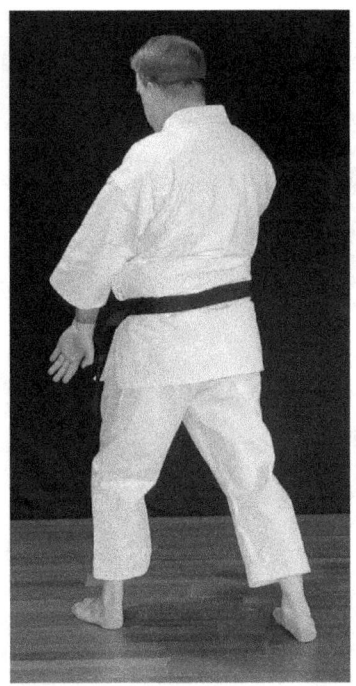

Rise Up in Stance while Left Hand Completes Gedan Harai Uke and Right Hand Shotei Oshi

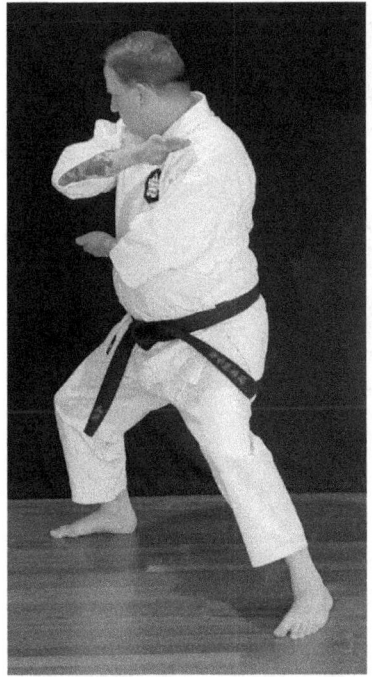

Bring Right Leg Around into Shiko Dachi, Placing Both Open Hands Right Palm Down, Left Palm Up (Tenchi no Kamae)

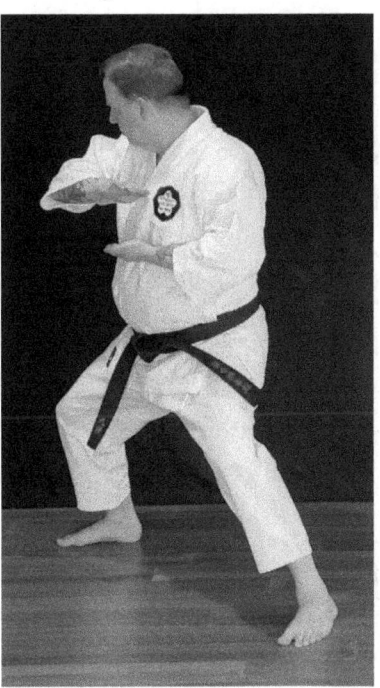

Pull Back Slightly on Both Arms

Sepai

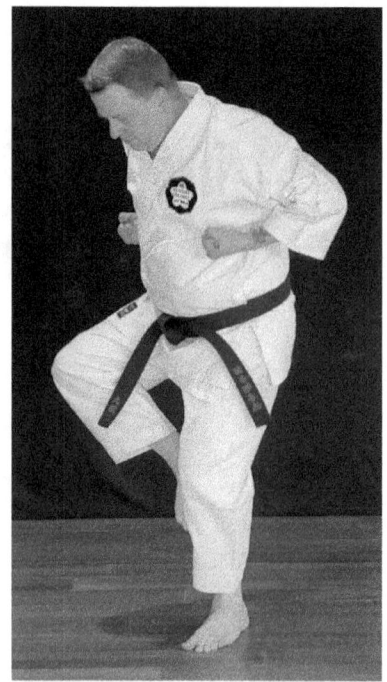

Pull Fists Back into Chamber while Completing Right Ashi Barai

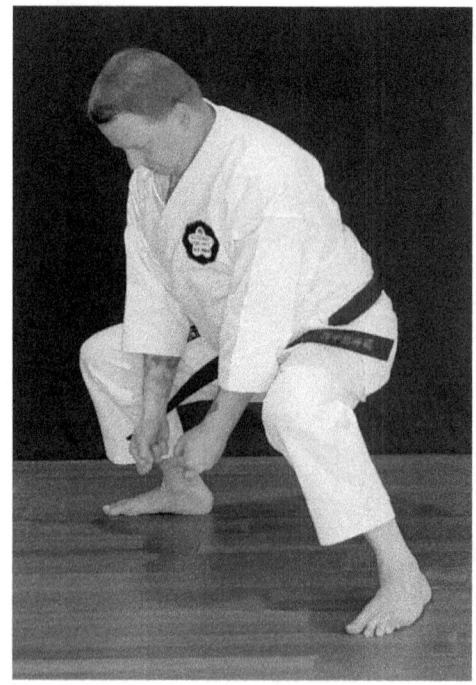

Complete Morote Nakadakaken Uchi Downward

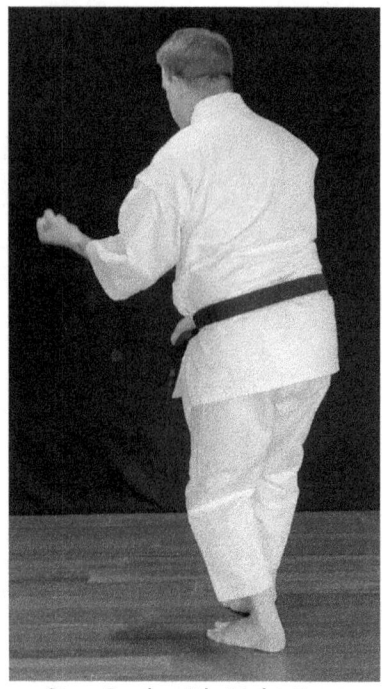

Step Back with Right Foot

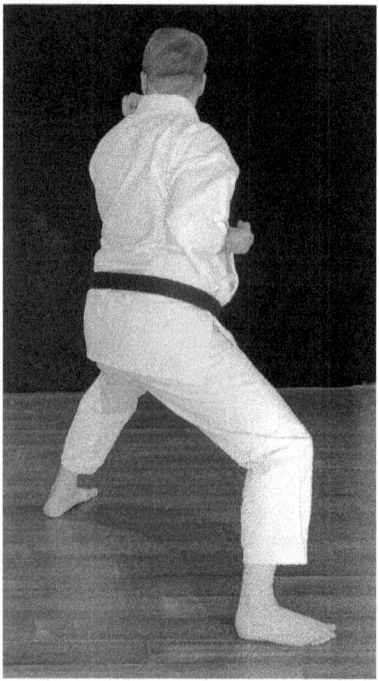

Land in Shiko Dachi on Same Angle, Begin Left Gedan Yoko Tettsui Uchi

Sepai

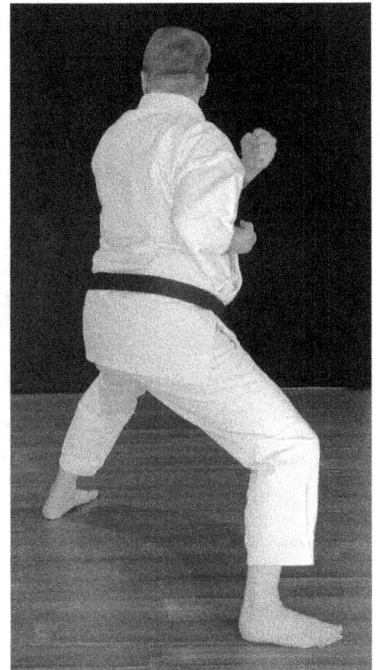 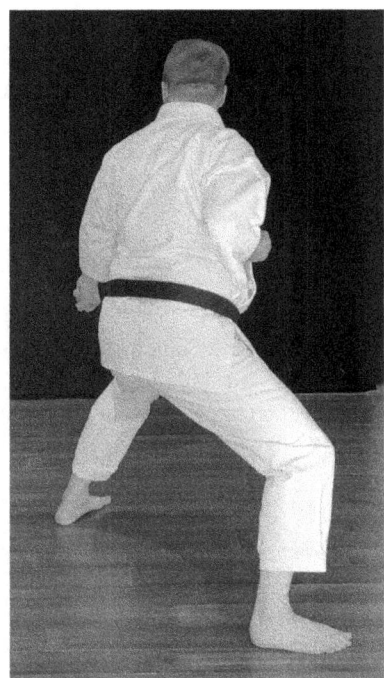

Gedan Yoko Tettsui Uchi (cont.)

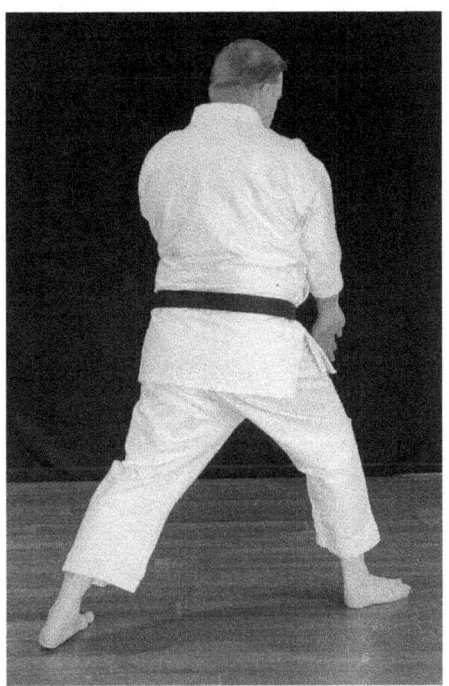 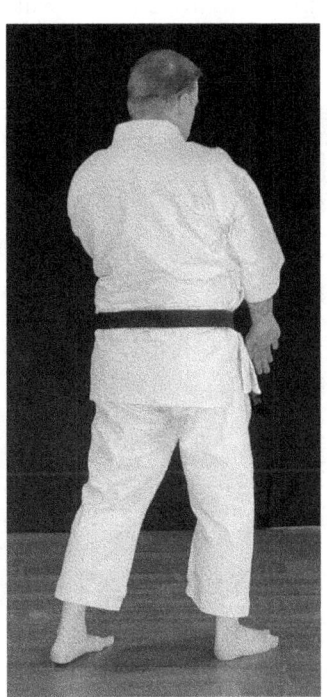

Right Step into Low Zenkutsu
Dachi on 135° Angle

Drag Left Foot Up while Right Hand
Completes Gedan Harai Uke and
Left Hand Shotei Oshi

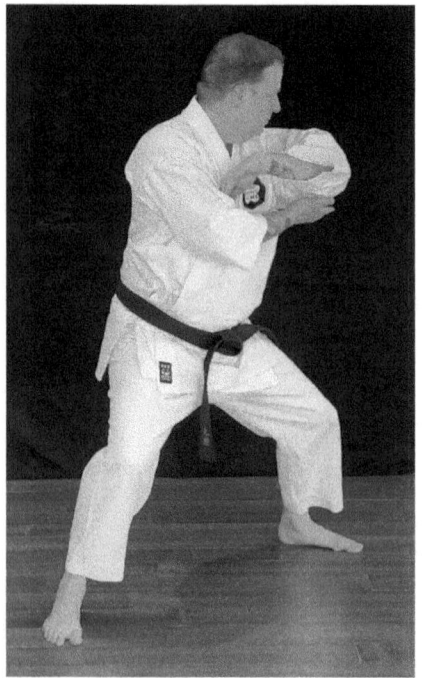

Bring Left Leg Around into Shiko Dachi, Placing Arms in Tenchi no Kamae

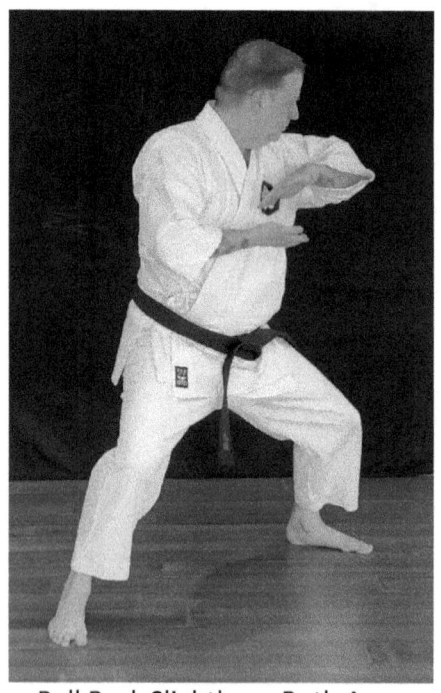

Pull Back Slightly on Both Arms

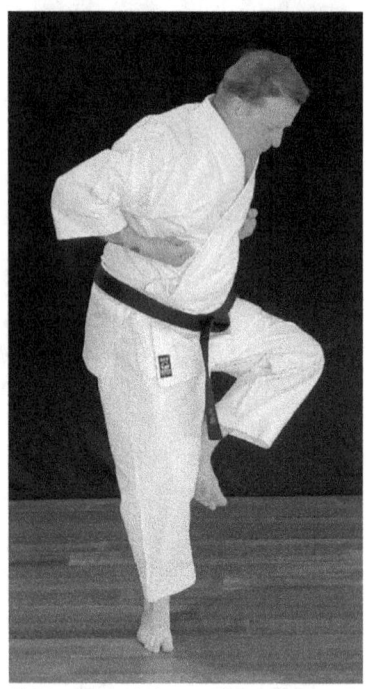

Pull Fists Back into Chamber While Performing Right Ashi Barai

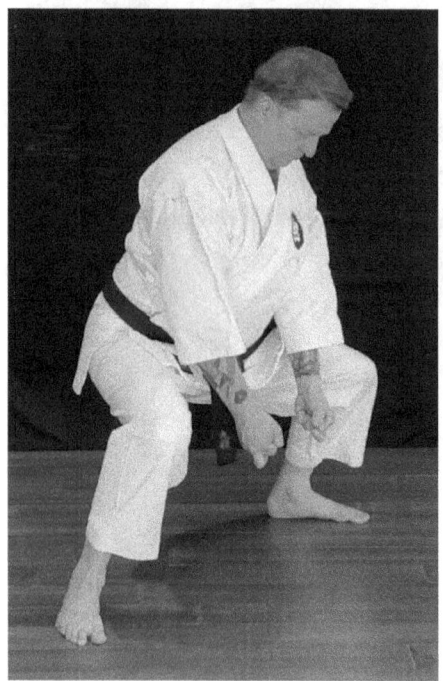

Complete Morote Nakadakaken Uchi Downward

Sepai

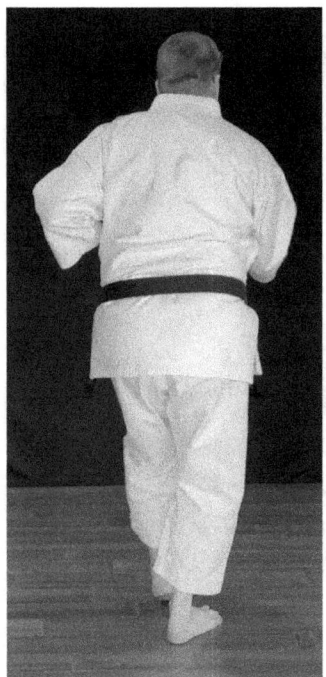

Step Back with Left Foot

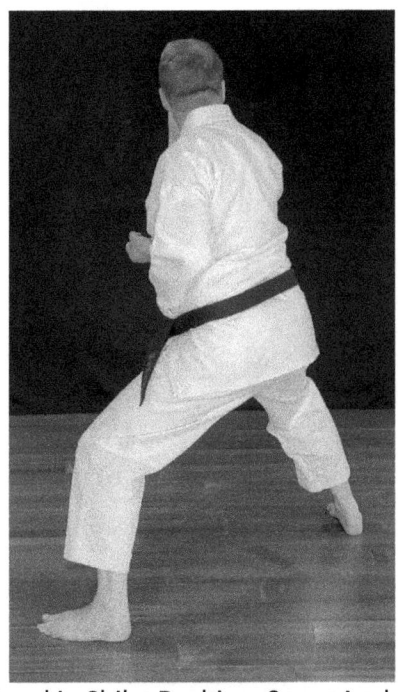

Land in Shiko Dachi on Same Angle, Begin Right Gedan Yoko Tettsui Uchi

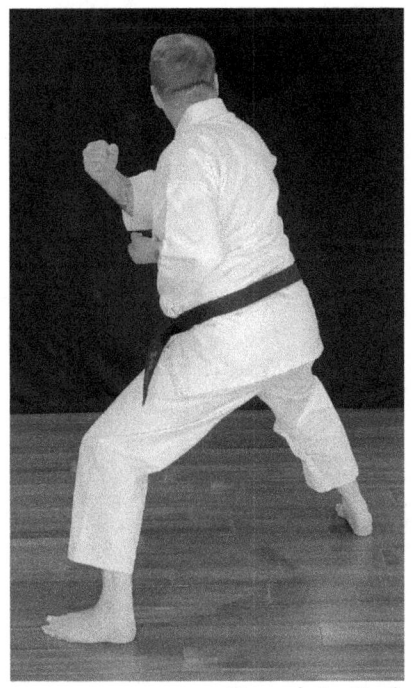

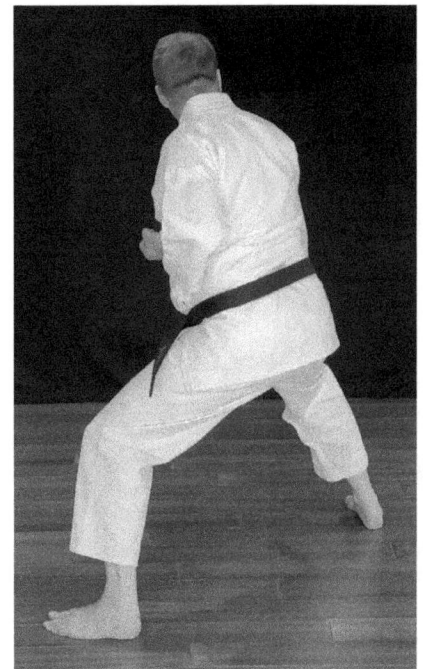

Complete Gedan Yoko Tettsui Uchi (cont.)

Sepai

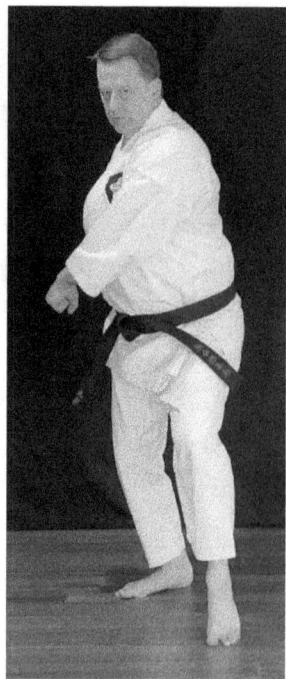

Right Foot Step Over Right Facing Forward, Drag Left Foot into Neko Ashi Dachi, Put Both Fists Across the Right Side of the Body

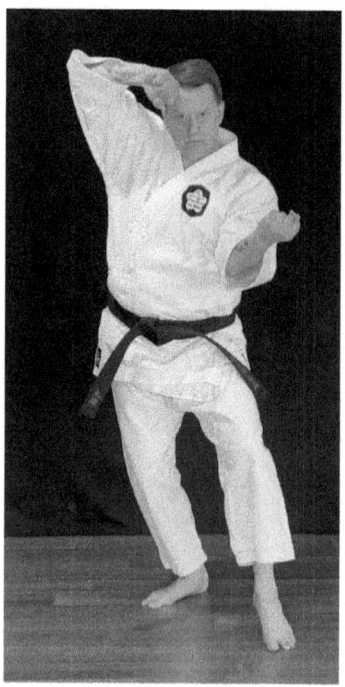

Complete Left Chudan Uke and Right Jodan Furi Zuki Simultaneously

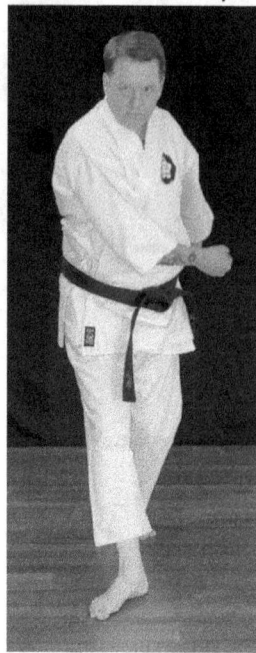

Right Step Up, Put Both Fists Across the Left Side of the Body

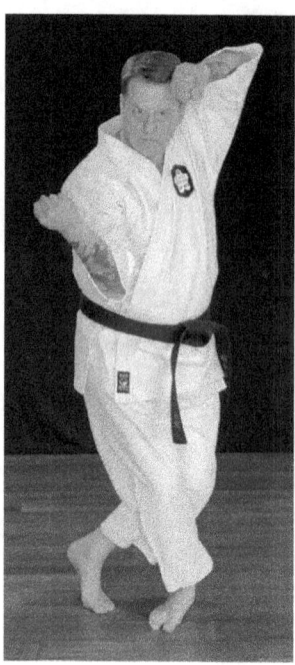

Left Foot Crosses Behind Right Foot, Complete Right Chudan Uke and Left Jodan Furi Zuki Simultaneously

Sepai

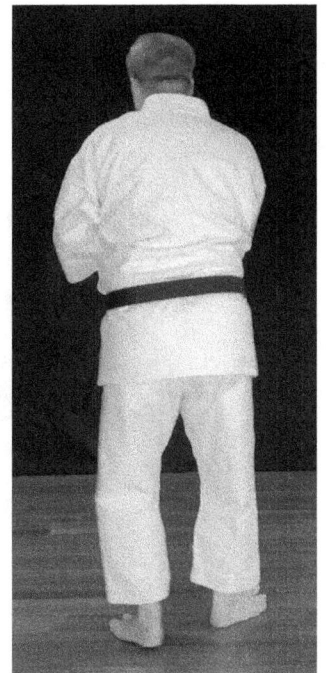
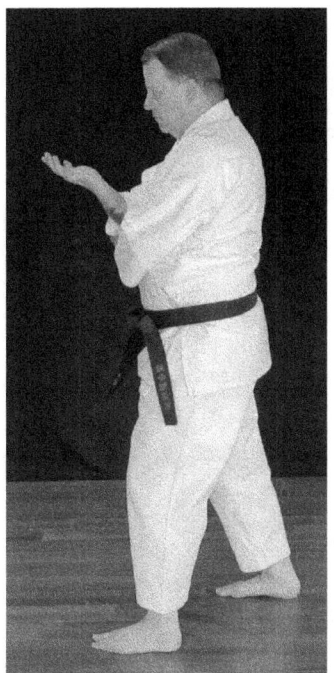

Pivot on Both Feet to 270° Angle, Begin Left Hari to Hiki Uke

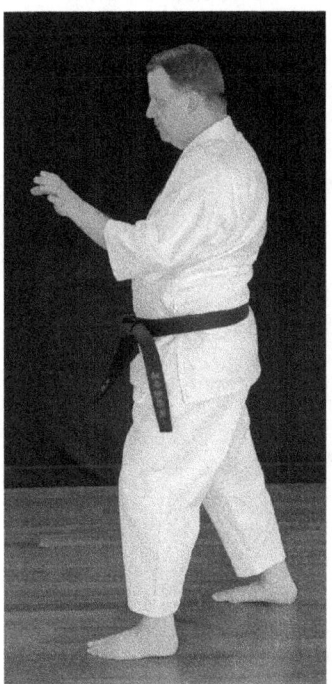
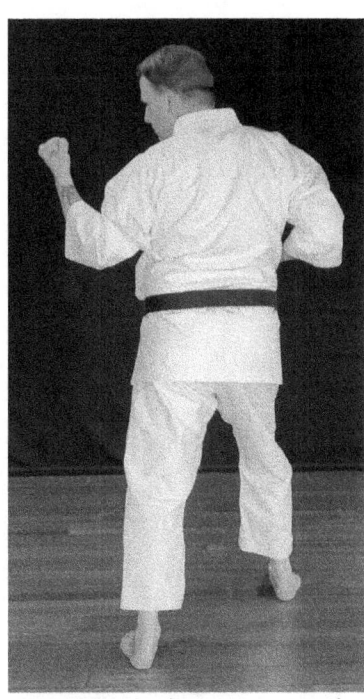

Complete Left Hari to Hiki Uke

Pivot Right (Towards Rear), Begin Left Gedan Furi Uchi

Sepai

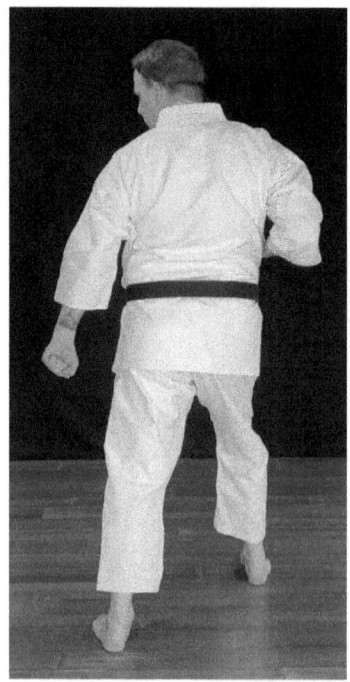

Complete Left Gedan Furi Uchi

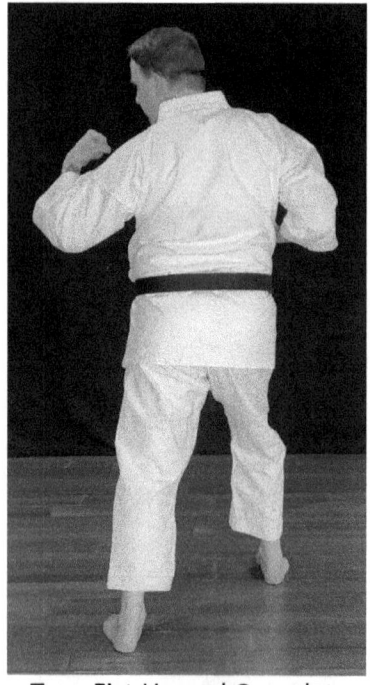

Turn Fist Up and Complete Left Uraken Uchi

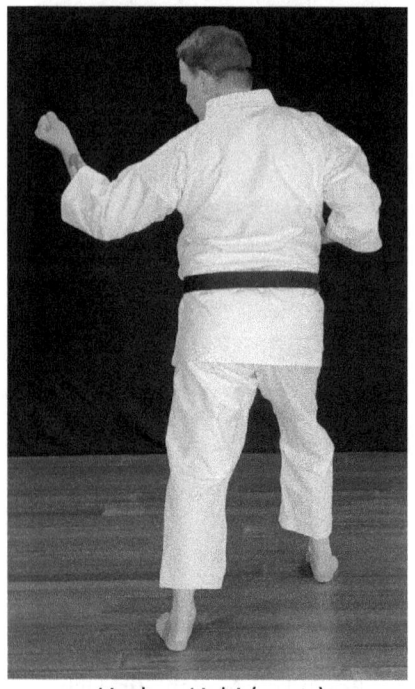

Uraken Uchi (cont.)

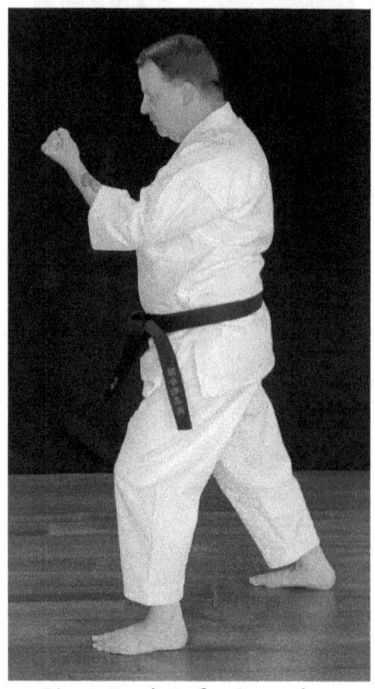

Pivot Back Left, Complete Right Chudan Uke

Sepai

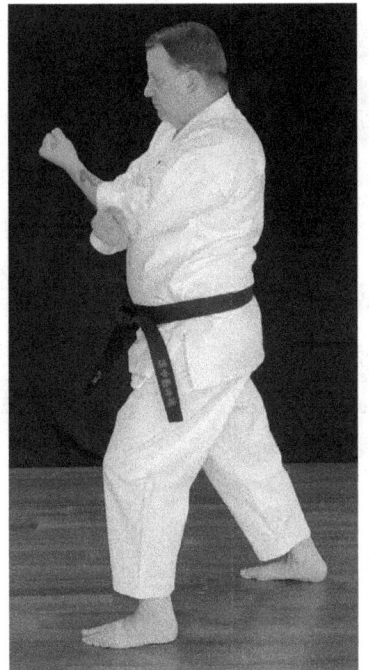
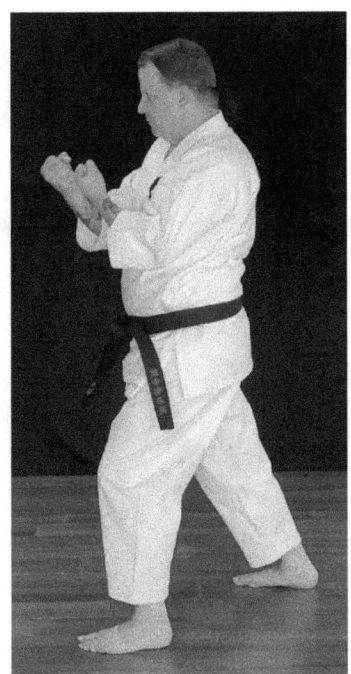

Right Chudan Uke (cont.)

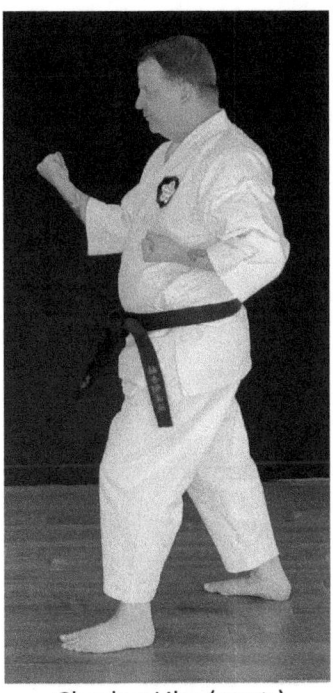
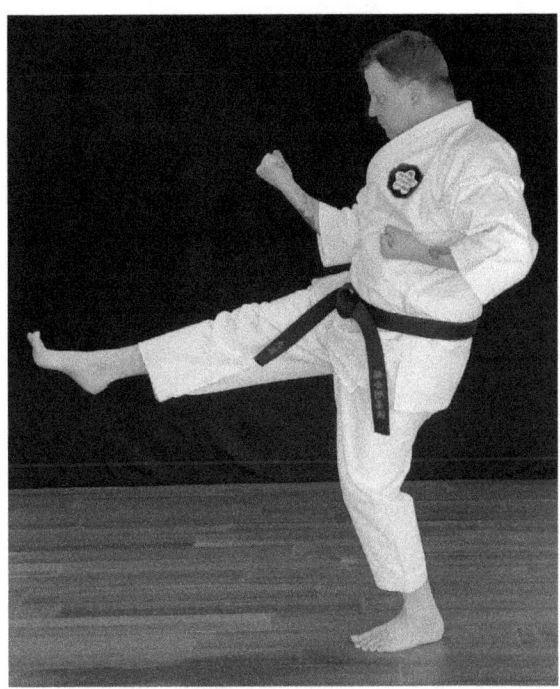

Chudan Uke (cont.) Complete Right Gedan Mae Keage Geri

Sepai

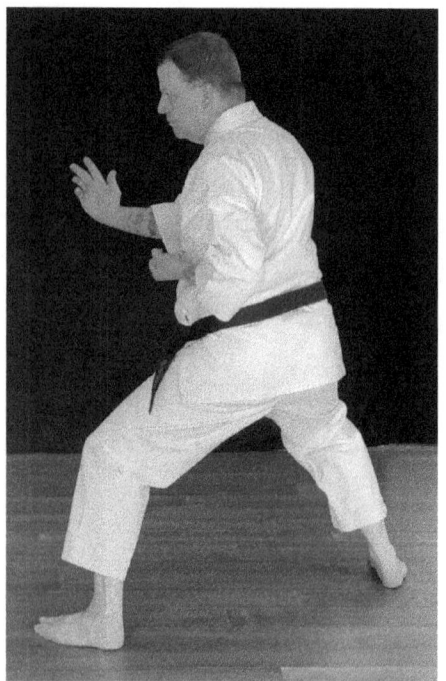
Land in Shiko Dachi on 225° Angle

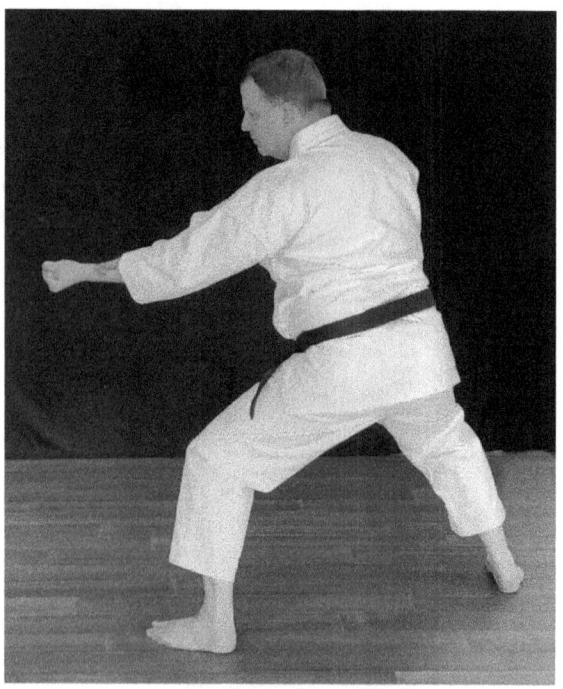
Complete Left Ura Zuki

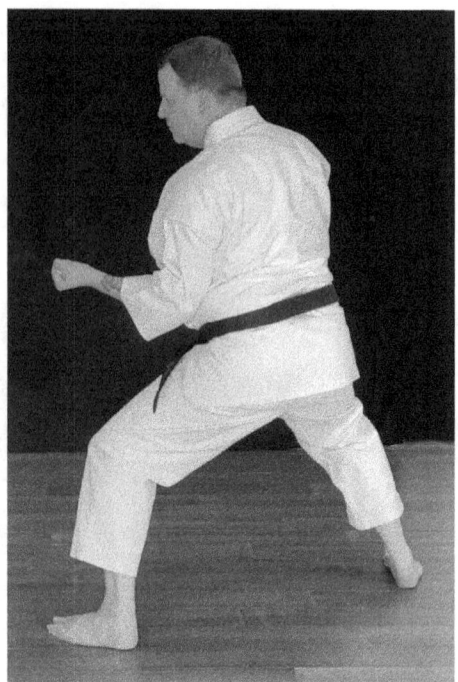
Left Ura Zuki (cont.)

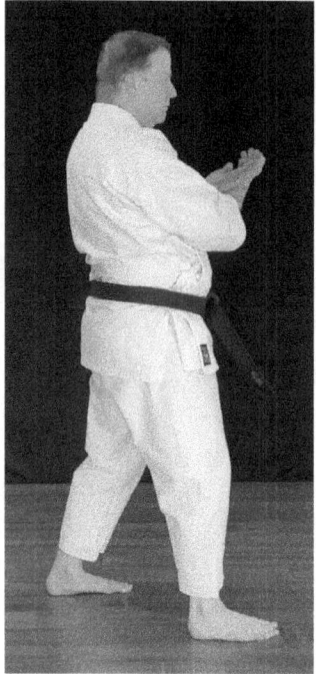
Pivot to 90° Angle and Complete
Right Chudan Hari to Hiki Uke

Sepai

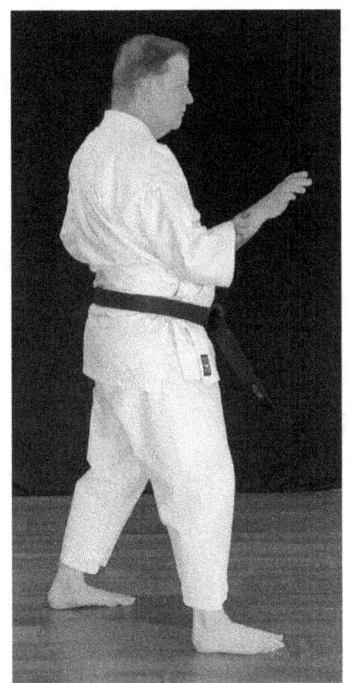

Chudan Hari to Hiki Uke (cont.)

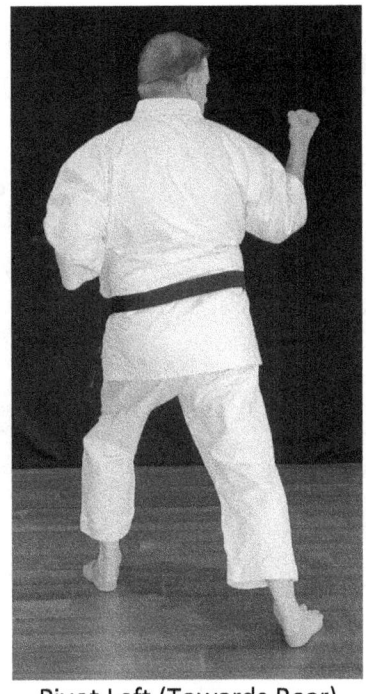

Pivot Left (Towards Rear), Begin Right Gedan Furi Uchi

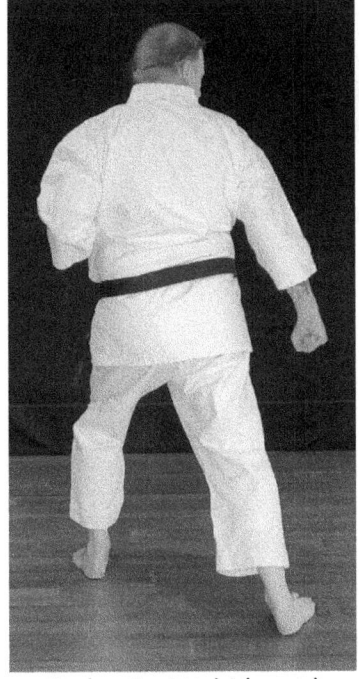

Gedan Furi Uchi (cont.)

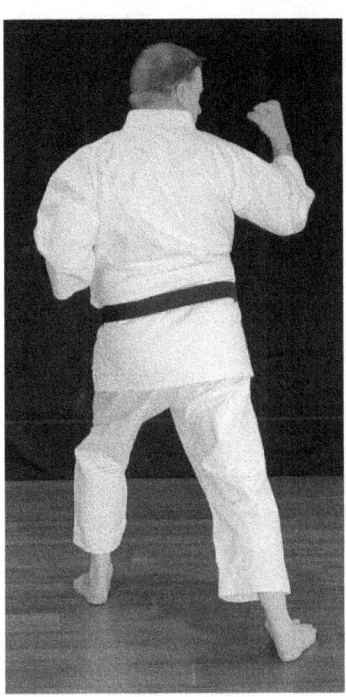

Turn Fist Up and Complete Right Uraken Uchi

Sepai

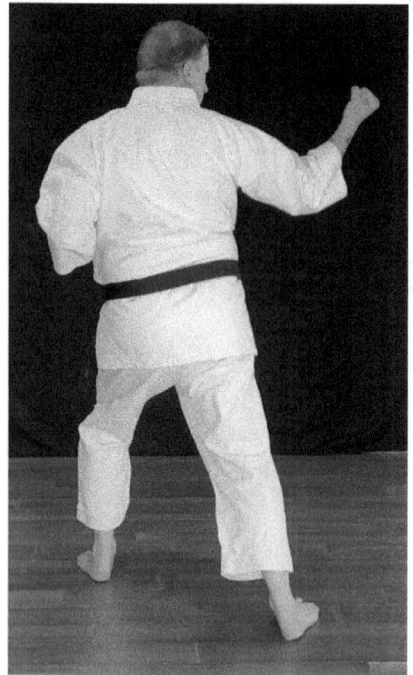
Uraken Uchi (cont.)

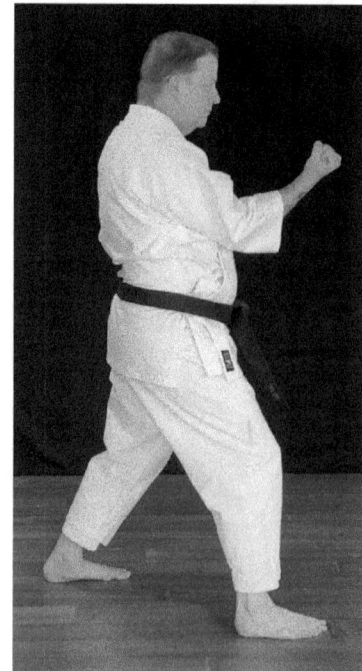
Pivot Back Right

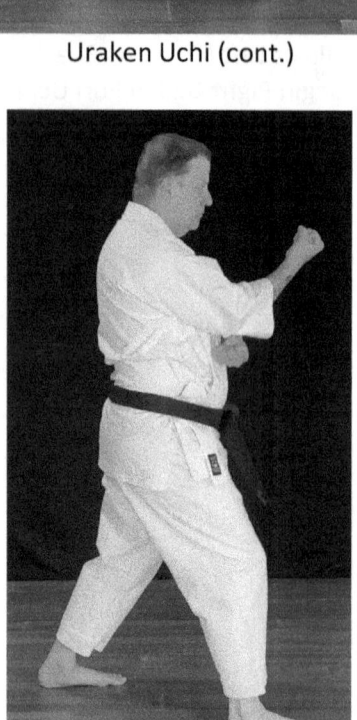

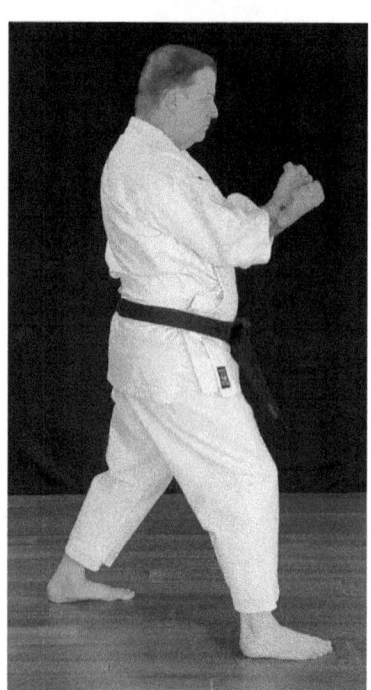
Complete Left Chudan Uke

Sepai

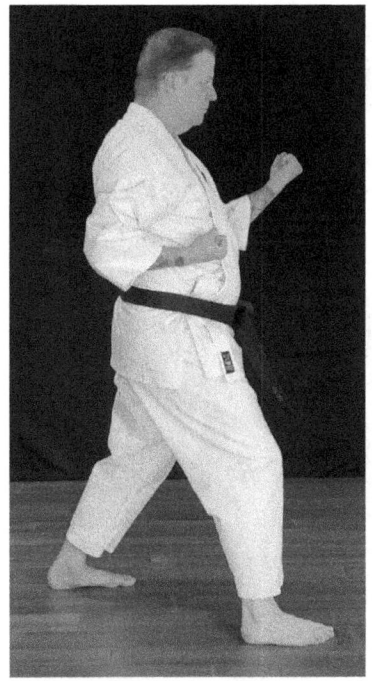
Chudan Uke (cont.)

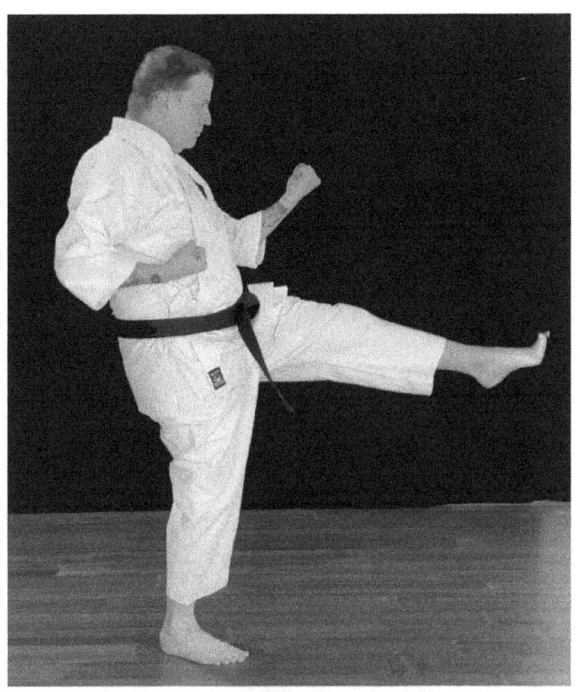
Complete Left Gedan Mae Keage Geri

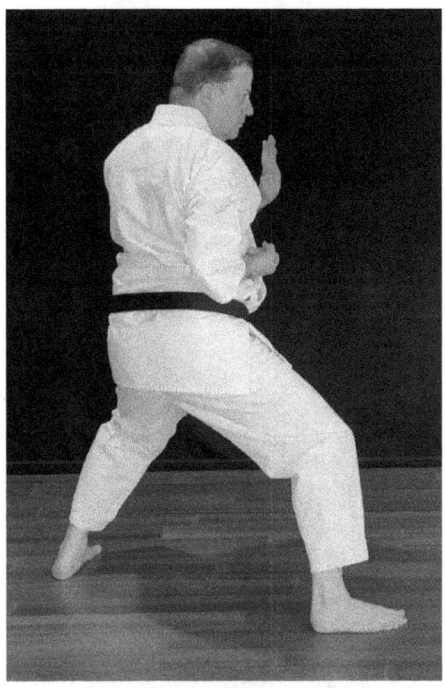
Land in Shiko Dachi on 135° Angle

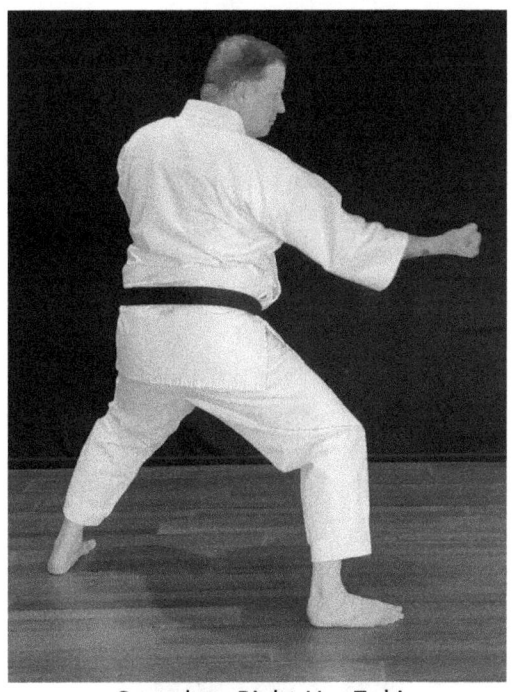
Complete Right Ura Zuki

Sepai

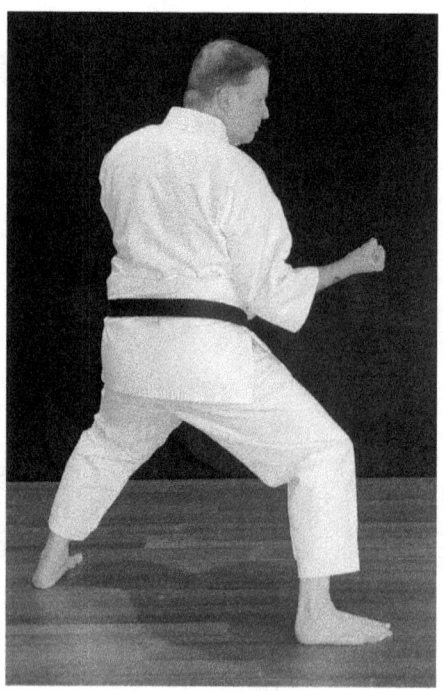

Ura Zuki (cont.)

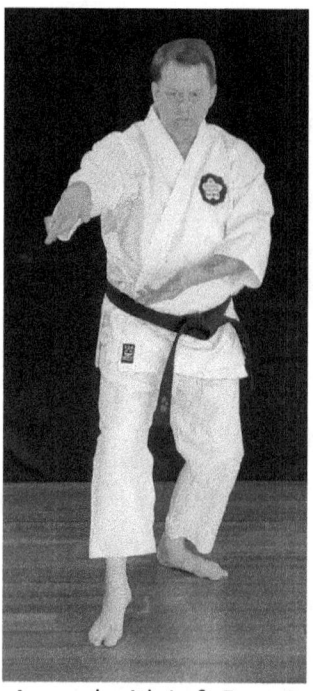

Step Around with Left Foot Facing Forward, Drag Right Foot into Neko Ashi Dachi, Move Hands into Tenchi no Kamae

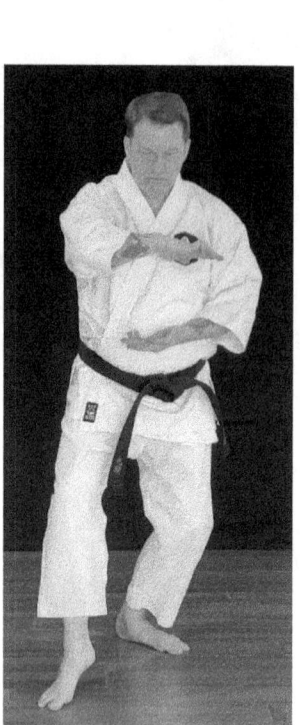

Tenchi no Kamae

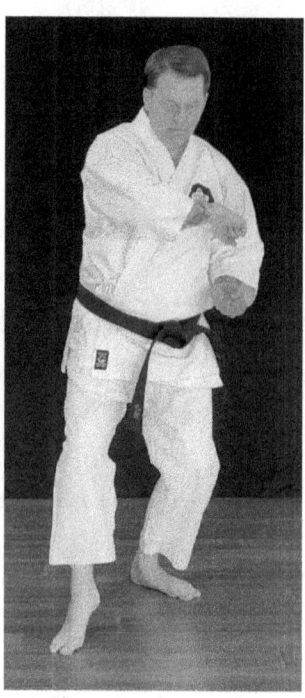

Close Both Hands, Begin Circling Fists

Sepai

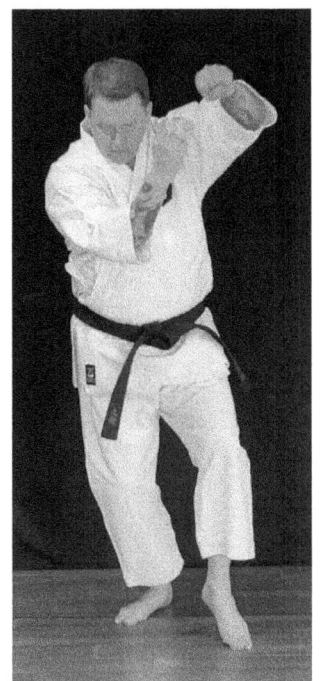 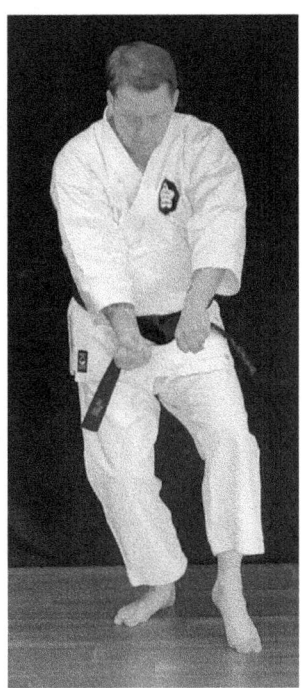

Step Back, Turn Fists Around and Down

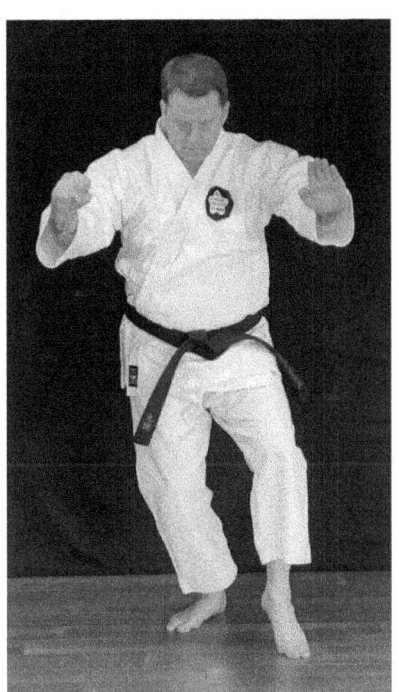 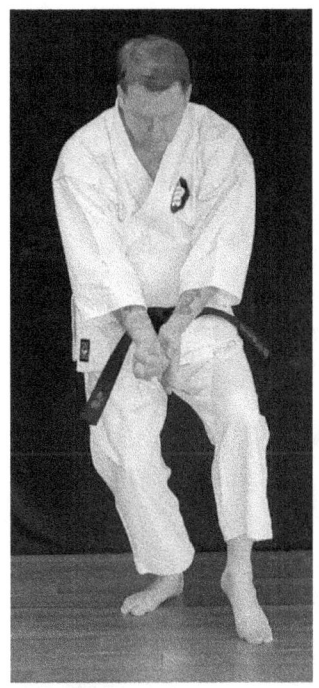

With an Arc Motion, Complete Tettsui Uchi with
Right Hand into Open Left Hand

Sepai

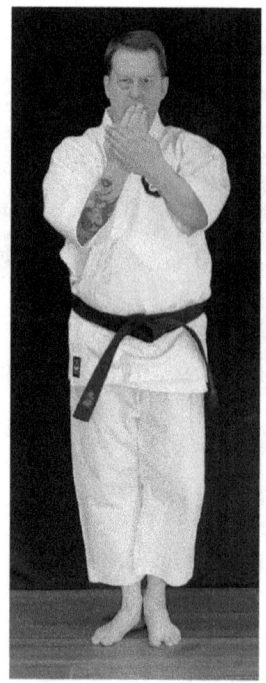

Bring Left Foot Back, Guard Throat

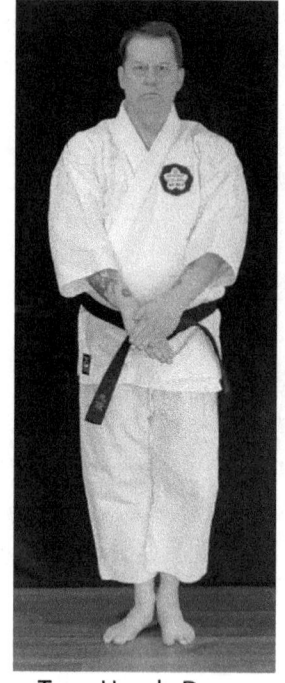

Turn Hands Down to Guard Groin

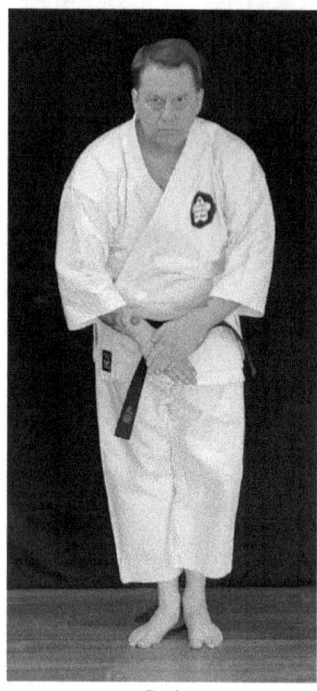

Rei

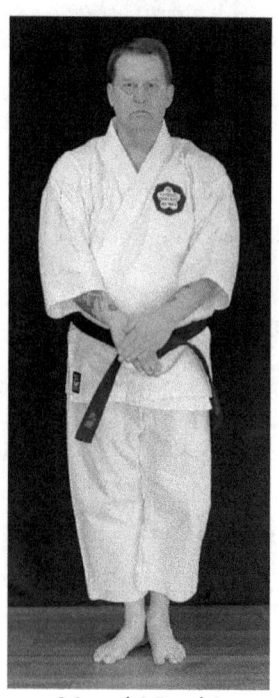

Musubi Dachi

Sepai

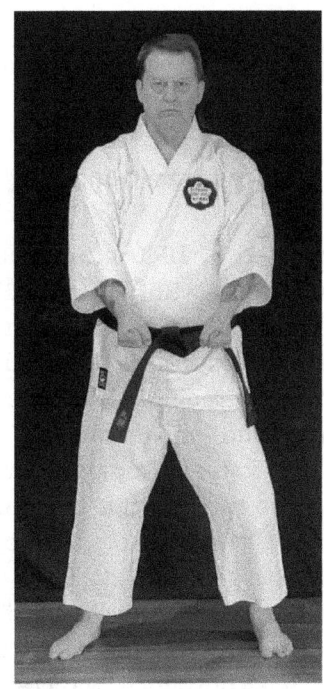

Heiko Dachi

Ketsugo Goju-Ryu Katas
When does non-traditional become traditional?

Gekisai Dai Ichi was created in 1940 by Chojun Miyagi but is considered a traditional kata. Shodai started training with Toguchi in 1955, only fifteen years later. There is no doubt that Gekisai Ichi, Gekisai Ni, and Tensho are considered traditional because they are katas that were not part of Nana-Te, but the newly created Goju-Ryu, founded by Chojun Miyagi. They are traditional katas to Goju-Ryu. As for traditional, I do not think there are "traditional" and "non-traditional" katas. It is accurate to say that Goju-Ryu Karate simply has twelve katas. If someone trains in Goju-Ryu Karate in any form, he will eventually learn those twelve katas. The Ketsugo Goju-Ryu variation has an additional sixteen. If a student trains in Ketsugo Goju-Ryu Karate and learns the entire system, he will learn twenty-eight katas in all.

When Shodai was in Okinawa, he learned all the katas Seikichi Toguchi was teaching during the late 1950's. This included the twelve traditional Goju-Ryu katas and many supplementary katas that Seikichi Toguchi was creating at the time. When Shodai came back to America and began to promote Goju-Ryu Karate-Do, he found that the traditional katas on their own did not attract enough students, at least not in the way he needed to grow the system. Even just attracting students to the "mystical art of the Orient" was a chore. In 1950's Okinawa, students were satisfied with tradition. In America it was not so easy. Even in the late 1960's, martial arts tournaments were the way to get noticed. Katas in tournaments were flashy and acrobatic. Shodai needed to adapt to the American way if he was going to attract American students.

First, he made slight changes to the low rank traditional katas (Gekisai Ichi and Gekisai Ni), then he started making up his own katas to include things he wanted to see in katas. It was not an easy task, but he was determined to make up katas he felt had a traditional base but could be competitive as well. He would create nine open hand katas and six weapons katas. There are currently ten open hand Ketsugo Goju-Ryu katas and in this chapter, we will explore five of them.

Kihon Ichi

Kihon Ichi means "basic one." Kihon Ichi is the first kata in the KGJKA system. The kata follows the standard plus sign (+) embusen (pattern,) uses all closed hands, and only contains two low kicks to the groin. It also includes the turning step from Sanchin. Kihon Ichi is the first kata learned in the Ketsugo Goju-Ryu Karate system.

Below is the method by which Ketsugo Goju-Ryu performs Kihon Ichi kata. Complete details about each move are not included, as this is simply a demonstration.

These are the Japanese terms used for this kata. Bear in mind, karate terms are not completely streamlined. There are terms that were used in the middle of the 20th Century that are no longer used today. Oftentimes there are more than one term that can be used for the same technique. The important thing is not what it is called, but the technique itself.

Barai - Sweeping Block	**Mae Keage Geri** – Front Snap Kick
Chudan - Middle	**Musubi Dachi** - Attention Stance, Toes Out
Dachi – Stance	
Gedan – Low	**Rei** – Bow (Respect)
Gyaku Zuki - Reverse Punch	**Shiko Dachi** - Straddle Leg Stance
Hajime – Command to Begin	**Tsuki/-Zuki** - Punch
Heiko Dachi - Parallel Stance	**Uchi** – Strike
Jodan - High	**Uke** – Block (Receive)
	Yoi – Ready Command

Kihon Ichi

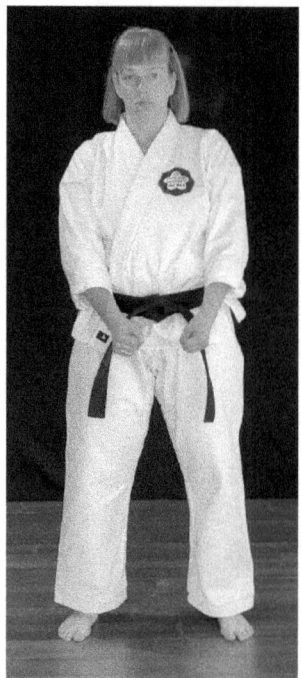

Heiko Dachi

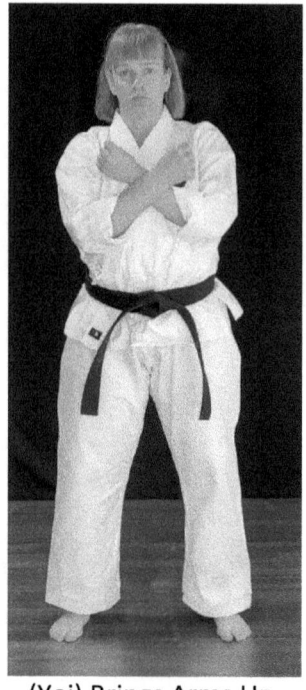

(Yoi) Brings Arms Up, Crossed at the Wrist

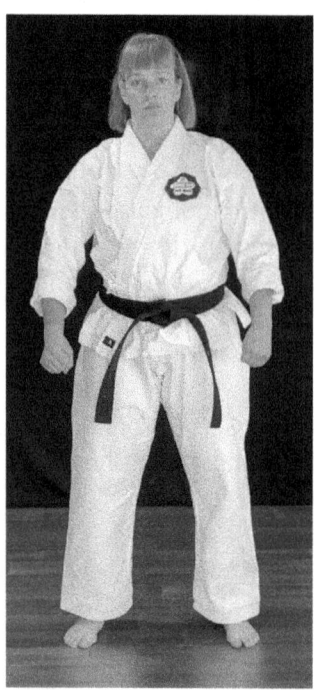

Bring Arms Down

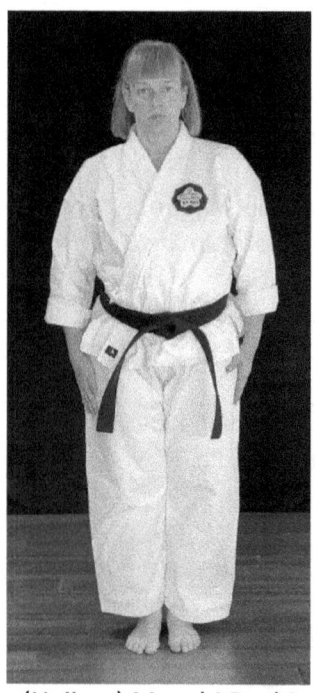

(Hajime) Musubi Dachi

Kihon Ichi

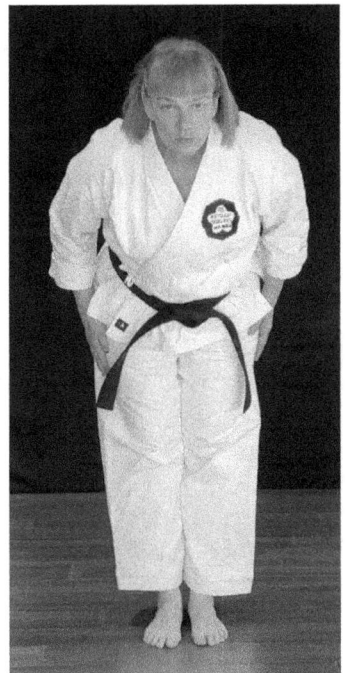
Rei

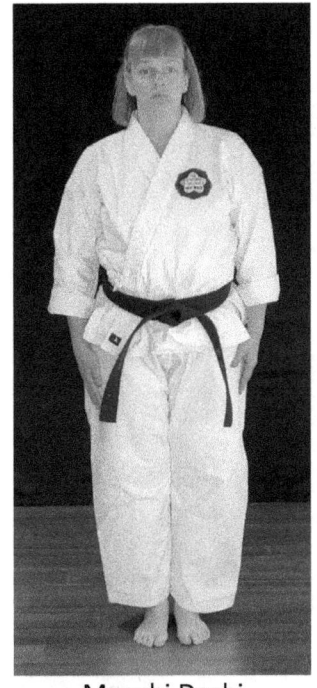
Musubi Dachi

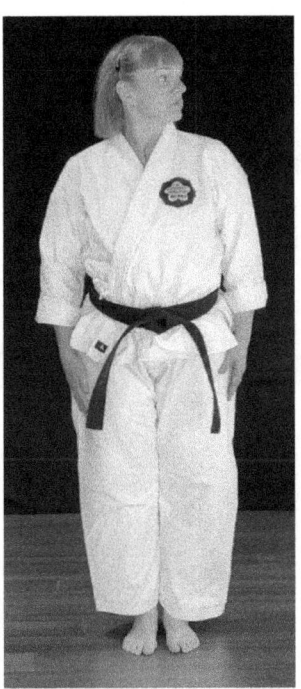
Look Left

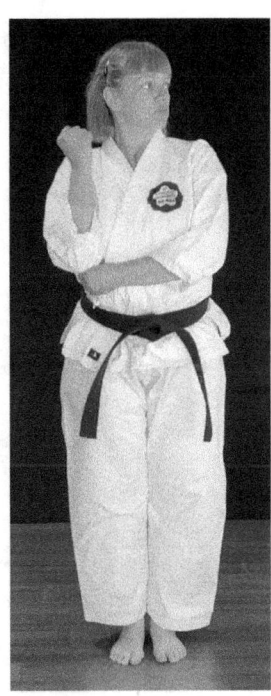
Chamber Left Fist Under Right Elbow

Kihon Ichi

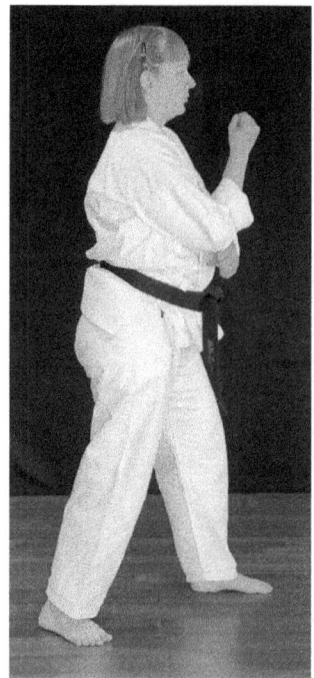
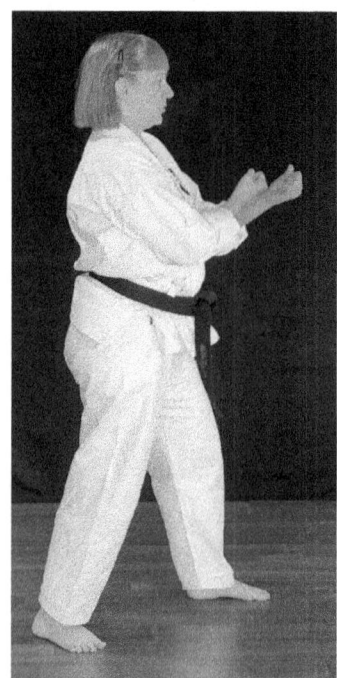

Pivot Left, Complete Left Chudan Uke

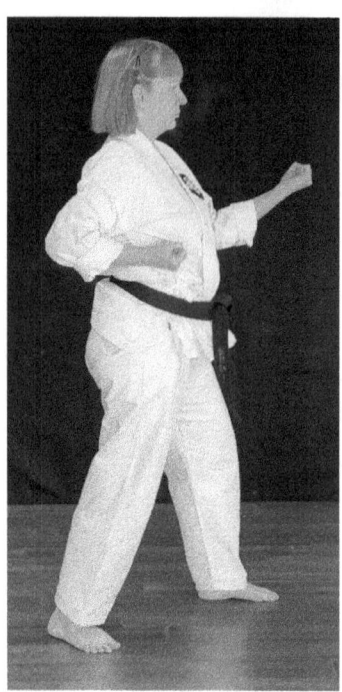
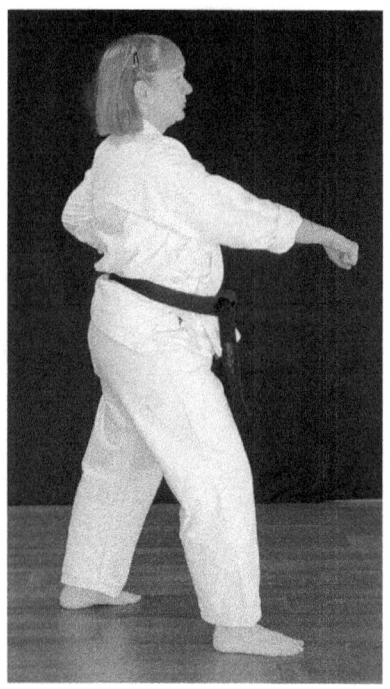

Chudan Uke (cont.)

Step, Complete Right Chudan Zuki

Kihon Ichi

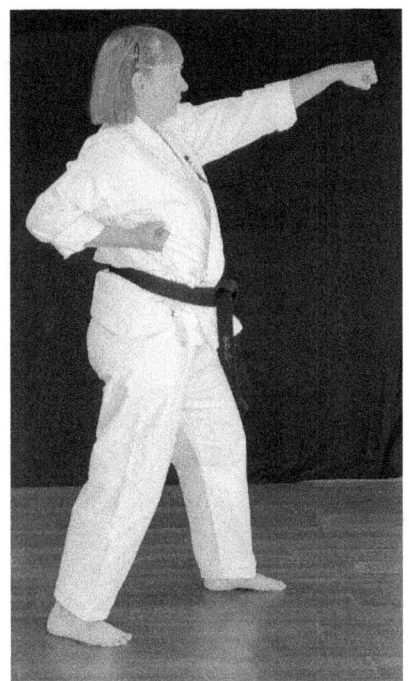

Step, Complete Left
Jodan Zuki

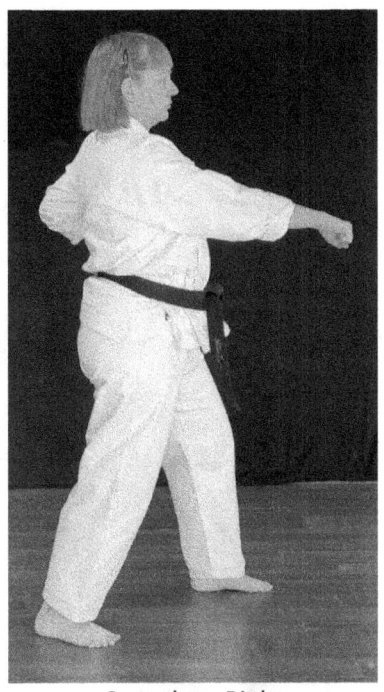

Complete Right
Chudan Zuki

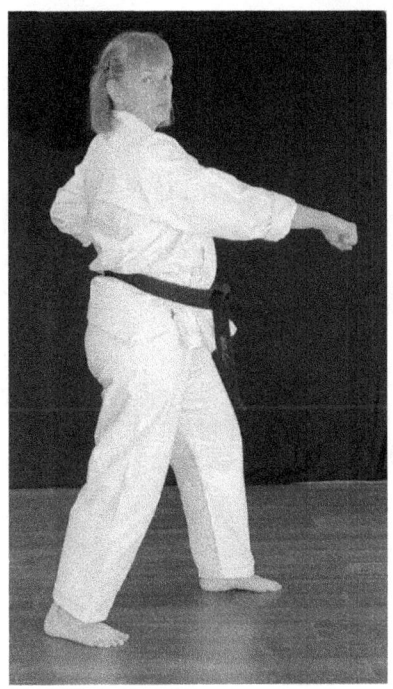

Look Right (Front)

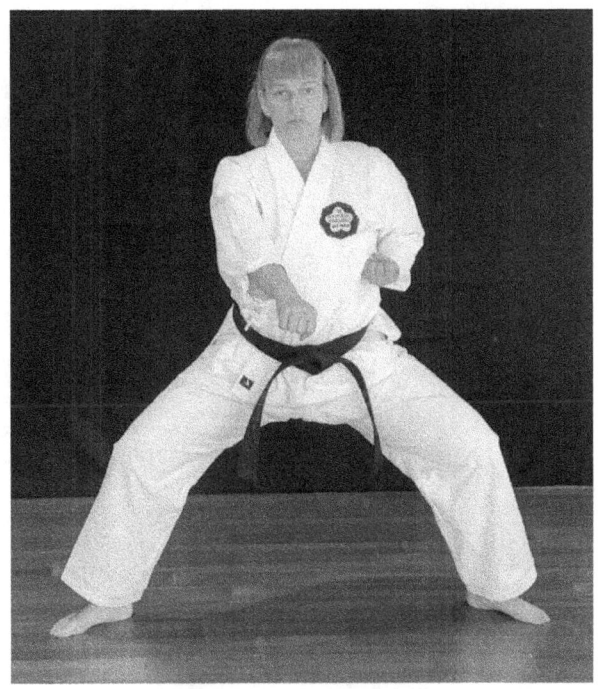

Left Foot Step Back into
Shiko Dachi Facing Forward

Kihon Ichi

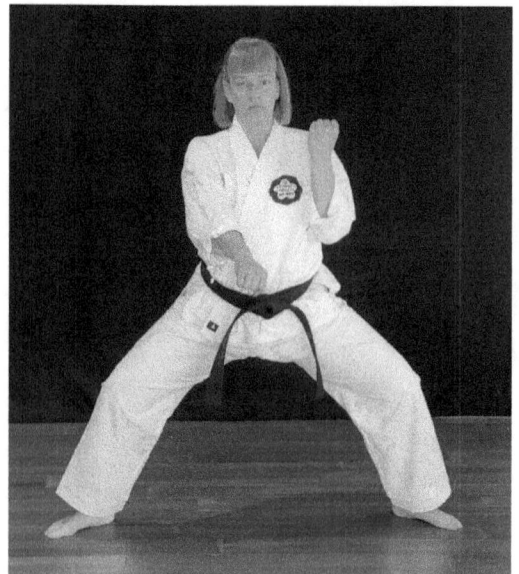
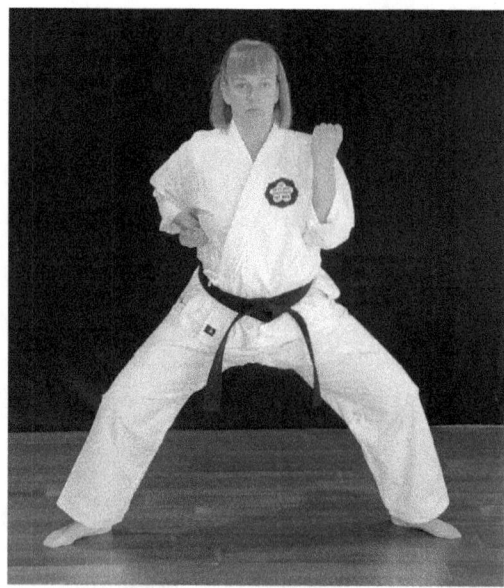

Complete Left Gedan Barai

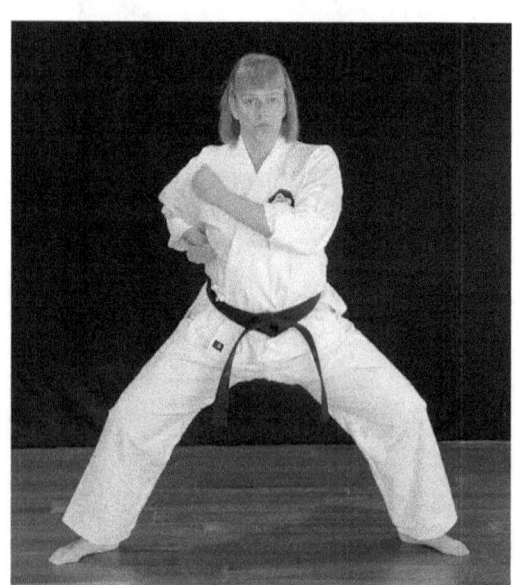
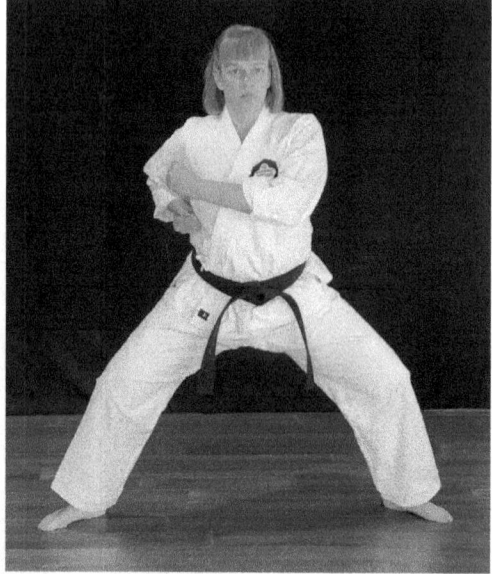

Gedan Barai (cont.)

Kihon Ichi

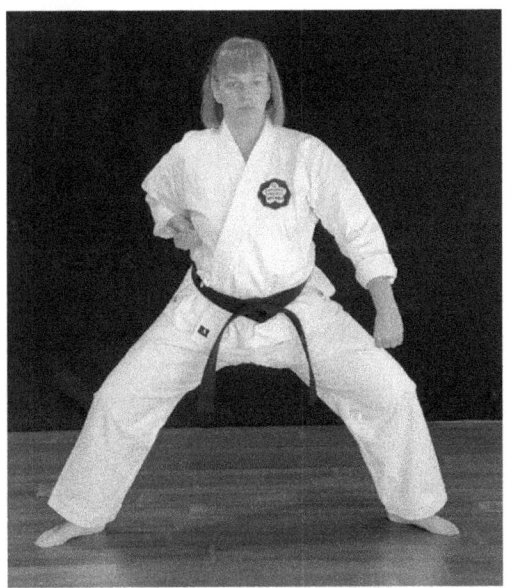
Gedan Barai (cont.)

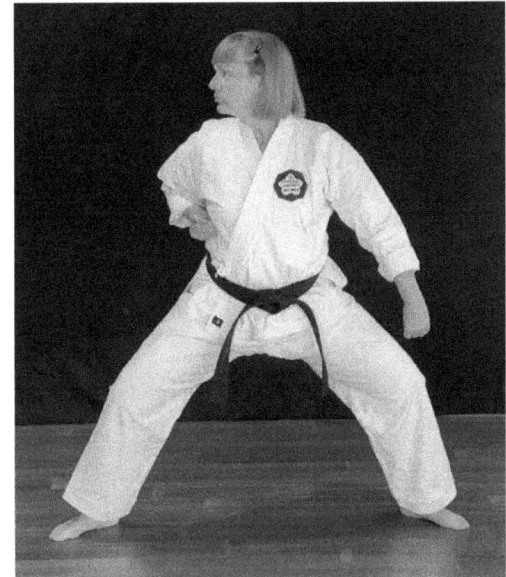
Right

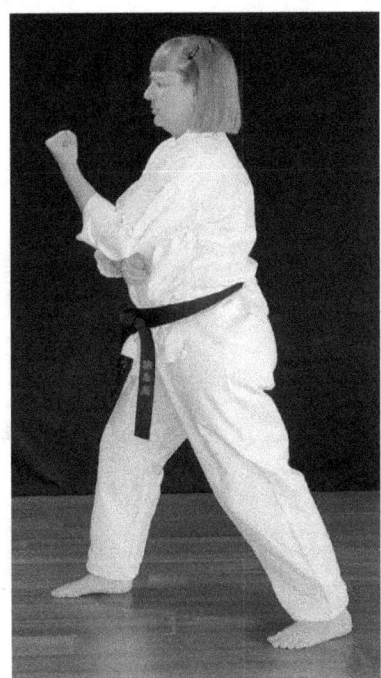
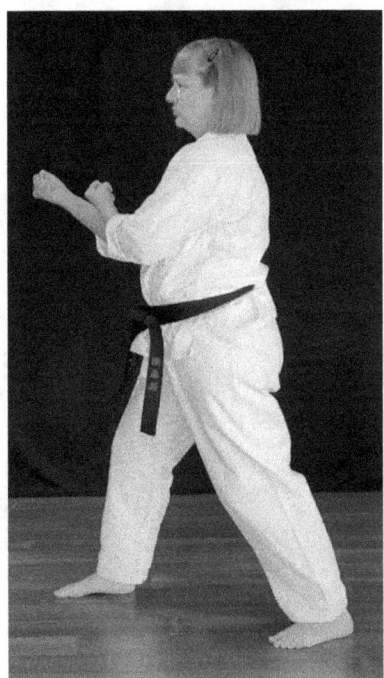
Pivot Right, Complete Right Chudan Uke

Kihon Ichi

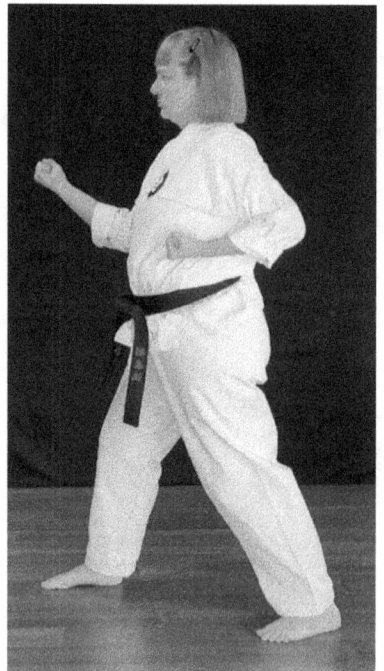

Chudan Uke (cont.)

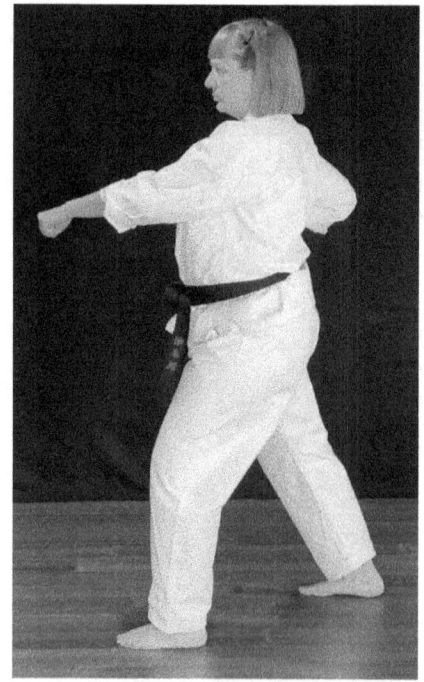

Step, Complete Left Chudan Zuki

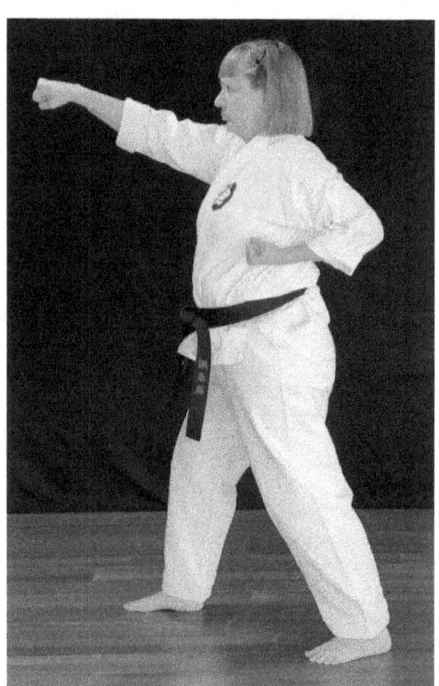

Step, Complete Right Jodan Zuki

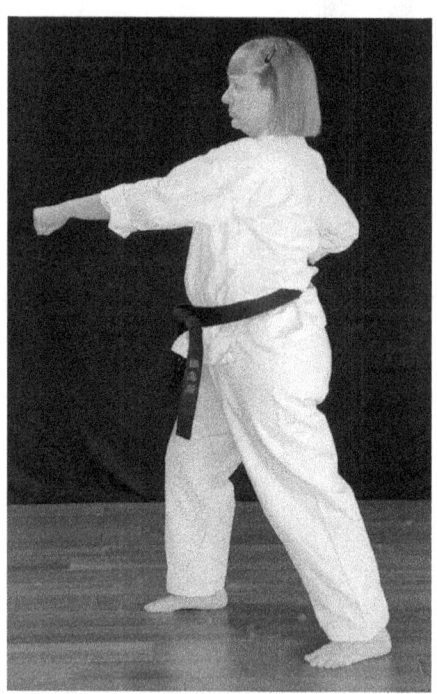

Complete Left Chudan Zuki

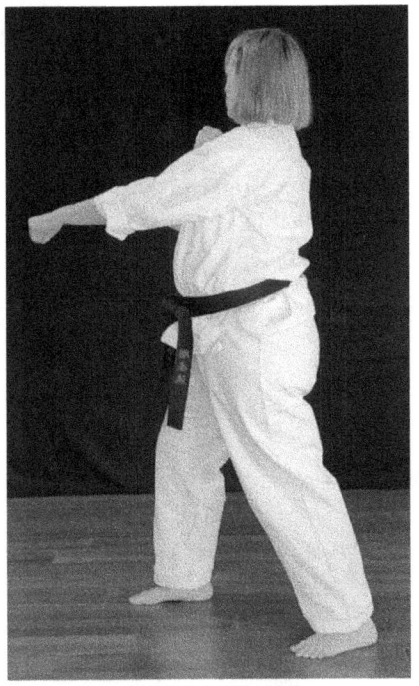

Look Right, Chamber
Right Hand on Top of Left Arm

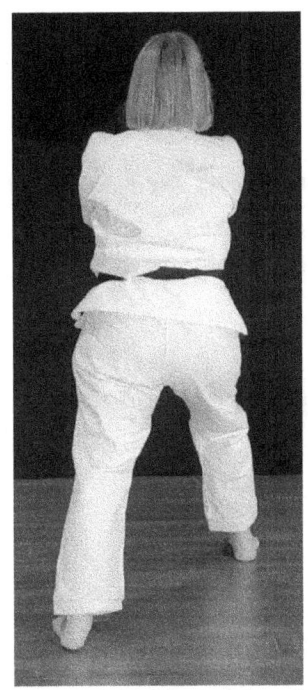

Pivot Right (Facing Rear)

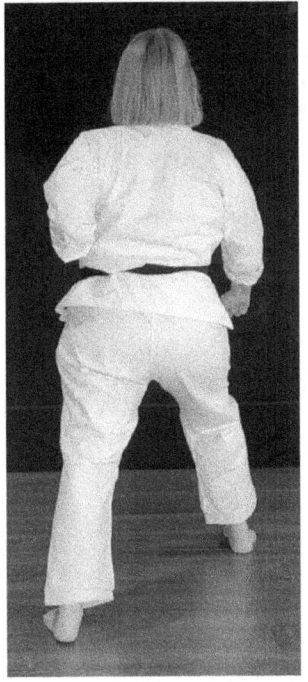

Complete Right Gedan Uke

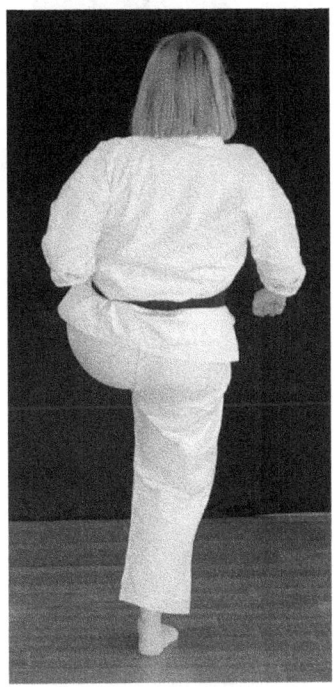

Complete Gedan Mae
Keage Geri (kiai)

Kihon Ichi

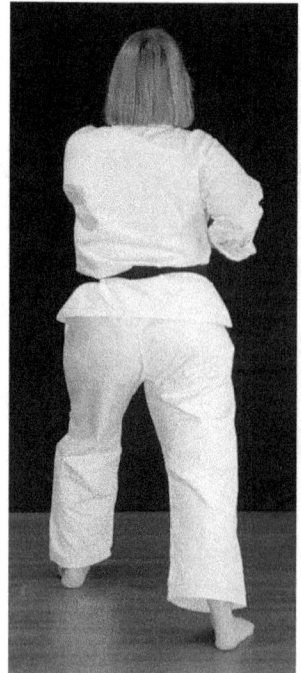
Complete Left Chudan Zuki

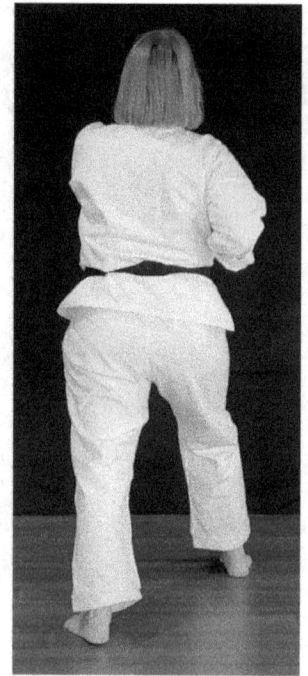
Step

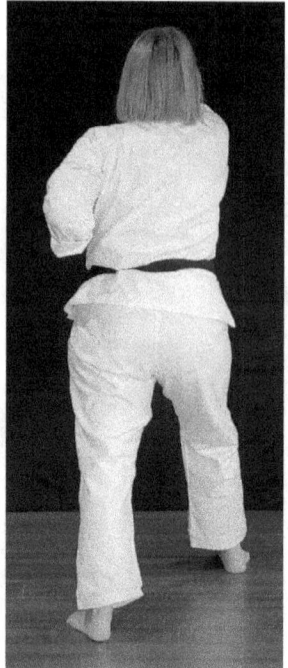
Complete Three Punches in Succession: Jodan Zuki

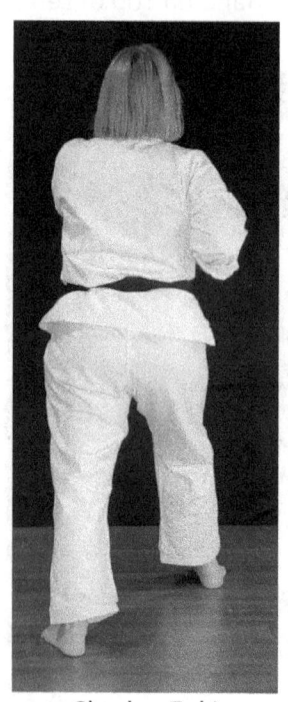
Chudan Zuki

Kihon Ichi

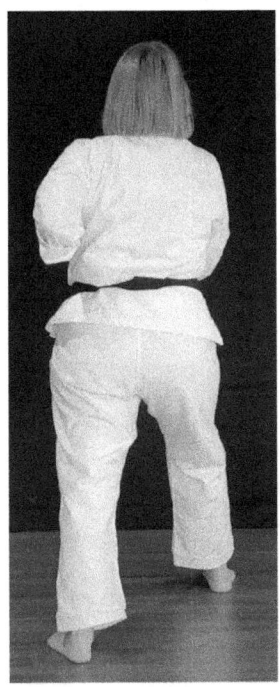
Gedan Zuki

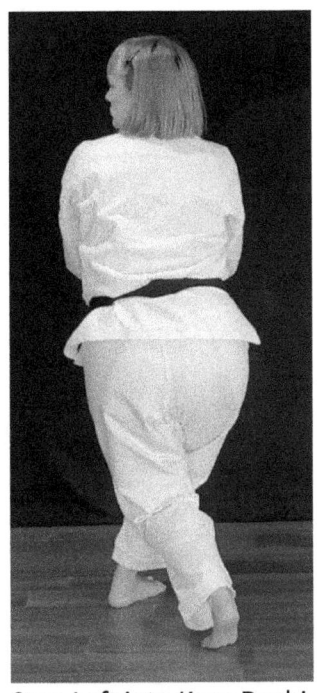
Step Left into Kosa Dachi,
Chamber Left Hand
Under Right Elbow

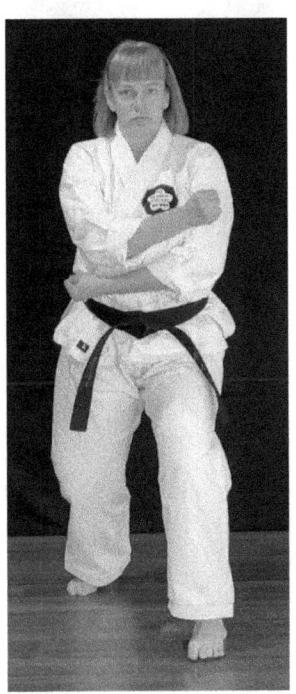

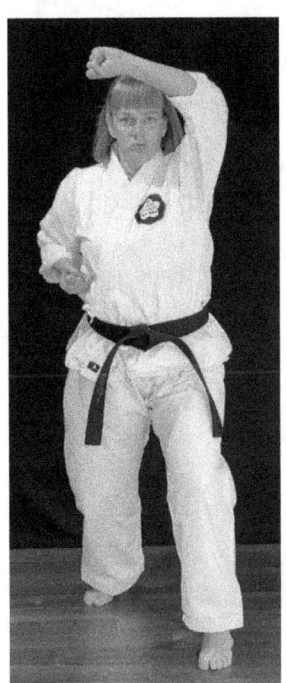

Pivot to Forward Facing, Complete Jodan Age Uke

Kihon Ichi

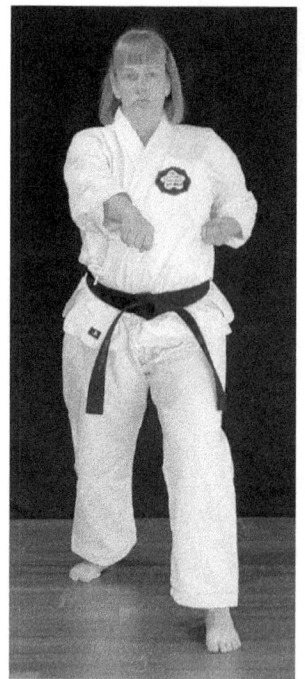

Complete Chudan Gyaku Zuki

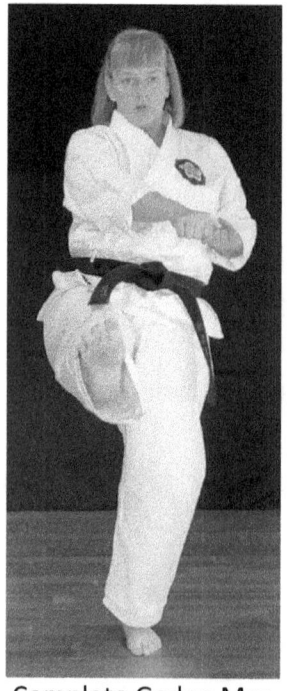

Complete Gedan Mae Keage Geri (kiai)

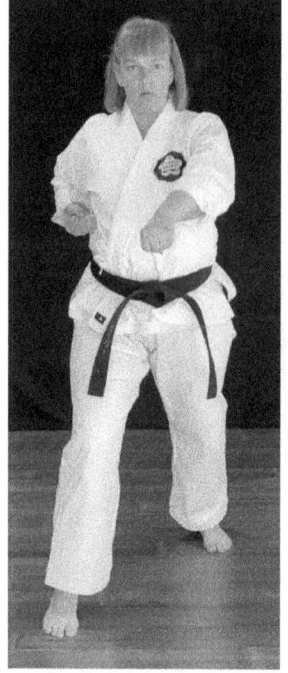

Complete Chudan Gyaku Zuki

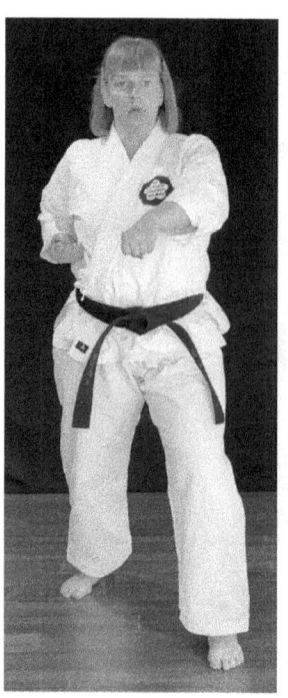

Step

Kihon Ichi

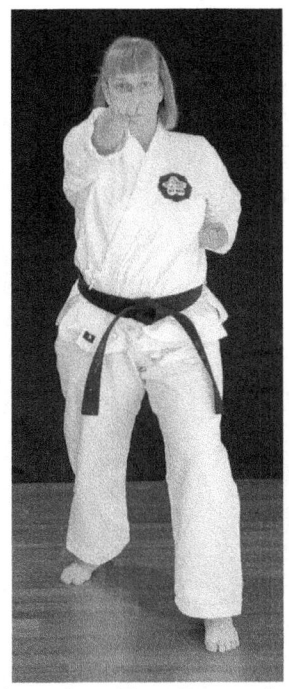
Complete Two Successive Punches: Jodan Zuki

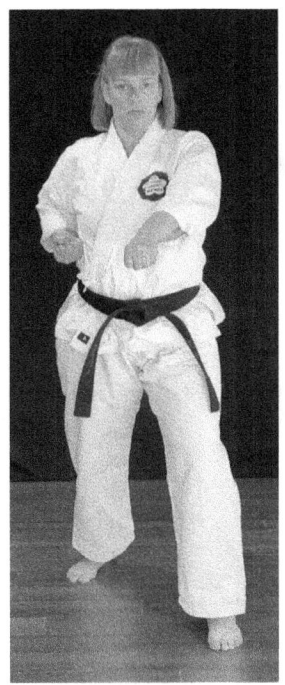
Chudan Zuki

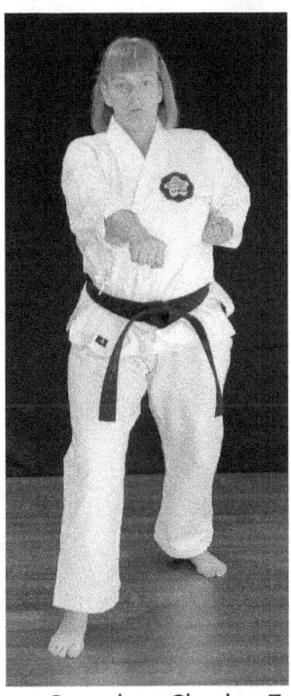
Step, Complete Chudan Zuki

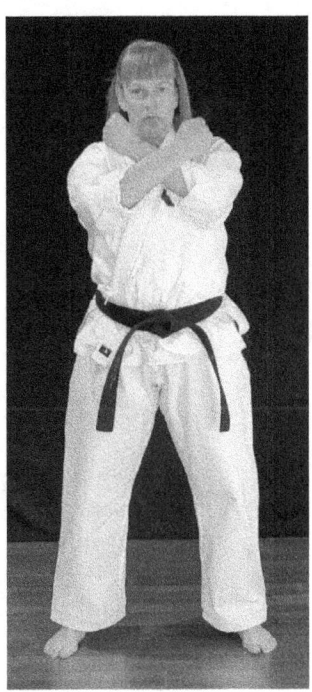
Step Back into Heiko Dachi while Completing Juji Uke

Kihon Ichi

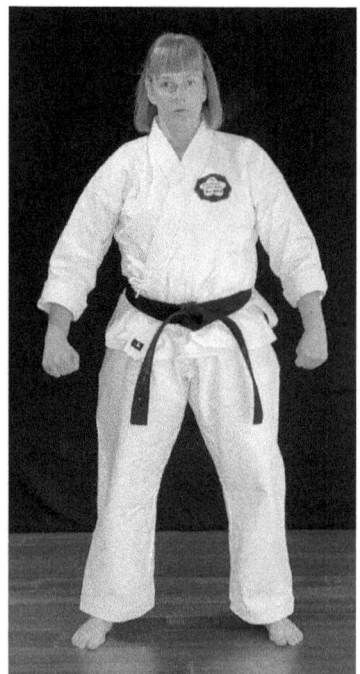
Bring Arms Down

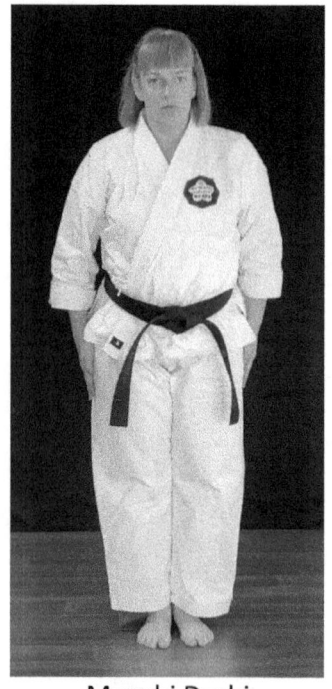
Musubi Dachi

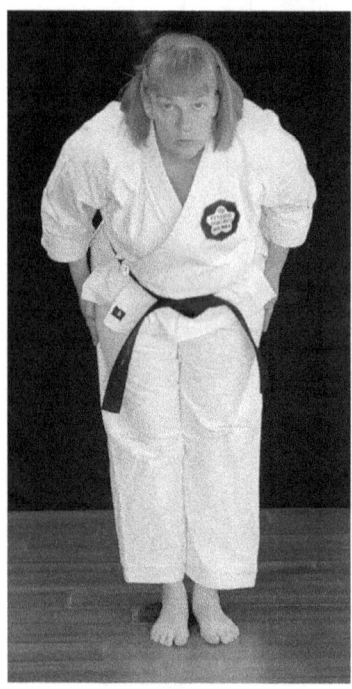
Rei

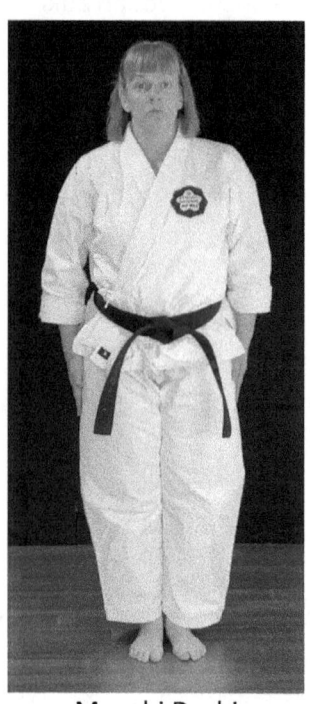
Musubi Dachi

Kihon Ichi

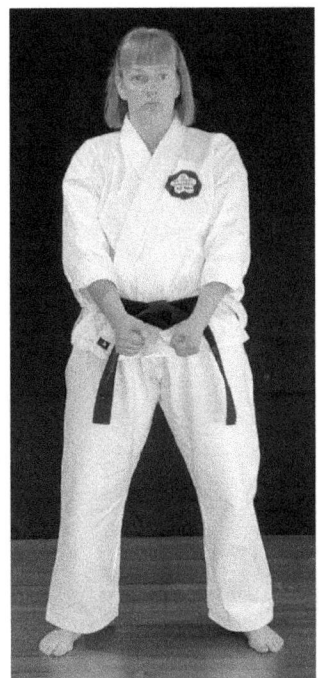

Heiko Dachi

Gekisai San

Gekisai San means "attack and smash three." The fact is, Shodai never learned Seikichi Toguchi's version of Gekisai San, which was not yet designed when Shodai left Okinawa in 1960, so he created his own version as the final kata in the Gekisai series. It adds neko ashi dachi and ippon ken strikes, open hand chest blocks and open hand elbow strikes. It also contains elements from Toguchi's Gekiha Ni kata, which he did learn, but did not include in the Ketsugo Goju-Ryu system.

Below is the method by which Ketsugo Goju-Ryu performs Gekisai San kata. Complete details about each move are not included, as this is simply a demonstration. It should be emphasized that is Ketsugo Goju-Ryu's version of Gekisai San, not the Shoreikan version.

These are the Japanese terms used for this kata. Bear in mind, karate terms are not completely streamlined. There are terms that were used in the middle of the 20th Century that are no longer used today. Oftentimes there are more than one term that can be used for the same technique. The important thing is not what it is called, but the technique itself.

Gekisai San

Age - Rising	**Musubi Dachi** - Attention Stance, Toes Out
Barai - Sweeping Block	
Chudan - Middle	**Neko Ashi Dachi** - Cat Leg Stance
Dachi – Stance	**Nihon Nukite** – Two Finger Spear Hand
Empi - Elbow	
Gedan – Low	**Oshi** - Push
Gyaku Zuki - Reverse Punch	**Otoshi** - Dropping (Downward)
Hajime – Command to Begin	**Rei** – Bow (Respect)
Hari Uke – Open Hand Block (Palm Up)	**Shiko Dachi** - Straddle Leg Stance
Heiko Dachi - Parallel Stance	**Shotei** - Palm Heel
Hiki Uke – Open Hand Block (Palm Down)/Pulling Block	**Tettsui Uchi** – Hammer Fist Strike
	Tora Guchi – Wheel Block
Hiza Geri – Knee Joint Kick	**Tsukami Hiki** – Grab and Pull
Ippon Ken – Single Knuckle Fist	**Tsuki/-Zuki** - Punch
Jodan – High	**Uchi** – Strike
Kake Uke - Hook Block	**Uke** – Block (Receive)
Ko Uke - Back of Wrist Block	**Ura Zuki** – Inverted Strike
Mae Keage Geri – Front Snap Kick	**Uraken Uchi** - Back Fist Strike
Morote Chudan Uke – Double Chest Block	**Yoi** – Ready Command
	Zenkutsu Dachi - Forward Leaning Stance

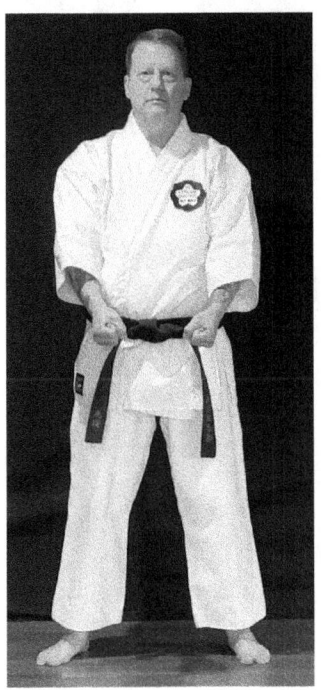

Heiko Dachi

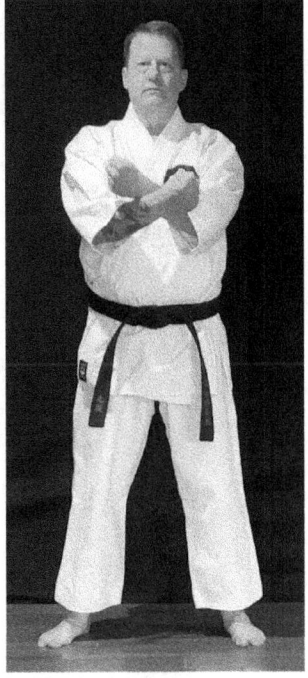

(Yoi) Brings Arms Up, Crossed at the Wrist

Gekisai San

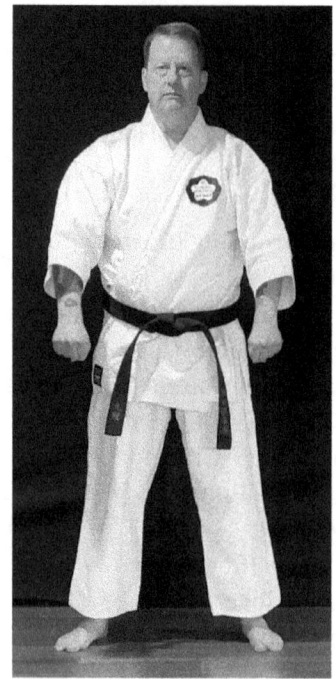
Bring Arms Down

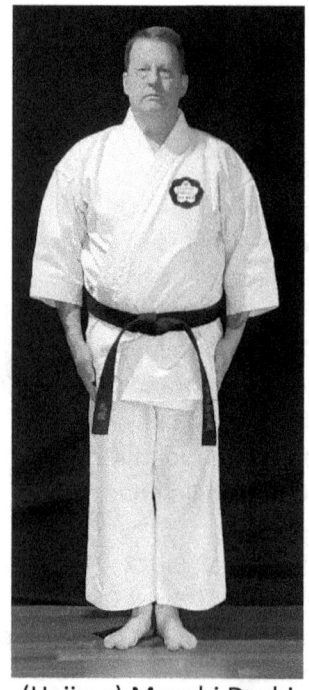
(Hajime) Musubi Dachi

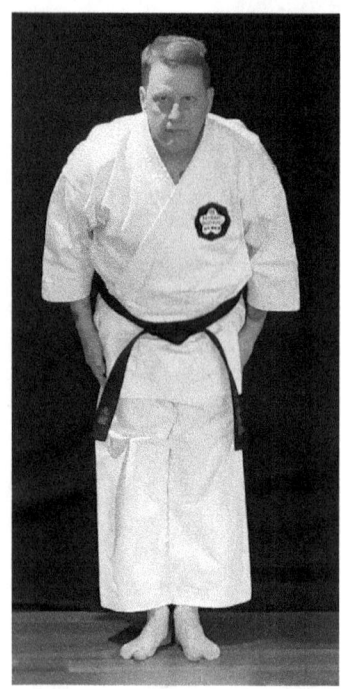
Rei

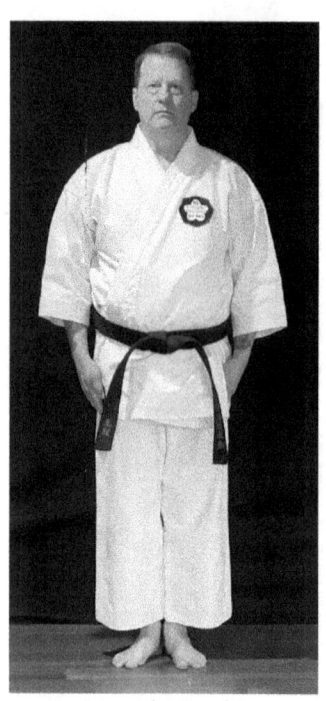
Musubi Dachi

Gekisai San

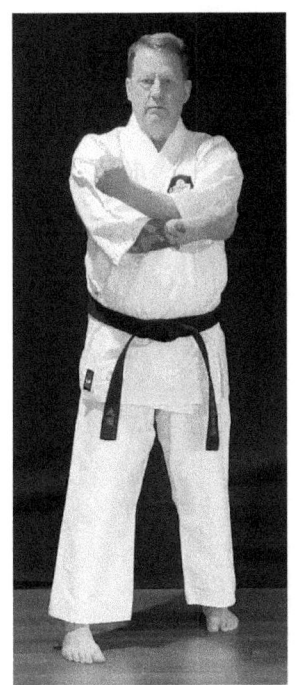 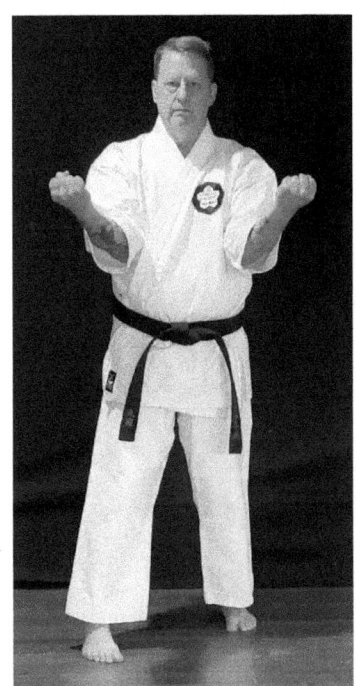

Step while Completing Morote Chudan Uke

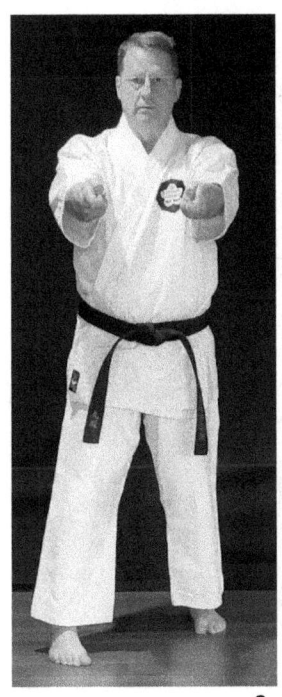 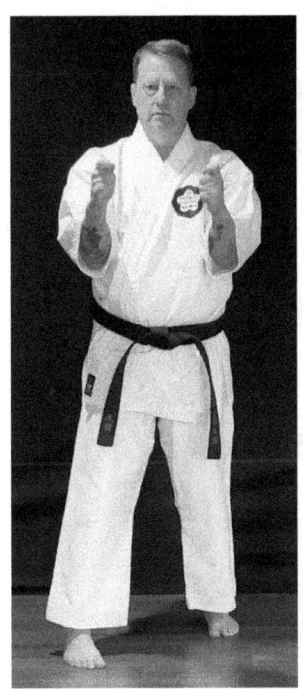

Set with Morote Ippon Ken

Gekisai San

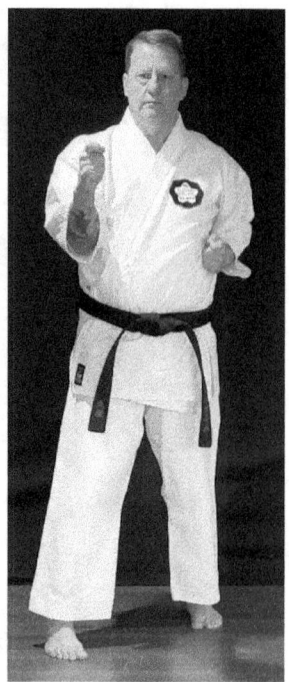
Chamber Left Hand

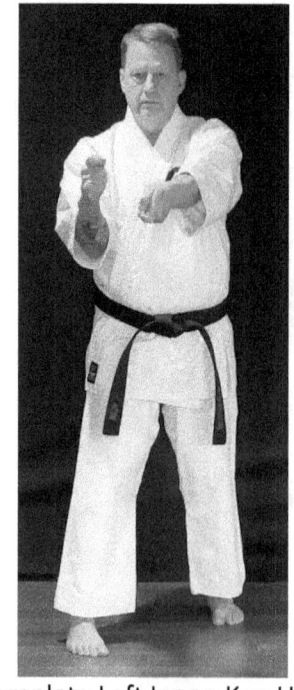
Complete Left Ippon Ken Uchi

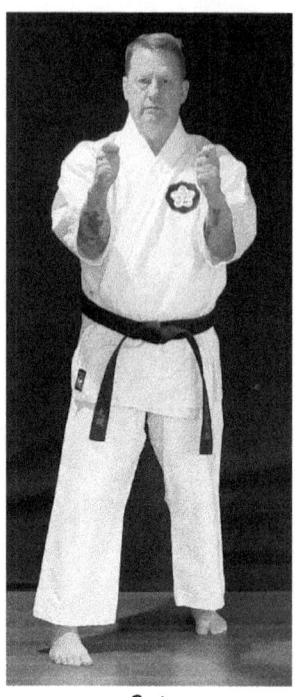
Set

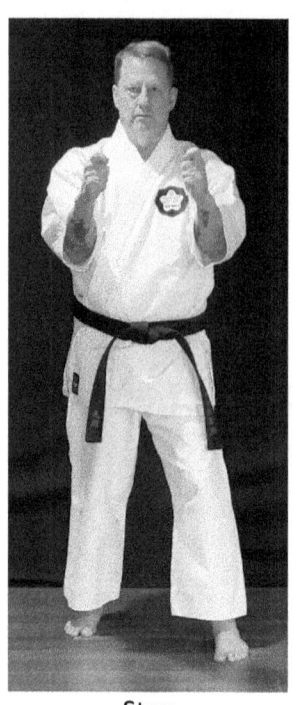
Step

Gekisai San

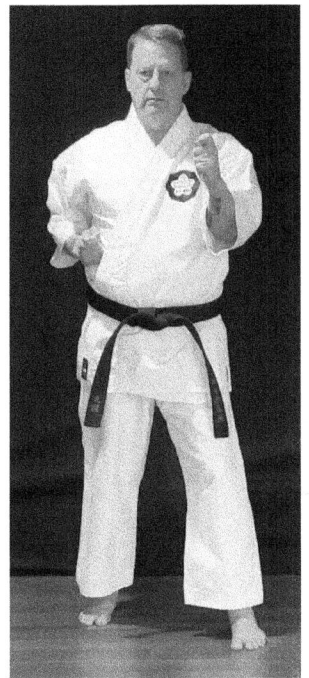
Chamber Right Hand

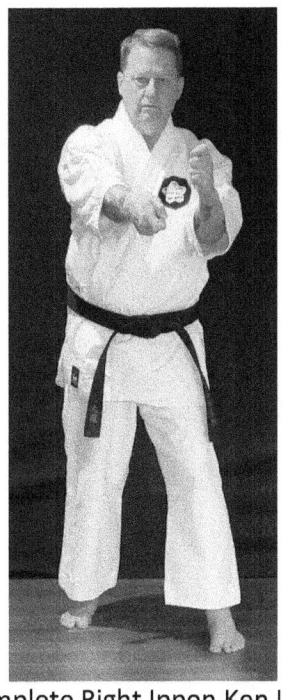
Complete Right Ippon Ken Uchi

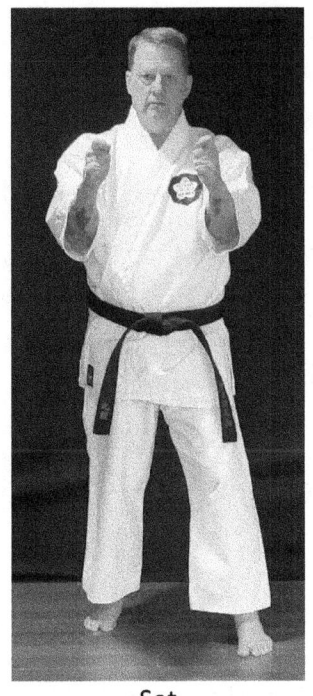
Set

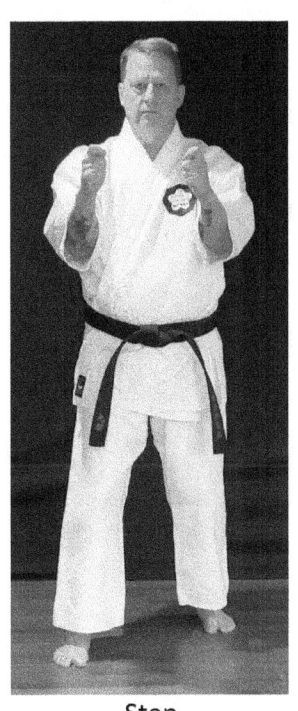
Step

Gekisai San

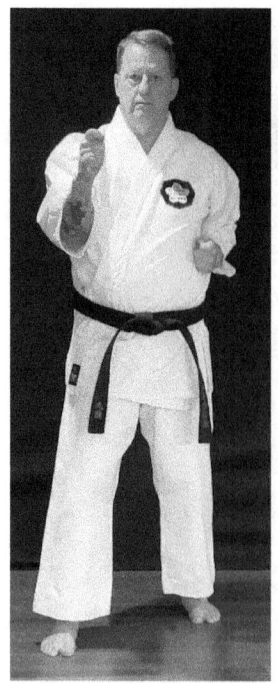

Chamber Left Hand

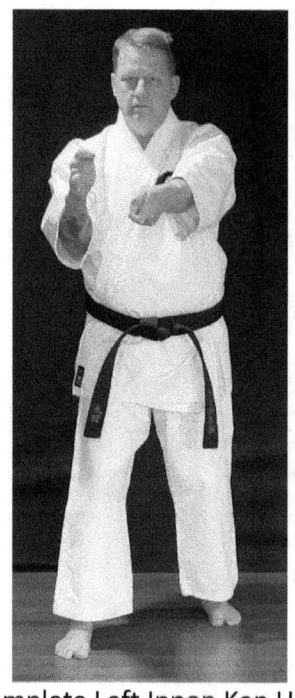

Complete Left Ippon Ken Uchi

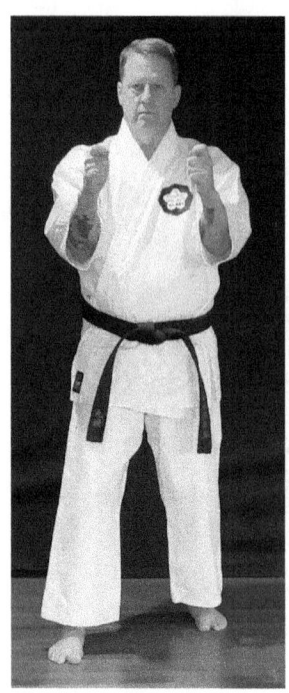

Set

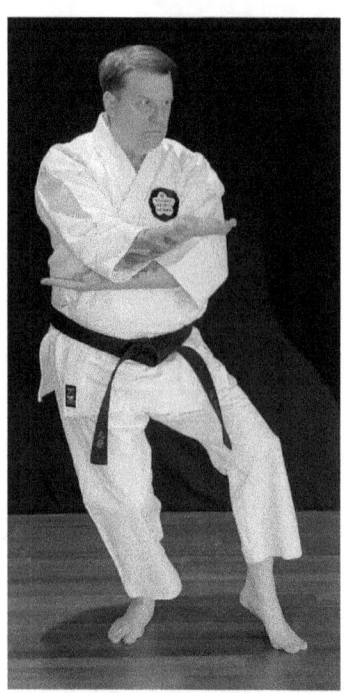

Right Foot Step Back on
45° Angle into Neko
Ashi Dachi, Prepare Left Hari Uke

Gekisai San

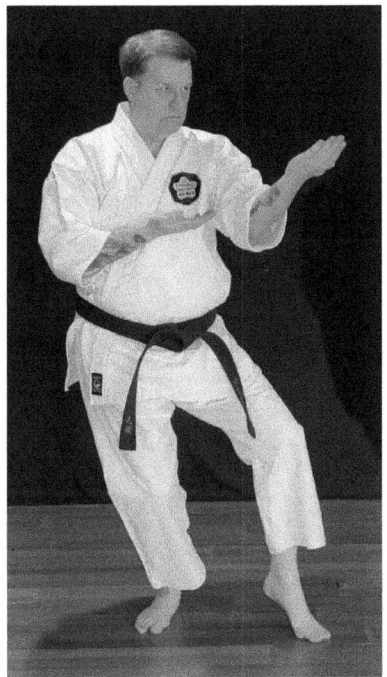
Hari Uke

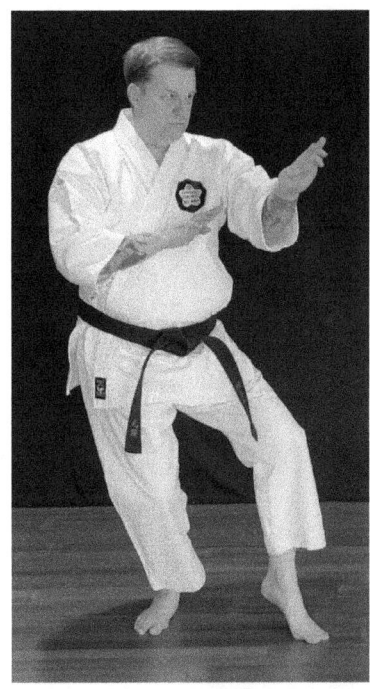
Turn Hands Over, Nihon Nukite

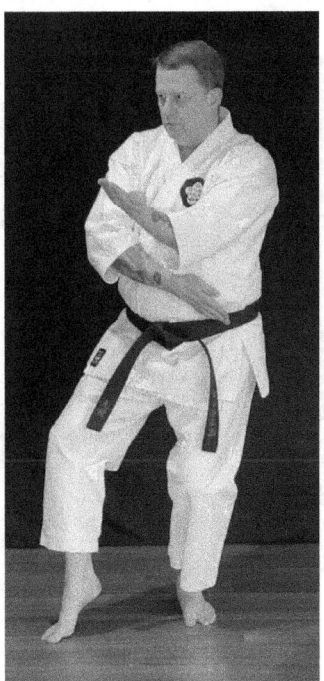
Left Foot Step Back on 315° Angle into Neko Ashi Dachi, Prepare Hari Uke

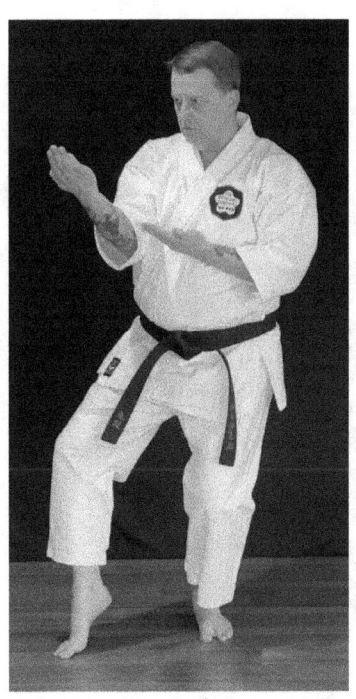
Hari Uke

Gekisai San

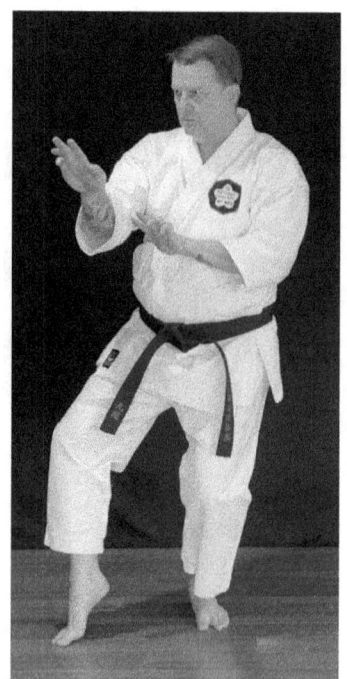
Turn Hands Over, Nihon Nukite

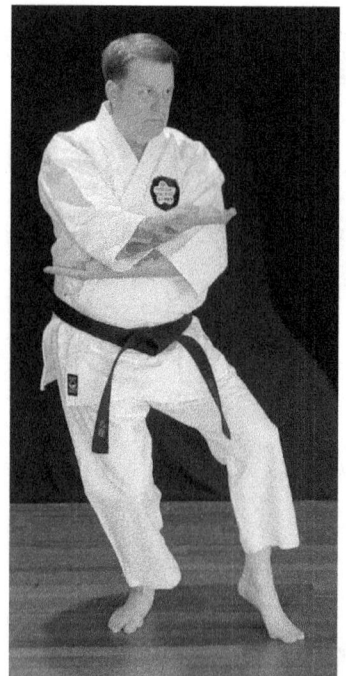
Right Foot Step Back on 45° Angle into Neko Ashi Dachi, Prepare Hari Uke

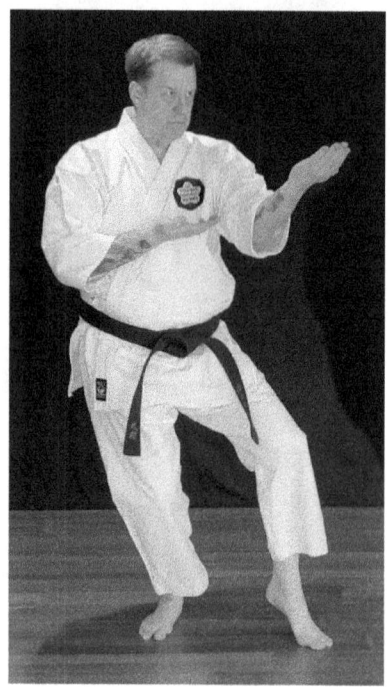
Hari Uke

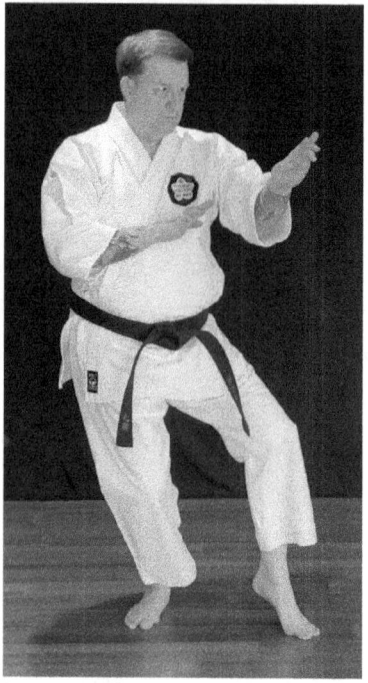
Turn Hands Over, Nihon Nukite

Gekisai San

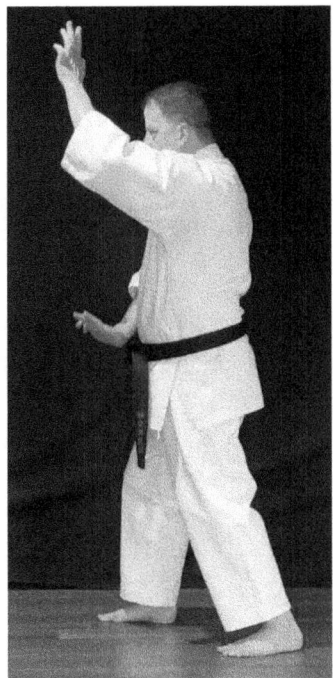

Pivot Right, Raise Left Arm Above Head, Drop Right Hand

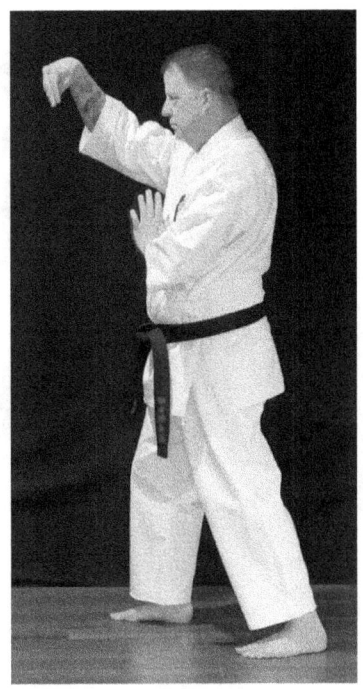

Complete Left Chudan Shotei Otoshi Uke & Right Jodan Age Ko Uke

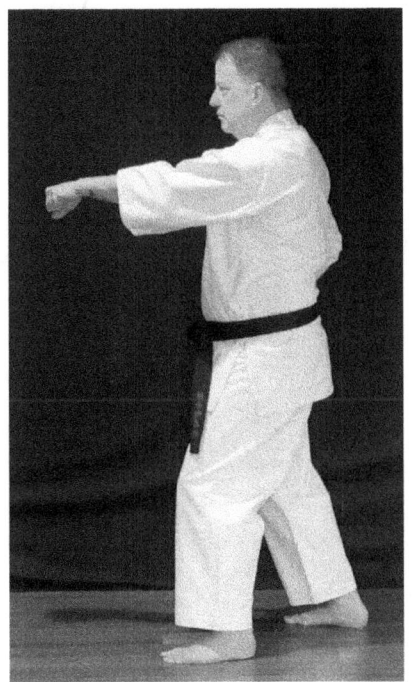

Step, Complete Left Chudan Zuki (Pause One Beat)

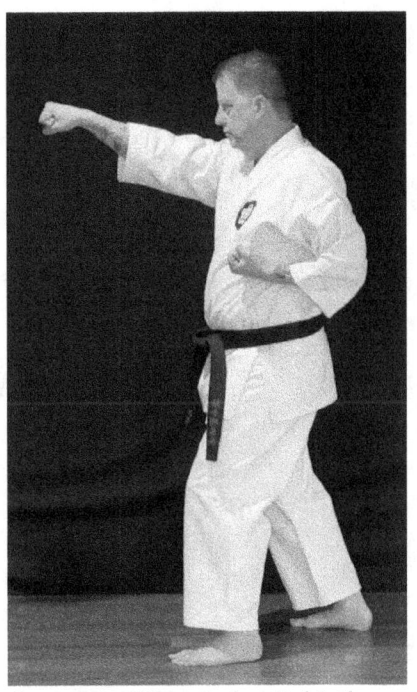

Complete Right Jodan Zuki, then..

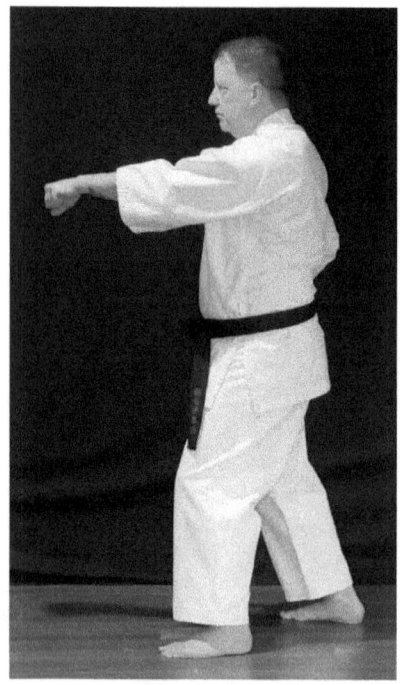
...an Immediate Left Chudan Zuki

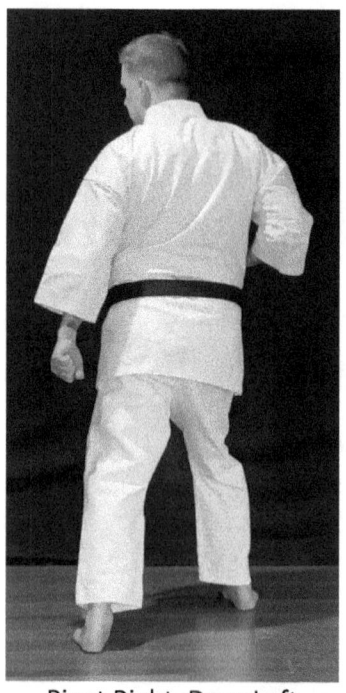
Pivot Right, Drop Left Arm Down and Back Slightly

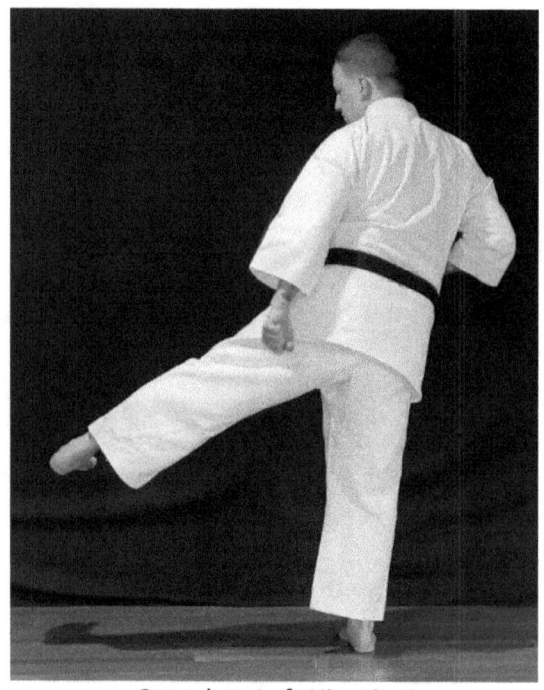
Complete Left Hiza Geri

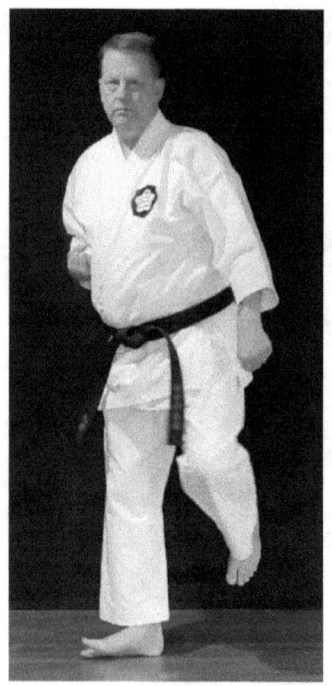
Without Setting Left Foot Down, Pivot Back Facing Forward

Gekisai San

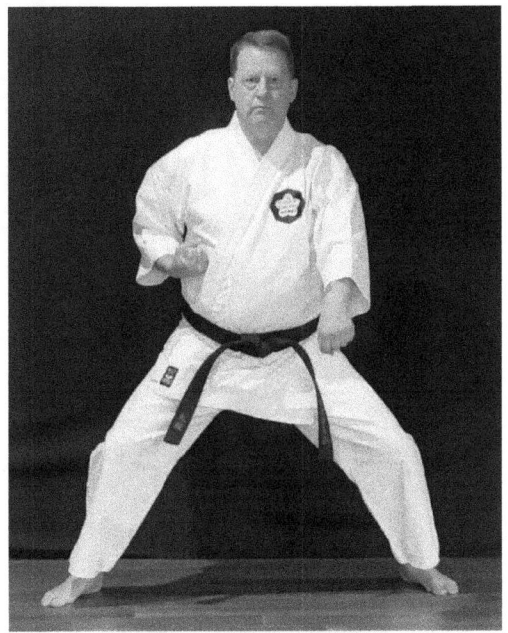
Land in Shiko Dachi

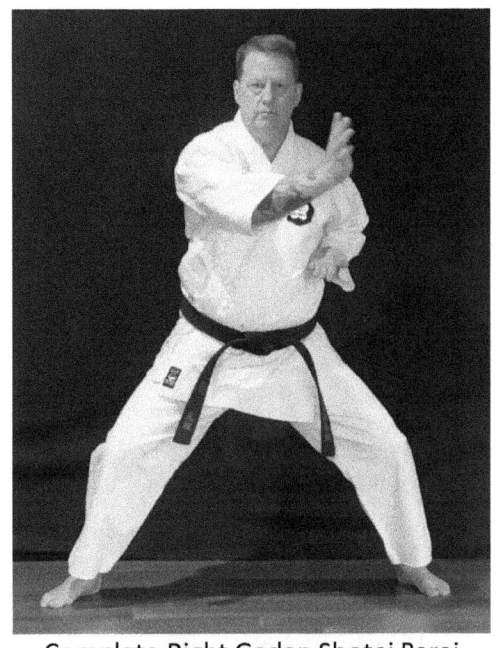
Complete Right Gedan Shotei Barai

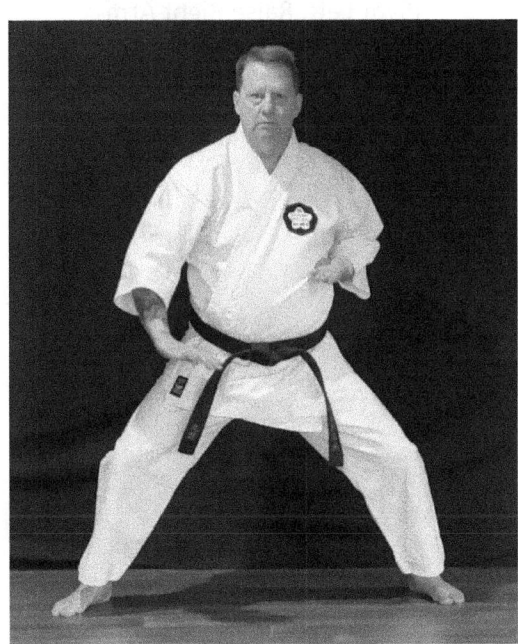
Gedan Shotei Barai (cont.)

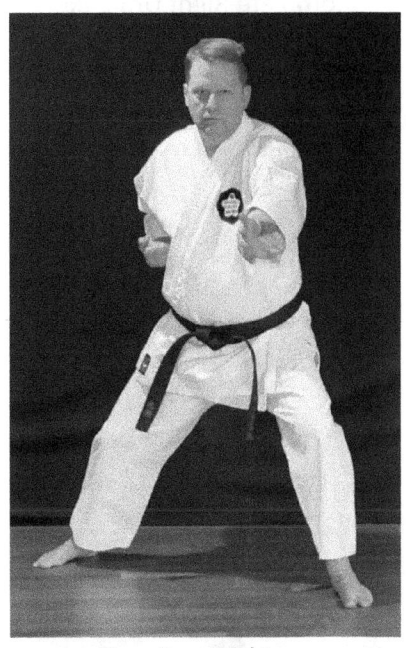
Step Forward Low,
Left Tsukami Hiki

Gekisai San

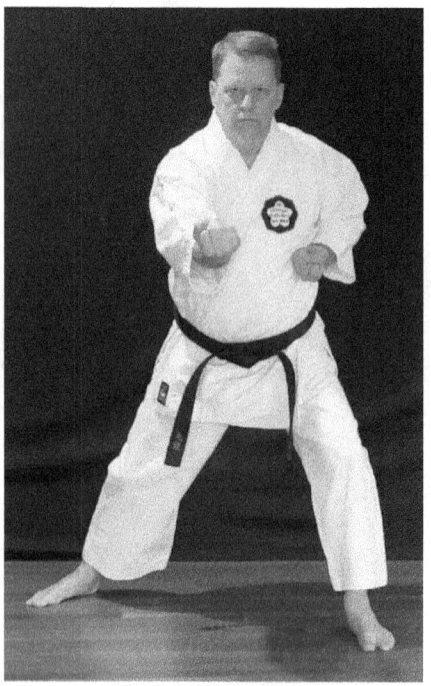

Complete Right Ura Zuki

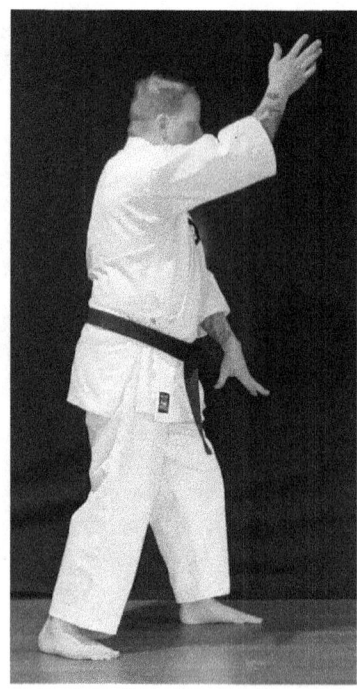

Pivot Left, Raise Right Arm Above Head, Drop Left Hand

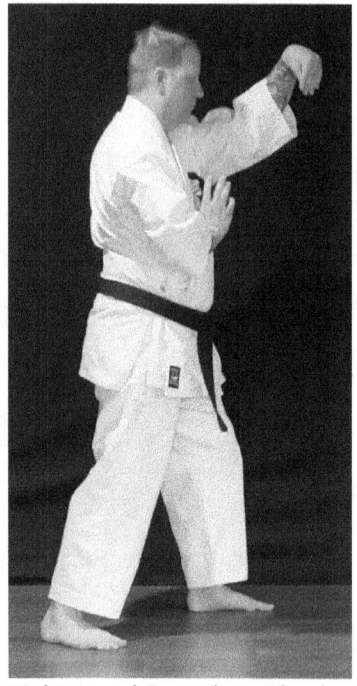

Right Hand Complete Chudan Shotei Otoshi Uke & Left Hand Jodan Age Ko Uke

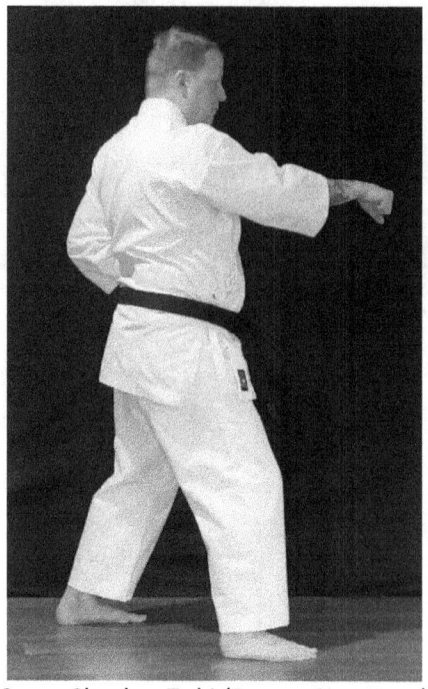

Step, Chudan Zuki (Pause One Beat)

Gekisai San

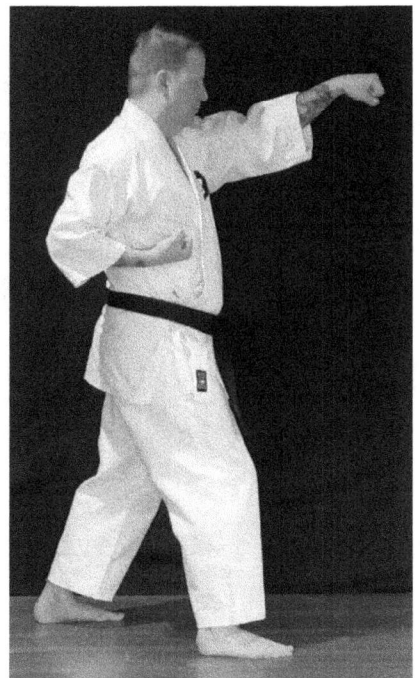
Complete Left Jodan Zuki, then..

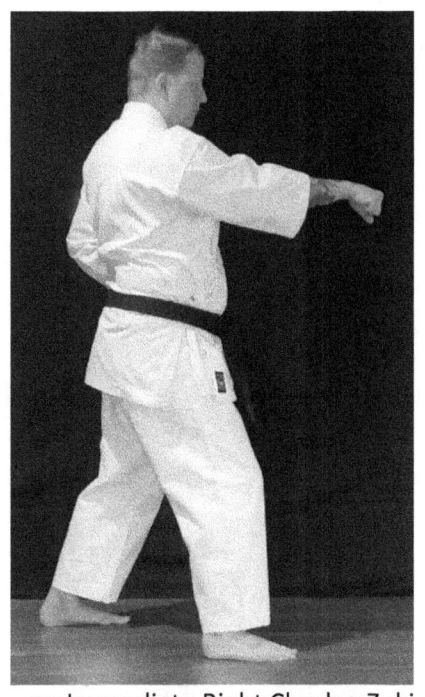
...an Immediate Right Chudan Zuki

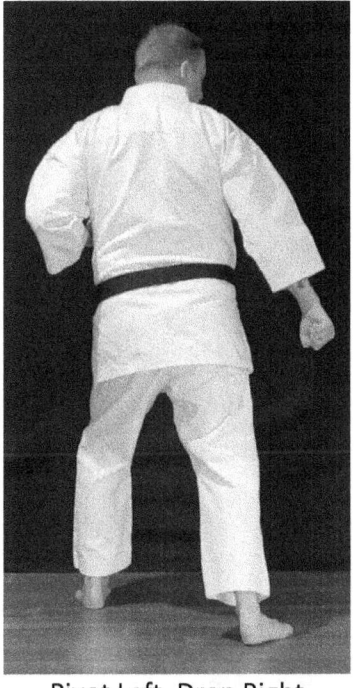
Pivot Left, Drop Right Arm Down and Back Slightly

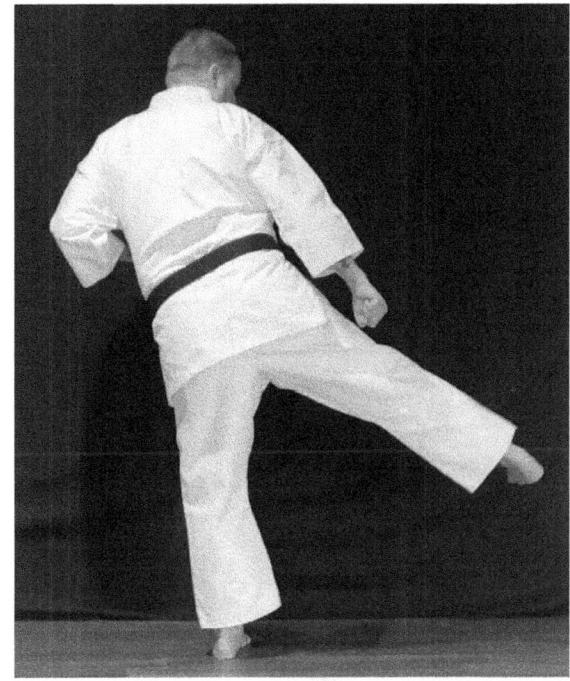
Complete Right Hiza Geri

Gekisai San

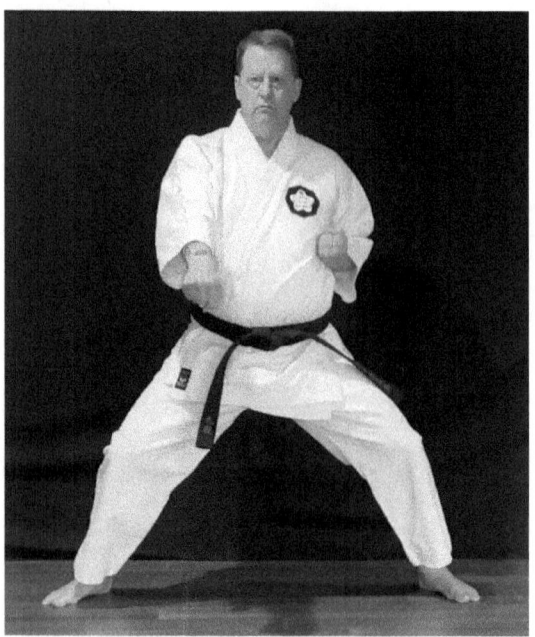

Without Setting Right Foot Down,
Pivot Back Facing Forward,
Land in Shiko Dachi

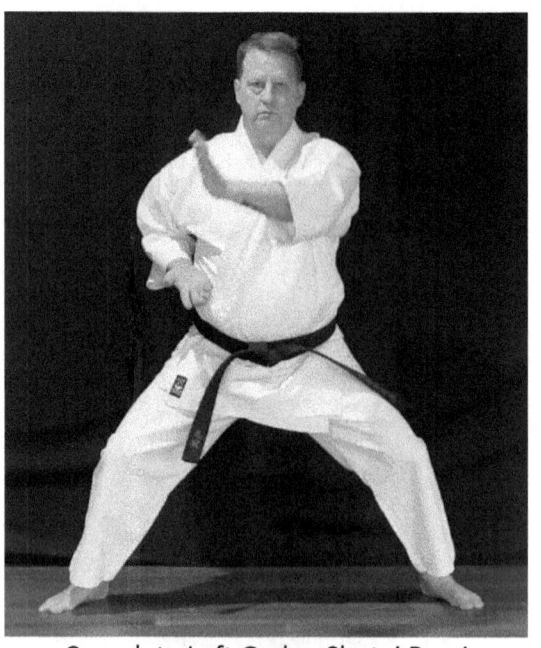

Complete Left Gedan Shotei Barai

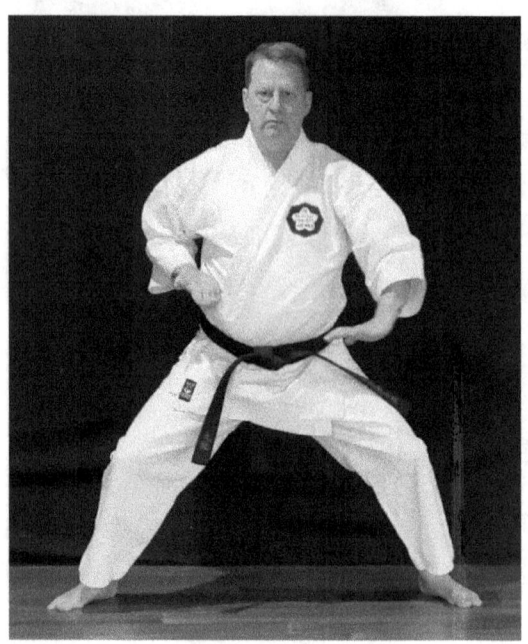

Gedan Shotei Barai (cont.)

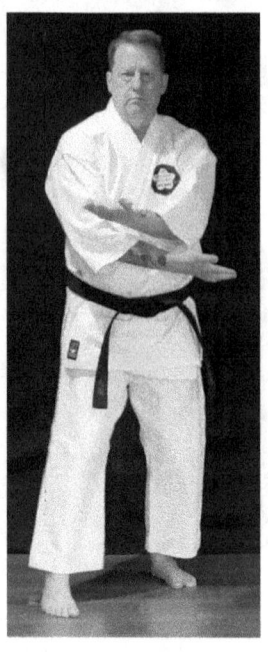

Right Step Forward,
Begin Right Chudan
Hari Uke

Gekisai San

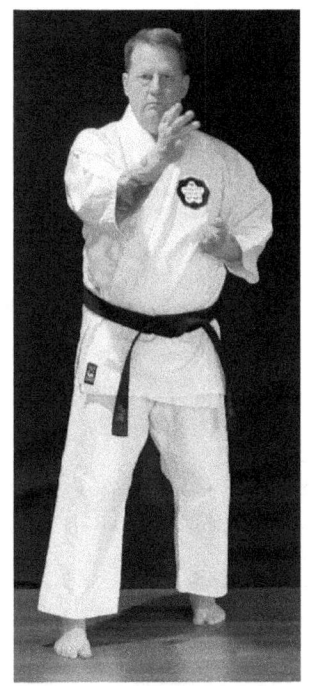 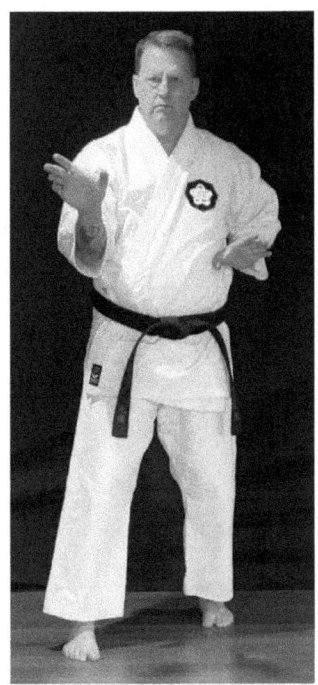

Complete Right Chudan Hari Uke to Hiki Uke

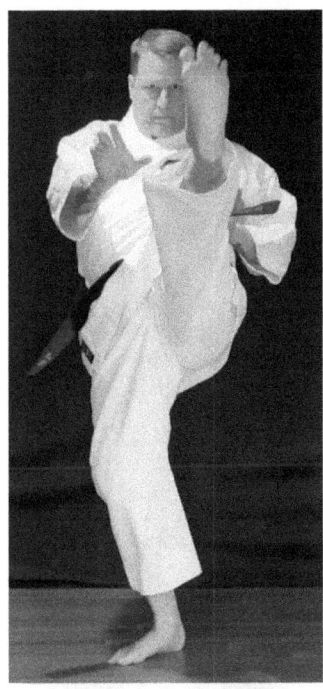 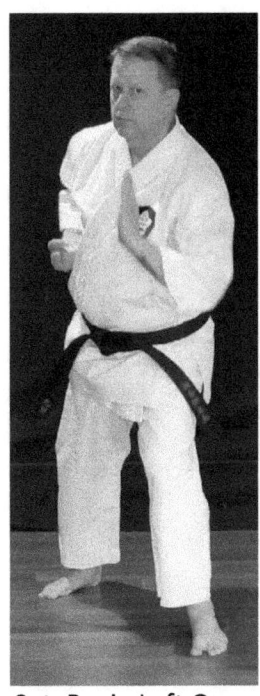

Complete Left Jodan
Mae Keage Geri (kiai)

Set, Begin Left Open
Handed Age Empi Uchi

Gekisai San

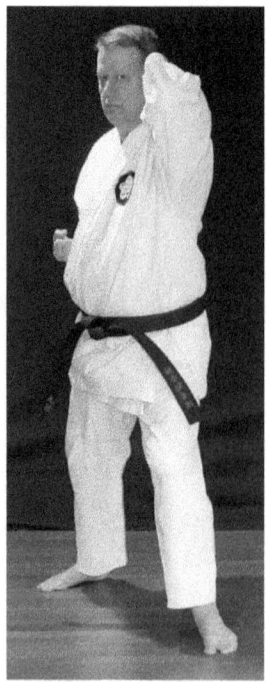
Age Empi Uchi (cont.)

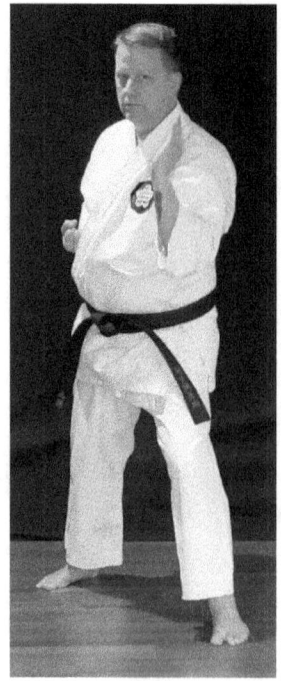
Bring Elbow Down

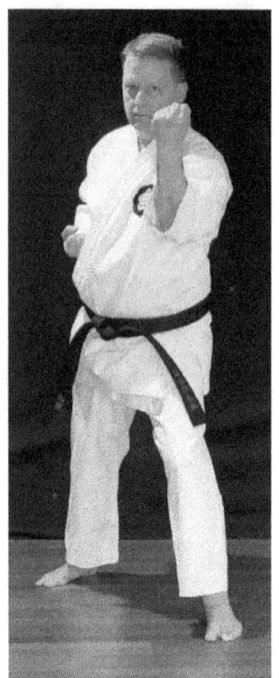
Complete Left Uraken Uchi

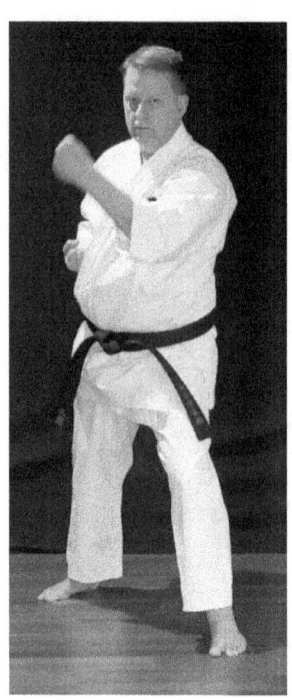
Complete Left Gedan Barai

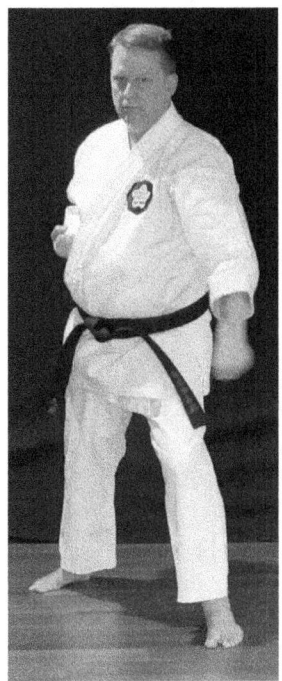

Gedan Barai (cont.)

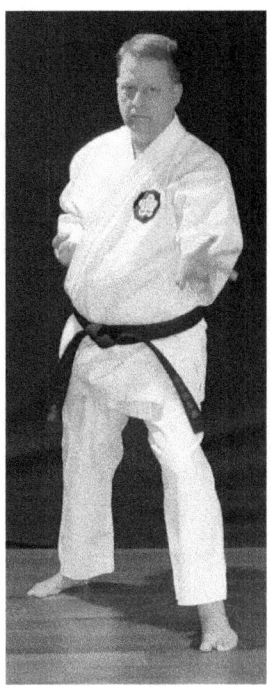

Reach Around and Grab
Opponent's Wrist (Tsukami Hiki)

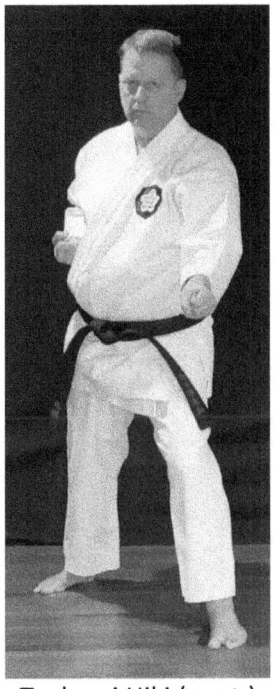

Tsukami Hiki (cont.)

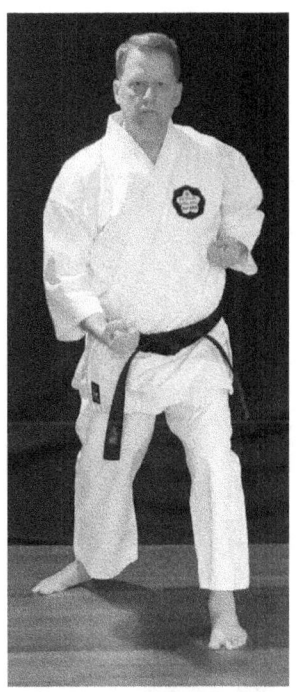

Twist Hips Facing Forward,
Complete Right Age Zuki

Gekisai San

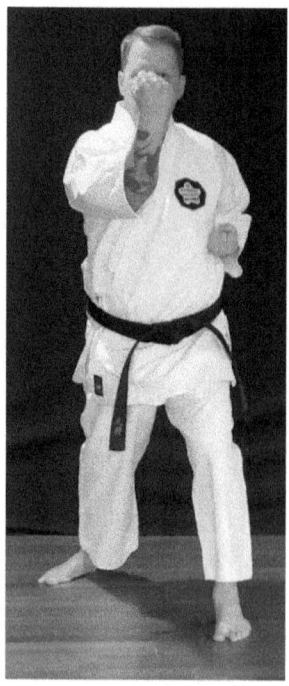

Age Zuki (cont.)

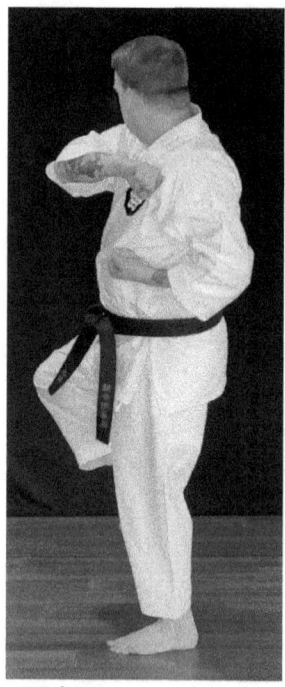

Bring Right Foot and Right Hand to Chamber Facing Rear, Looking Rear and Facing Side

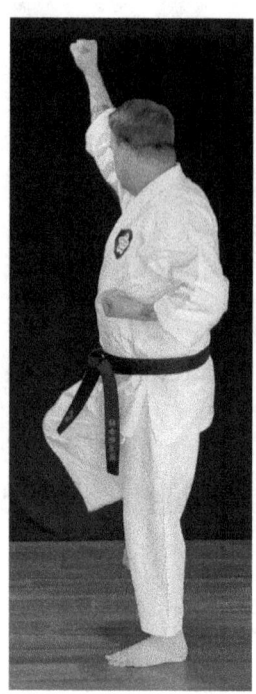

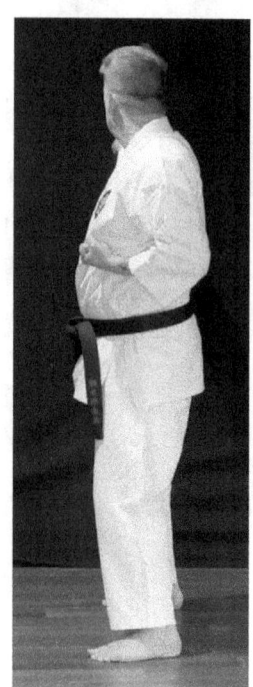

Complete Right Otoshi Tettsui Uchi

Gekisai San

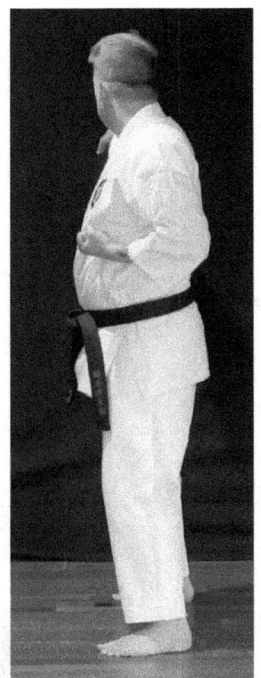
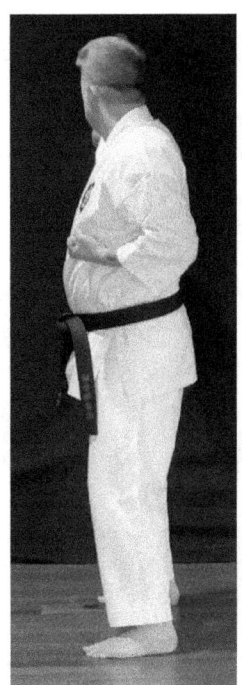

Complete Right Tsukami Hiki

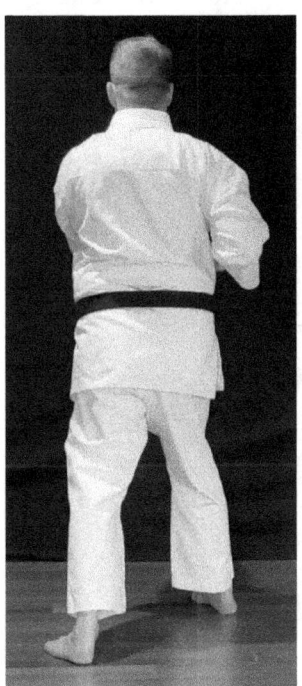
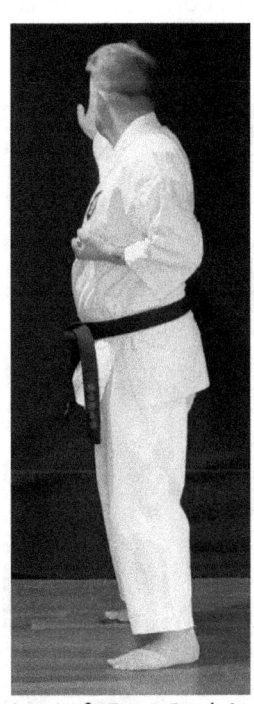

Twist Hips Facing Rear, Pull
Back with Right Hand while Completing
Left Ura Zuki

Bring Left Foot Back into
Heiko Dachi, Oshi

Gekisai San

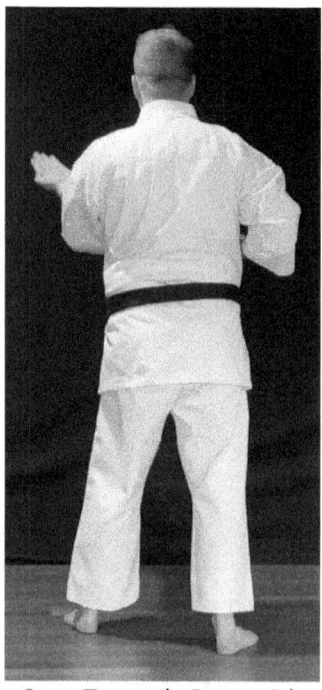

Step Towards Rear with Left Foot, Complete Left Chudan Hari Uke

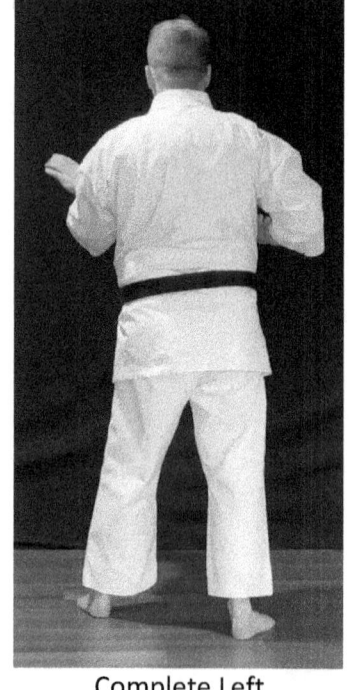

Complete Left Chudan Hiki Uke

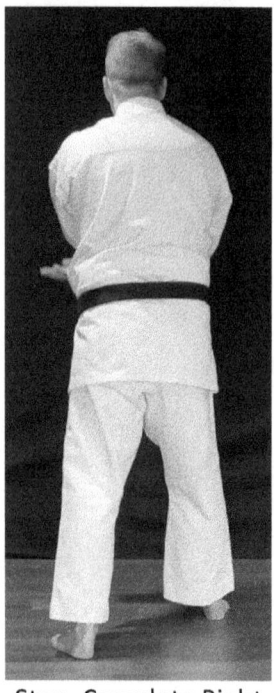

Step, Complete Right Chudan Hari Uke

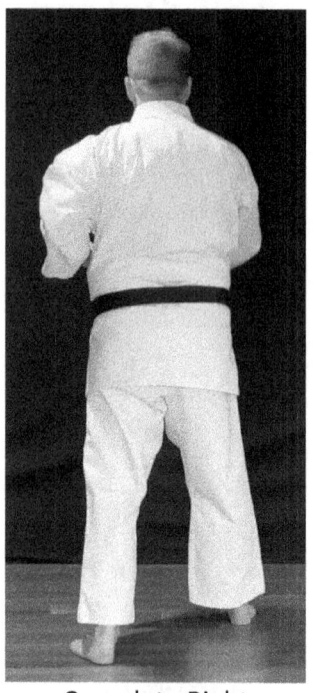

Complete Right Chudan Hiki Uke

Gekisai San

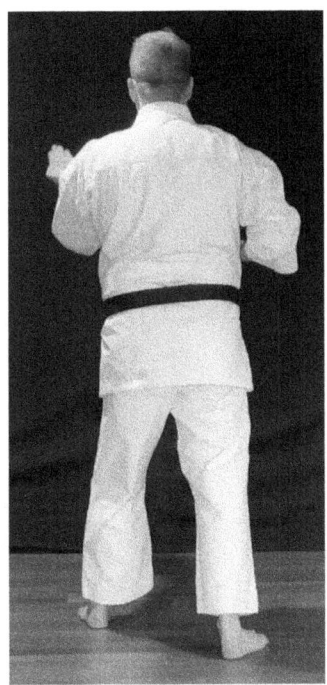

Step Back, Complete Left
Chudan Hari Uke

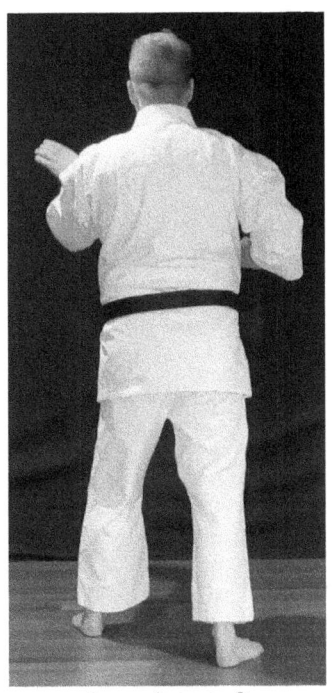

Complete Left
Chudan Hiki Uke

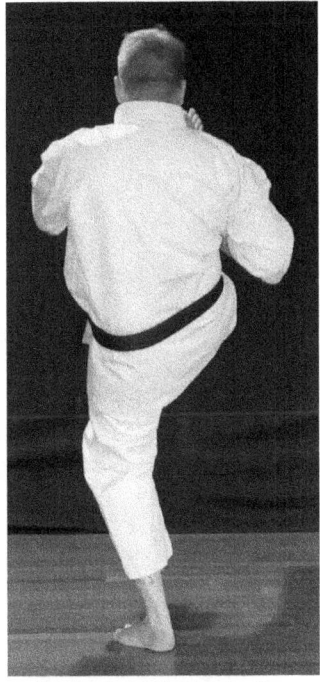

Complete Right Jodan
Mae Keage Geri (kiai)

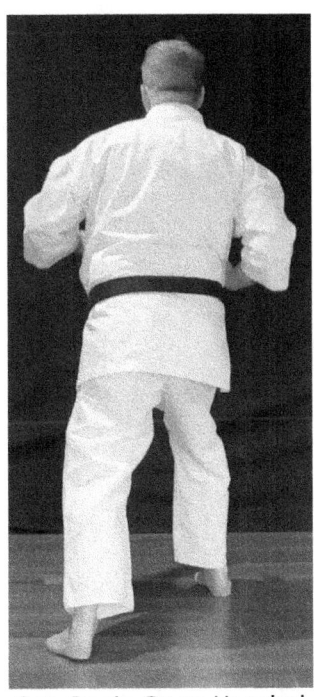

Set, Begin Open Handed
Right Age Empi Uchi

Gekisai San

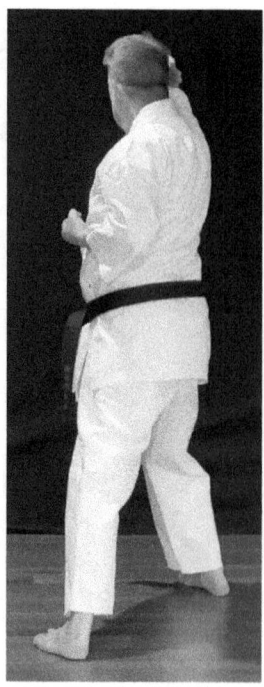

Age Empi Uchi (cont.)

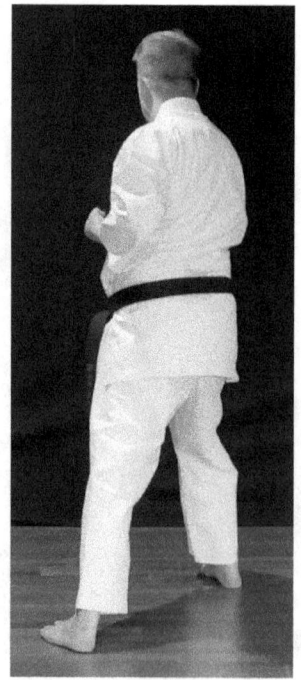

Bring Elbow Down,
Complete Right Uraken Uchi

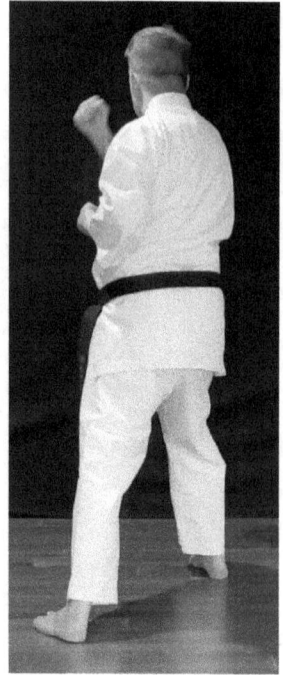

Complete Right Gedan Barai

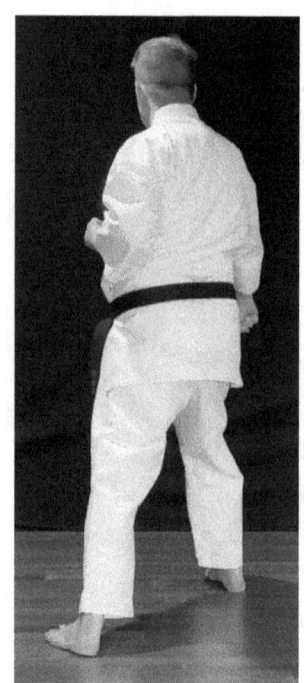

Gekisai San

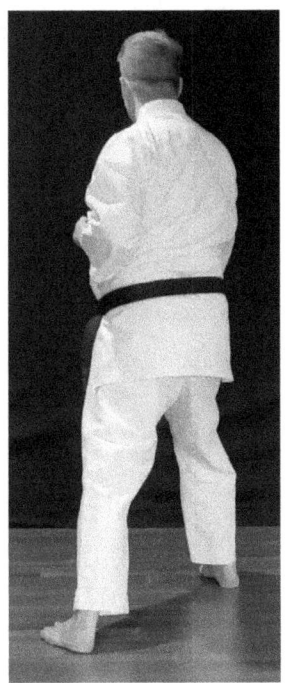

Reach Around and Grab
Opponent's Wrist
(Tsukami Hiki)

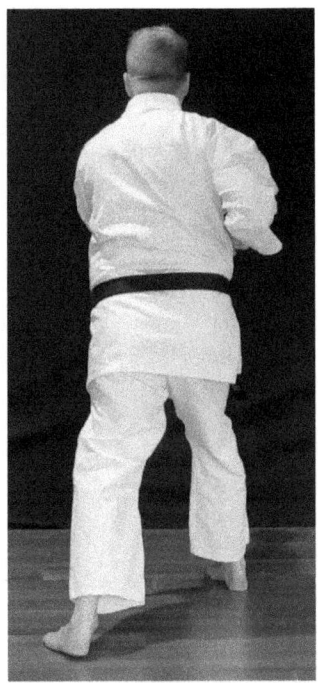

Twist Hips Facing Forward,
Pull Back Left Hand into
Chamber while Completing
Ura Zuki

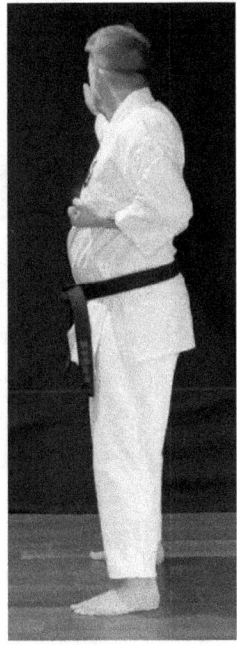

Bring Left Foot Back into
Heiko Dachi, Oshi

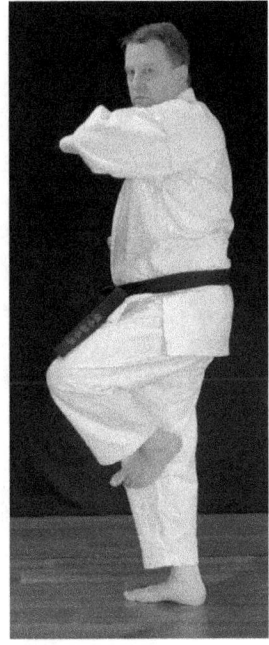

Bring Left Foot and Left Hand to Chamber
Facing Front, Looking Forward and Facing
Side

Gekisai San

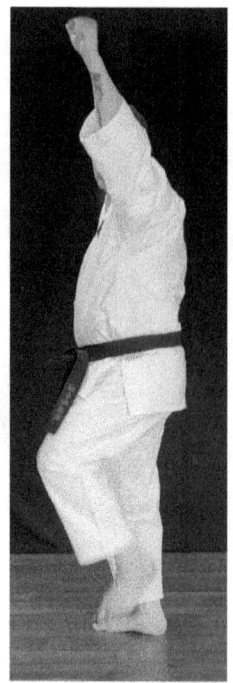
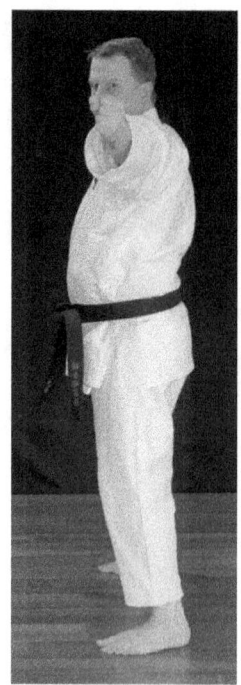

Complete Left Otoshi Tettsui Uchi

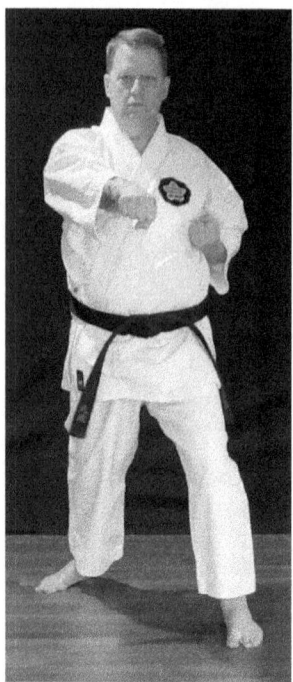

Bring Left Foot Out, Facing
Forward, Complete
Gyaku Zuki (kiai)

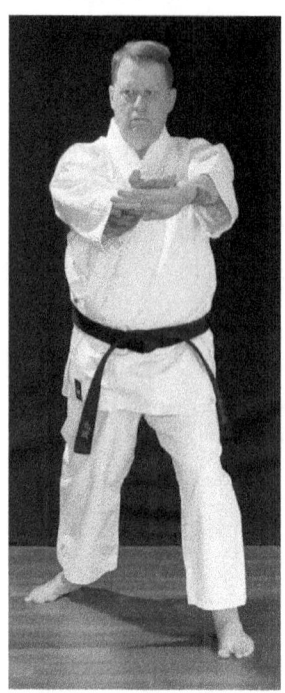

Turn Left Hand Palm Down
in Front, Place Right Hand
Palm Up on Top,
Look Front Right

Gekisai San

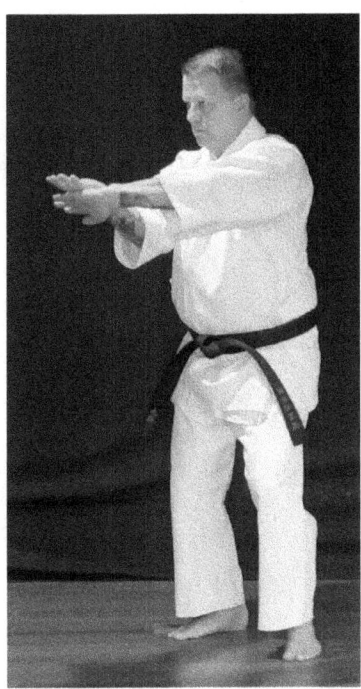

Move Hands to Angle while Stepping Back Facing 315° into Neko Ashi Dachi

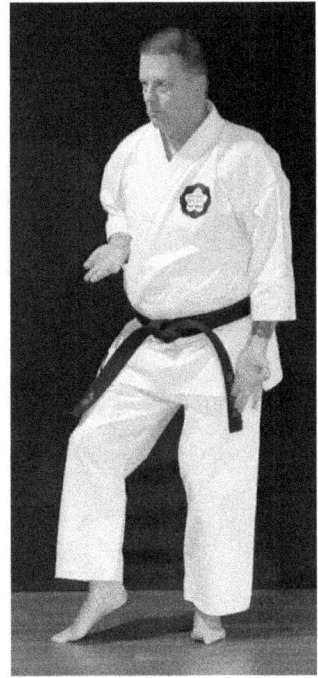

Land in Neko Ashi Dachi while Bringing Right Hand Straight into Chamber and Left Kake Uke

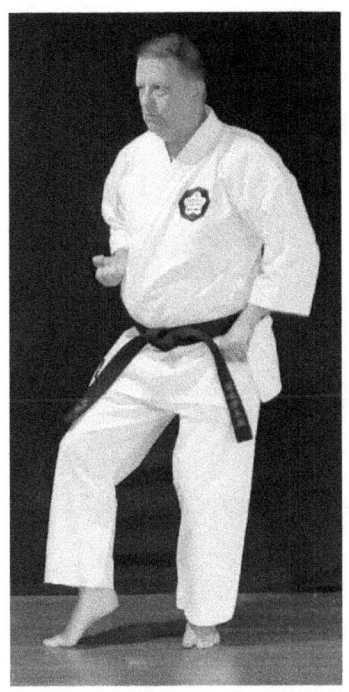

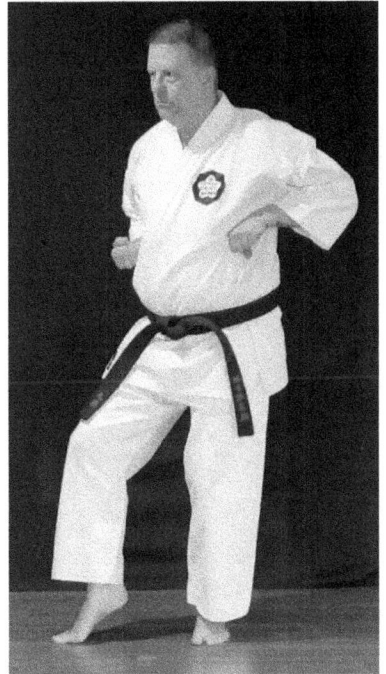

Turn Left Hand Over into a Fist, Pull Up to Chamber as Right Hand Closes into a Fist

Gekisai San

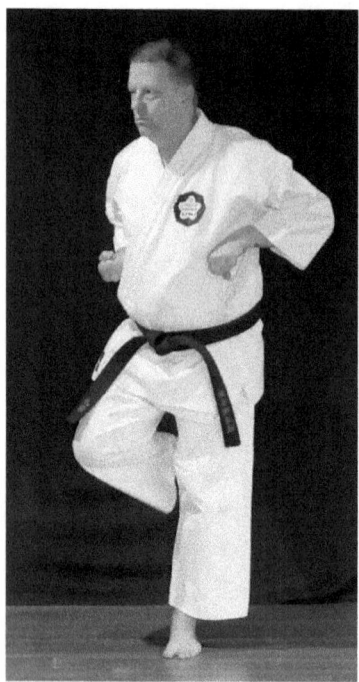

Pick up Right Leg

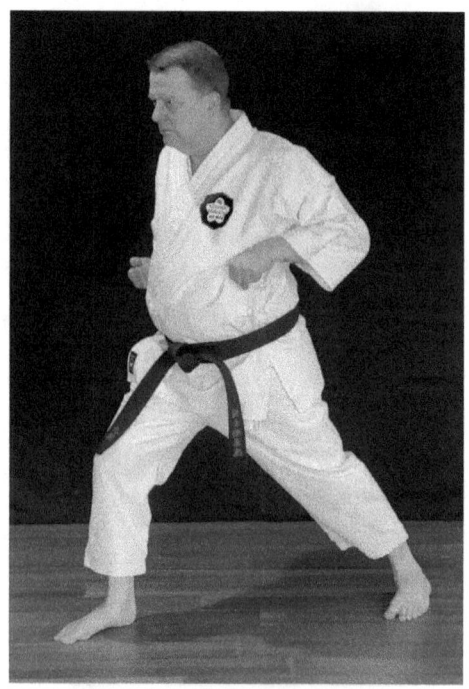

Step into Zenkutsu Dachi

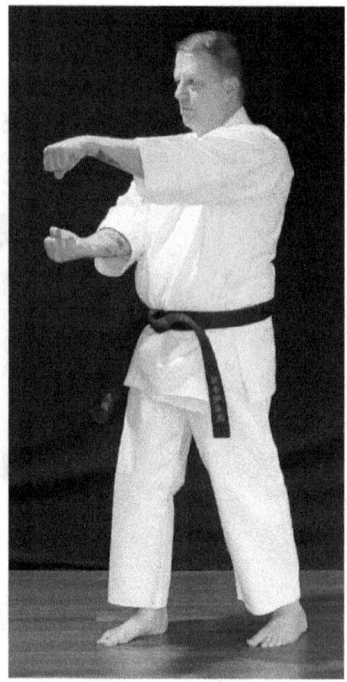

Drag Left Foot Up while
Completing Centerline
Morote Uchi (kiai)

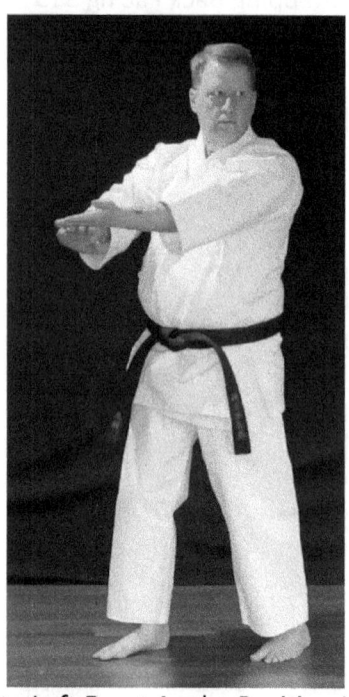

Look to Left Front Angle, Position Hands
with Right Hand Palm Down
and Left Arm Straight with Open
Hand Palm Up on Top

Gekisai San

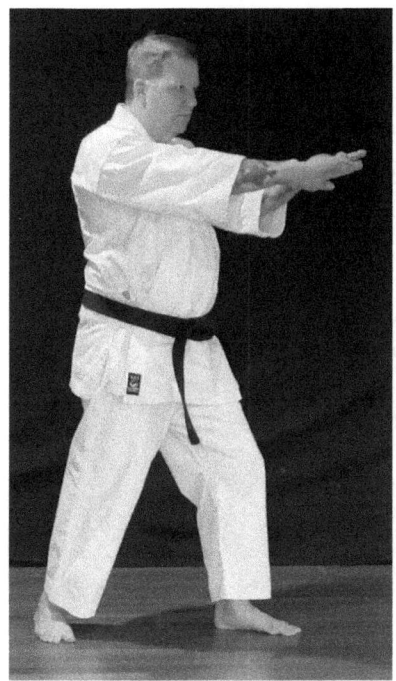

Pivot to Forward Left
Facing 45° Angle

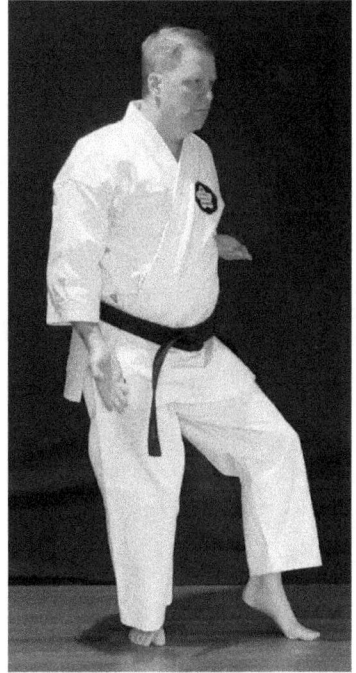

Land in Neko Ashi Dachi
while Bringing Left Hand
Straight into Chamber
and Right Kake Uke

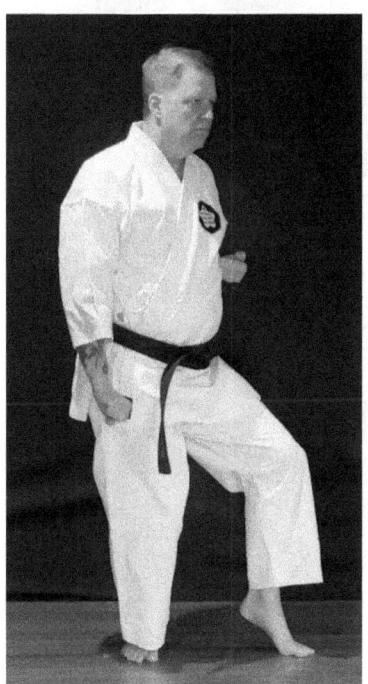

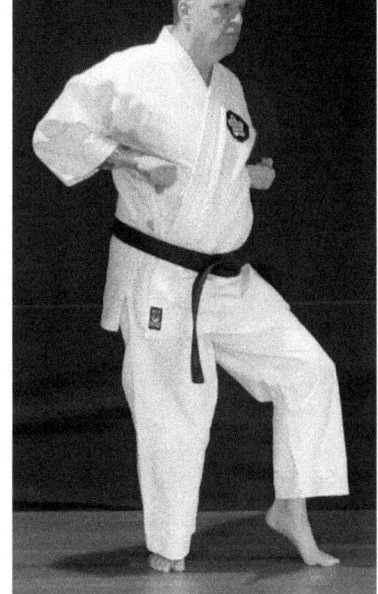

Turn Right Hand Over into a Fist, Pull Up to Chamber
as Left Hand Closes into a Fist

Gekisai San

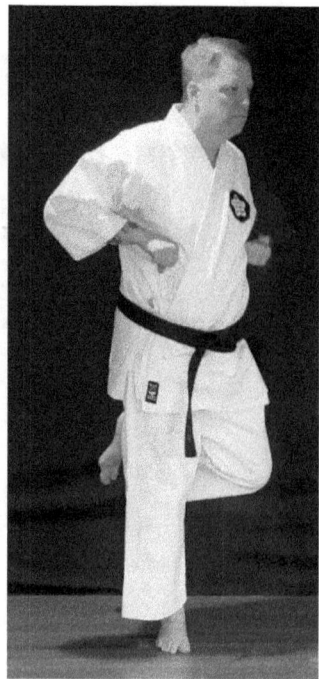
Bring Left Leg Up

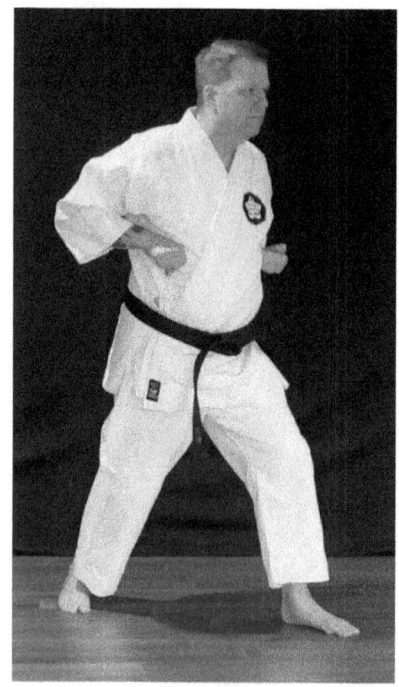
Left Step into Zenkutsu Dachi

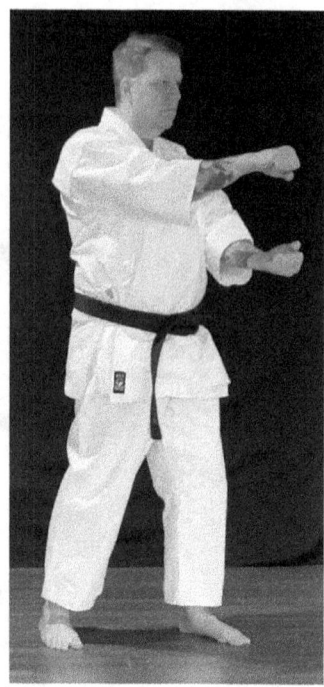
Drag Left Foot Up while Completing Centerline Morote Uchi (kiai)

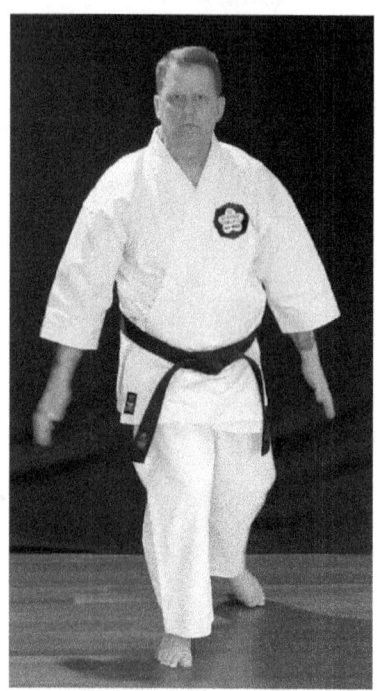
Step Back with Left Foot, Bring Arms Down and Around

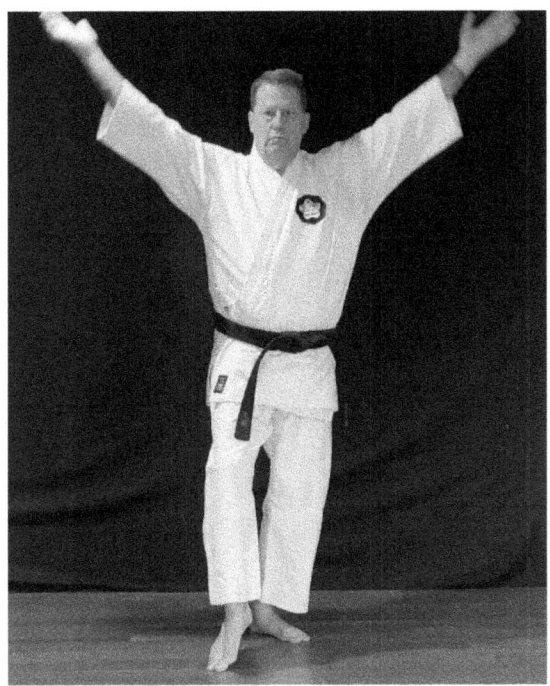
Bring Arms Around (cont.)

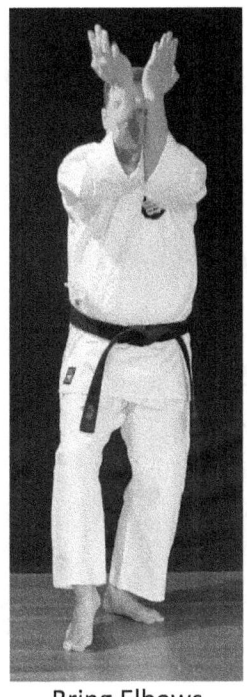
Bring Elbows Together and Down

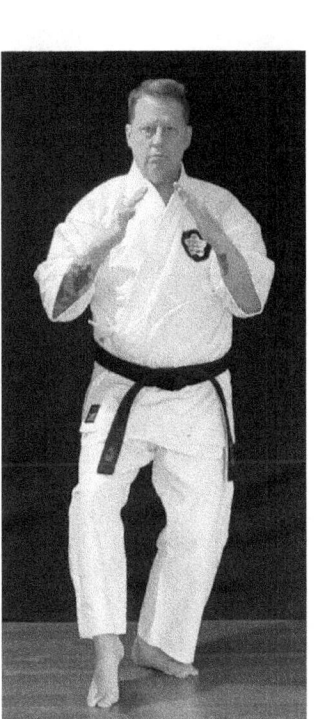
Set with Elbows Down and Hands Separated

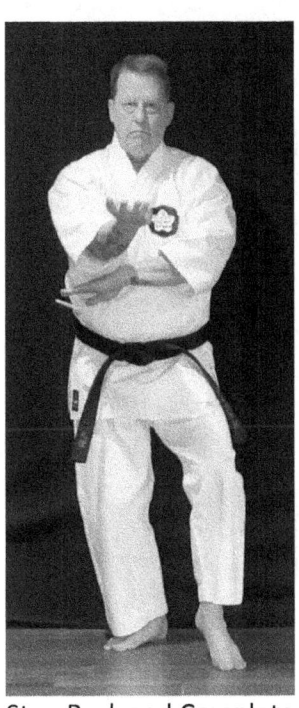
Step Back and Complete Tora Guchi

Gekisai San

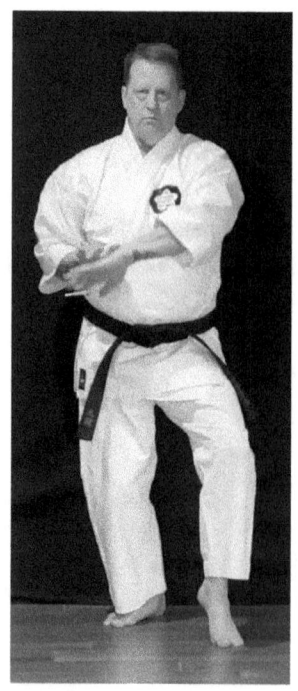
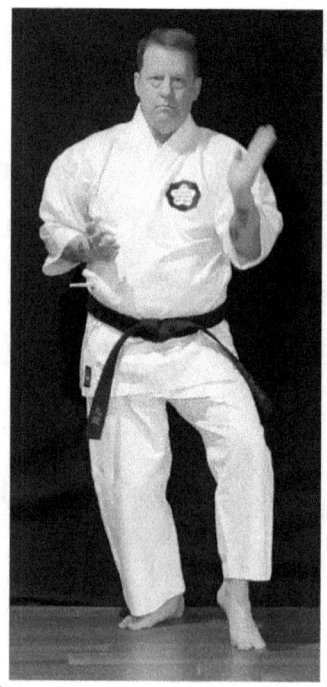

Tora Guchi (cont.)

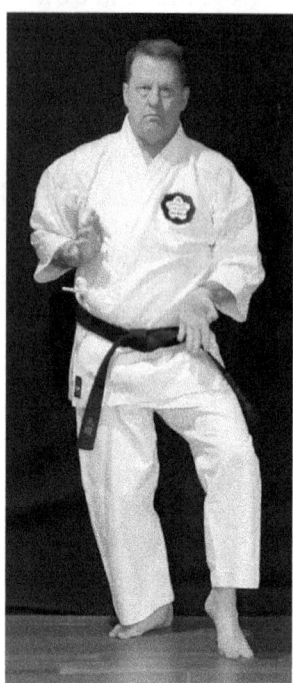
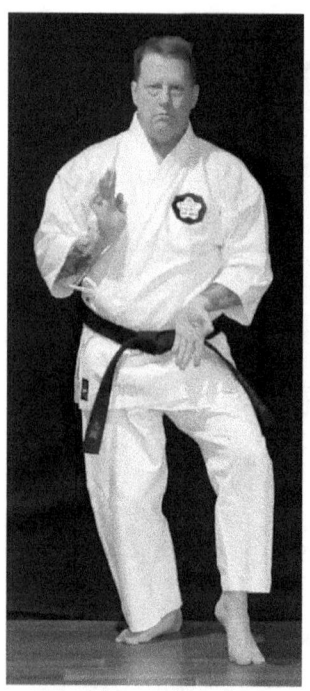

Tora Guchi (cont.)

Complete Centerline
Morote Shotei Uchi

Gekisai San

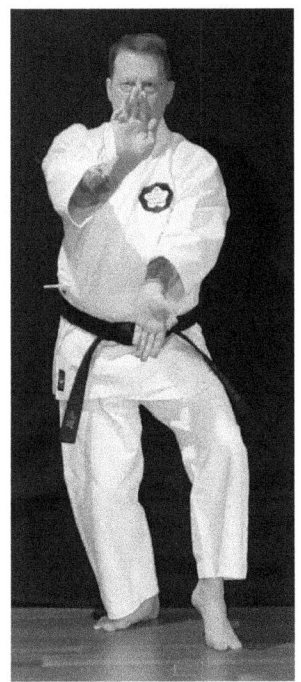

Centerline Morote
Shotei Uchi (cont.)

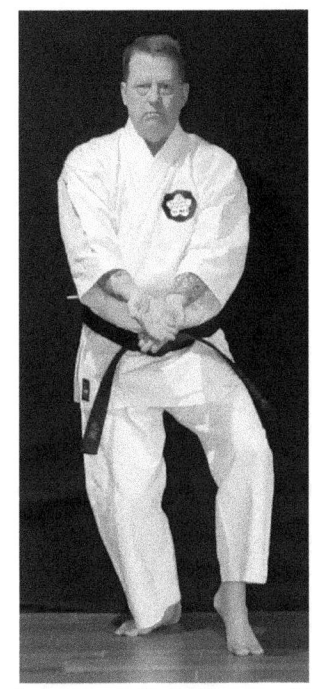

Bring Hands Together and Up

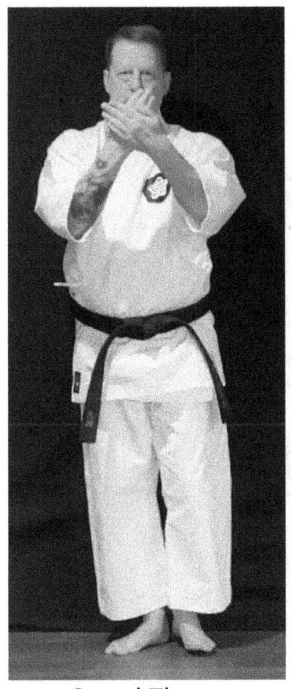

Guard Throat

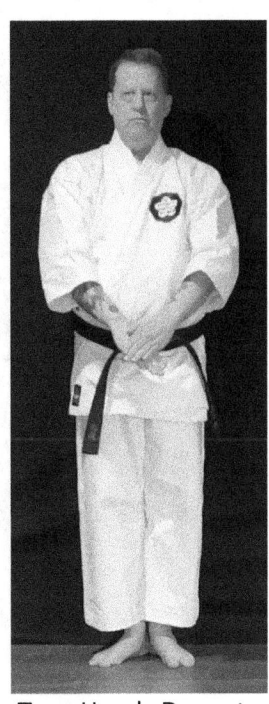

Turn Hands Down to
Guard Groin

Gekisai San

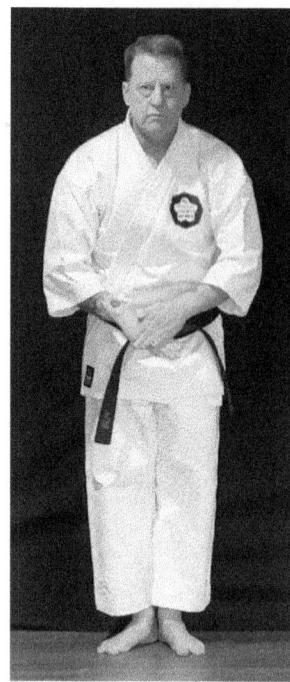

Rei

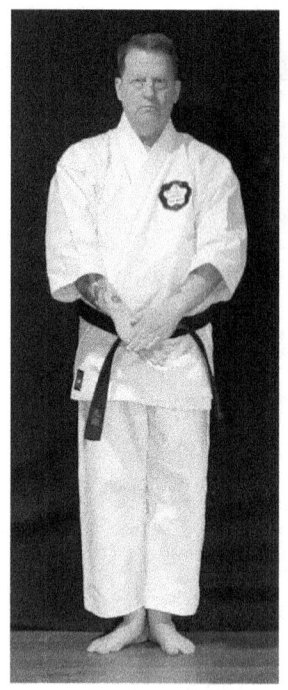

Musubi Dachi

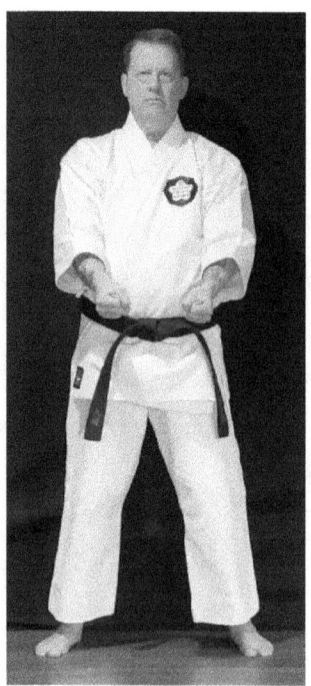

Heiko Dachi

Hon'nogeki

Hon'nogeki means "instinctive attack." The newest kata in the system, this is the author's kata as directed by Shodai to create in 2016. It emphasizes multiple angled attacks and contains a spinning elbow strike and multiple arm breaks. It also contains a crescent kick turning into a side kick. The author created Hon'nogeki after a directive from Shodai. I was asked to create a kata for inclusion to the system. A few months after the assignment in 2016 it was demonstrated to Shodai as Hon'nogeki (instinctive attack.) The idea was for the moves to be obvious instead of hidden. Shodai enjoyed hidden moves, but this kata would be different. Shodai made a few suggestions but ultimately gave his approval for the kata to be added.

Below is the method by which Ketsugo Goju-Ryu performs Hon'nogeki kata. Complete details about each move are not included, as this is simply a demonstration.

These are the Japanese terms used for this kata. Bear in mind, karate terms are not completely streamlined. There are terms that were used in the middle of the 20th Century that are no longer used today. Oftentimes there are more than one term that can be used for the same technique. The important thing is not what it is called, but the technique itself.

Barai - Sweeping Block	**Morote Chudan Uke** – Double Chest Block
Chudan - Middle	
Dachi – Stance	**Musubi Dachi** - Attention Stance, Toes Out
Empi - Elbow	
Gedan – Low	**Neko Ashi Dachi** - Cat Leg Stance
Geri - Kick	**Oshi** - Push
Haito Uchi – Ridge Hand Strike	**Otoshi** - Dropping (Downward)

Hon'nogeki

Hajime – Command to Begin	**Rei** – Bow (Respect)
Heiko Dachi - Parallel Stance	**Sanchin Dachi** – Hourglass Stance
Hiki Uke – Open Hand Block (Palm Down)/Pulling Block	**Shiko Dachi** - Straddle Leg Stance
Hiraken - Second Knuckles Fist	**Shotei** - Palm Heel
Hiza Geri – Knee Joint Kick	**Shuto Uchi** – Chop Strike
Hiza Uchi – Strike (Using the Knee)	**Tettsui Uchi** – Hammer Fist Strike
Jodan – High	**Tsuki/-Zuki** - Punch
Kake Geri - Hook Kick	**Uchi** – Strike
Kake Uke - Hook Block	**Uke** – Block (Receive)
Keage Geri – Snap Kick	**Ura Mawashi Empi Uchi** – Spinning Elbow Strike
Kokutsu Dachi – Rear Leaning Stance	**Ushiro** – Rear (Back)
Kote Uchi – Forearm Strike	**Ushiro Mawashi Geri** – Spinning Hook Kick
Mae – Front	**Uraken Uchi** - Back Fist Strike
Mawashi Geri – Roundhouse Kick	**Yoi** – Ready Command
Mikazuki Geri – Crescent Kick	**Yoko** - Side
	Zenkutsu Dachi - Forward Leaning Stance

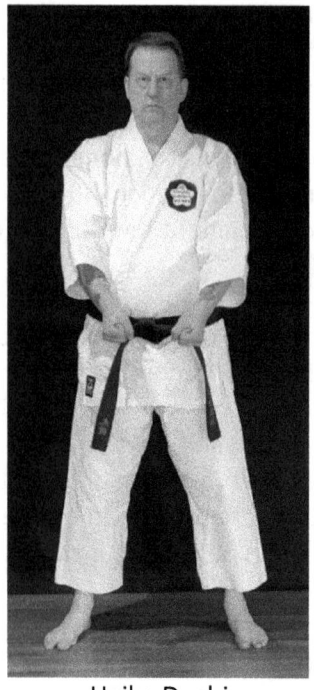

Heiko Dachi

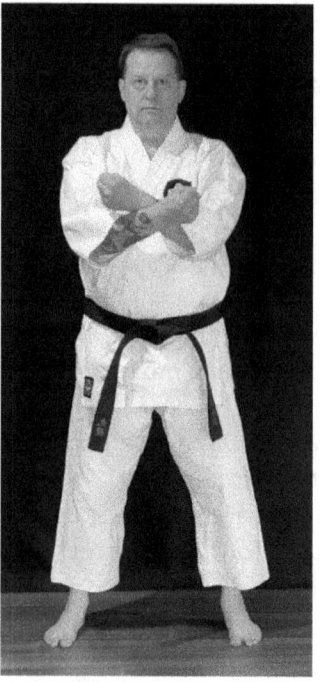

(Yoi) Brings Arms Up, Crossed at the Wrist

Hon'nogeki

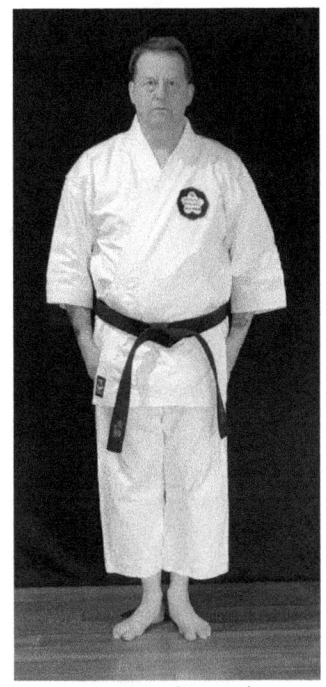
Hajime (Begin)

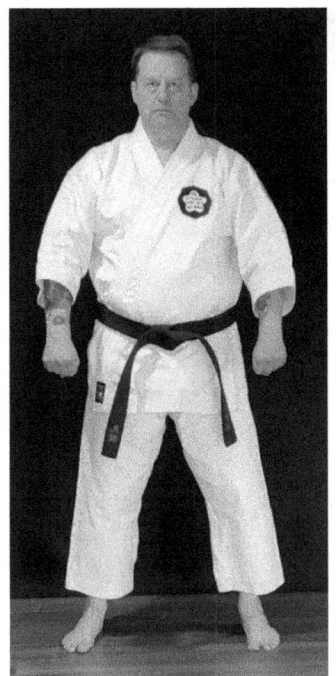
Bring Arms Down

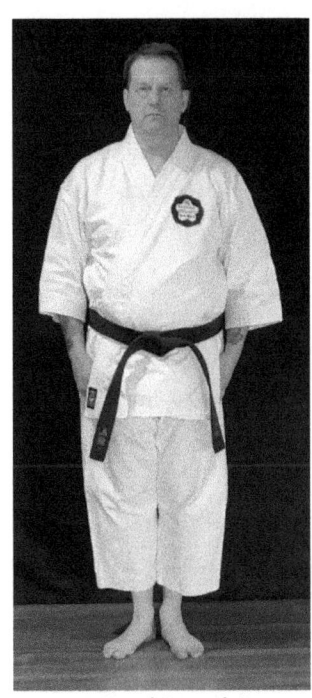
Musubi Dachi

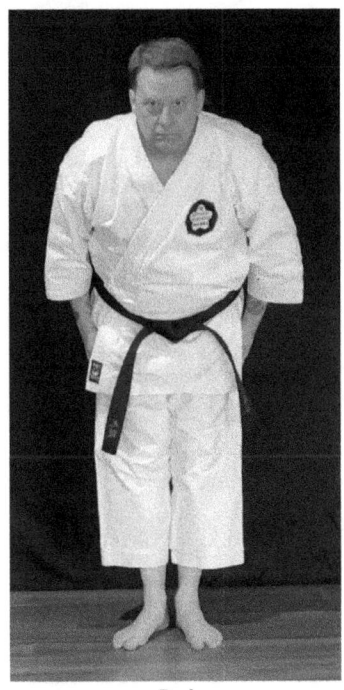
Rei

Hon'nogeki

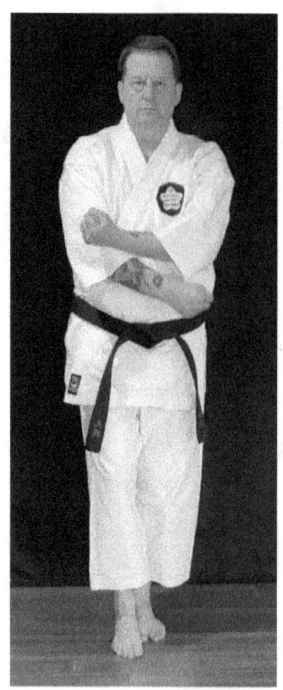 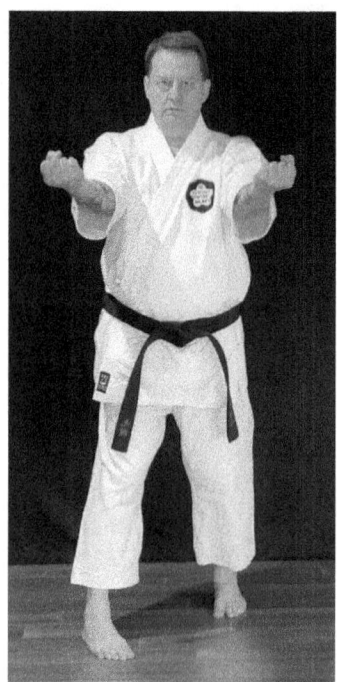

Step in Sanchin Dachi, Complete Slow Morote Chudan Uke

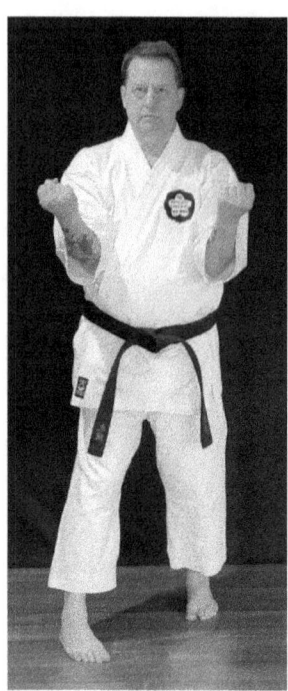 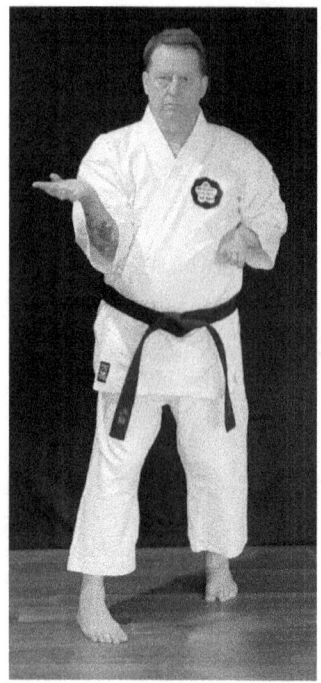

Set   Begin Right Gedan Shotei Barai

Hon'nogeki

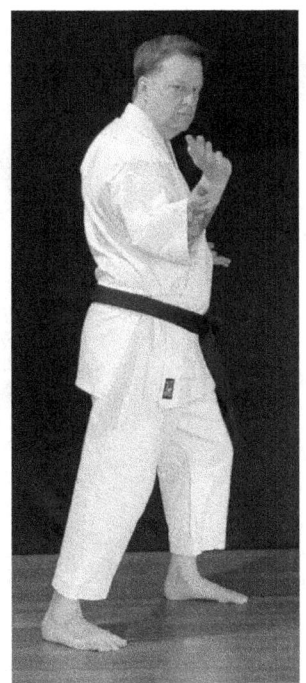 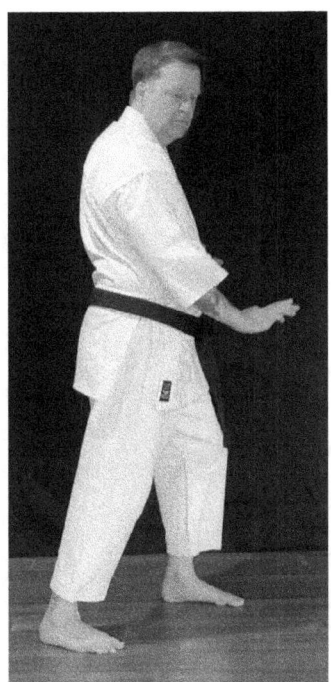

Pivot Left, Complete Right Gedan Yoko Shotei Barai (cont.)

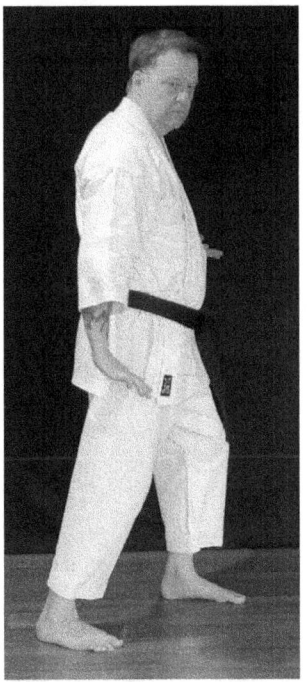 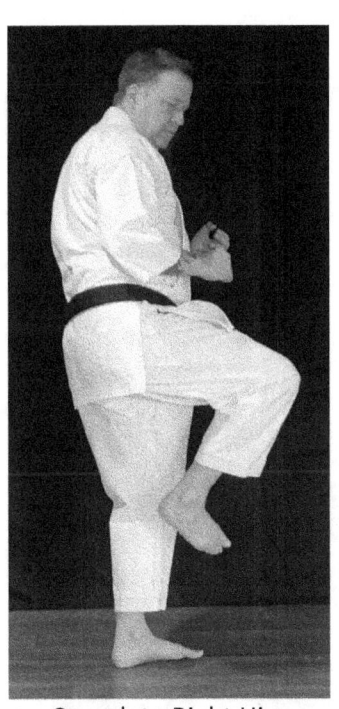

Gedan Yoko Shotei Barai (cont.)   Complete Right Hiza Geri on 45° Angle

Hon'nogeki

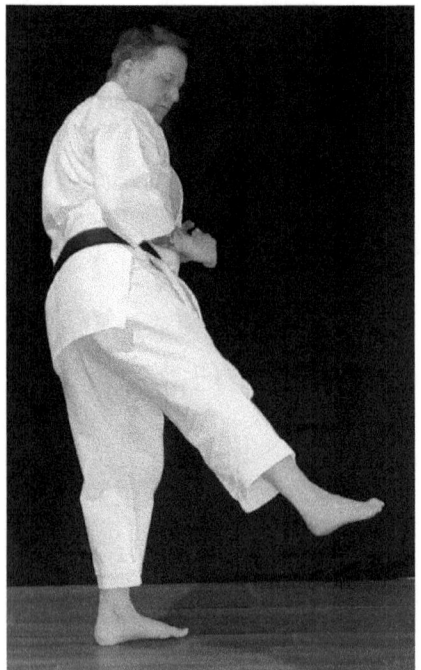

Hiza Geri (cont.)

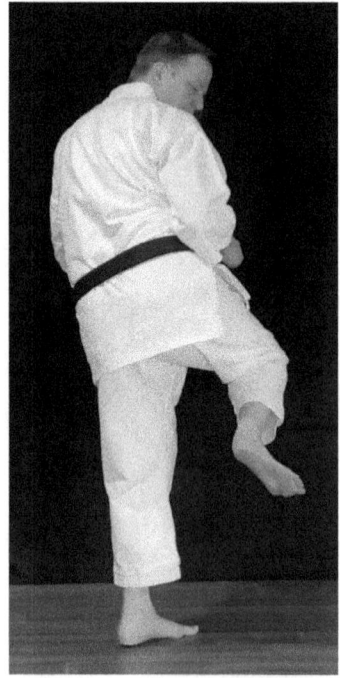

Without Putting Leg Down, Chamber Leg

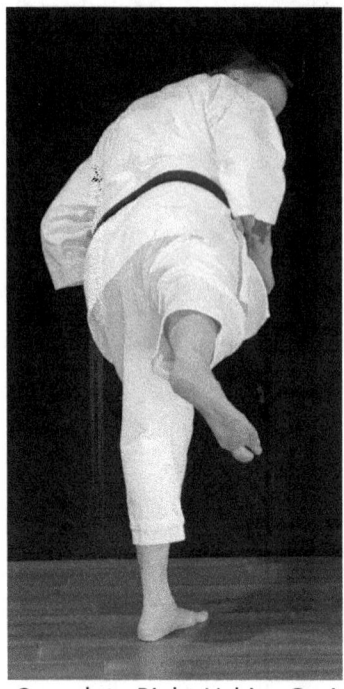

Complete Right Ushiro Geri

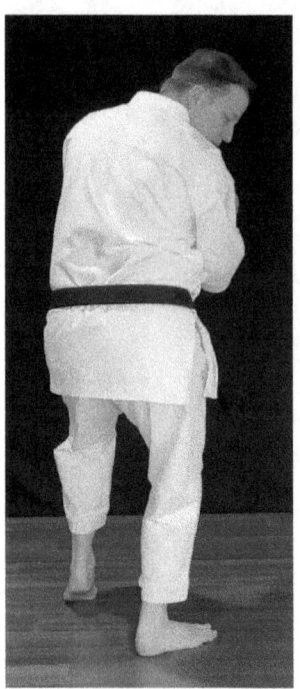

Set Back in Neko Ashi Dachi, Begin Right Ushiro Empi Uchi

Hon'nogeki

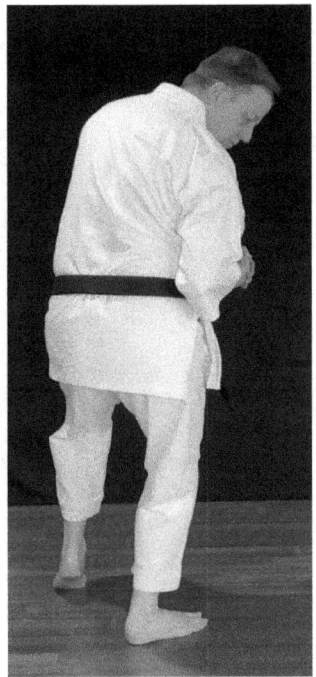
Ushiro Empi Uchi (cont.)

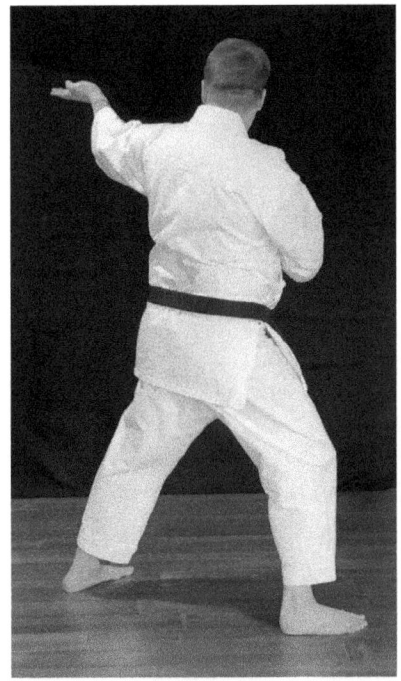
Step Out on 45° Angle in Kokustu Dachi,
Left Kake Uke on 225° Angle

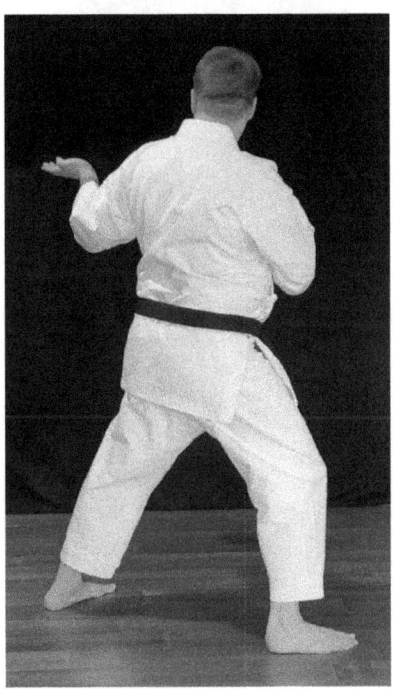
Kake Uke (cont.)

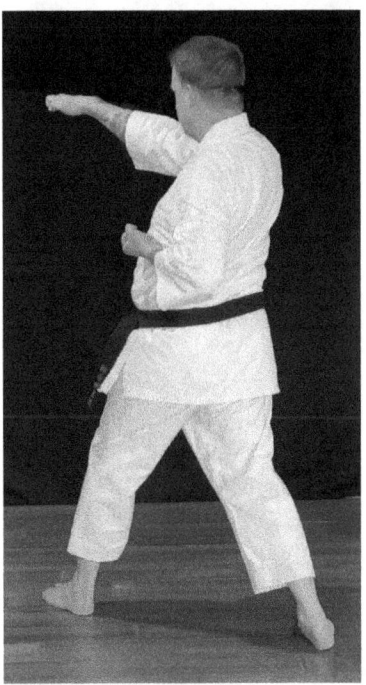
Pivot on Same Angle,
Complete Right Hiraken Uchi

Hon'nogeki

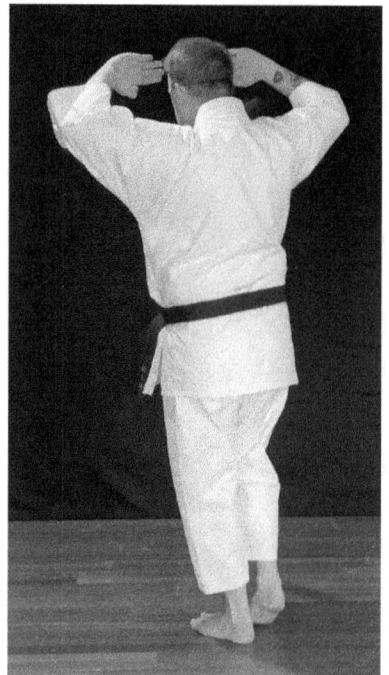 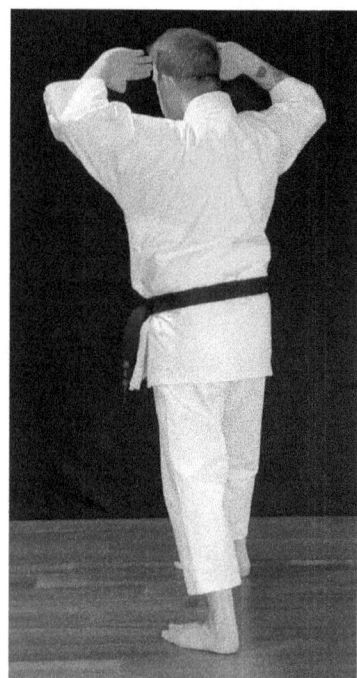

Step while Chambering for Morote Shuto Uchi

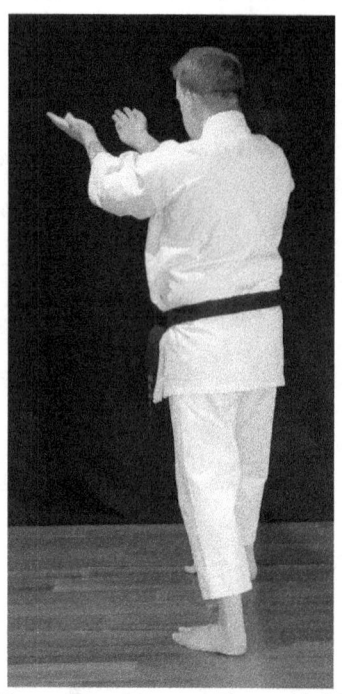 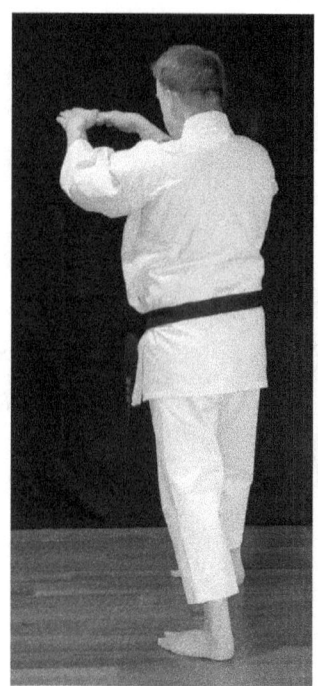

Complete Morote Shuto Uchi   Turn Palms Down

Hon'nogeki

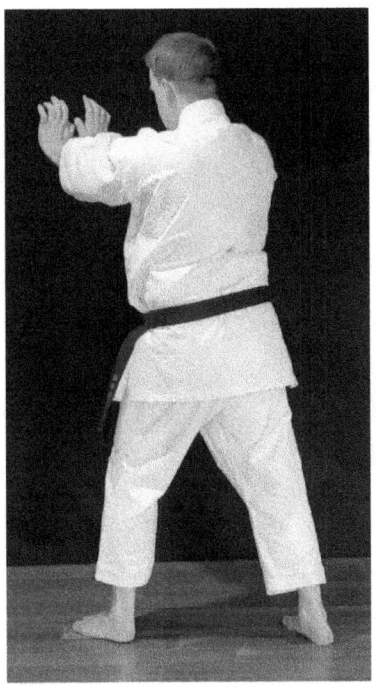
Step, Complete Morote Oshi

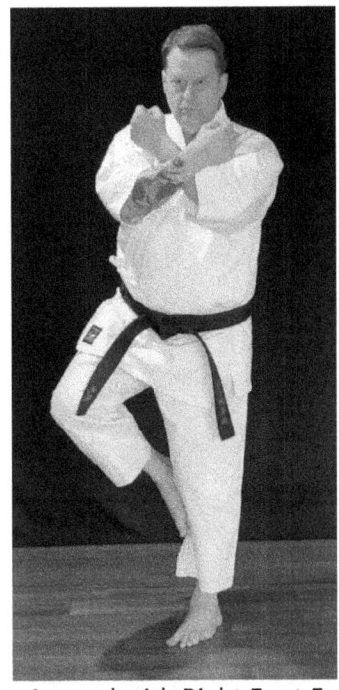
Step Around with Right Foot Facing Forward, Bring Hands Up

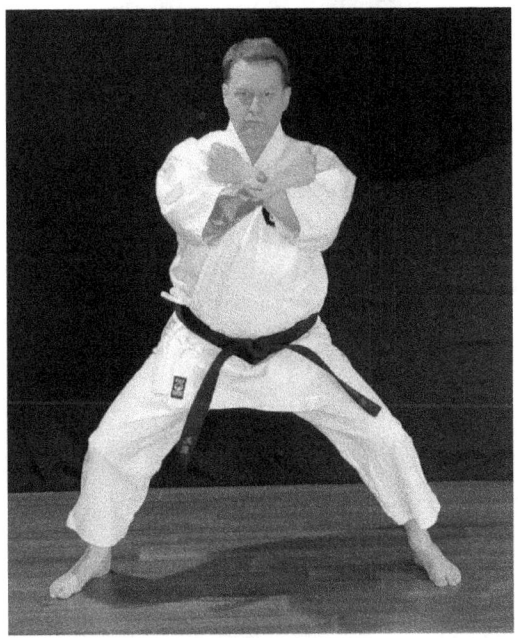
Come Down into Shiko Dachi

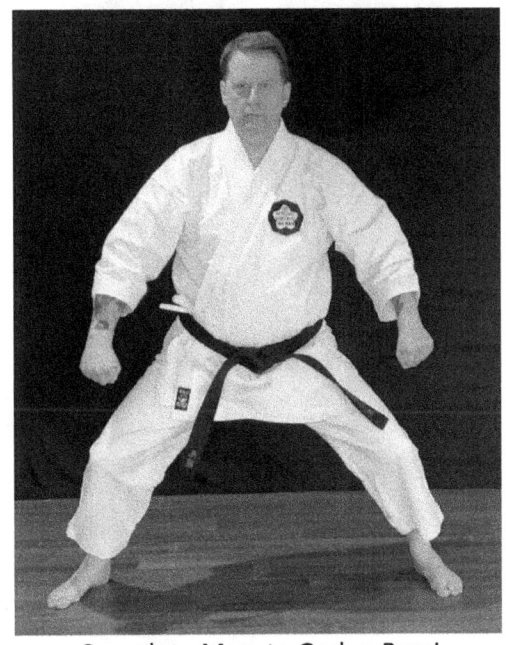
Complete Morote Gedan Barai

Hon'nogeki

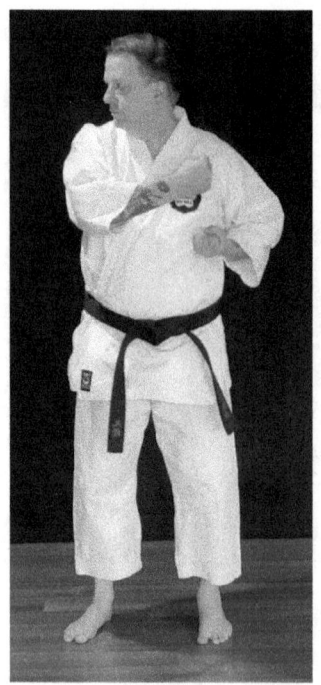 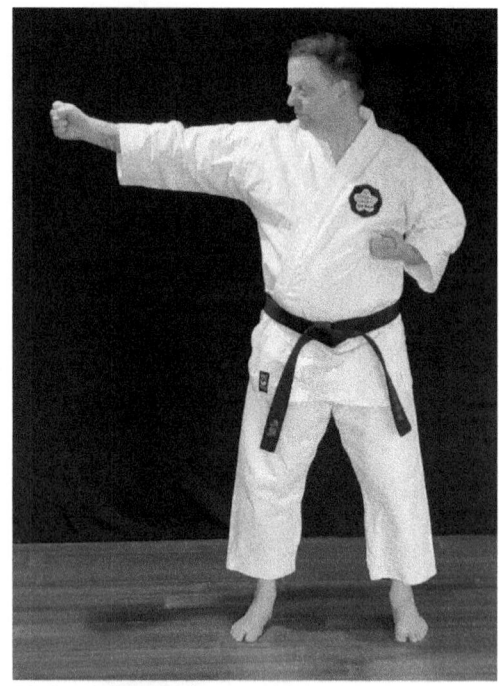

Slide Over Right, Complete Right Yoko Uraken Uchi

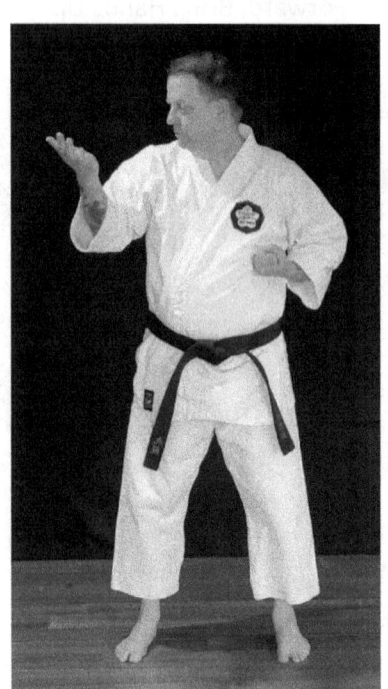 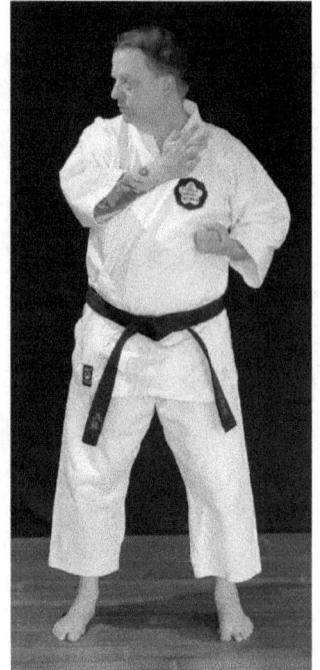

Chamber Shuto Uchi

Hon'nogeki

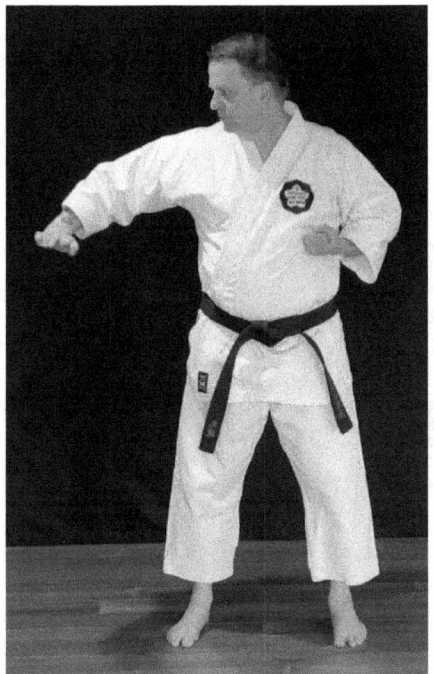
Complete Right Chudan Shuto Uchi

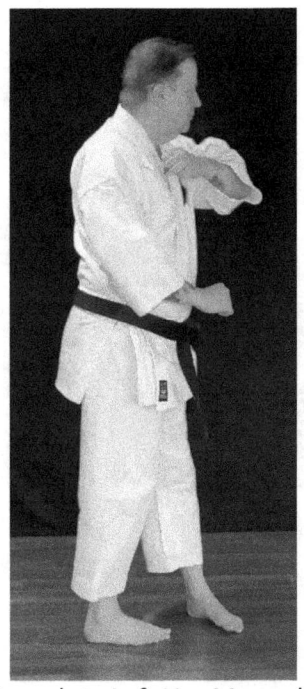
Complete Left Ura Mawashi Empi Uchi (Spinning Elbow)

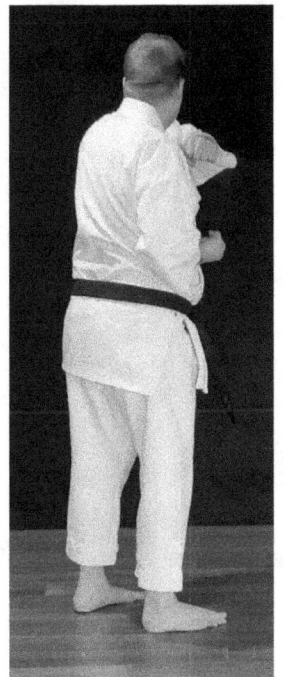
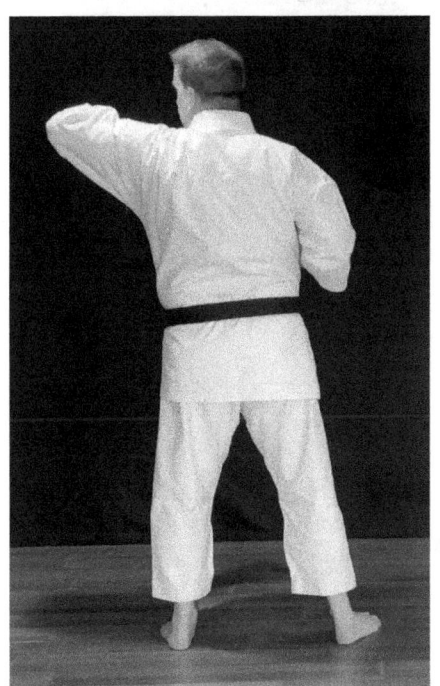
Ura Mawashi Empi Uchi (cont.)

Hon'nogeki

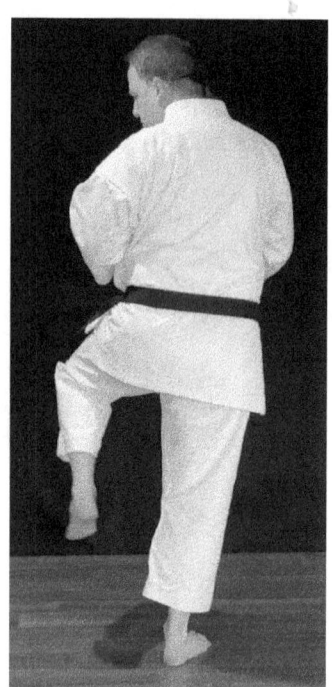
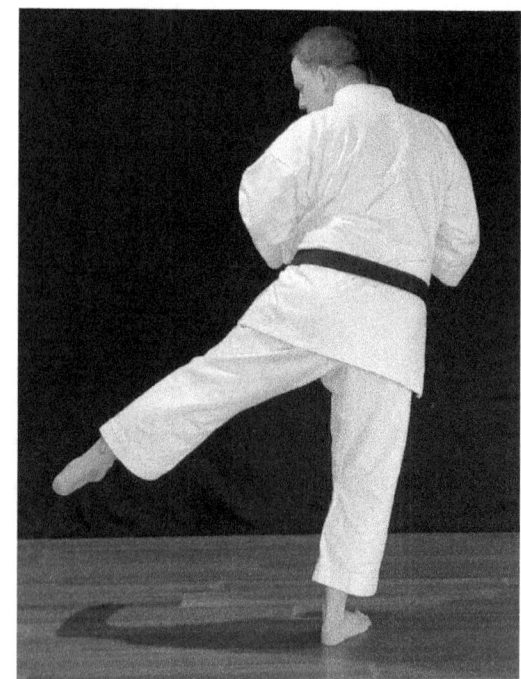

Complete Left Hiza Geri

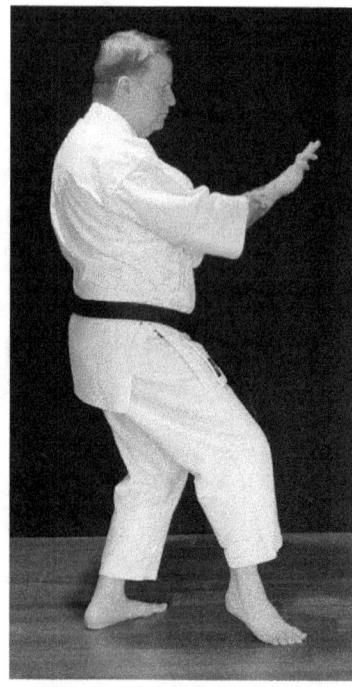

Set in Neko Ashi Dachi
Facing 90°

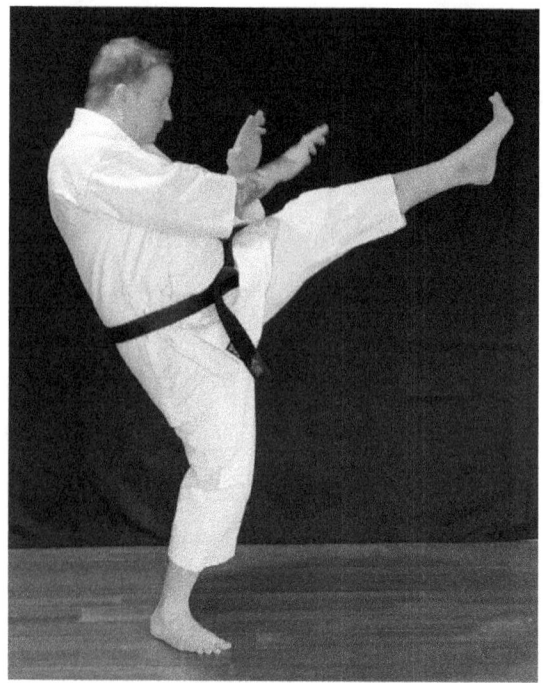

Complete Right Jodan Mae Keage Geri

Hon'nogeki

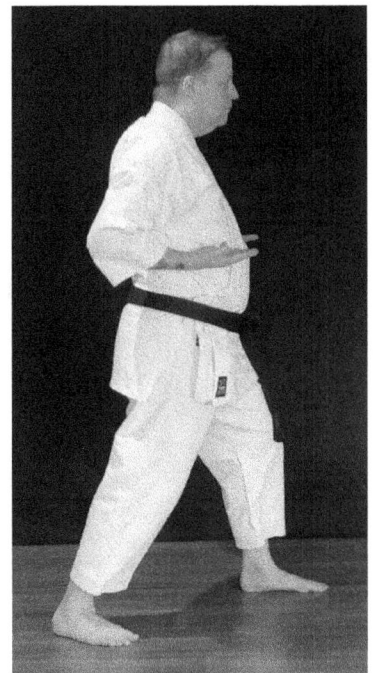 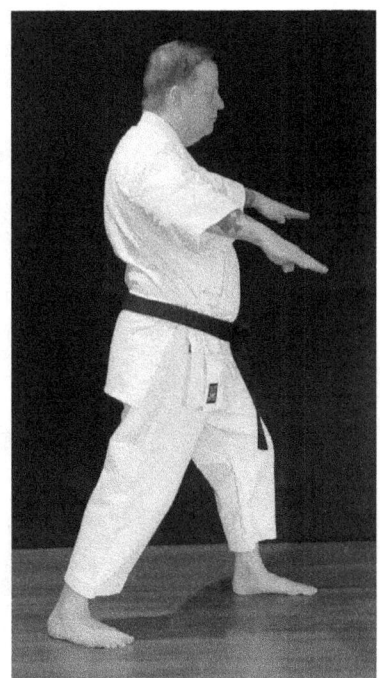

Land Kick, then Complete Morote Haito Uchi

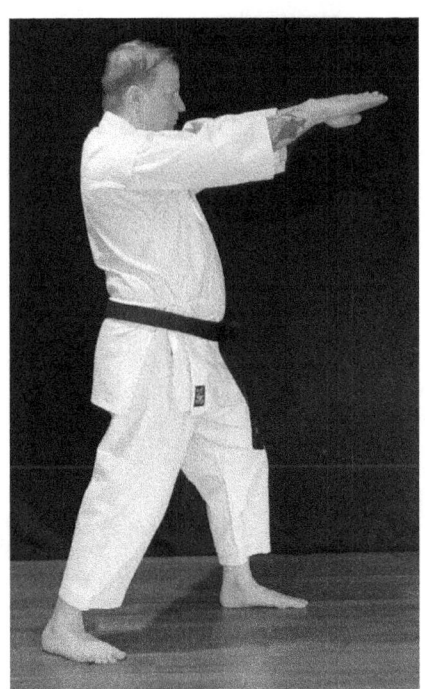 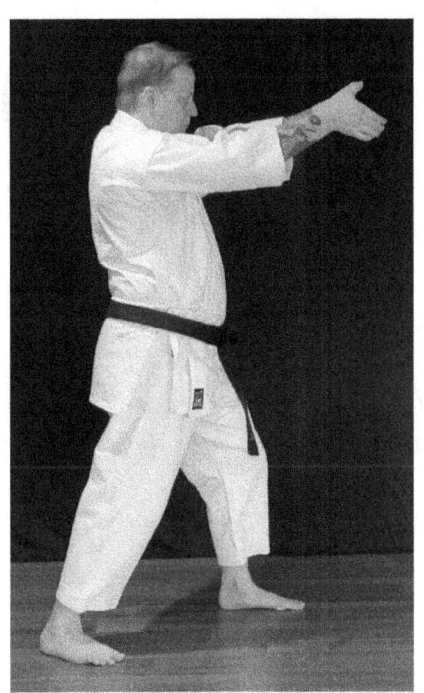

Morote Haito Uchi (cont.)   Turn Both Hands, Thumbs Up

Hon'nogeki

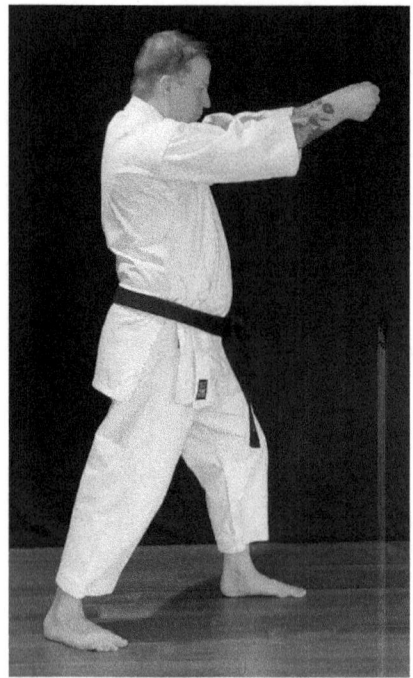
Close Hands

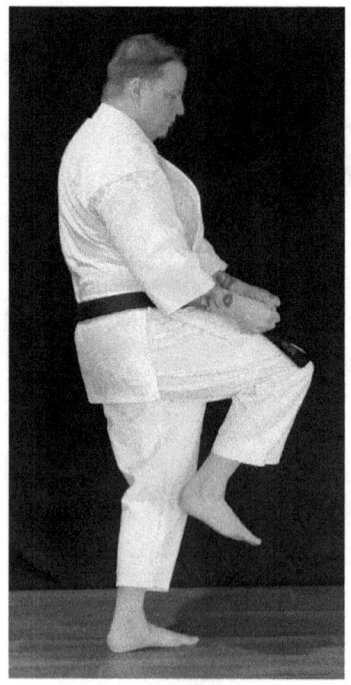
Complete Right Hiza Uchi

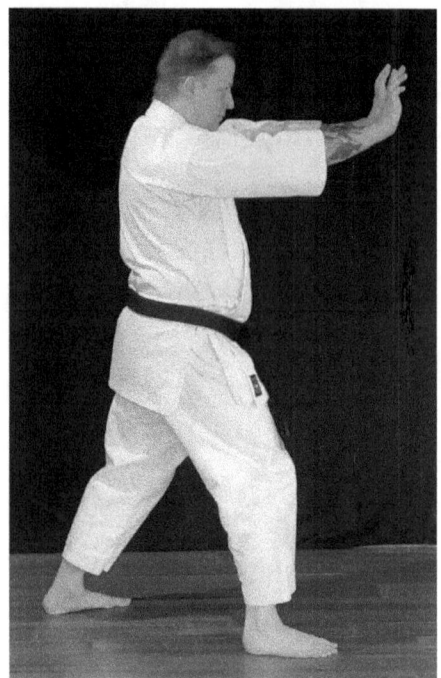
Step, Complete Morote Oshi

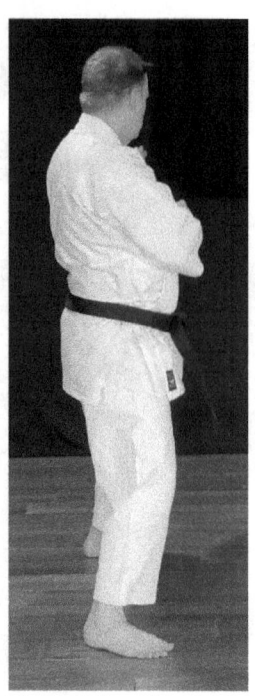
Bring Left Leg Up and Set Facing Rear, Open Hands

Hon'nogeki

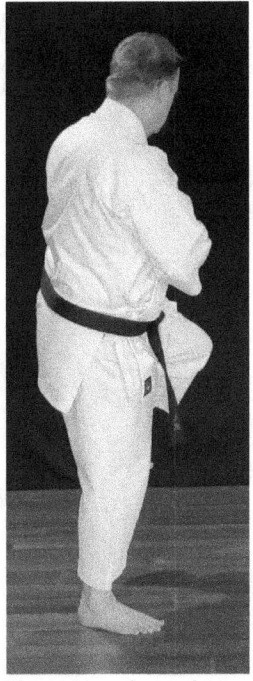
Close Hands and Hop Up for Hiza Geri

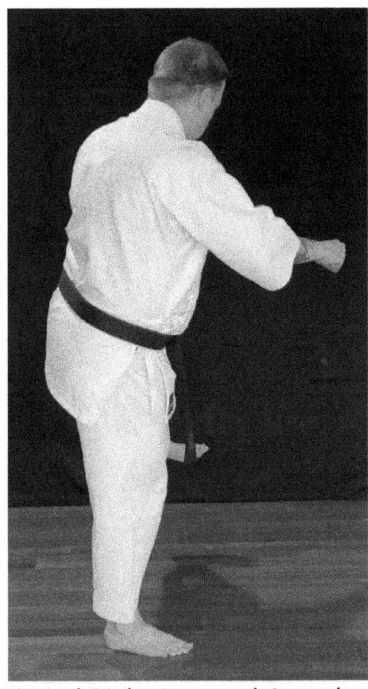
Extend Right Arm and Complete Left Hiza Geri

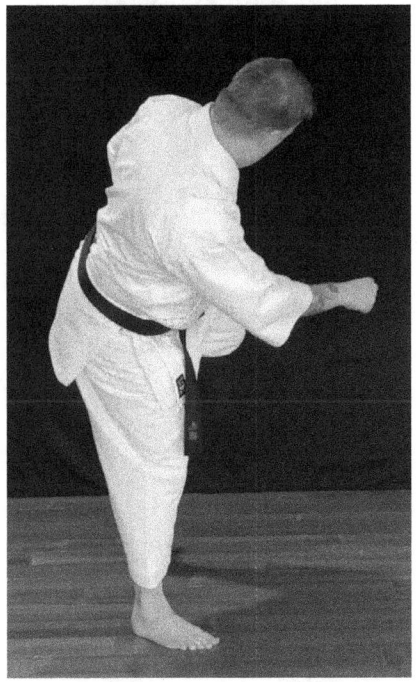

Without Putting Left Leg Down, Complete Left Kake Geri – Mid Height

Hon'nogeki

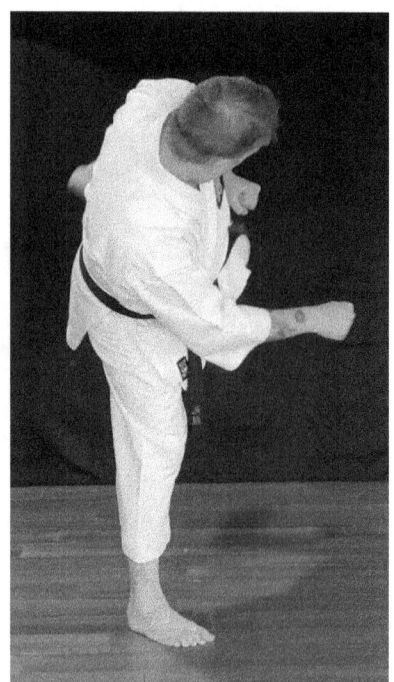 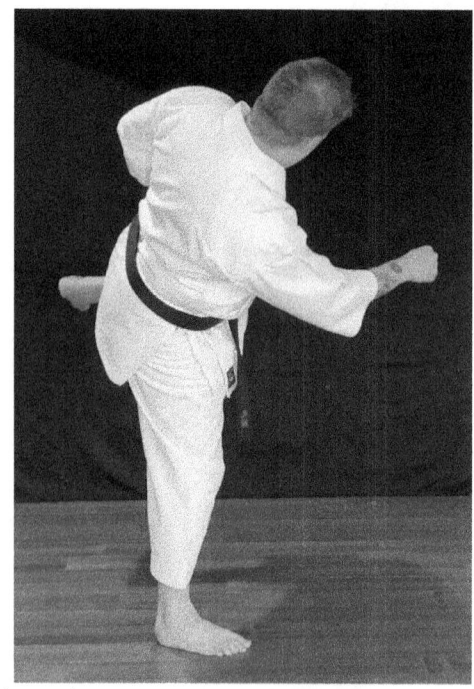

Kake Geri (cont.)

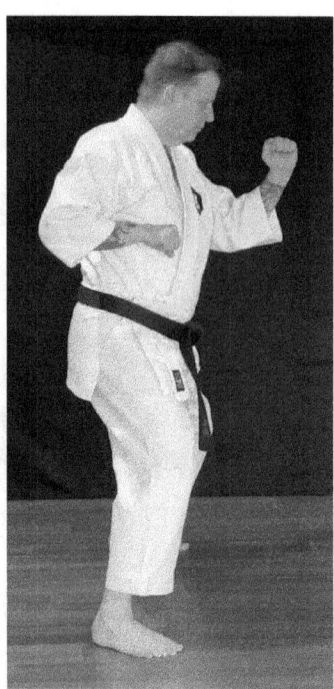

Come Down while Completing Left Kote Uchi and Bringing Right Hand to Chamber, Palm Down (kiai)

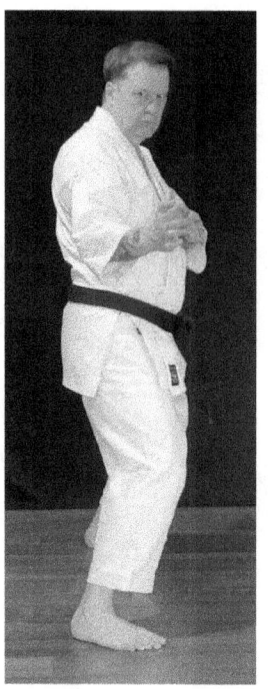

Move Hands to Set Facing Front, Open Hands

Hon'nogeki

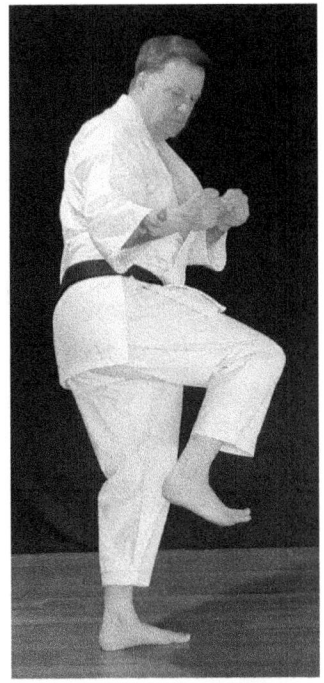
Close Hands and Hop Up for Hiza Geri

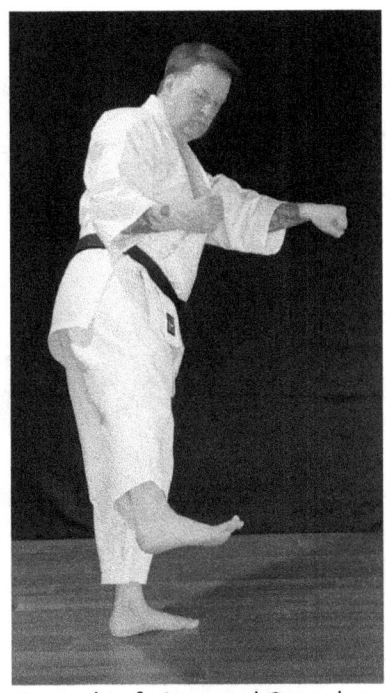
Extend Left Arm and Complete Right Hiza Geri

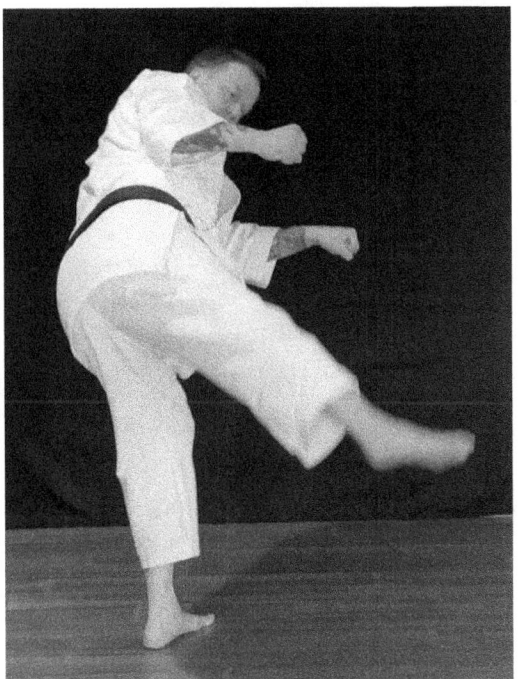
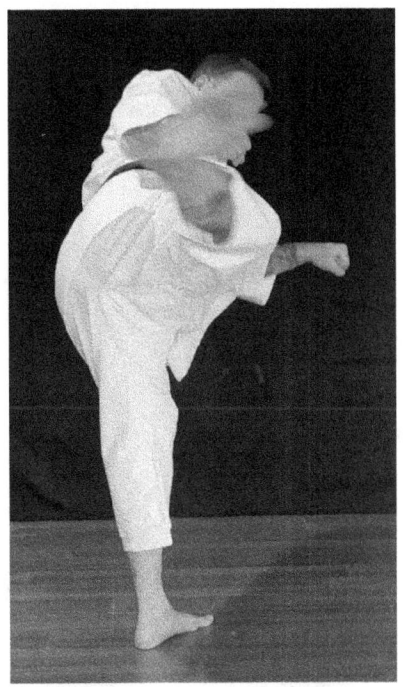
Without Putting Right Leg Down, Complete Right Kake Geri – Mid height

Hon'nogeki

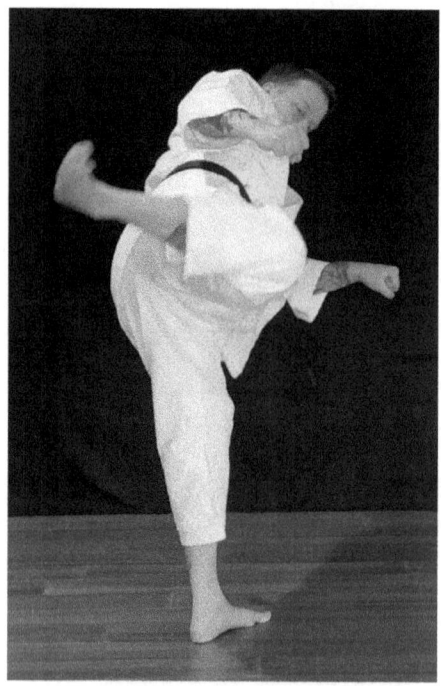
Kake Geri (cont.)

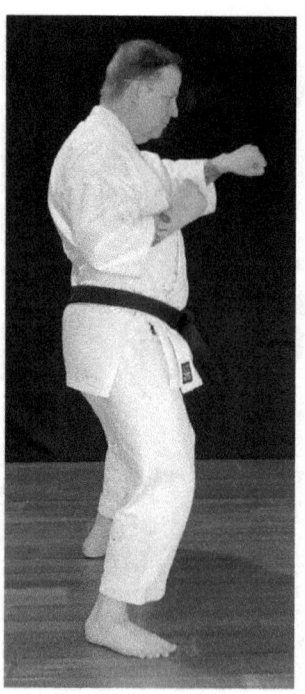
Come Down while Completing Right Kote Uchi and Bringing Right Hand to Chamber, Palm Down (kiai)

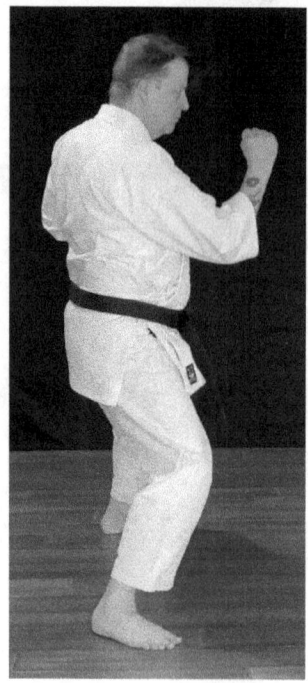
Complete Kote Uchi (kiai) (cont.)

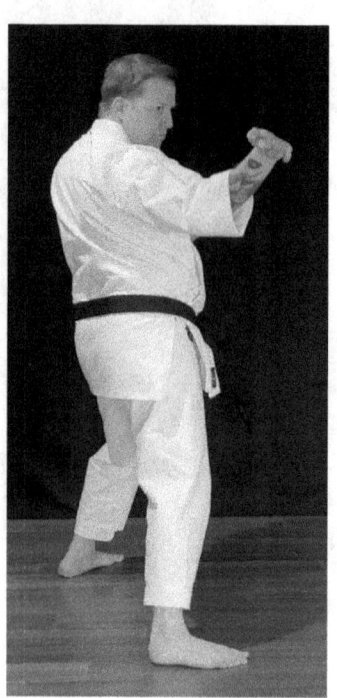
Step on 225° Angle in Kokustu Dachi, Kake Uke on 45° Angle

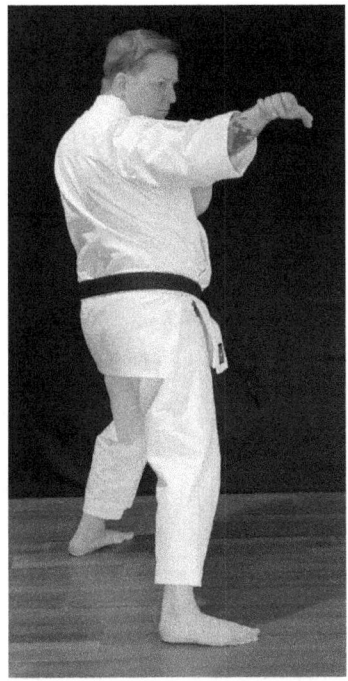

Complete Right Hiki Uke

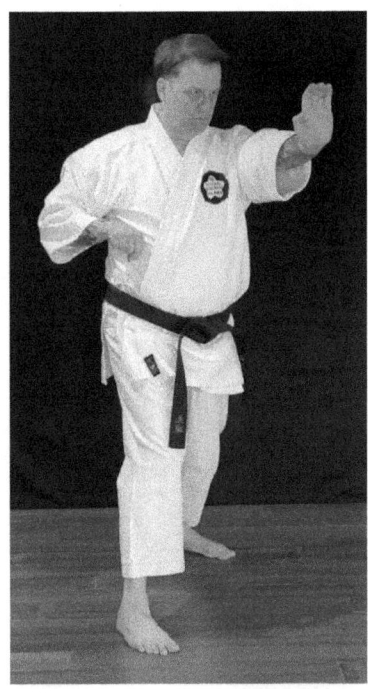

Pivot on 45° Angle while Pulling Right Hand Back into Chamber, Complete Left Shotei Uchi

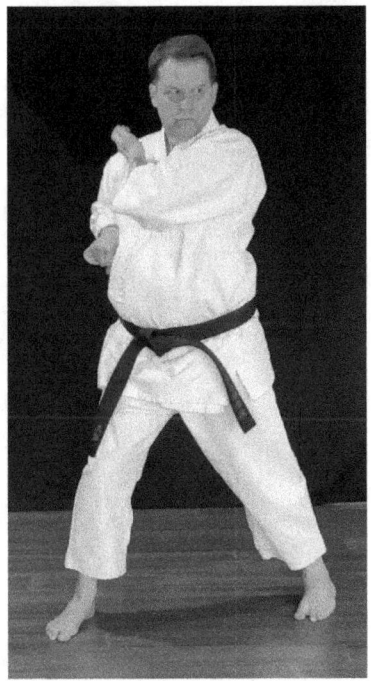

Step on 315° Angle in Kokutsu Dachi, Chamber Right Hand to Shuto Uchi, Looking Left

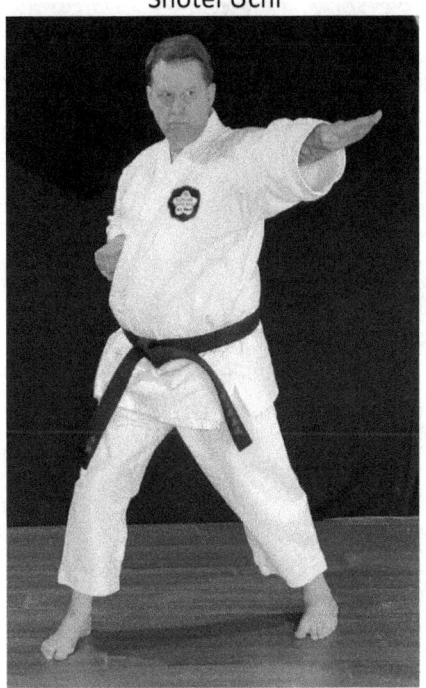

Complete Yoko Shuto Uchi at 45° Angle

Hon'nogeki

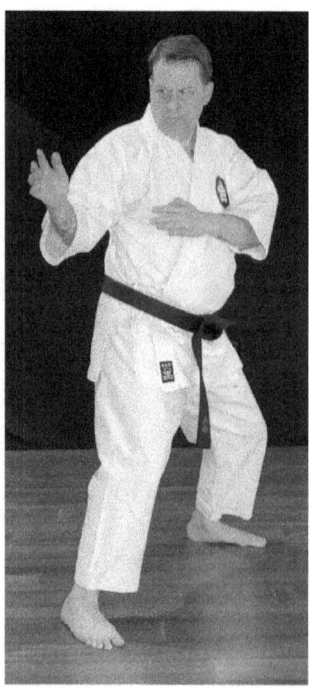
Bring Right Foot Up to Fighting Stance

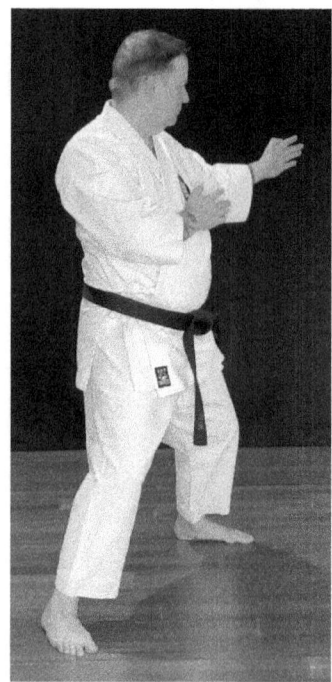
Move Hands to Set Facing 135°

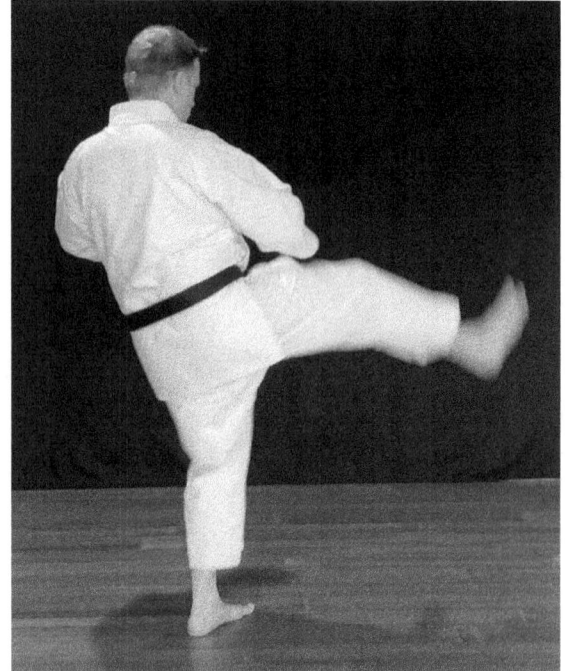

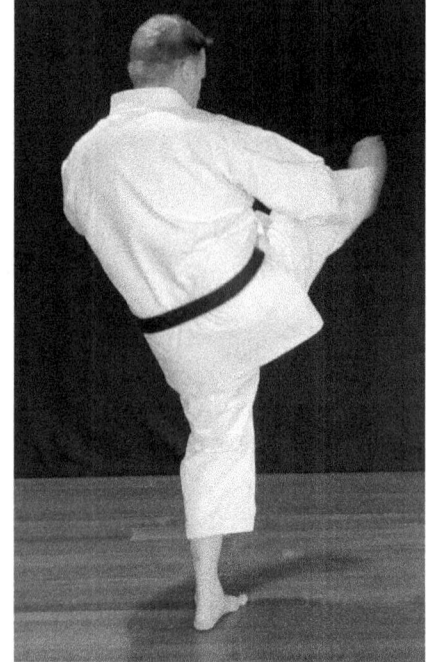

Complete Right Mikazuki Geri

Hon'nogeki

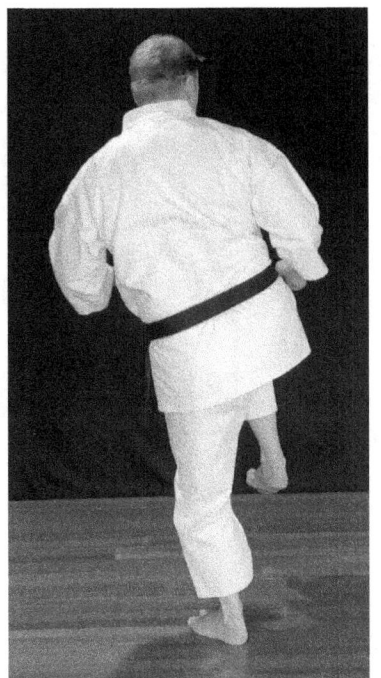

Mikazuki Geri (cont.)

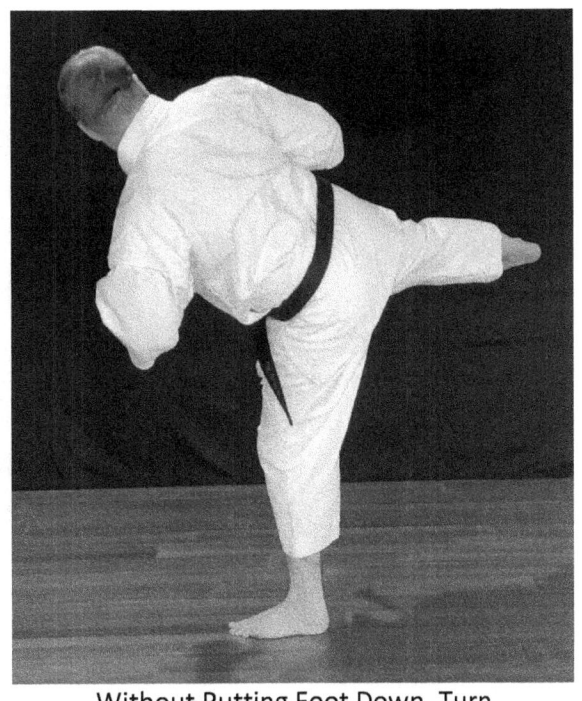

Without Putting Foot Down, Turn Kick into Right Chudan Yoko Keage Geri

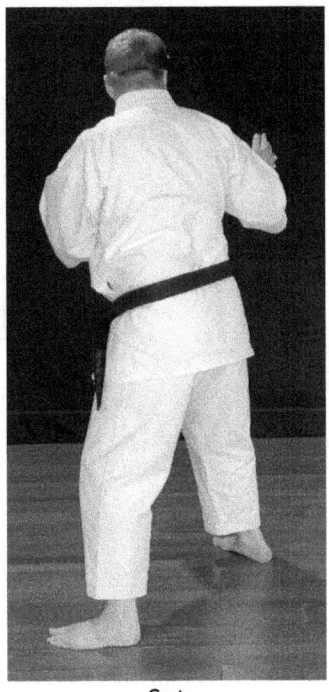

Set

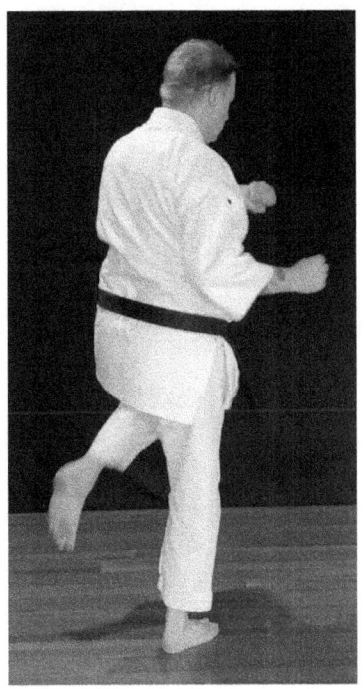

Complete Left Gedan Mawashi Geri

Hon'nogeki

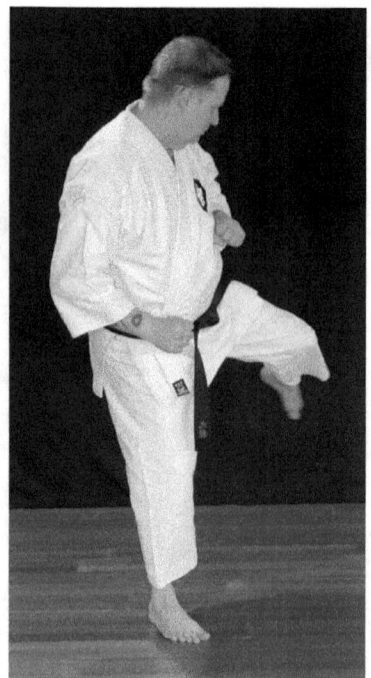
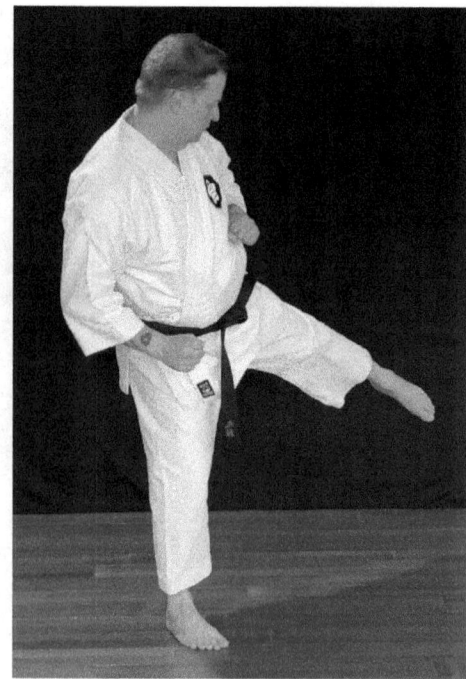

Gedan Mawashi Geri (cont.)

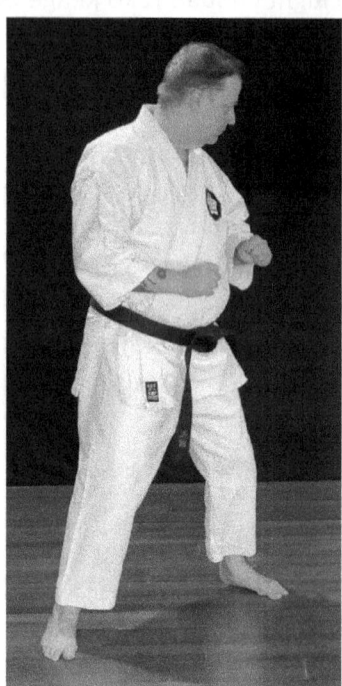

Set

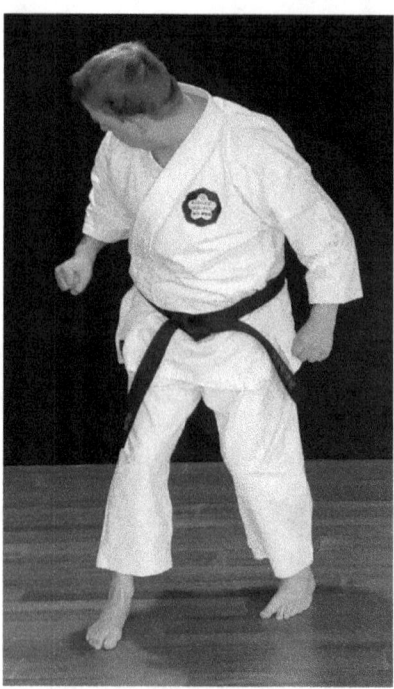

Pivot on Left Foot, Complete
Ushiro Mawashi Geri

Hon'nogeki

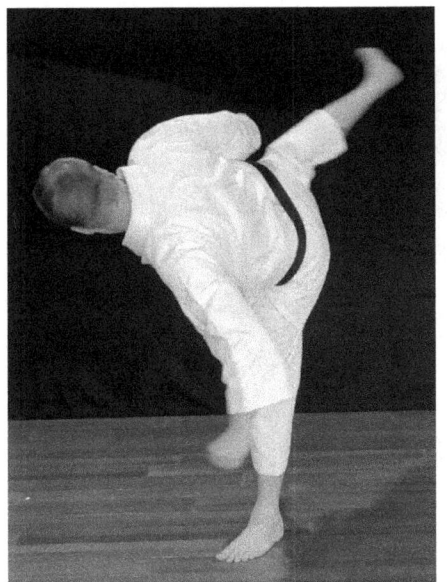
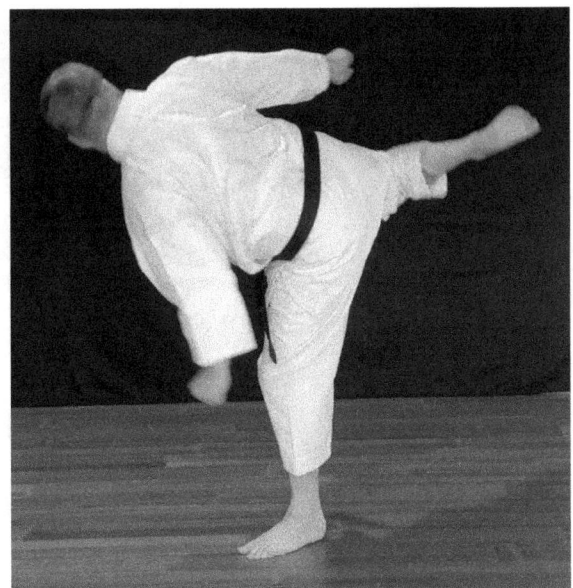

Ushiro Mawashi Geri (cont.)

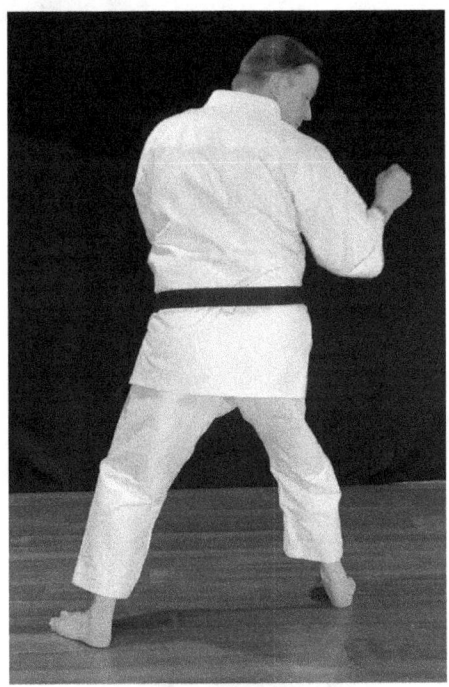

Look Over Right Shoulder

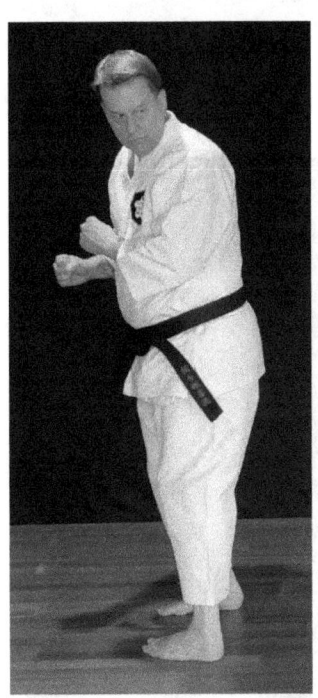

Slide Right Foot Over Left

Hon'nogeki

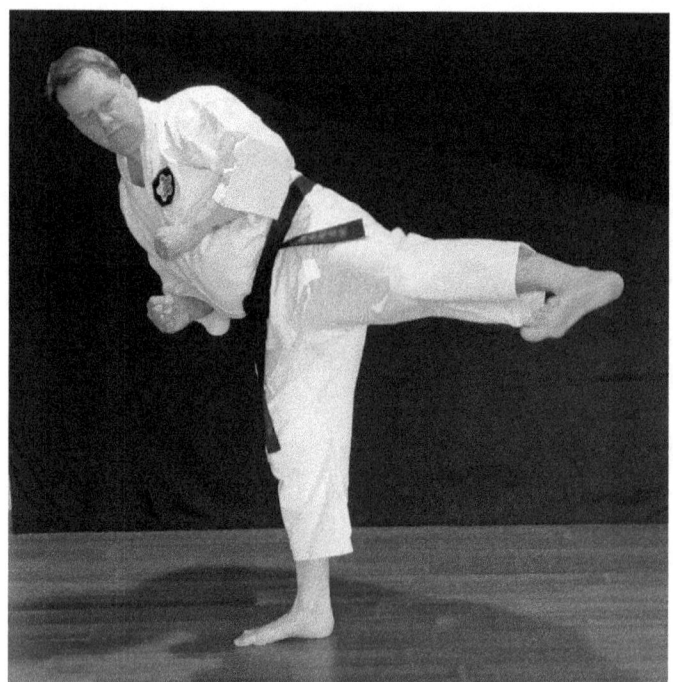
Complete Left Chudan Yoko Keage Geri on 45° Angle

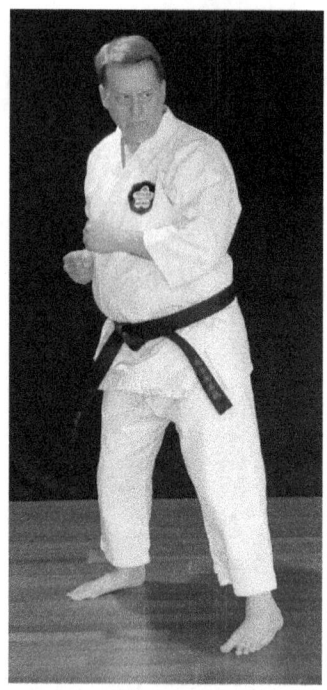
Set

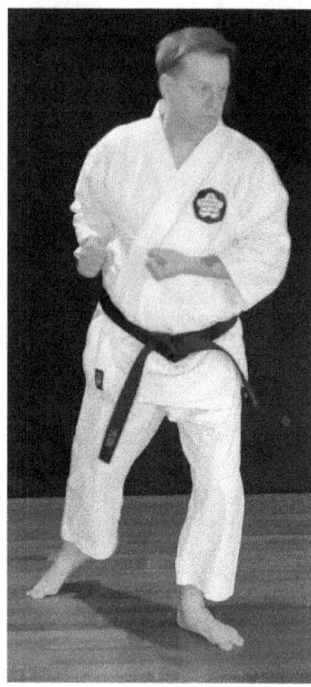

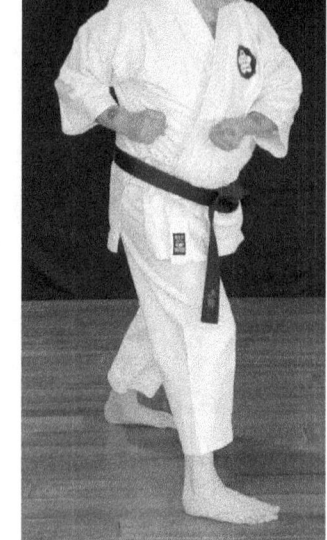

Step Around on Angle, Prepare for Empi Uchi

Hon'nogeki

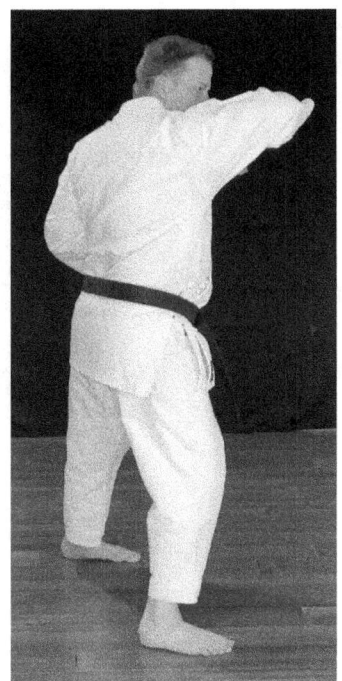
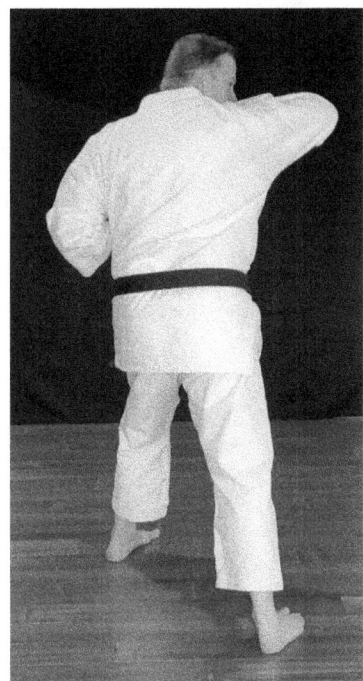

Complete Left Jodan Empi Uchi and Land Facing Rear

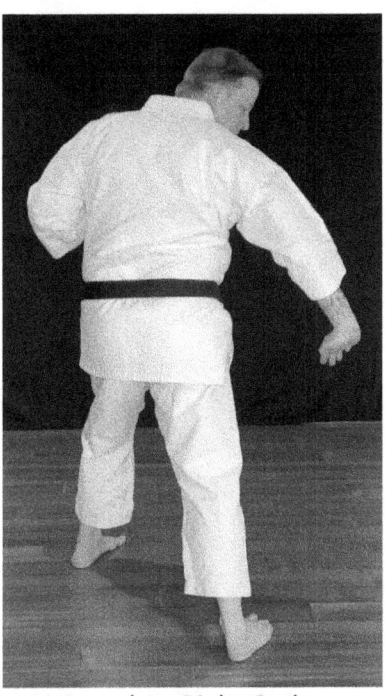
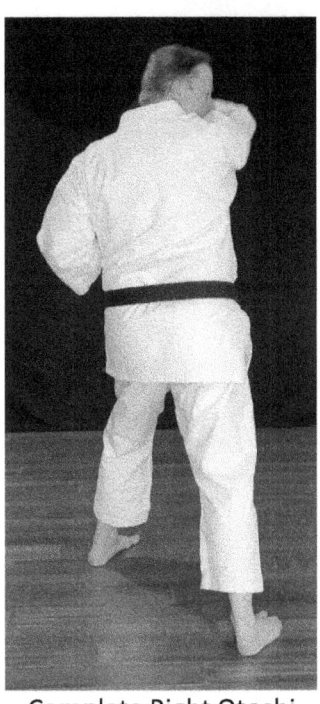

Complete Right Gedan
Shotei Uchi on 45° Angle

Complete Right Otoshi
Tettsui Uchi

Hon'nogeki

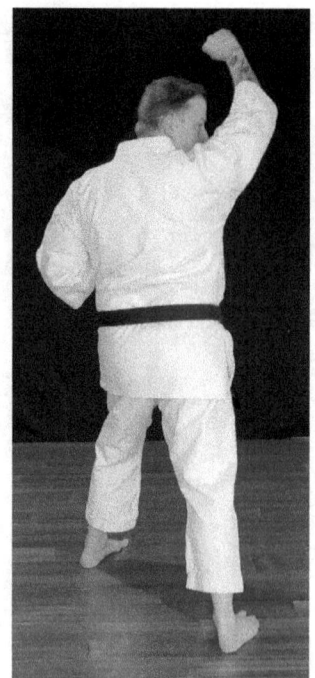 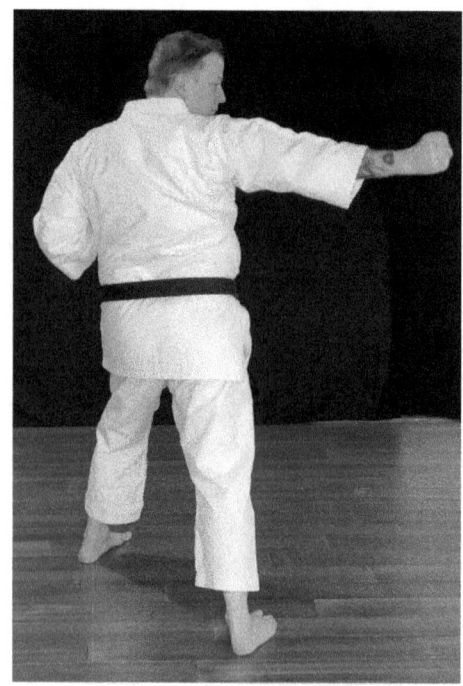

Otoshi Tettsui Uchi (cont.)

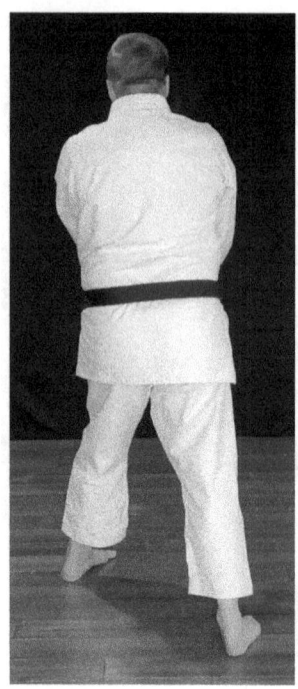 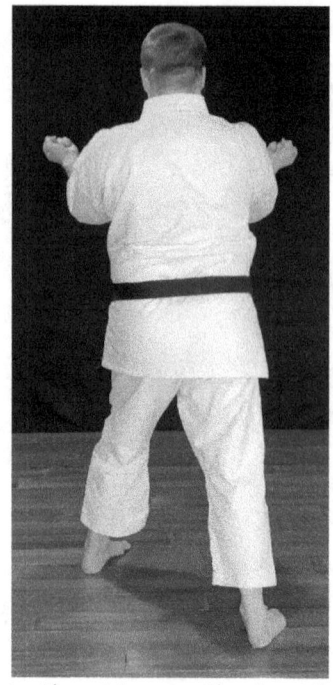

Pivot Towards Rear in Sanchin Dachi, Complete Slow Morote Chudan Uke

Hon'nogeki

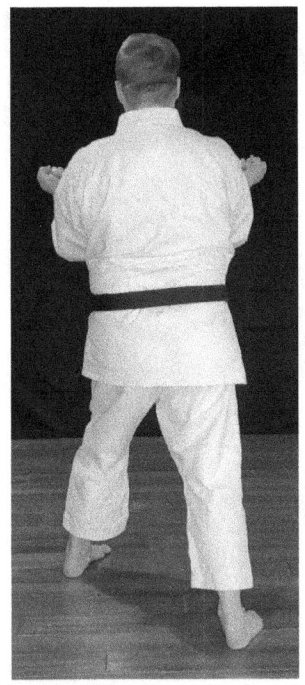
Morote Chudan Uke (cont.)

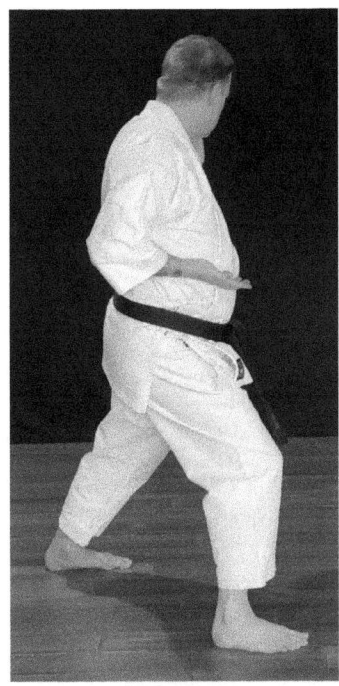
Pivot Left

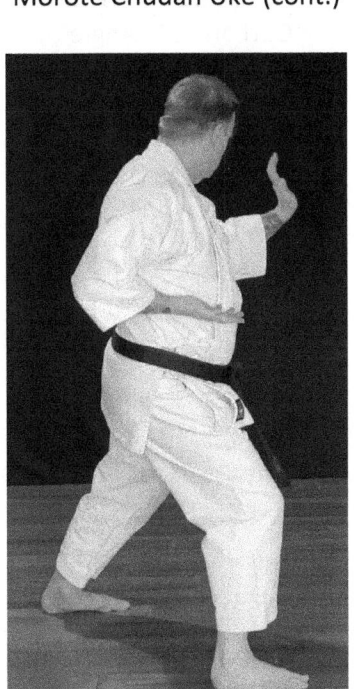
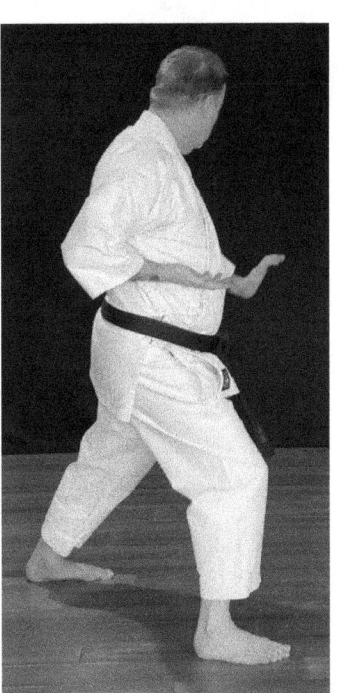
Complete Left Gedan Yoko Shotei Barai

Hon'nogeki

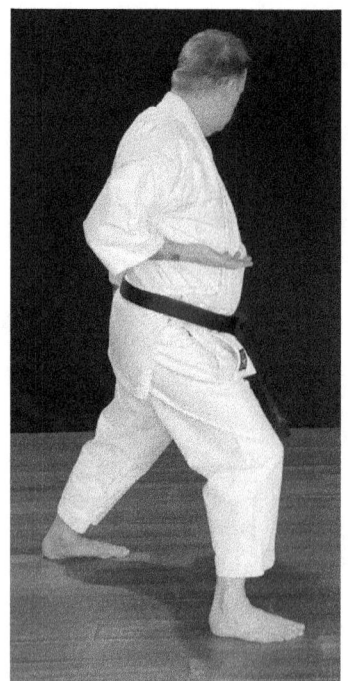
Gedan Yoko Shotei Barai (cont.)

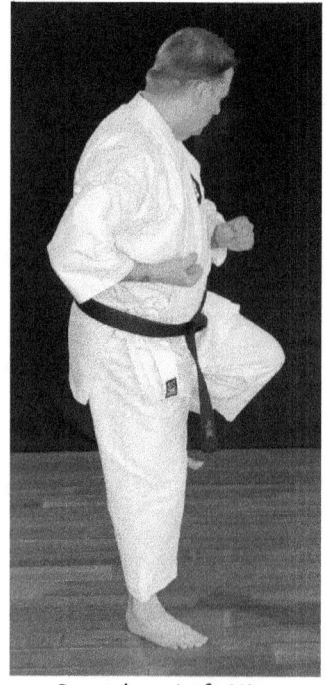
Complete Left Hiza Geri on 135° Angle

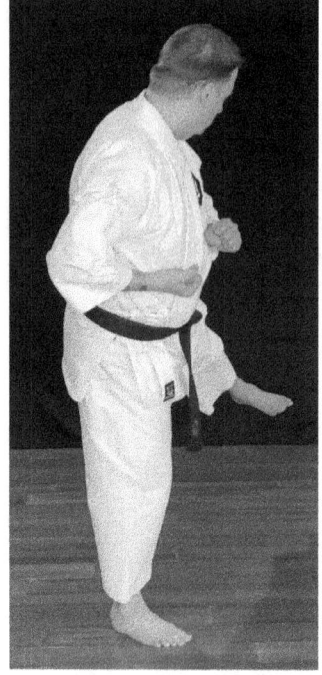
Hiza Geri (cont.)

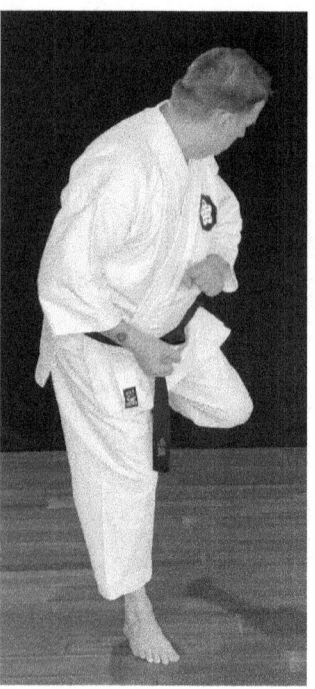
Without Putting Leg Down, Chamber

Hon'nogeki

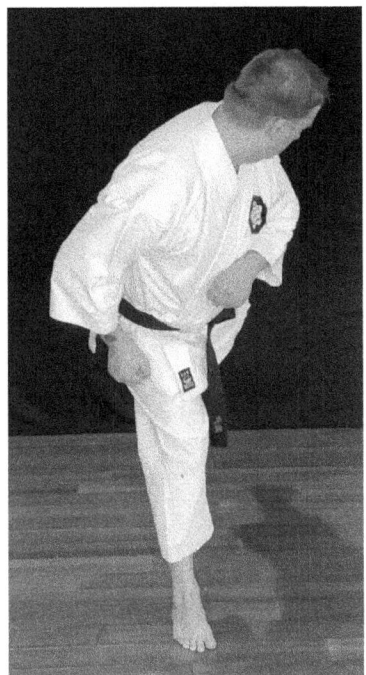

Complete Left Ushiro Geri

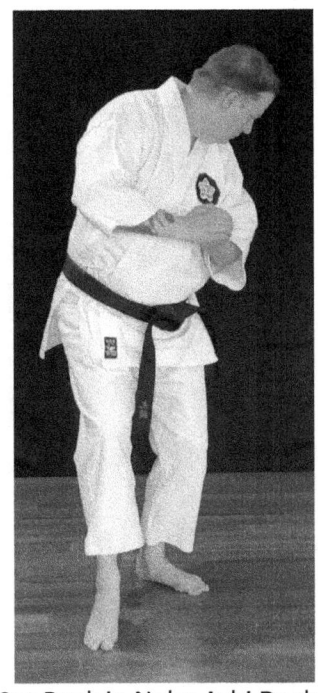

Set Back in Neko Ashi Dachi,
Begin Left Ushiro Empi Uchi

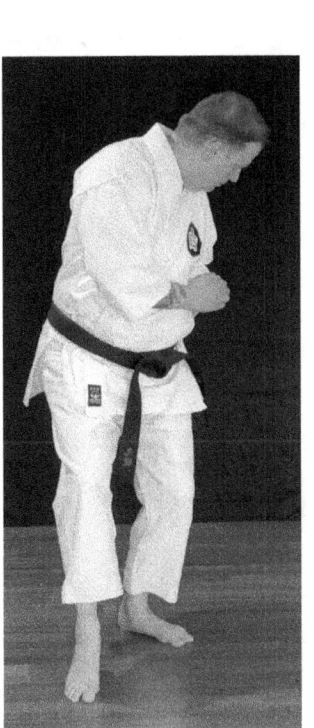

Ushiro Empi Uchi (cont.)

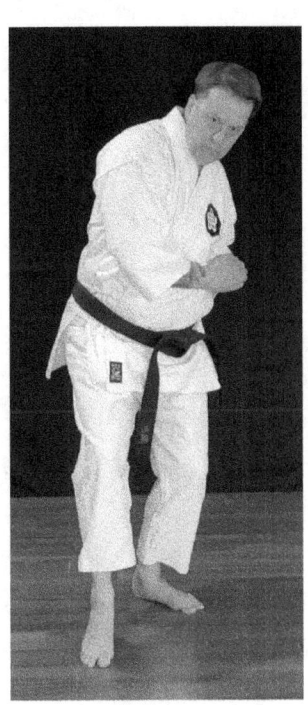

Look Forward

Hon'nogeki

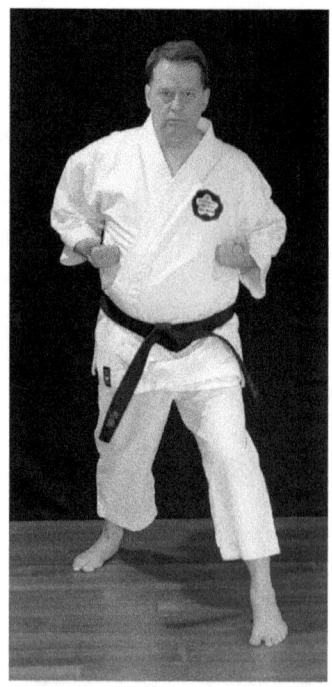
Step Back with Right Foot into Zenkutsu Dachi, Chamber Both Hands

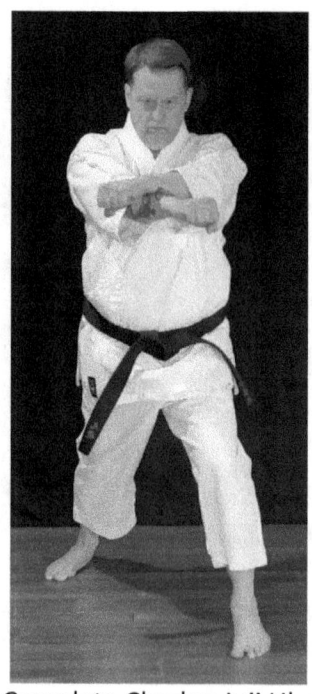
Complete Chudan Juji Uke

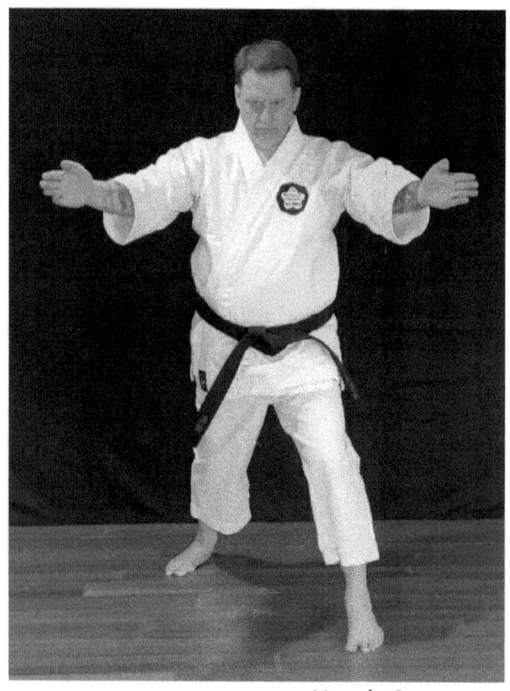

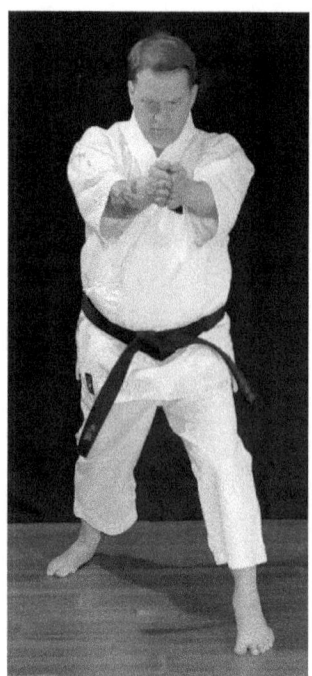

Hands Separate and Come Together

Hon'nogeki

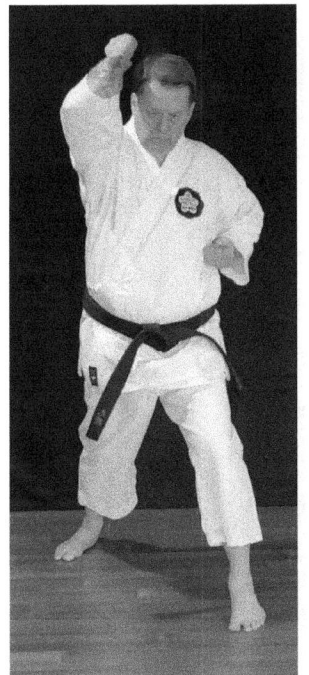 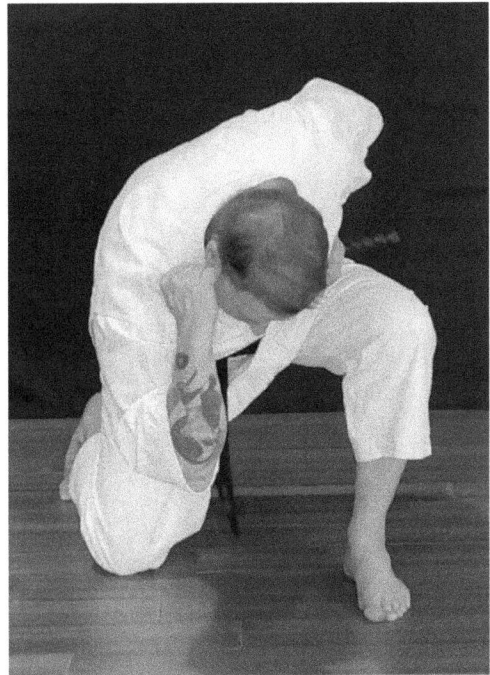

Lift Right Elbow Up, Otoshi Empi Uchi, Land on Right Knee (kiai)

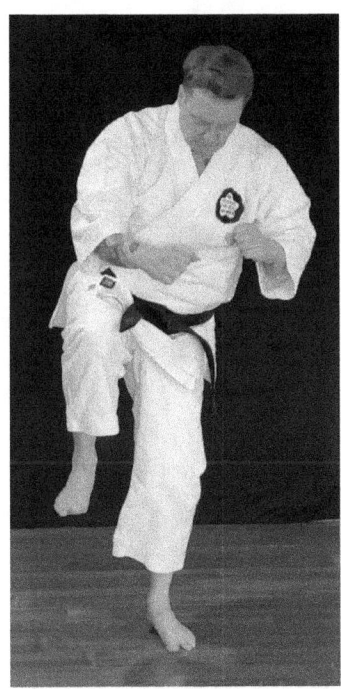 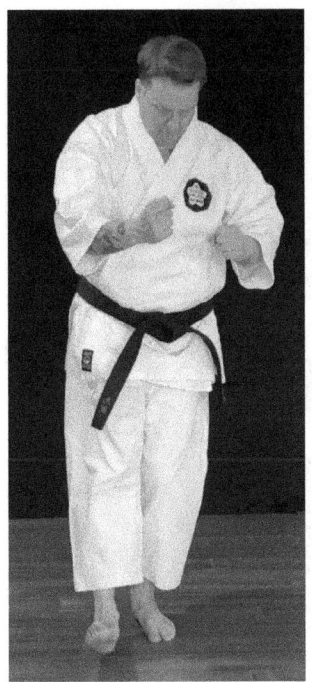

Stand Up, Complete Right Otoshi Kakato Geri

Hon'nogeki

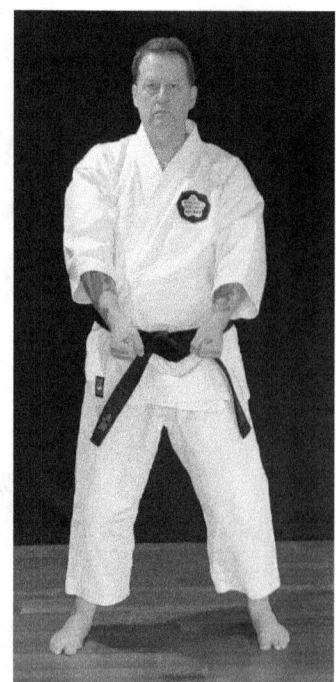
Heiko Dachi

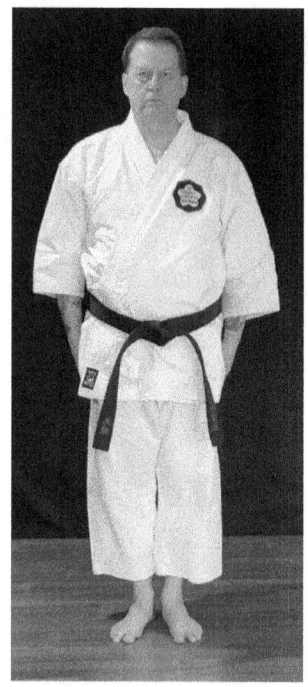
Musubi Dachi

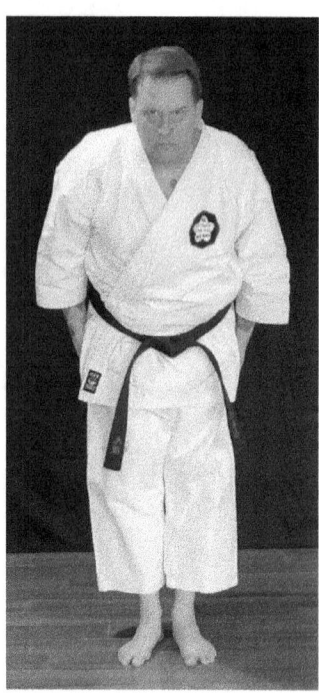
Rei

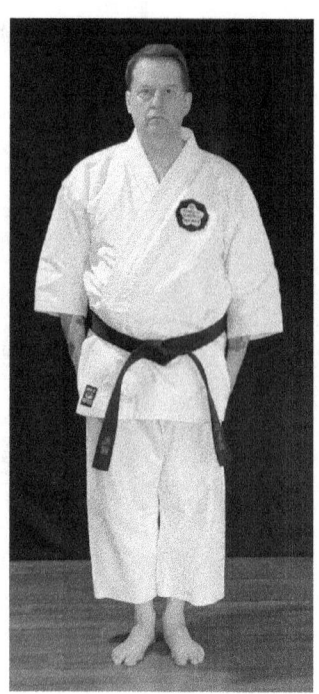
Musubi Dachi

Hon'nogeki

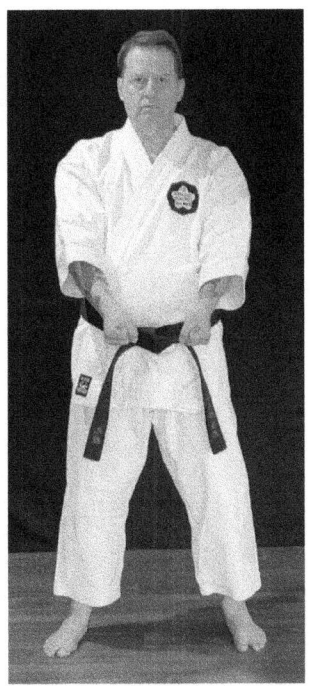

Heiko Dachi

Genshin

Genshin means "destroy defeat." Shodai created this as an early tournament kata. Genshin is a moderately long kata that includes the side kick-back fist combination ending in an otoshi tettsui uchi. It also contains the double shuto uchi from shiko dachi move in Kururunfa.

Below is the method by which Ketsugo Goju-Ryu performs Genshin kata. Complete details about each move are not included, as this is simply a demonstration.

These are the Japanese terms used for this kata. Bear in mind, karate terms are not completely streamlined. There are terms that were used in the middle of the 20th Century that are no longer used today. Oftentimes there are more than one term that can be used for the same technique. The important thing is not what it is called, but the technique itself.

Age – Rising	**Mae** – Front
Ashi Barai – Leg Sweep	**Mawashi Geri** – Roundhouse Kick
Barai - Sweeping Block	**Morote** – Double
Chudan - Middle	**Musubi Dachi** - Attention Stance, Toes Out
Dachi – Stance	
Empi – Elbow	**Neko Ashi Dachi** - Cat Leg Stance
Fumikomi Geri – Stamping Kick	**Odeko Ate** – Head Butt
Gedan – Low	**Otoshi** - Dropping (Downward)
Geri - Kick	**Rei** – Bow (Respect)
Hajime – Command to Begin	**Shiko Dachi** - Straddle Leg Stance
Hari Uke – Open Hand Block (Palm Up)	**Shuto Uchi** – Chop Strike
Heiko Dachi - Parallel Stance	**Tettsui Uchi** – Hammer Fist Strike
Hiki Uke – Open Hand Block (Palm Down)/Pulling Block	**Tsuki/-Zuki** - Punch
	Uchi – Strike
Hiraken - Second Knuckles Fist	**Uke** – Block (Receive)

Hiza Geri – Strike (To the Knee) **Hiza Uchi** – Strike (Using the Knee) **Jodan** – High **Juji Uke** – X Block **Keage Geri** – Snap Kick **Kote Uchi** – Forearm Strike	**Ura Zuki** – Inverted Punch **Uraken Uchi** – Back Fist Strike **Ushiro** – Rear (Back) **Ushiro Mawashi Geri** – Spinning Hook Kick **Yoi** – Ready Command **Yoko** - Side **Zenkutsu Dachi** - Forward Leaning Stance

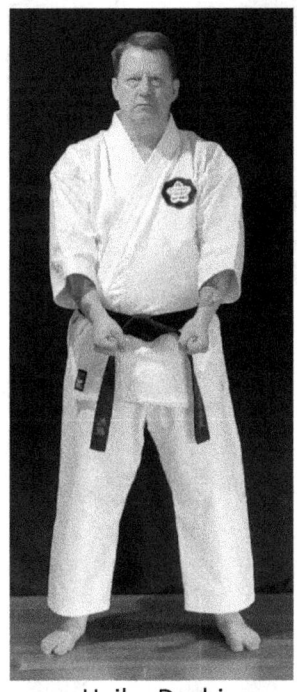

Heiko Dachi

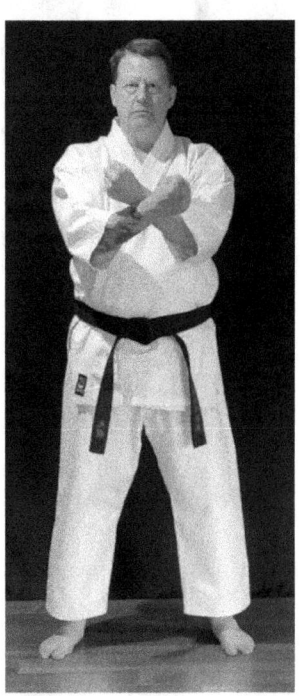

(Yoi) Brings Arms Up, Crossed at the Wrist

Genshin

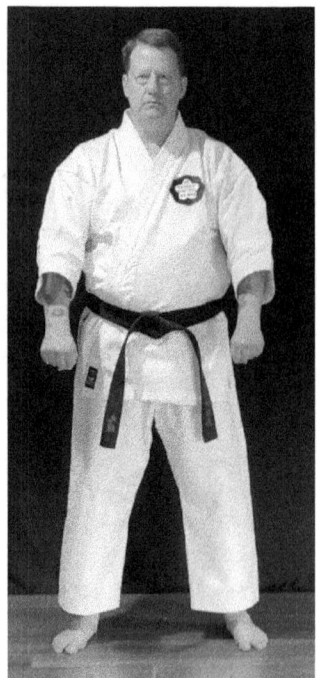
Bring Arms Down

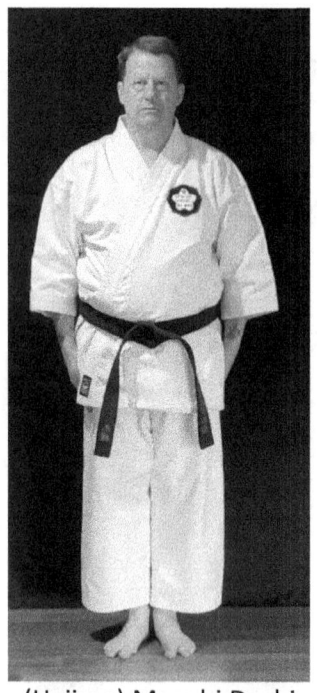
(Hajime) Musubi Dachi

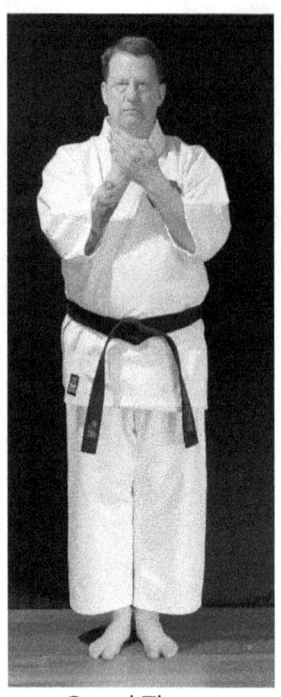
Guard Throat

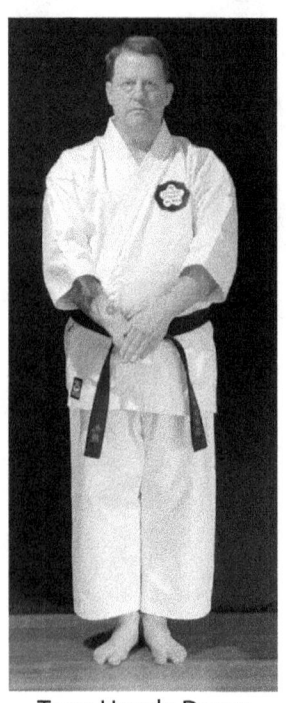
Turn Hands Down
to Guard Groin

Genshin

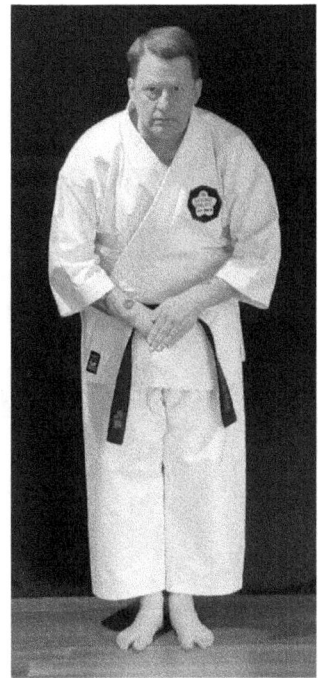

Rei

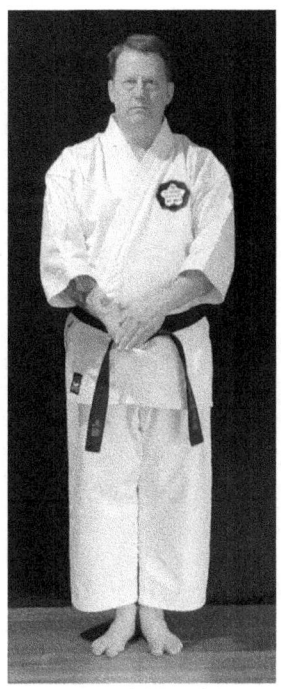

Musubi Dachi

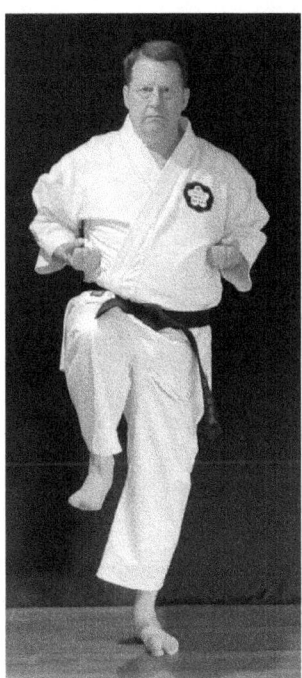

Lift Right Knee while Bringing Both Hands Back to Chamber

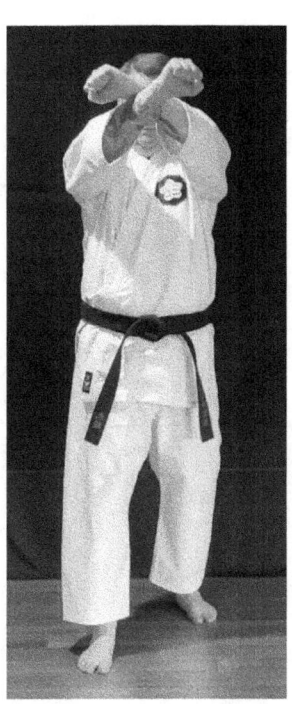

Complete Jodan Juji Uke

Genshin

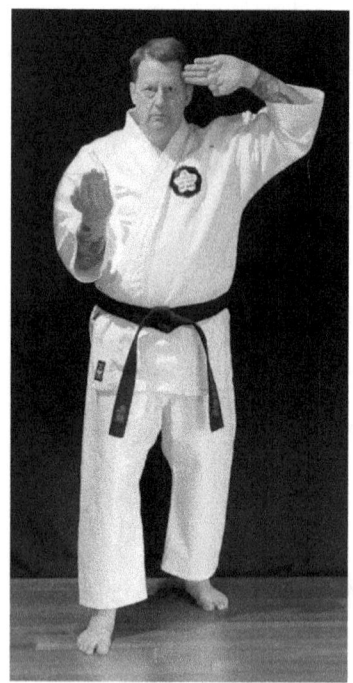

Chamber Hands for Shuto Uchi

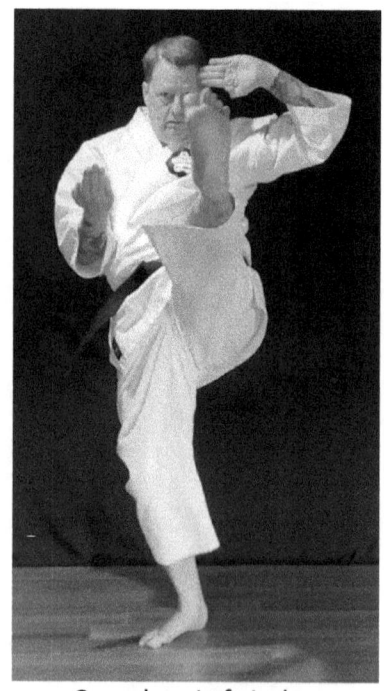

Complete Left Jodan Mae Keage Geri

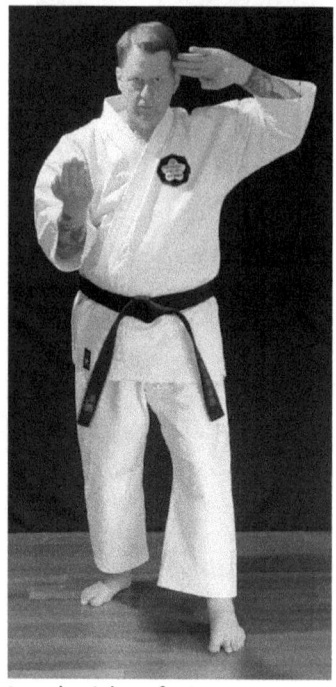

Land with Left Foot in Front

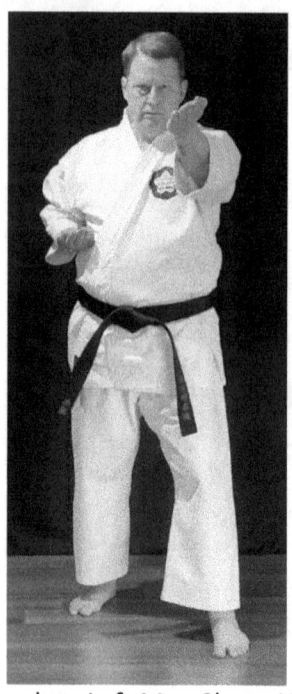

Complete Left Mae Shuto Uchi

Genshin

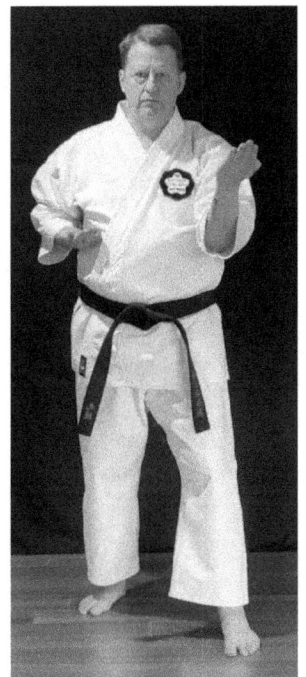
Set

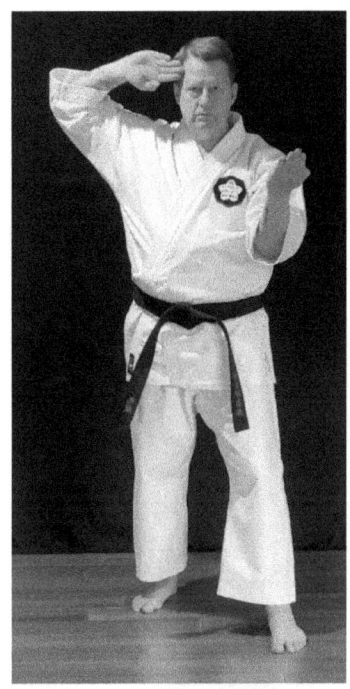
Chamber Hands for Shuto Uchi

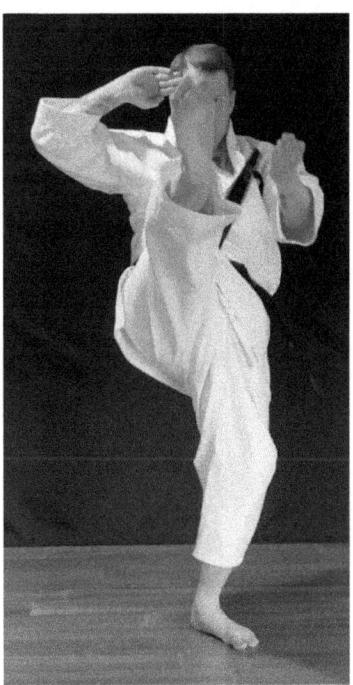
Complete Right Jodan
Mae Keage Geri

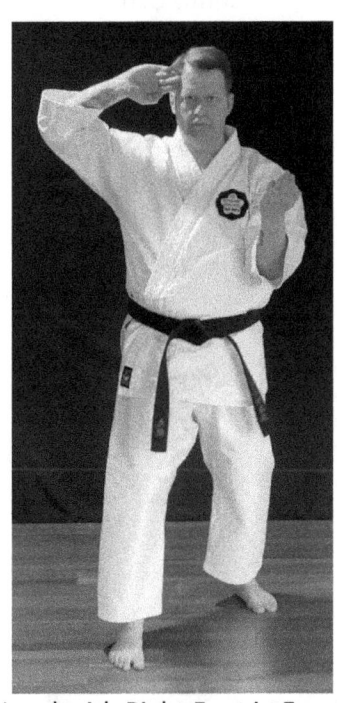
Land with Right Foot in Front

Genshin

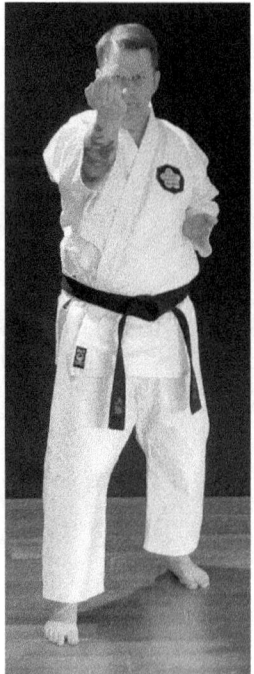

Complete Right Mae Shuto Uchi

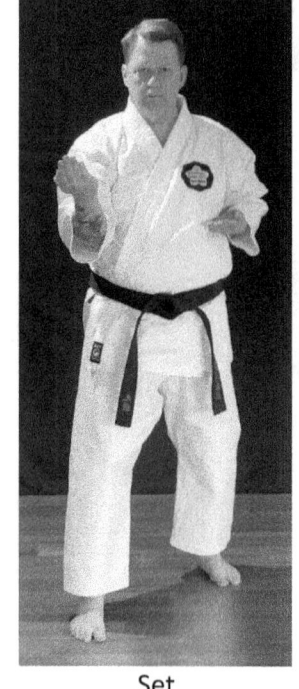

Set

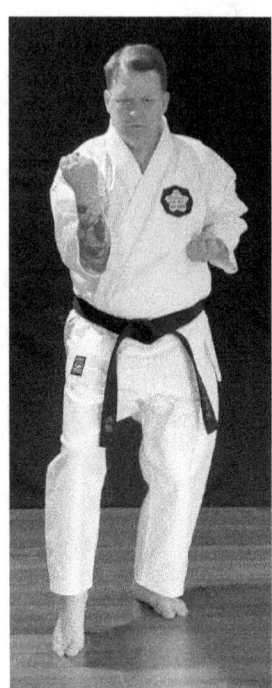

Close Hands and Drag Right Foot Back into Neko Ashi Dachi

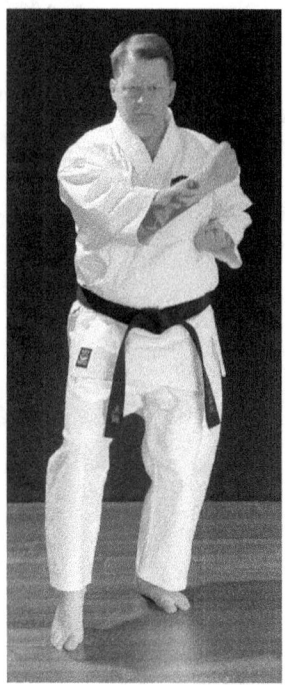

Complete Right Gedan Barai

Genshin

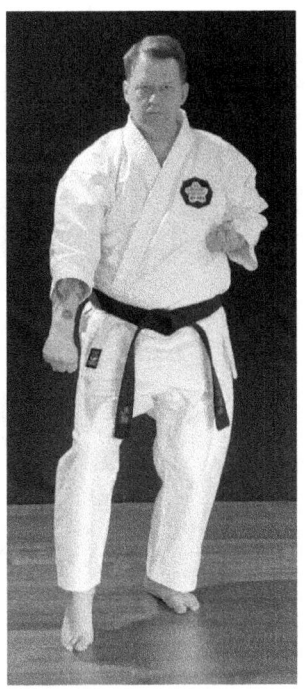

Gedan Barai (cont.)

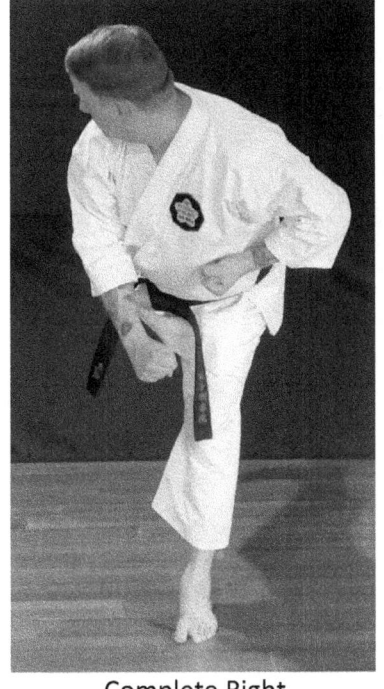

Complete Right
Ushiro Geri

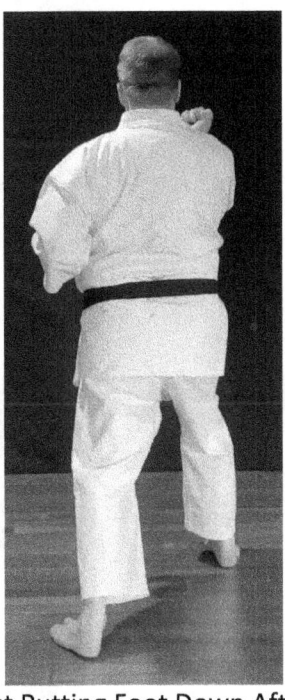

Without Putting Foot Down After Kick,
Spin Around on Left Foot 180°,
Land in Zenkutsu Dachi

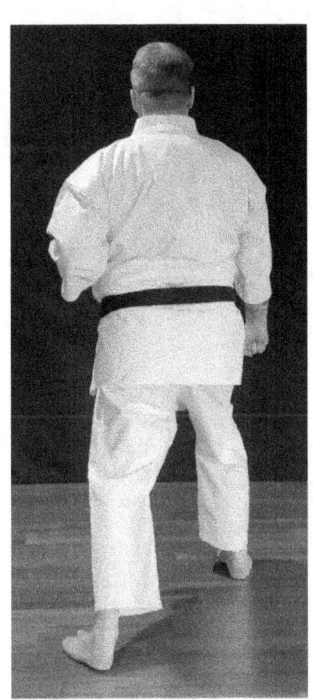

Complete Right Gedan Barai

Genshin

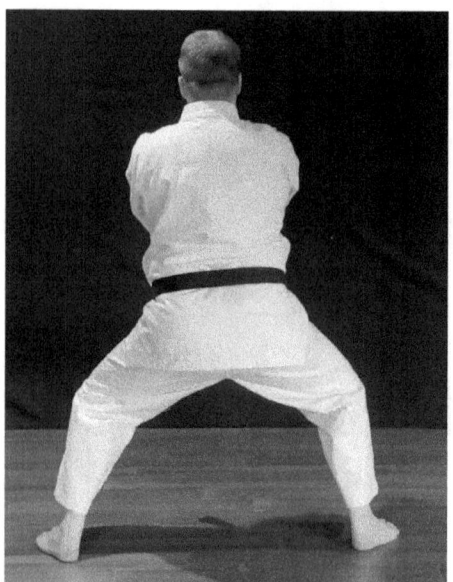
Bring Left Foot Up to Shiko Dachi with Arms Crossed Open in Front

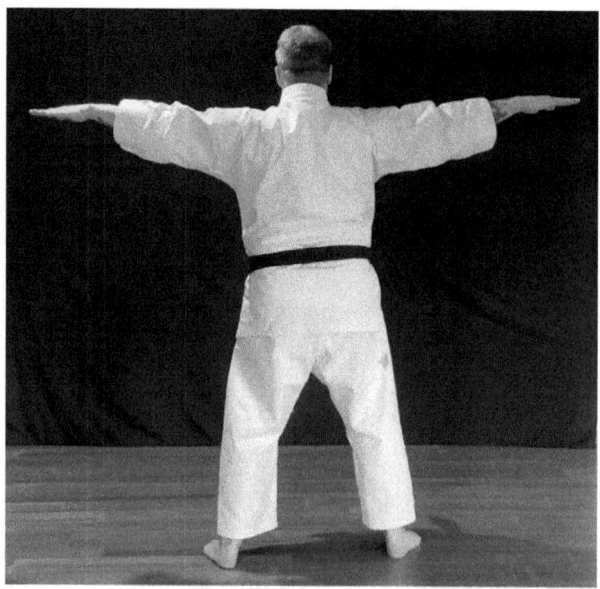
Rise Up to Heiko Dachi while Completing Morote Yoko Shuto Uchi

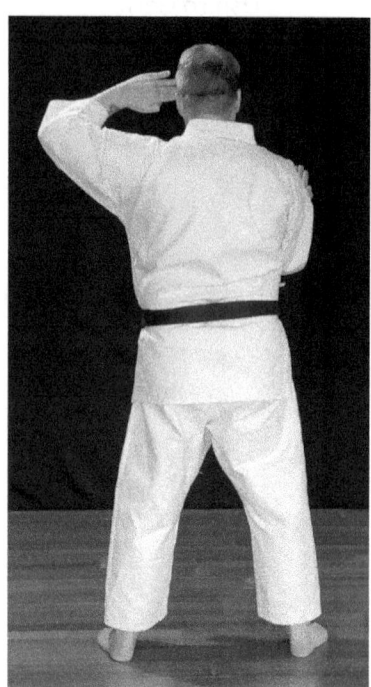
Chamber Hands for Shuto Uchi

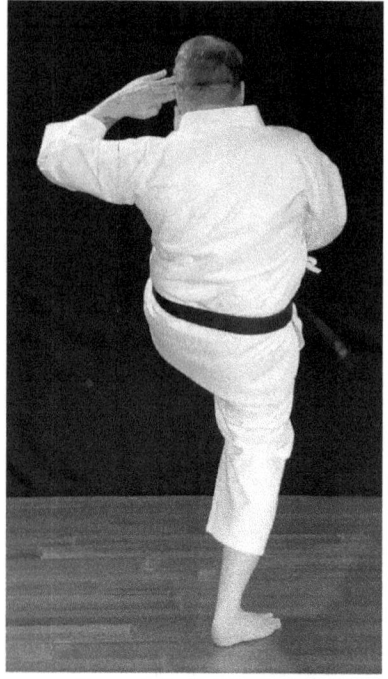
Complete Left Jodan Mae Keage Geri

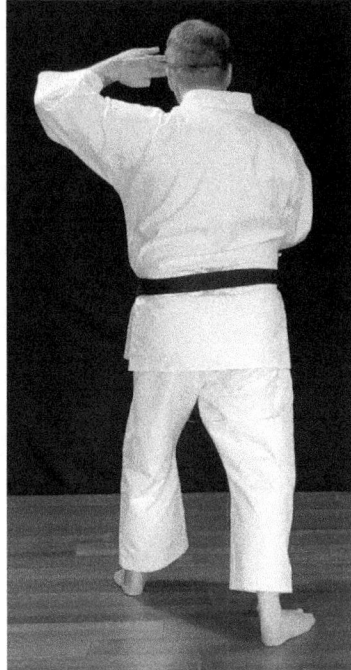
Land with Left Foot in Front

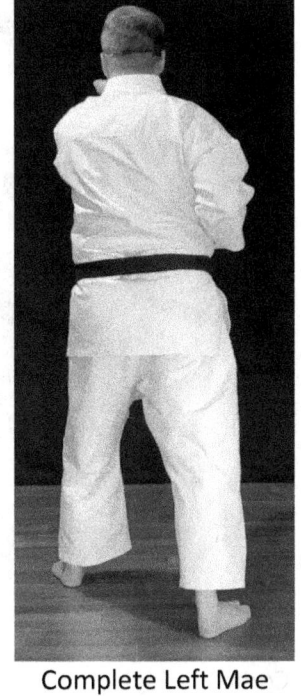
Complete Left Mae Shuto Uchi

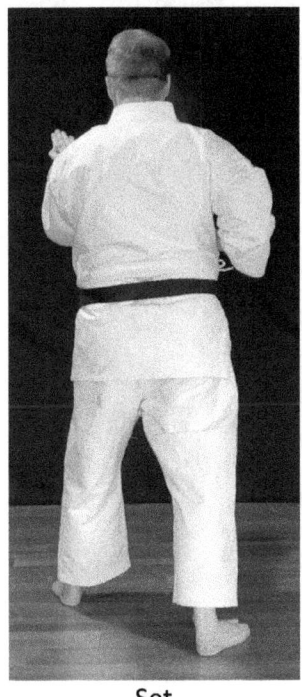
Set

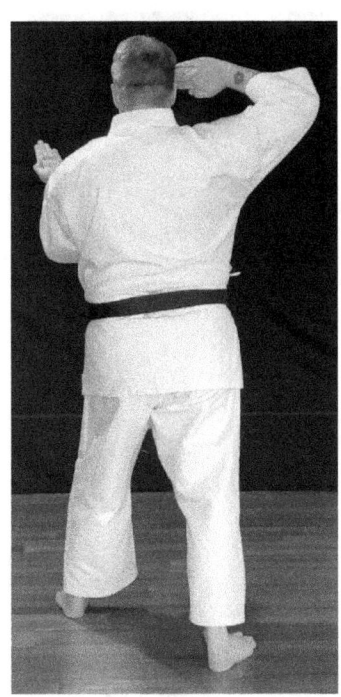
Chamber Hands for Shuto Uchi

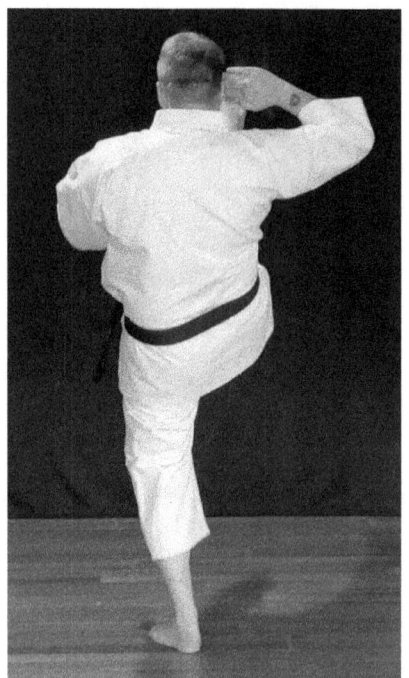

Complete Right Jodan
Mae Keage Geri

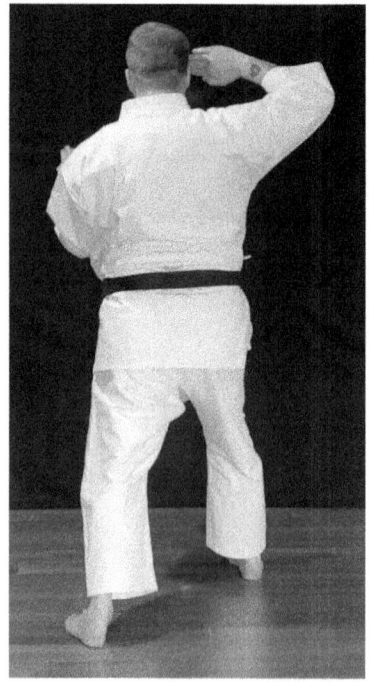

Land with Right Foot in Front

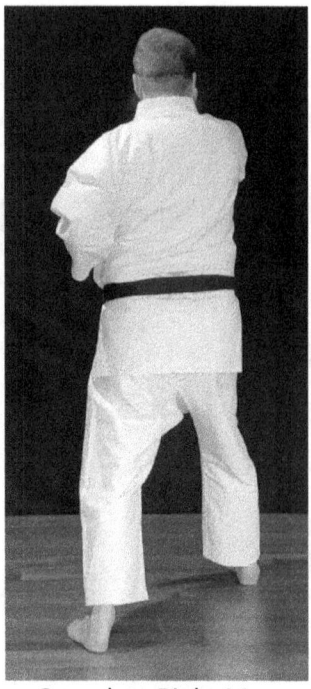

Complete Right Mae
Shuto Uchi

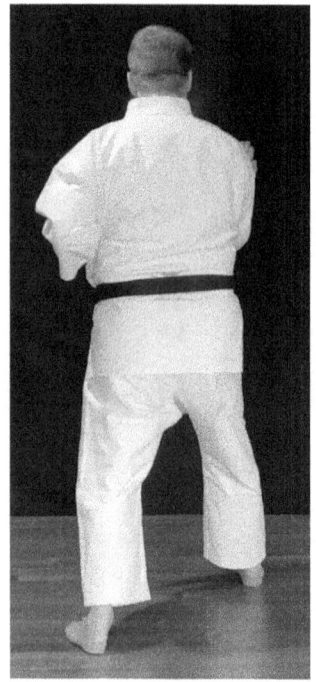

Set

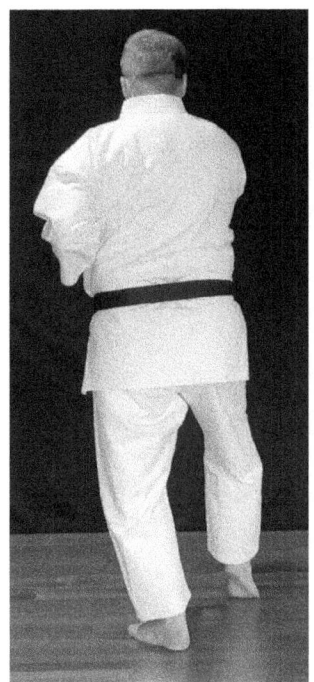

Close Hands and Drag Right
Foot Back into Neko Ashi Dachi

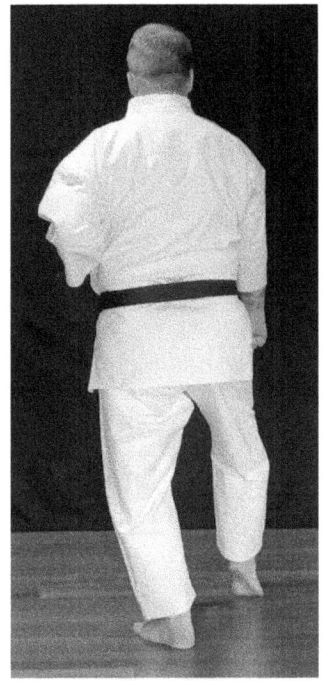

Complete Right
Gedan Barai

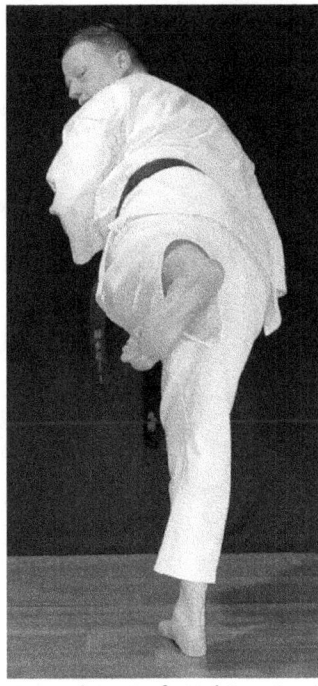

Complete Left Ushiro Geri

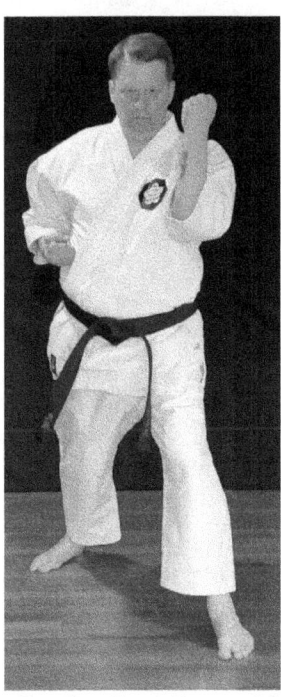

Without Putting Foot Down After Kick,
Spin Around on Right Foot 180°

Genshin

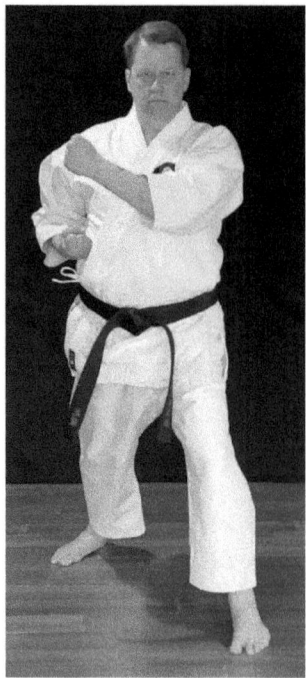
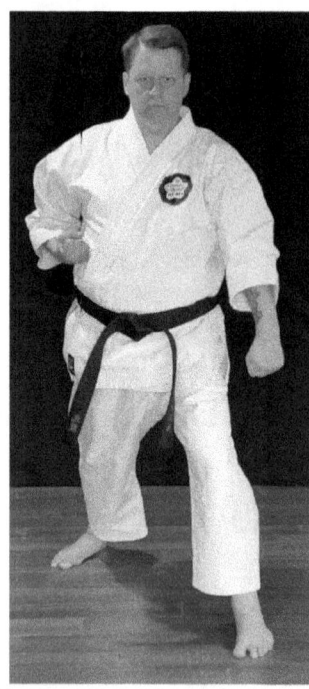

Complete Left Gedan Barai

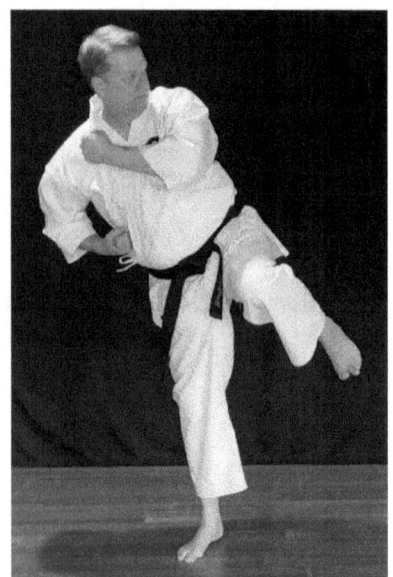

Look Left, Chamber
Leg and Hand

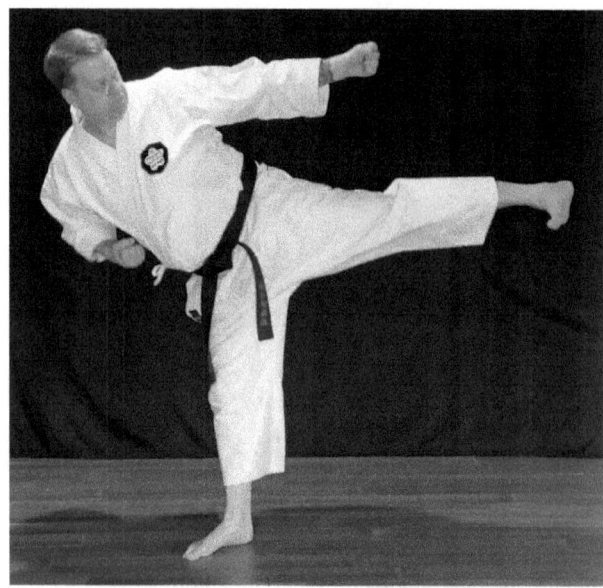

Complete Left Yoko Uraken Uchi
with Left Yoko Keage Geri

Genshin

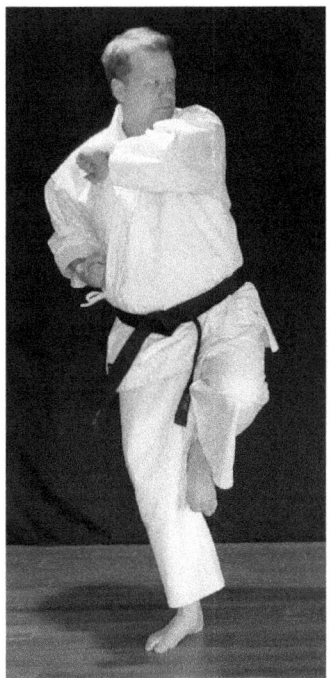

Without Putting Foot Down After Kick, Complete Left Ashi Barai and Chamber Left Hand

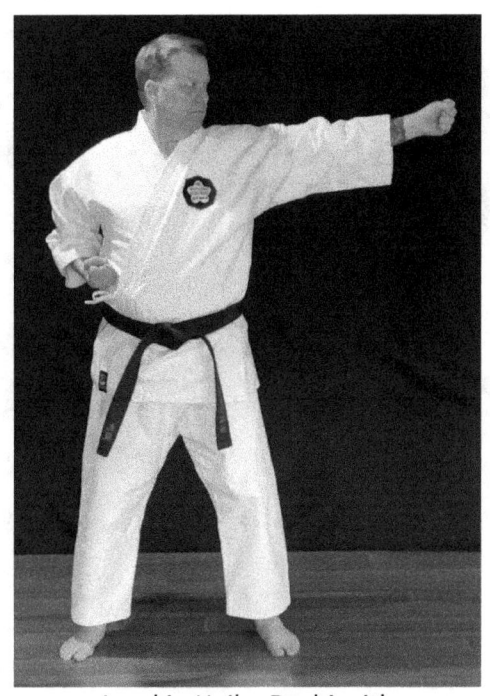

Land in Heiko Dachi with Left Otoshi Tettsui Uchi

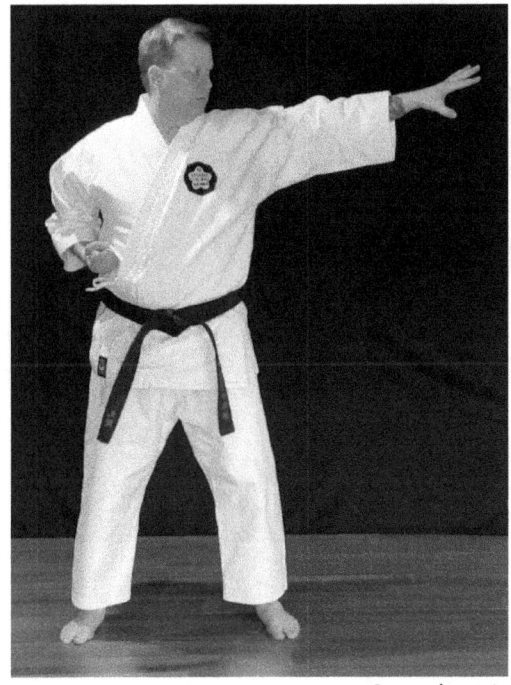
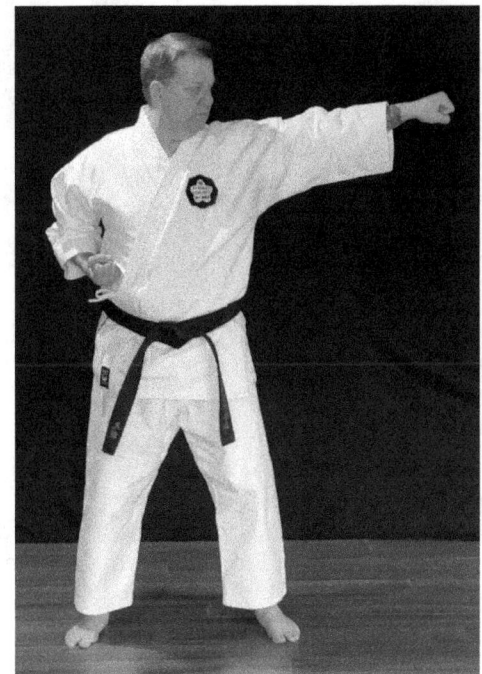

Complete Left Tsukami Hiki

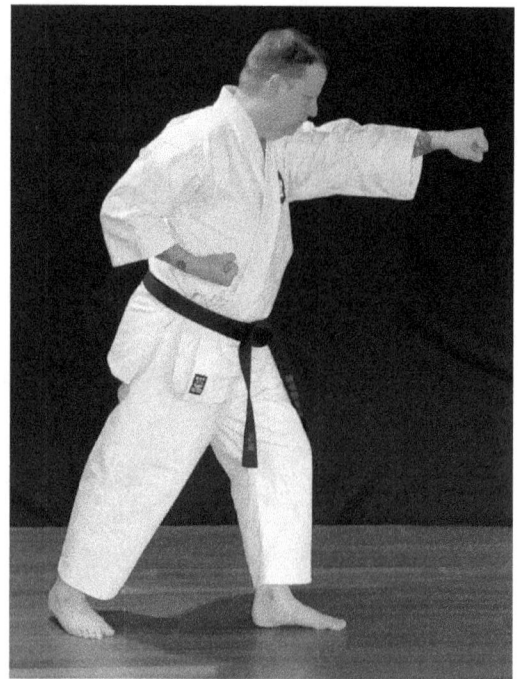 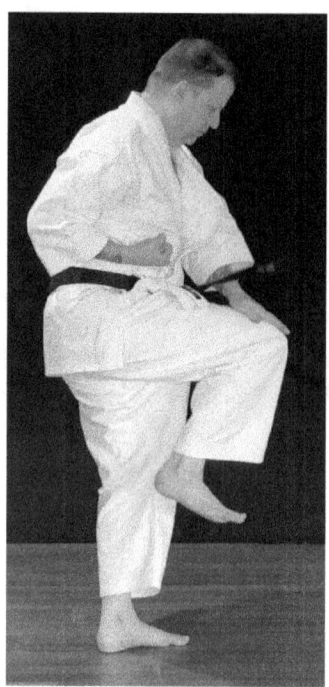

Pivot Left 90° and Pull Down to Knee

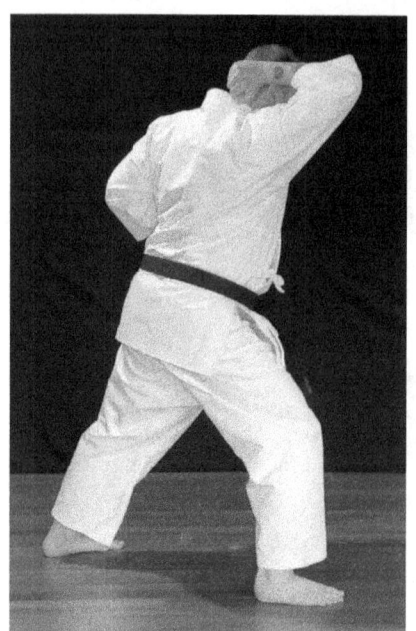 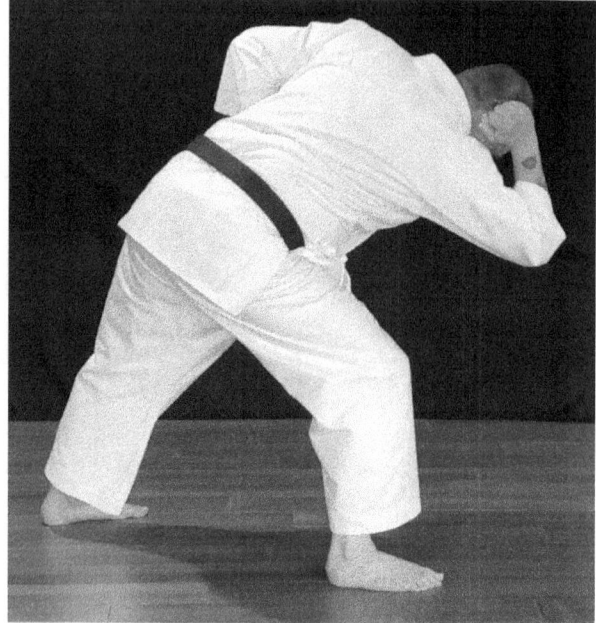

Step Forward, Complete Right Otoshi Empi Uchi

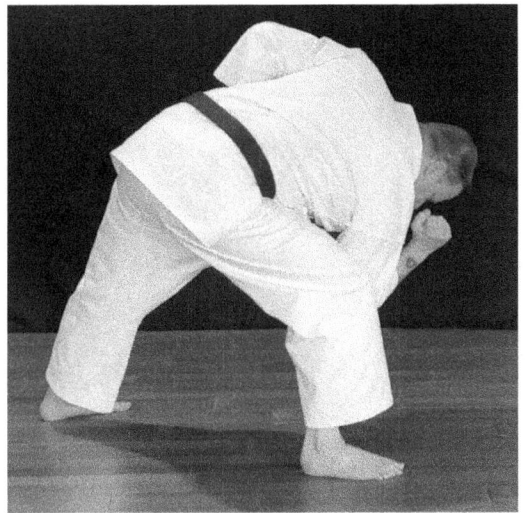
Otoshi Empi Uchi (cont.)

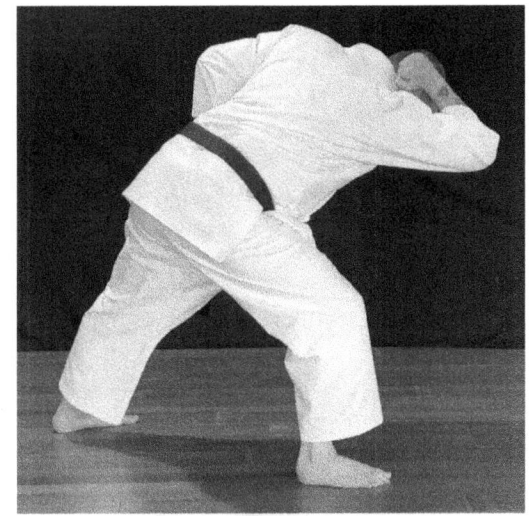
Lift Elbow

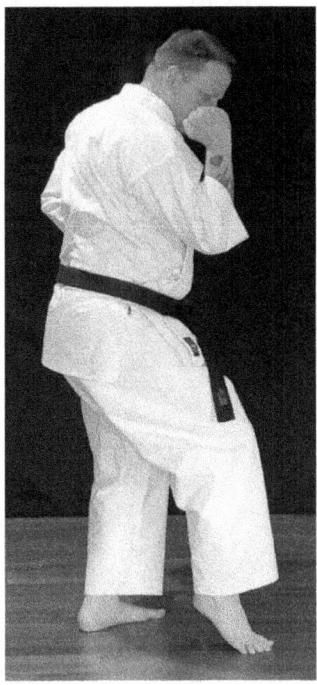
Come Up and Drag Right
Foot Back into Neko Ashi Dachi

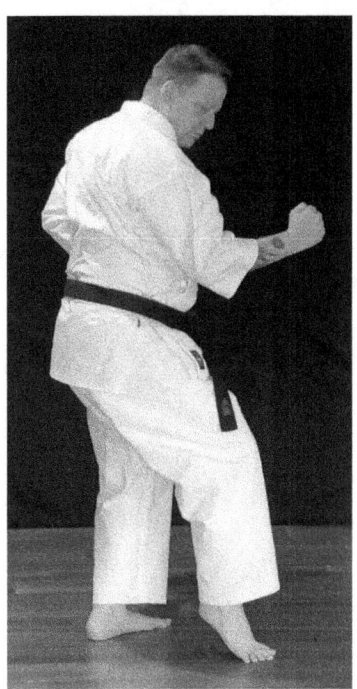
Complete Right
Gedan Yoko Barai

Genshin

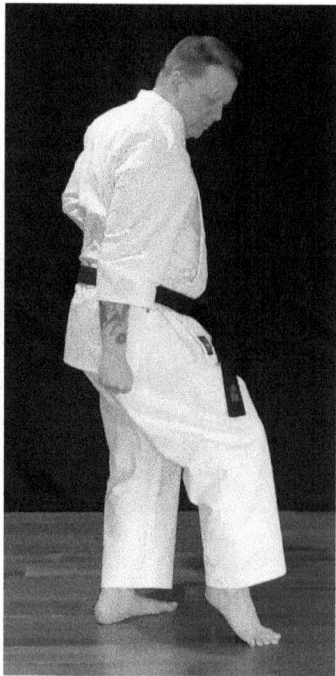
Gedan Yoko Barai (cont.)

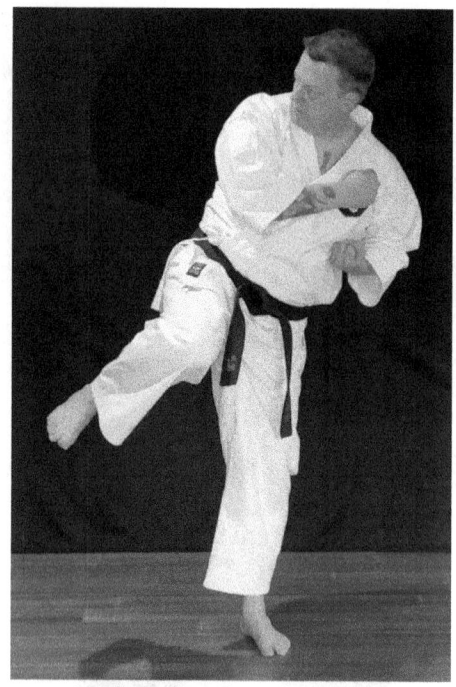
Look Right, Chamber Right Leg and Fist

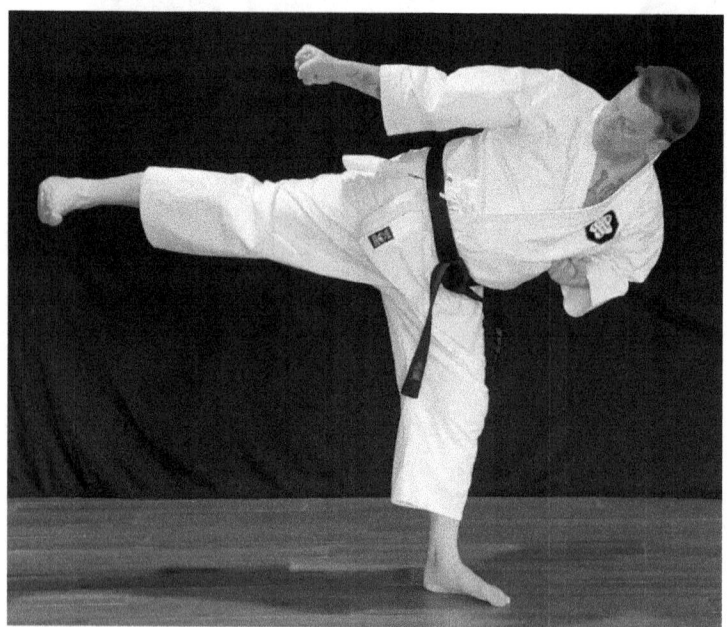
Complete Right Yoko Uraken Uchi with Right Yoko Keage Geri

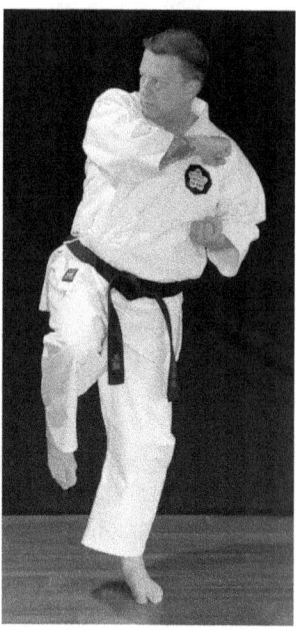
Without Putting Foot Down After Kick, Right Complete Right Ashi Barai and Chamber Right Hand

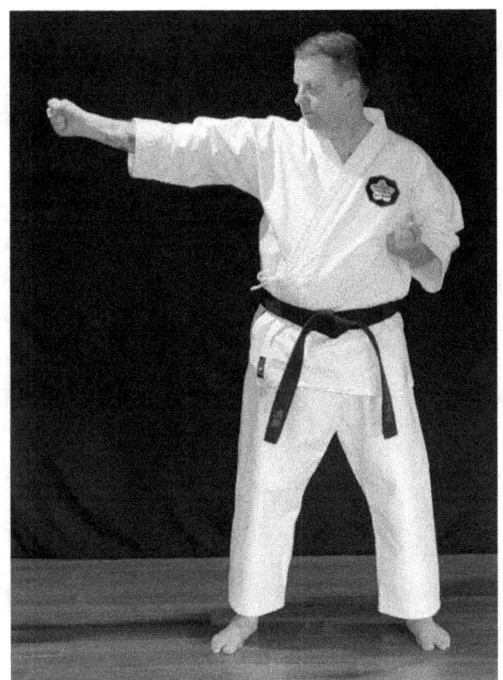
Land in Heiko Dachi with Otoshi Tettsui Uchi

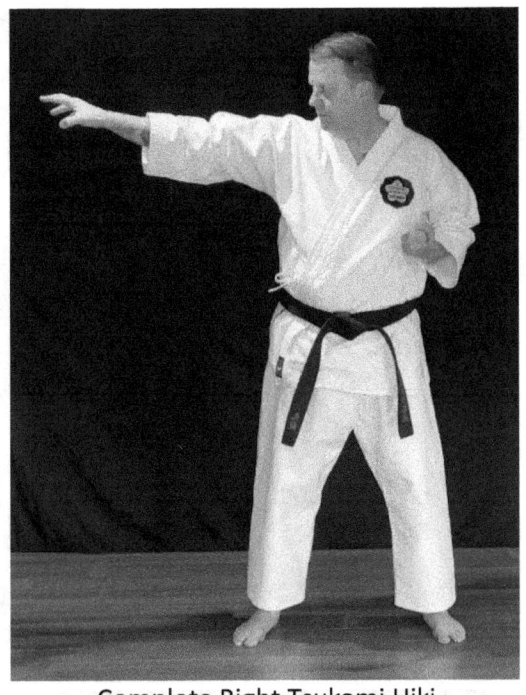
Complete Right Tsukami Hiki

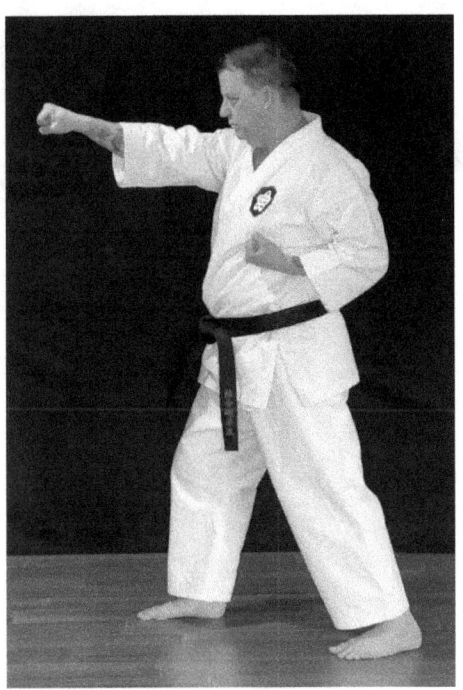
Complete Tsukami Hiki (cont.) while Pivoting Right

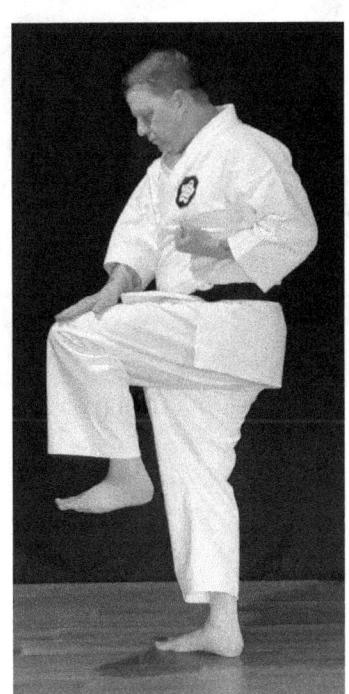
Pull Down to Knee

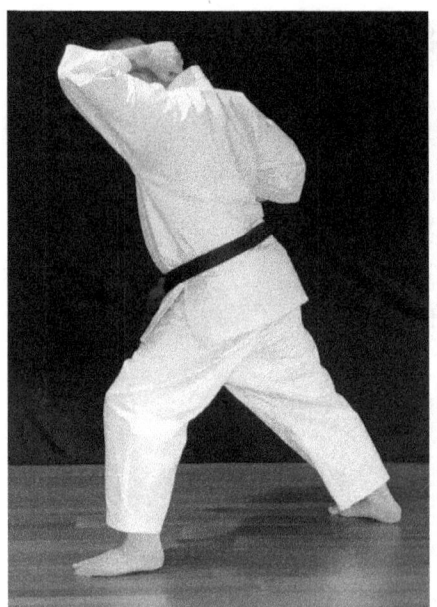 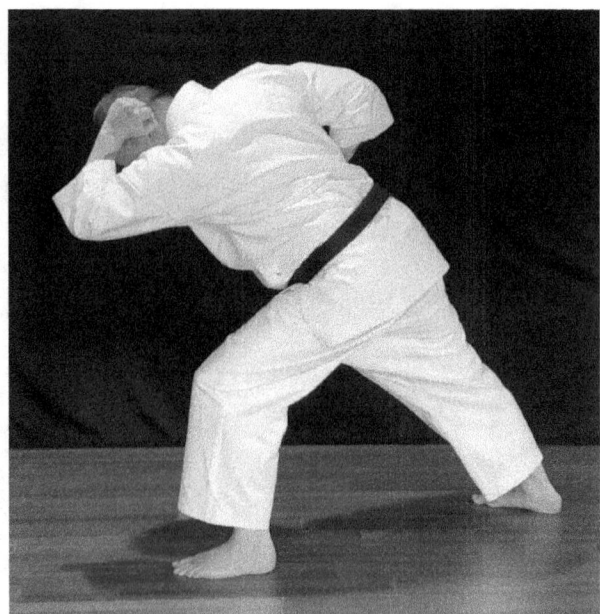

Step Forward, Complete Left Otoshi Empi Uchi

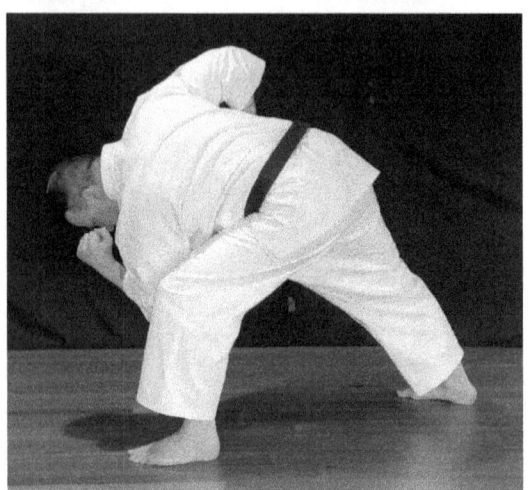 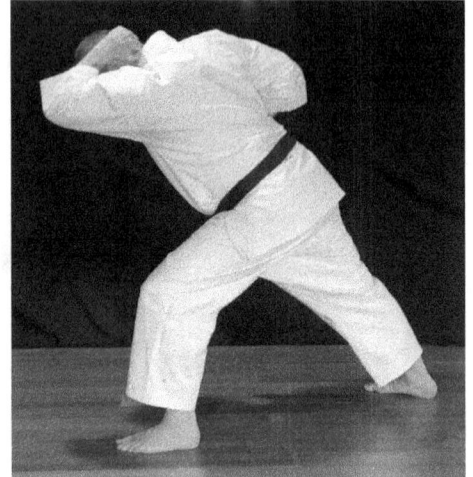

Otoshi Empi Uchi (cont.)   Lift Elbow

Genshin

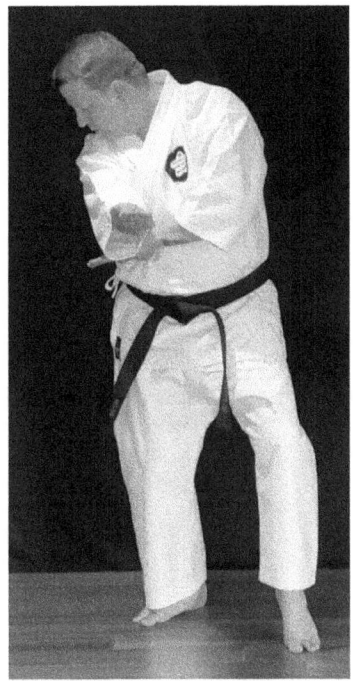

Step Around with Right Foot, Facing Forward into Neko Ashi Dachi, Right Arm Straight Out, Left Hand Across Torso

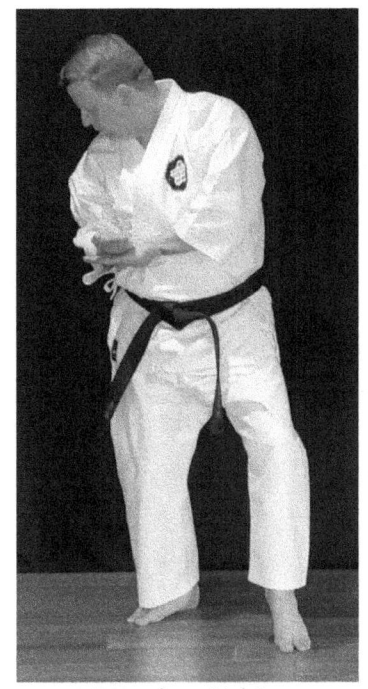

Complete Ushiro Empi Uchi

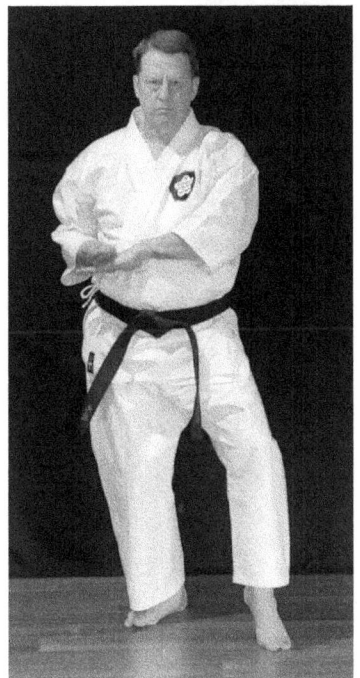
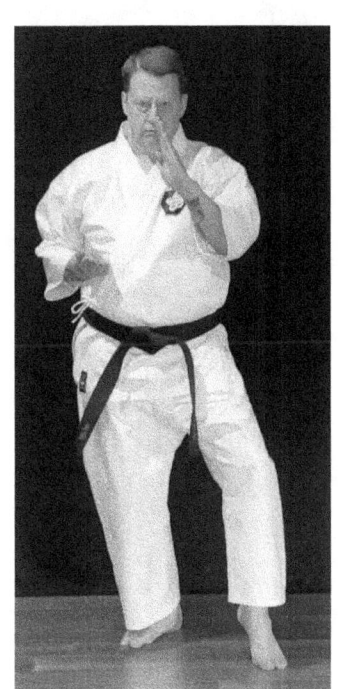

Complete Right Tora Guchi

Genshin

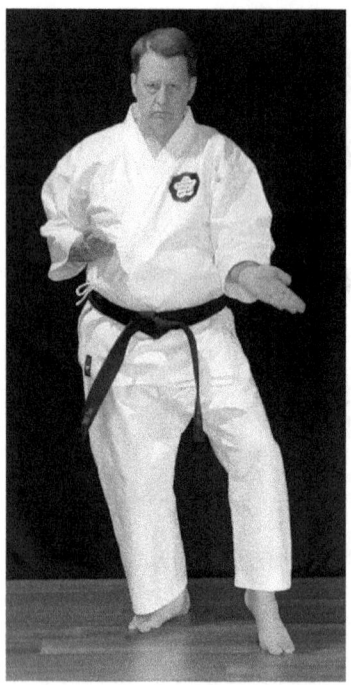 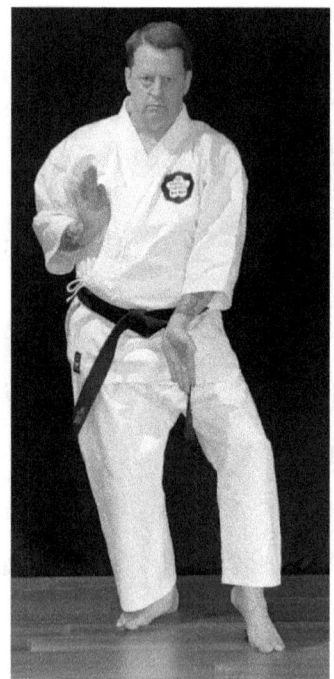

Tora Guchi (cont.)

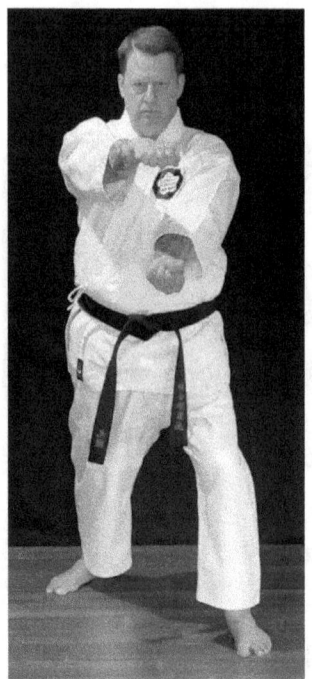

Left Step Forward, Complete
Centerline Morote Uchi
(Hiraken and Ura Zuki)

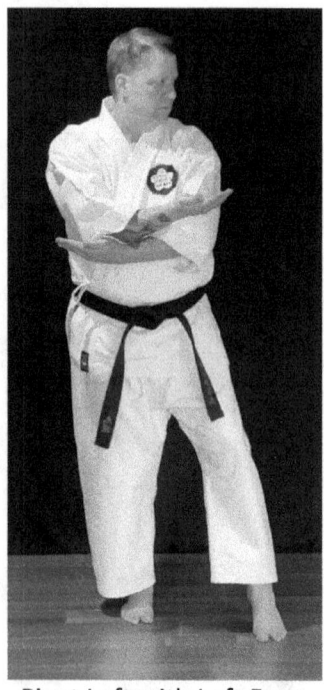

Pivot Left with Left Foot,
Preparing for Chudan Hari Uke

Genshin

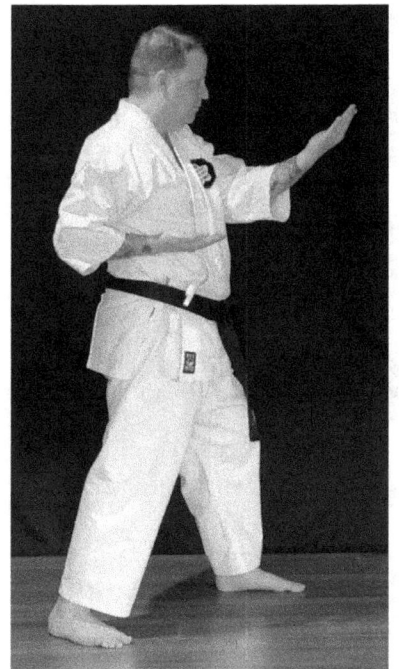
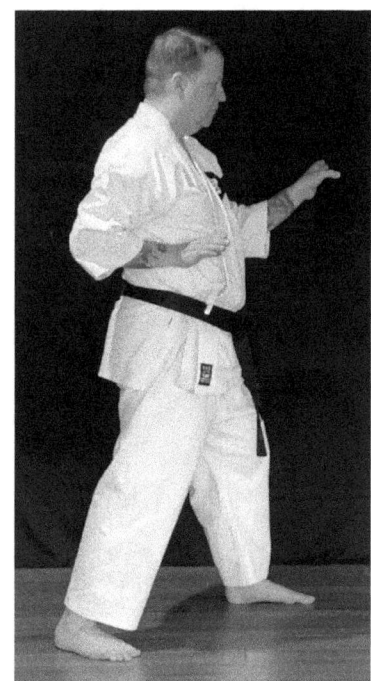

Complete Left Chudan Hari Uke into Hiki Uke

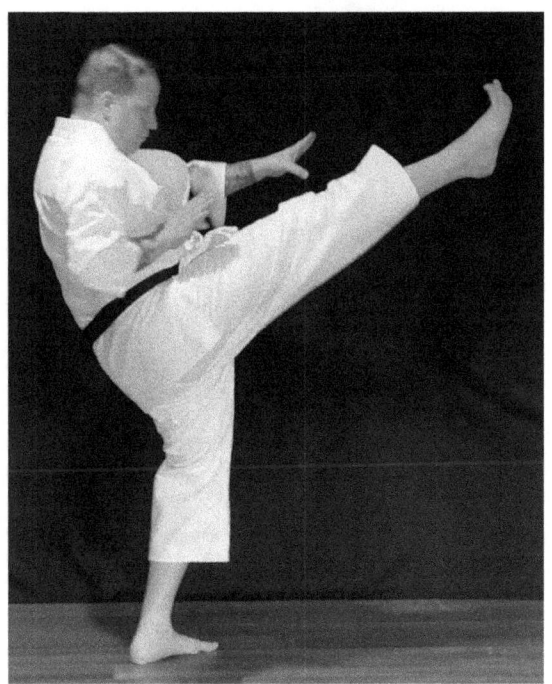

Complete Right Jodan Mae Keage Geri

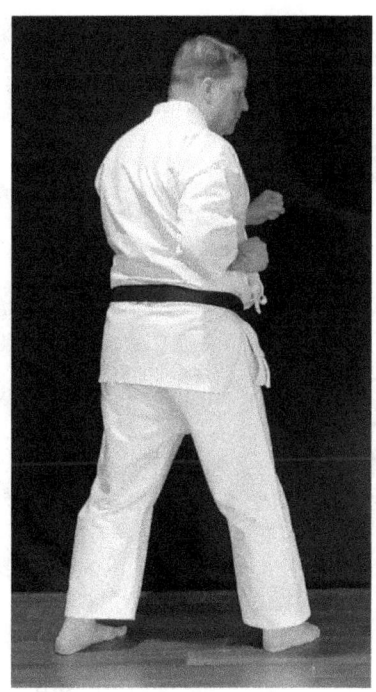

Set Down in Yoko Heiko Dachi

Genshin

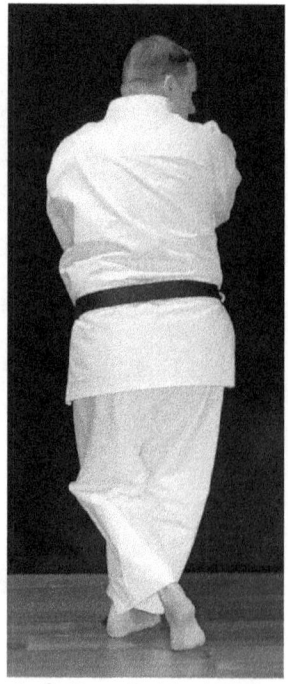
Left Step Behind Right

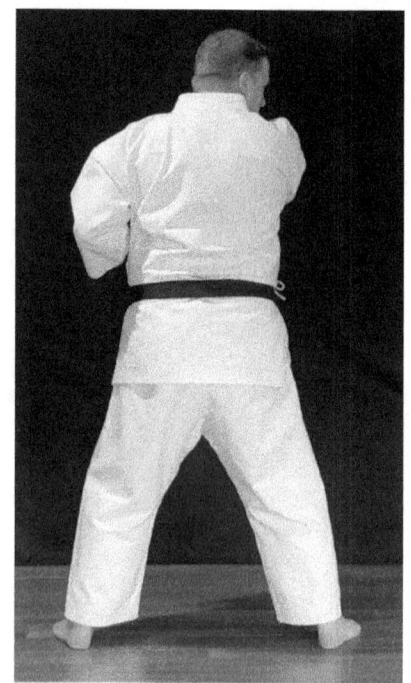
Set

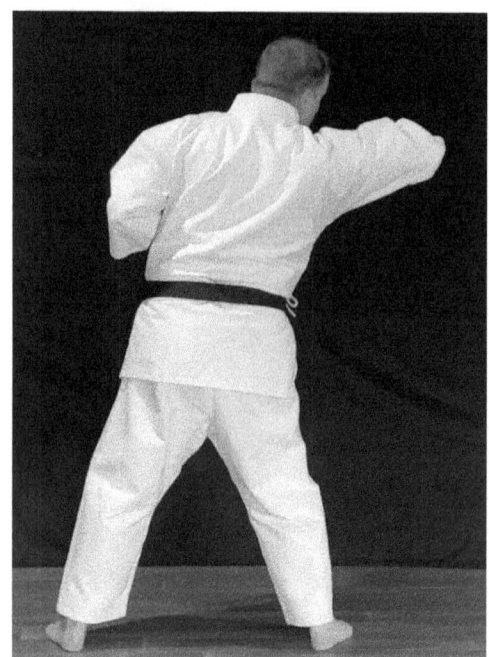

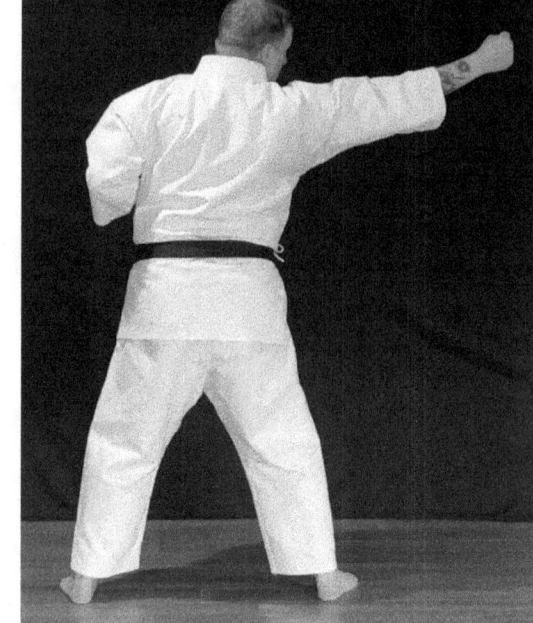
Complete Right Jodan Yoko Uraken Uchi

Genshin

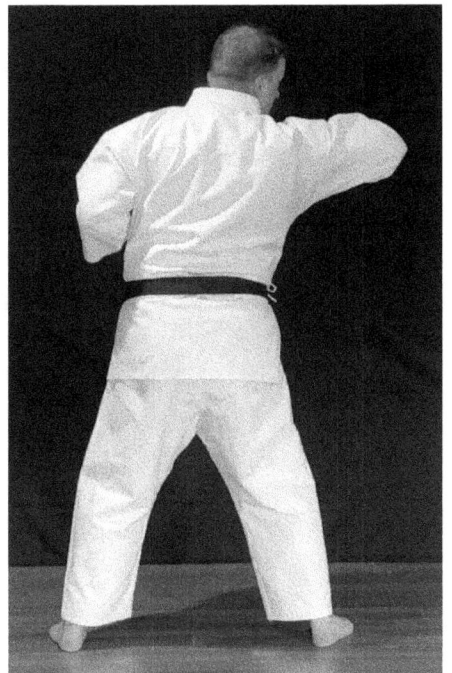
Re-Chamber Right Arm

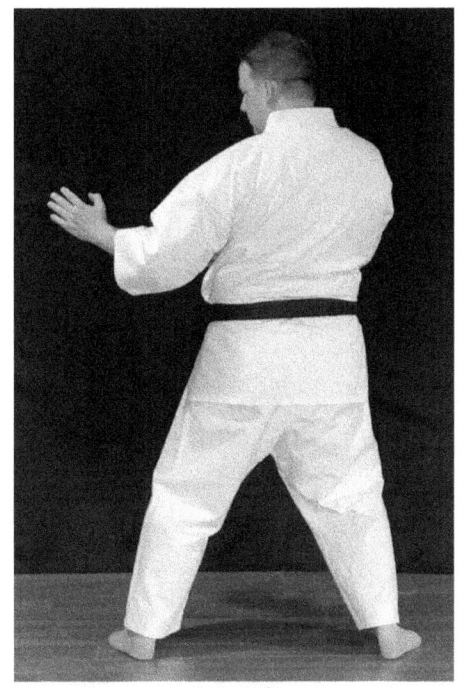
Set Left

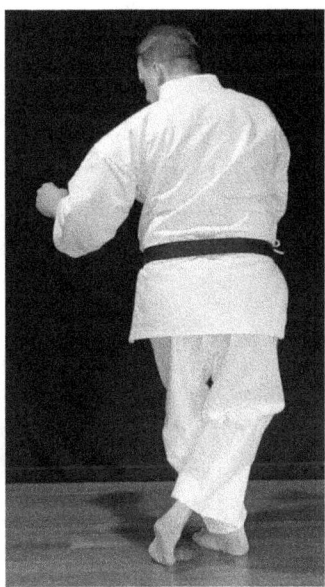
Right Step Behind Left

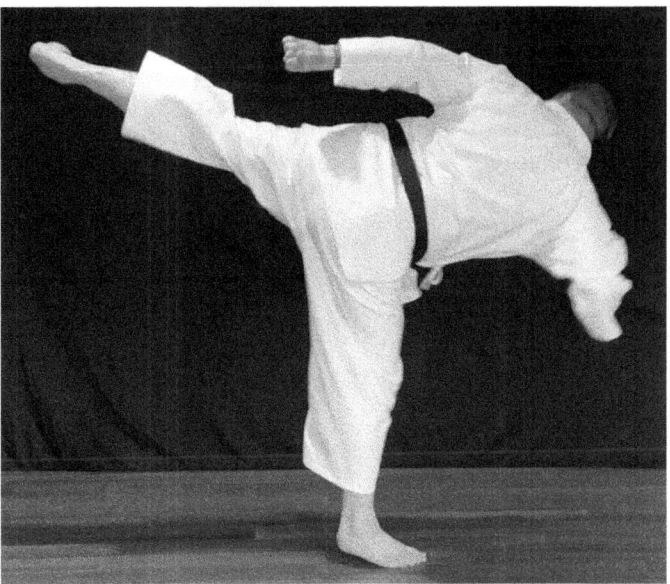
Complete Jodan Yoko Keage Geri

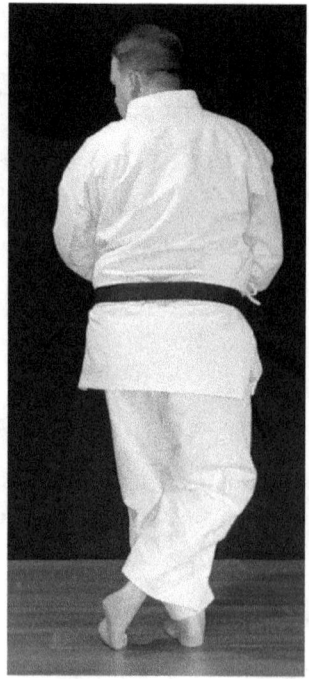
Set, Right Step Behind Left

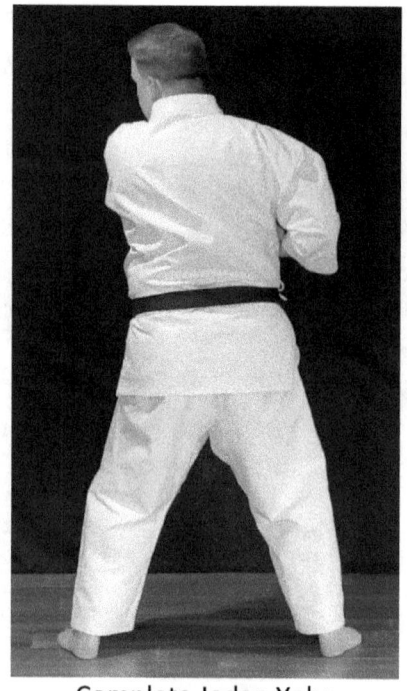
Complete Jodan Yoko Uraken Uchi

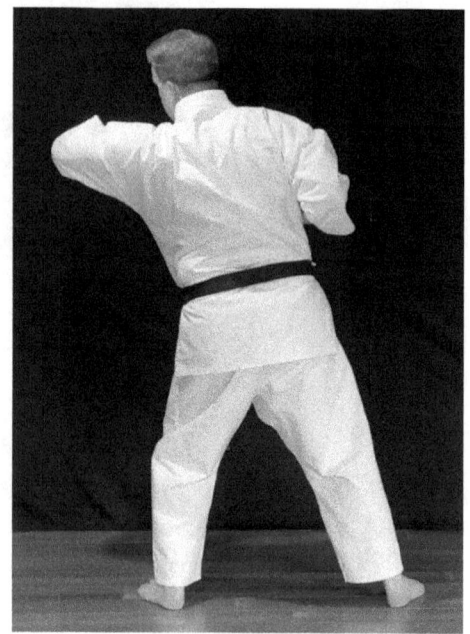
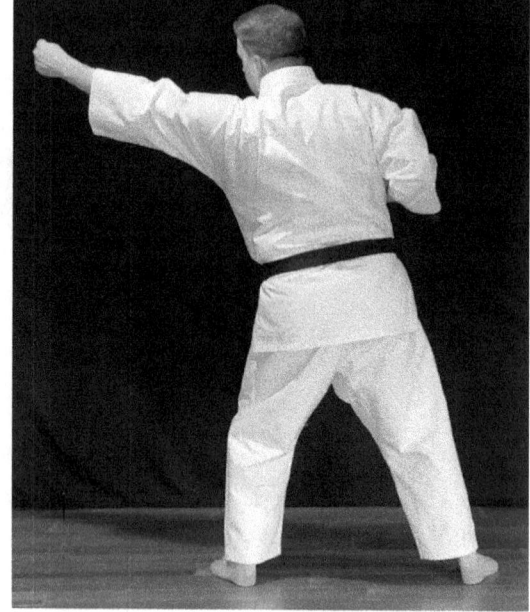
Jodan Yoko Uraken Uchi (cont.)

Genshin

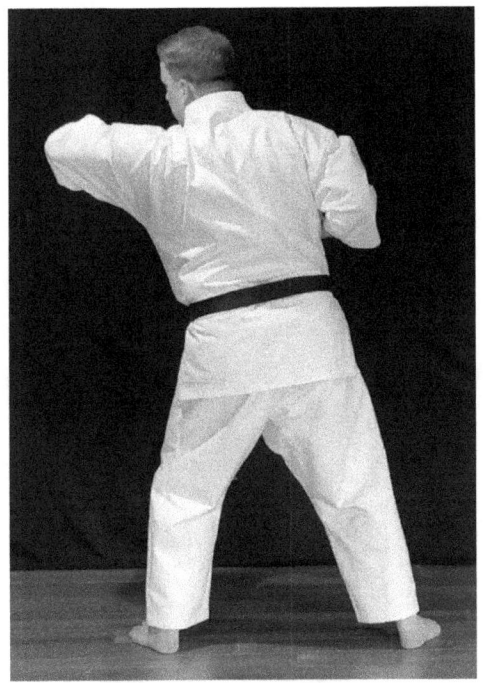
Re-Chamber Left Arm

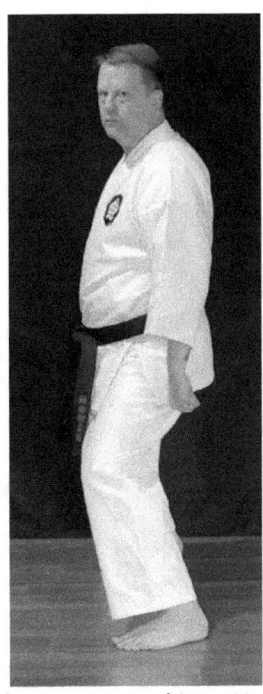
Bring Right Leg Around into Heiko Dachi Facing 270°, Drop Both Arms

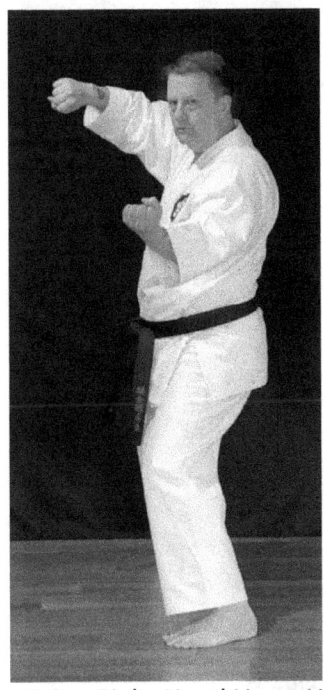

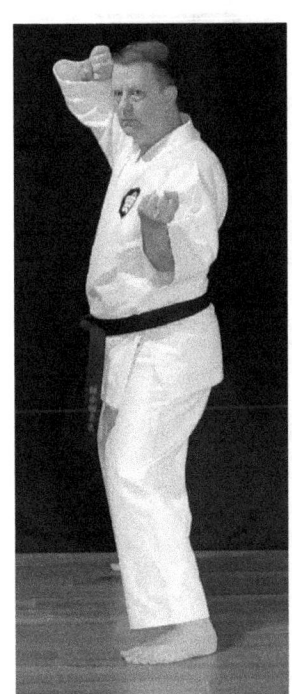
Bring Right Hand Up to Head, Left Hand Completes Chudan Yoko Uke

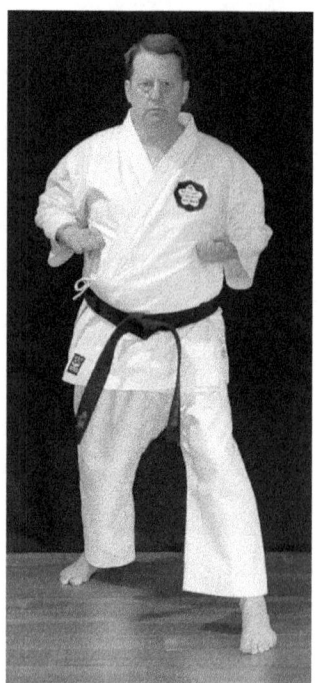 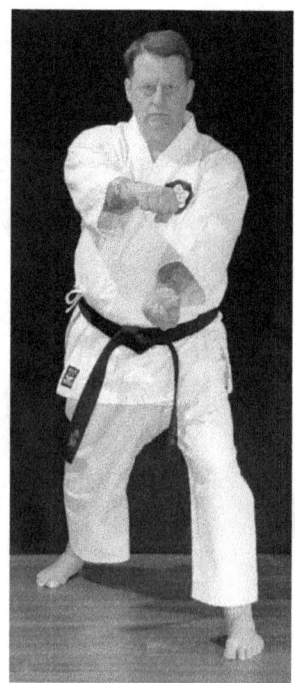

Drag Left Foot Out, Facing Forward,
Complete Centerline Morote Zuki

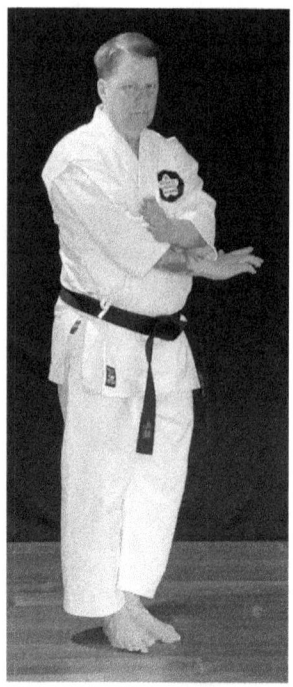 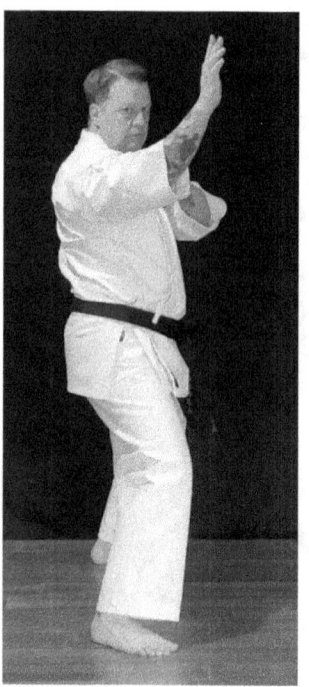

Step Back with Left Leg into Heiko Dachi
Facing 90° and Set with Open Hands

Genshin

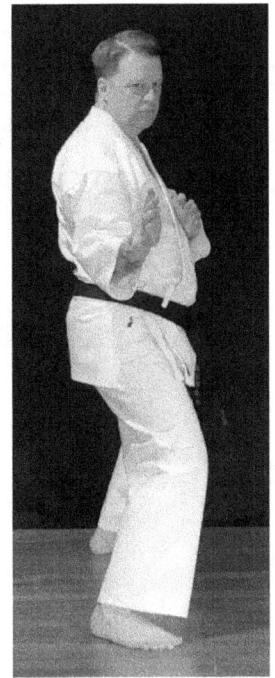
Set

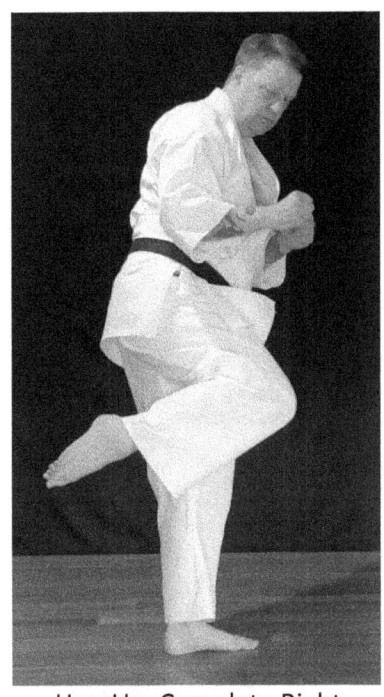
Hop Up, Complete Right Mawashi Hiza Geri

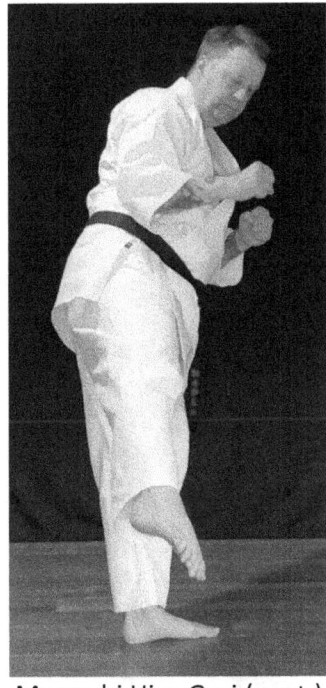
Mawashi Hiza Geri (cont.)

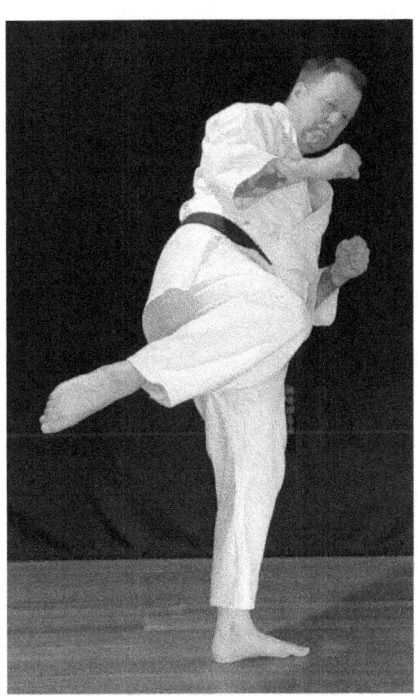
Without Putting Foot Down, Chamber for Second Mawashi Geri

Genshin

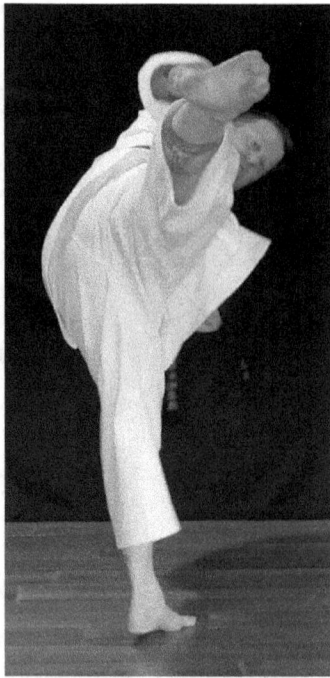

Complete Right Jodan
Mawashi Geri

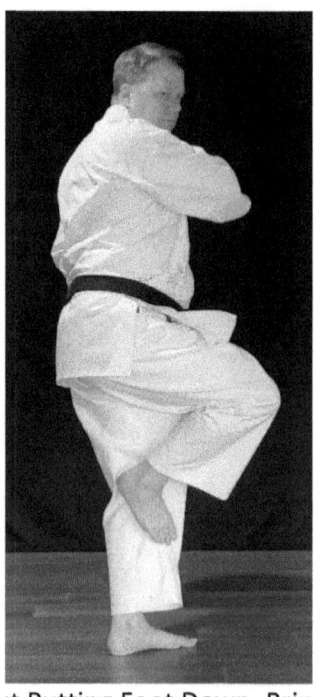

Without Putting Foot Down, Bring Right
Foot and Right Hand to Chamber Looking
Forward and Facing Left

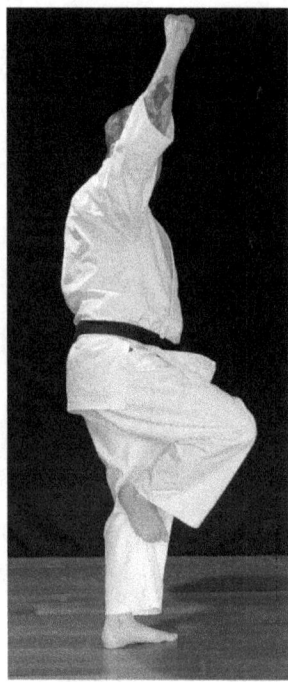

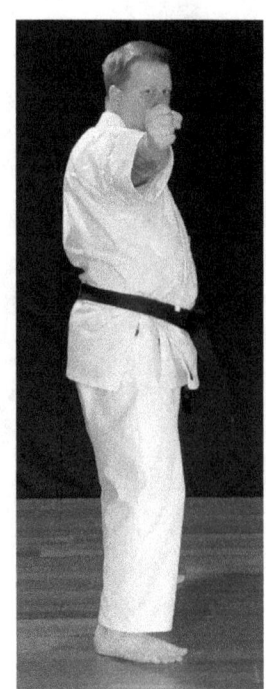

Complete Right Otoshi Tettsui Uchi with Right Fumikomi Geri

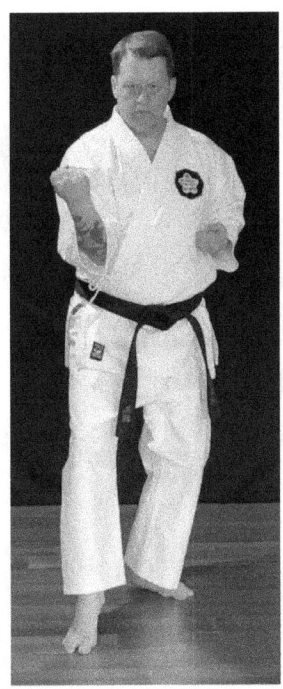

Slide Right Leg Back into Neko Ashi Dachi while Preparing for Gedan Barai

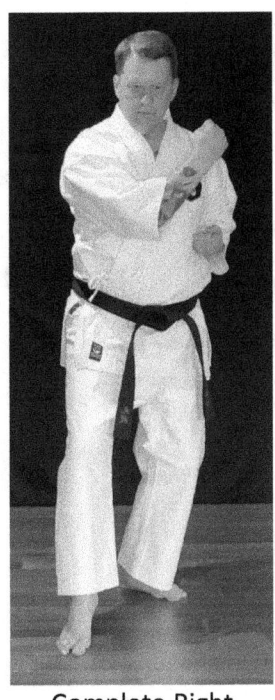

Complete Right Gedan Barai

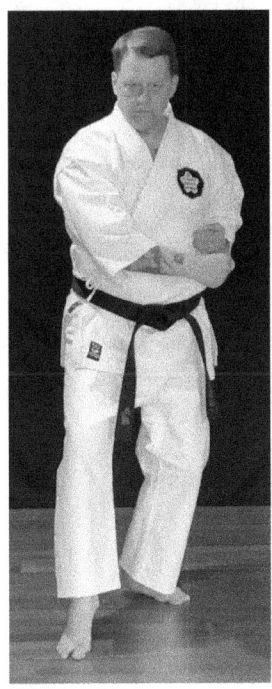
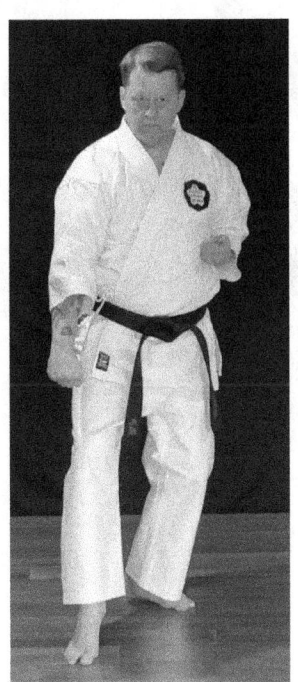

Gedan Barai (cont.)

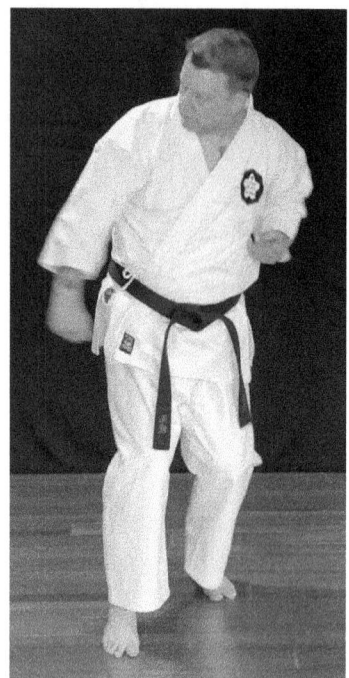 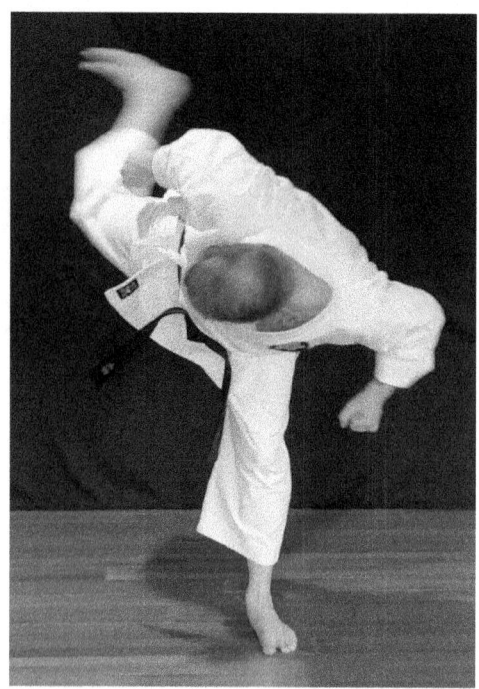

Complete Right Ushiro Mawashi Geri, 180°

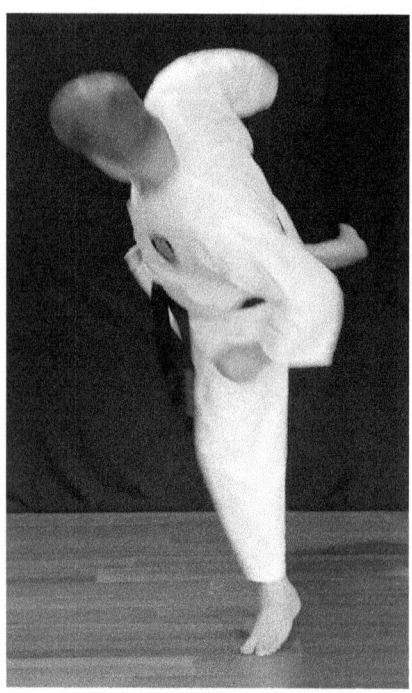 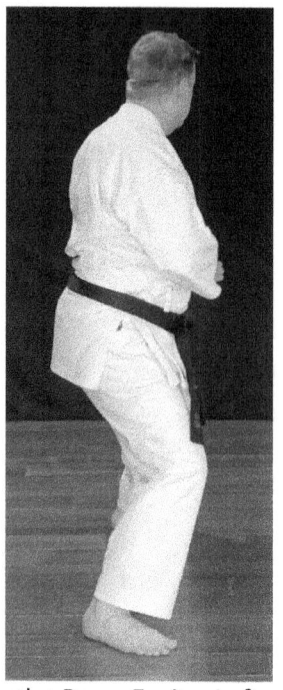

Ushiro Mawashi Geri (cont.), Set Looking to the Rear, Facing Left

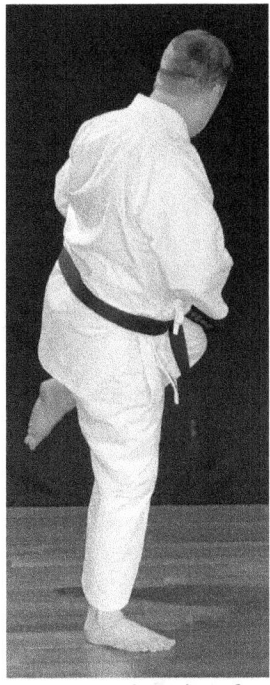

Hop Up, Chamber for
Mawashi Geri

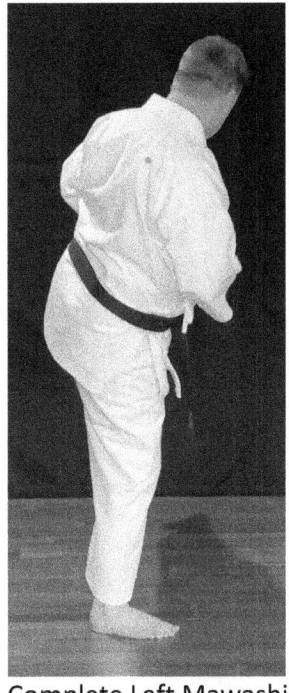

Complete Left Mawashi
Hiza Geri

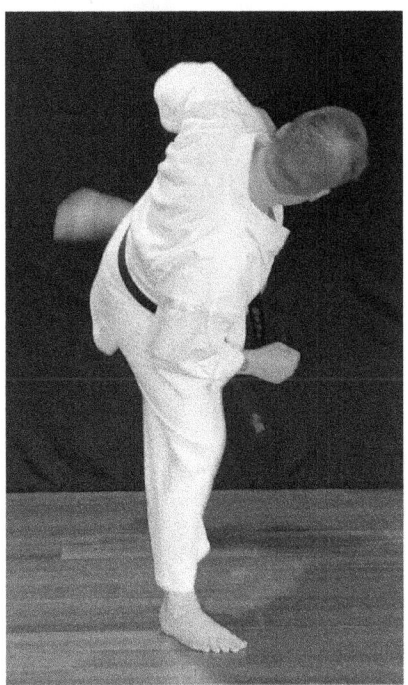

Without Putting Foot Down,
Chamber for Second Mawashi Geri

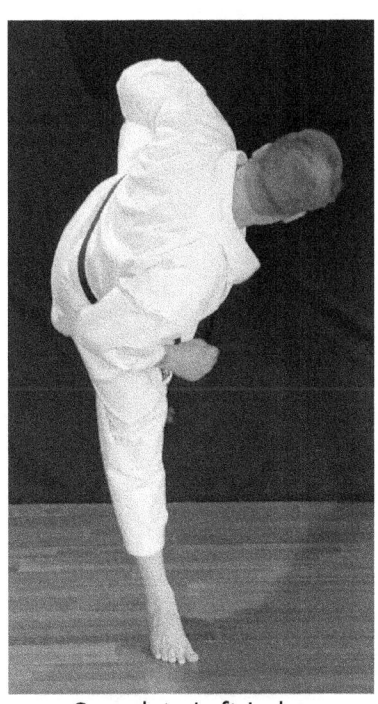

Complete Left Jodan
Mawashi Geri

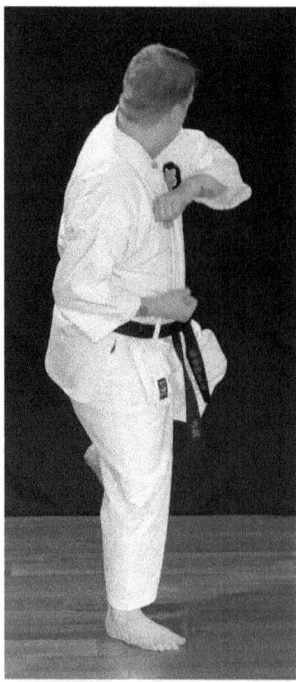

Without Putting Foot Down, Bring Left Foot and Left Hand to Chamber Looking to the Rear and Facing Left

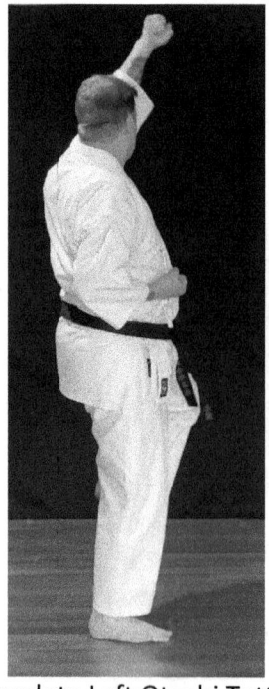

Complete Left Otoshi Tettsui Uchi with Left Fumikomi Geri

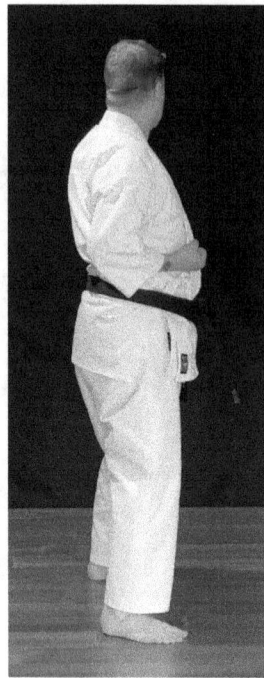

Complete Tettsui Uchi And Fumikomi Geri

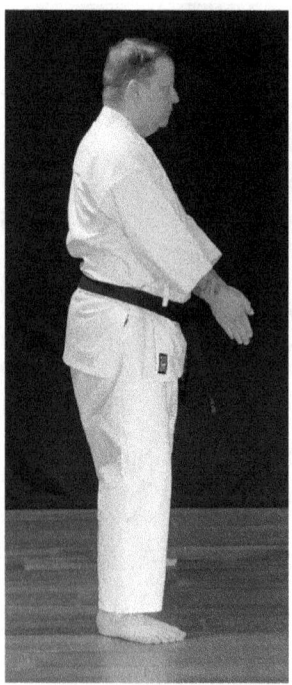

Face Back 90°, Drop and Put Hands Together

Genshin

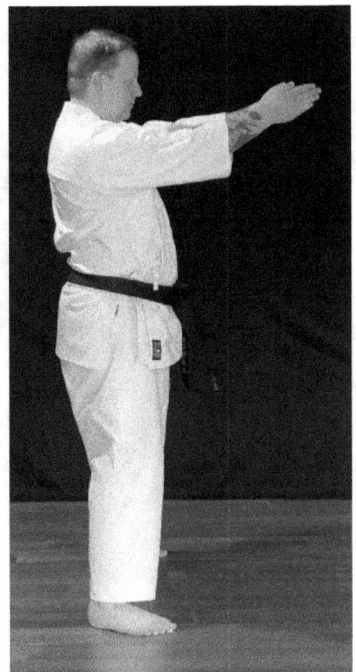
Bring Hands Up to Face Level

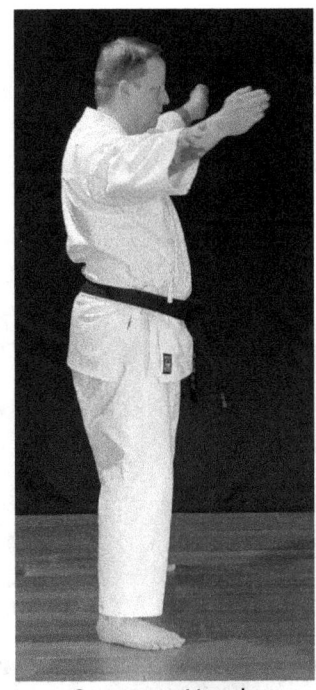
Separate Hands

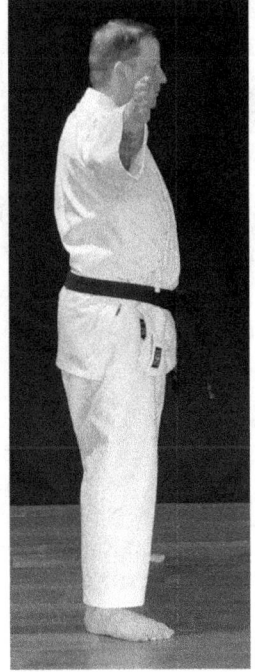
Separate Hands (cont.)

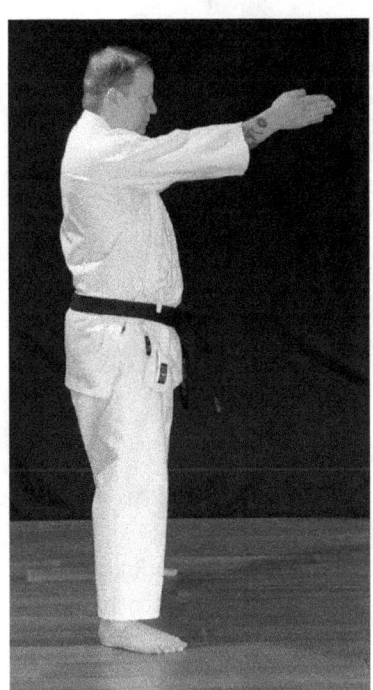
Close Hands Together

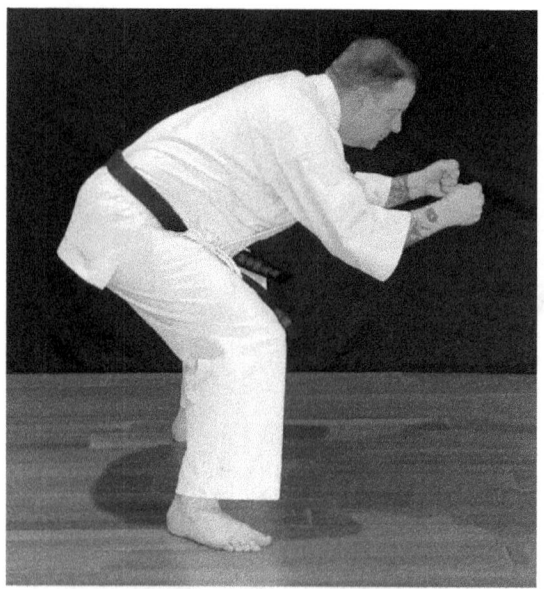
Open Hands, Slide Arms Down, Grab

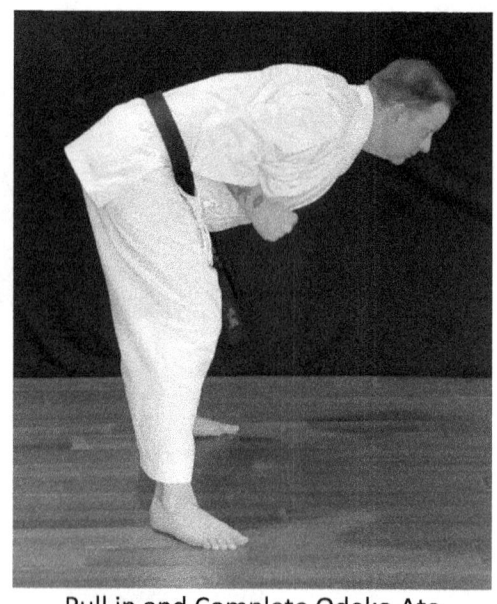
Pull in and Complete Odeko Ate

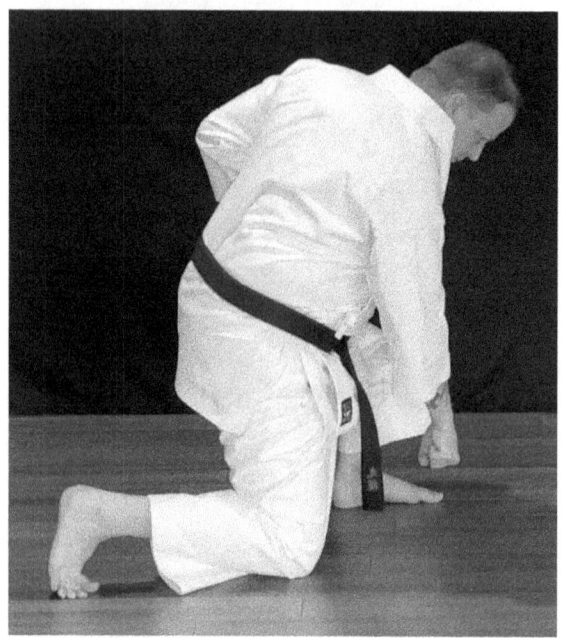
Drop Down to Right Knee,
Complete Right Otoshi Zuki (kiai)

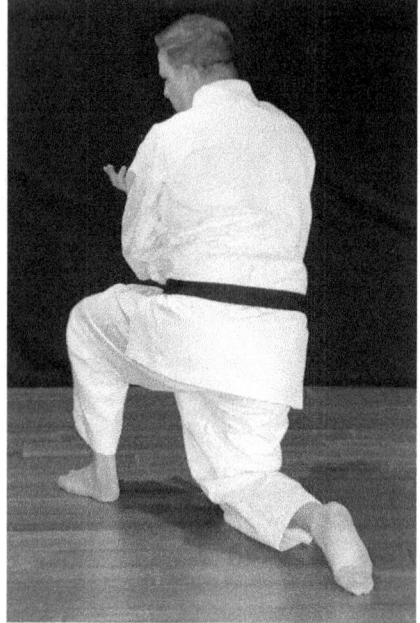
Pivot on Right Knee
to 270° Angle

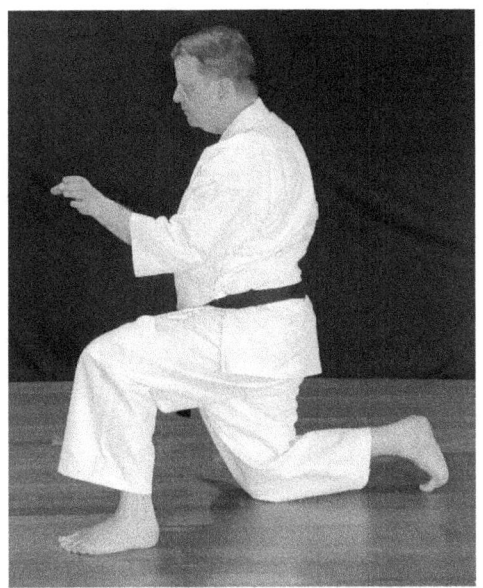
Complete Right Hari to Hiki Chudan Uke

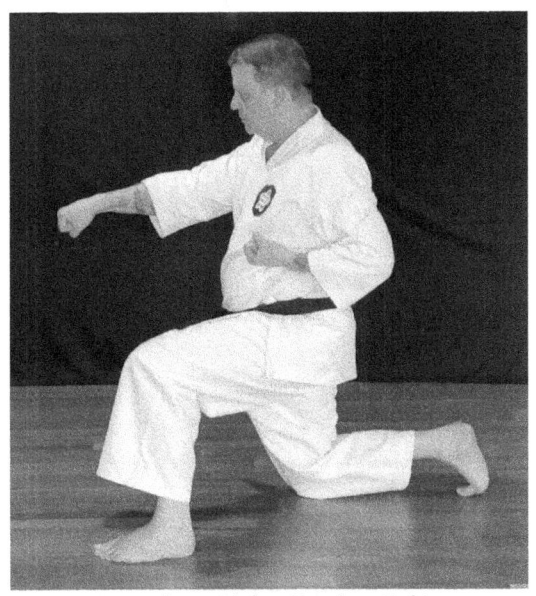
Complete Right Chudan Zuki...

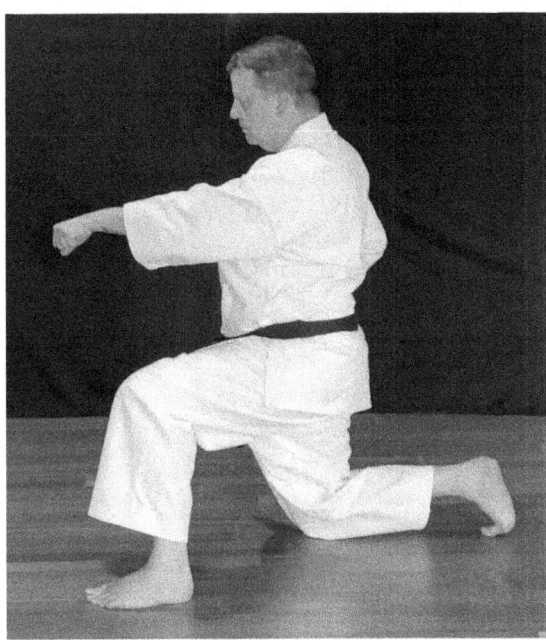
...then an Immediate Left Chudan Zuki

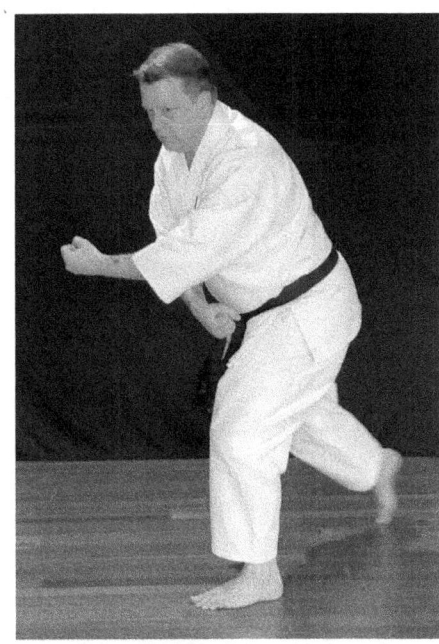
Come Up and Step Around with Right Foot Facing Forward

Genshin

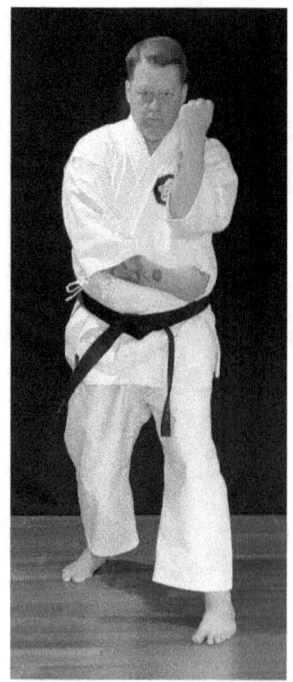 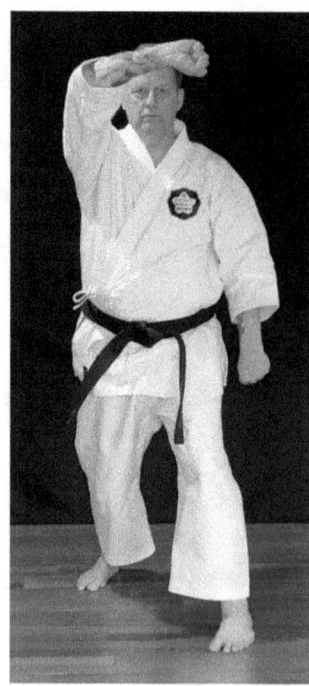

Once Set, Perform Left Gedan Barai and Right Jodan Age Uke Together

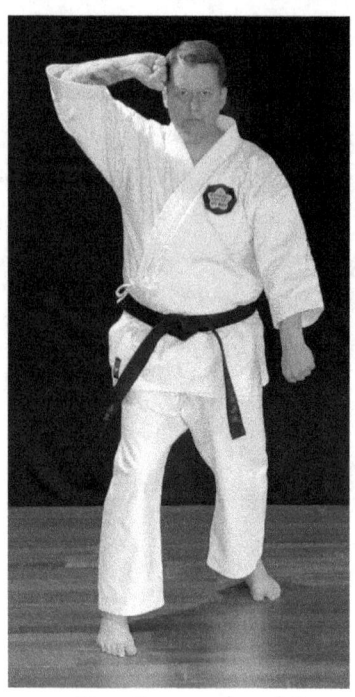 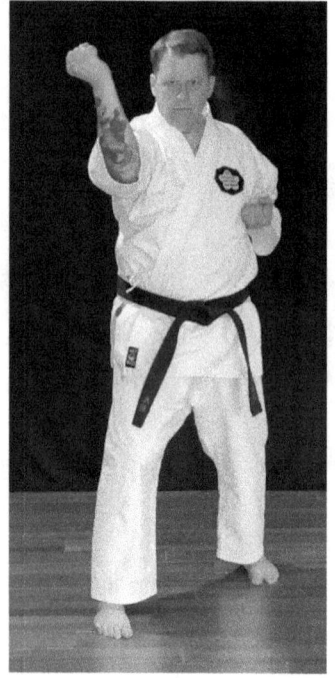

Step Forward and Complete Right Jodan Mae Tettsui Uchi (kiai)

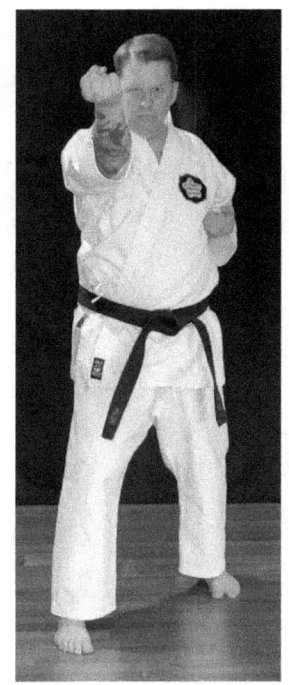 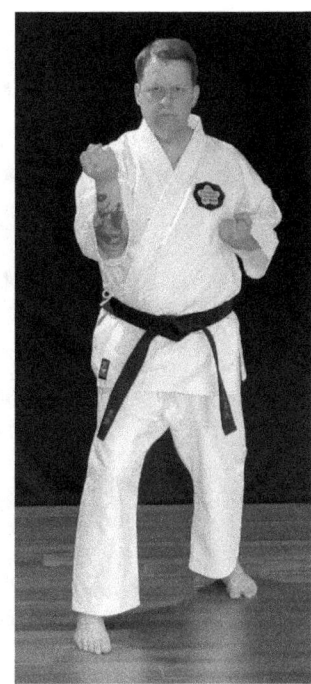

Tettsui Uchi (kiai) (cont.)

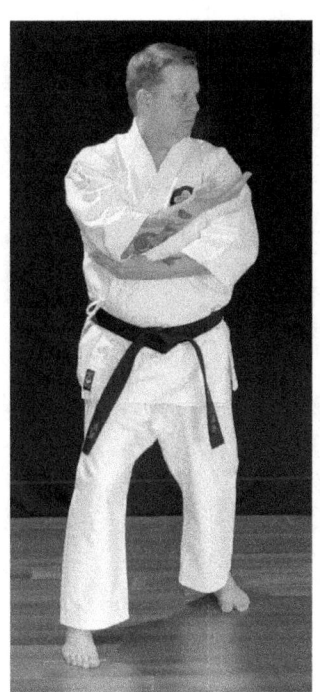 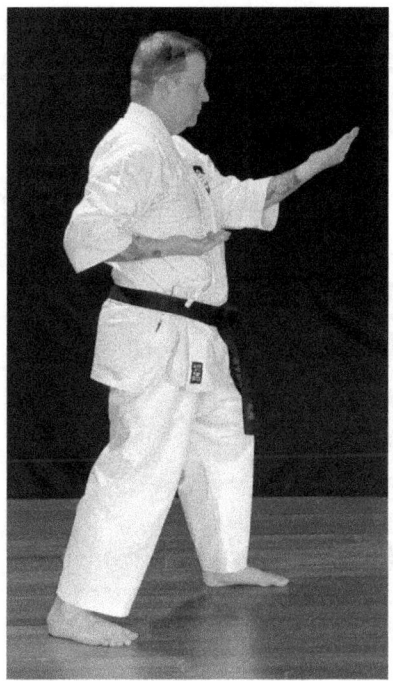

Pivot Left, Complete Left Chudan Hari Uke...

Genshin

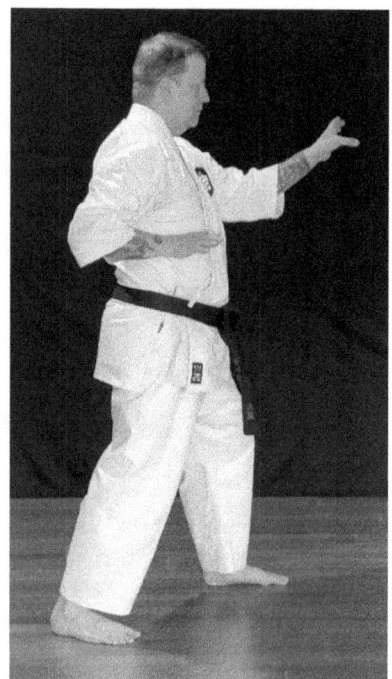 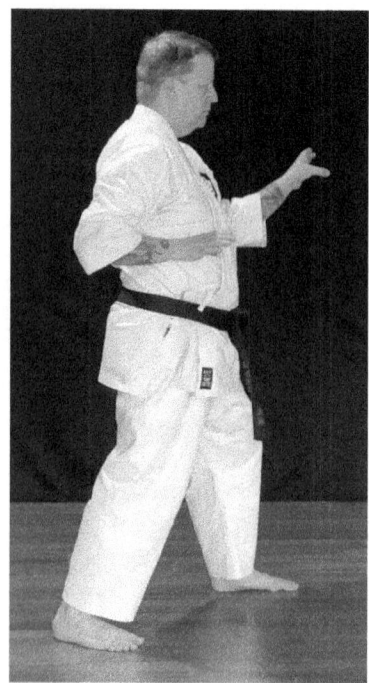

...Turning into Left Chudan Hiki Uke

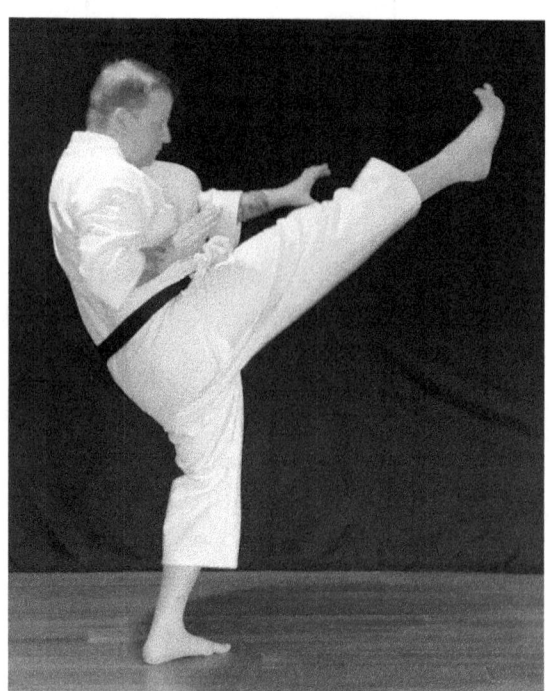 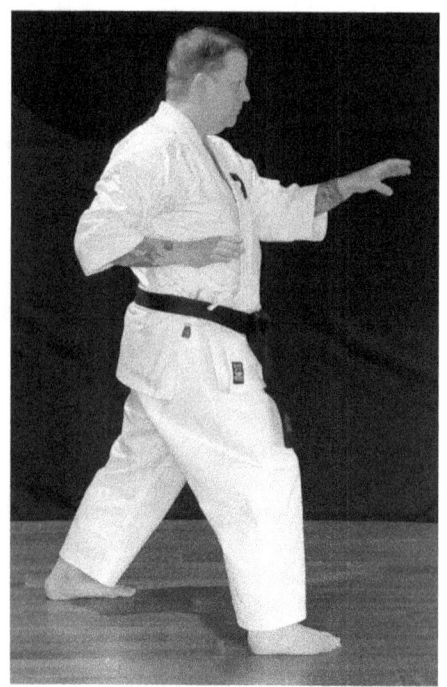

Complete Right Jodan Mae Keage Geri   Set

Genshin

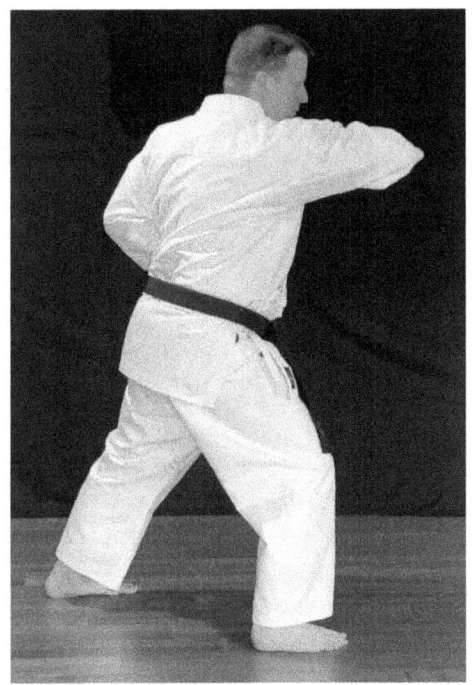

Complete Right Chudan Kote Uchi

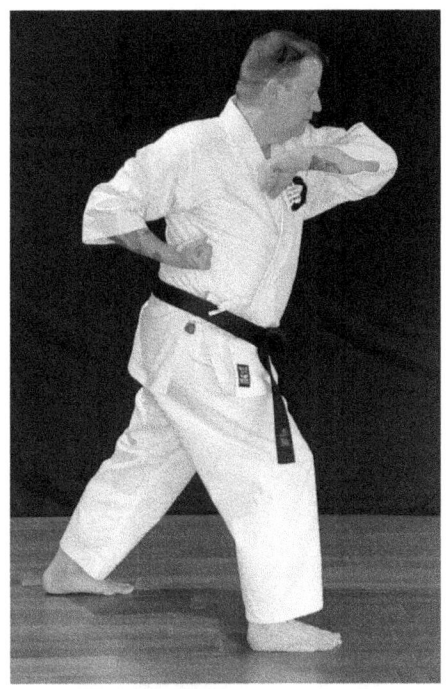

Complete Left Chudan Empi Uchi

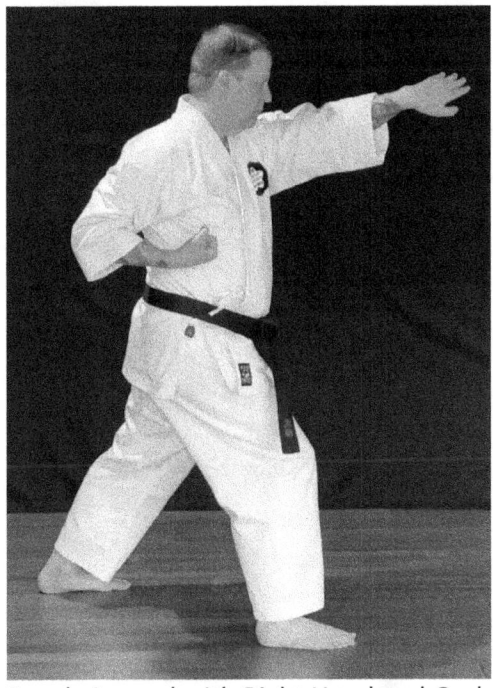

Reach Around with Right Hand and Grab Behind Opponent's Neck

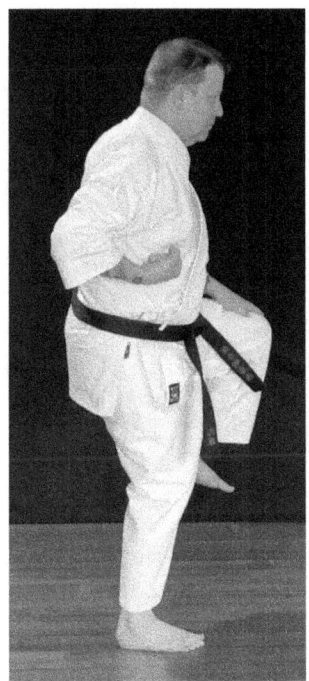

Pull Down to Hiza Uchi

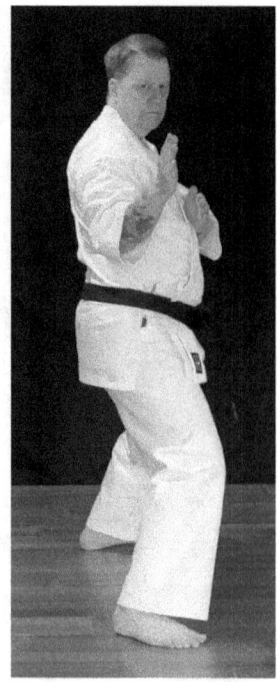

Left Foot Set Back into Yoko Heiko Dachi with Open Hands, Right Side Forward Forward

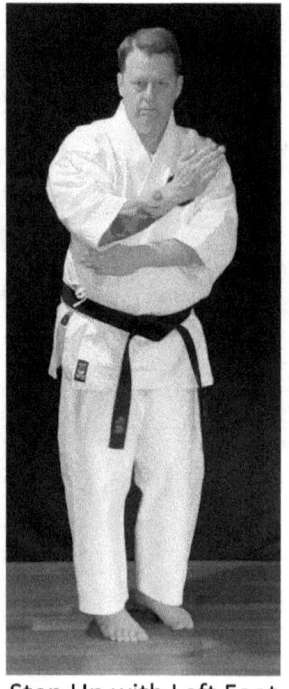

Step Up with Left Foot

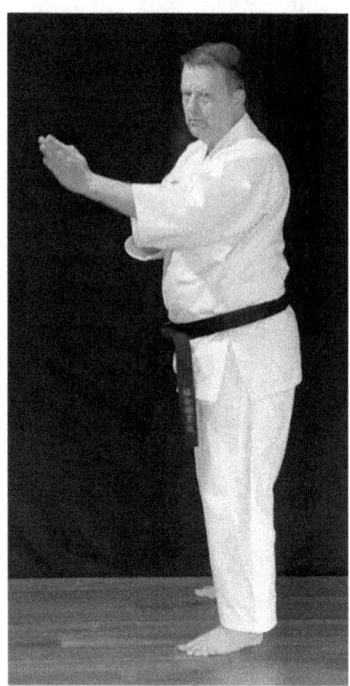

Step Back with Right Foot

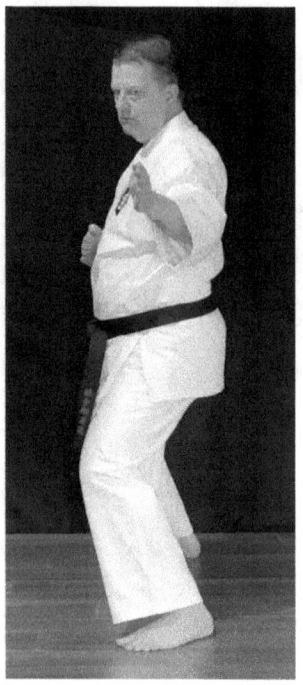

Set into Yoko Heiko Dachi with Open Hands with Open Hands, Left Side Forward

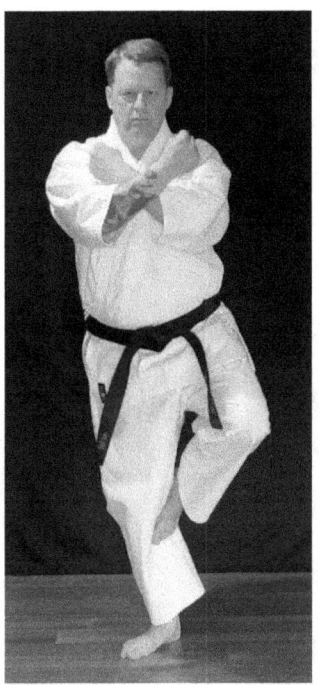
Step Back with Right Foot into Heiko Dachi with Arms Crossed and Foot Chambered in Ashi Barai

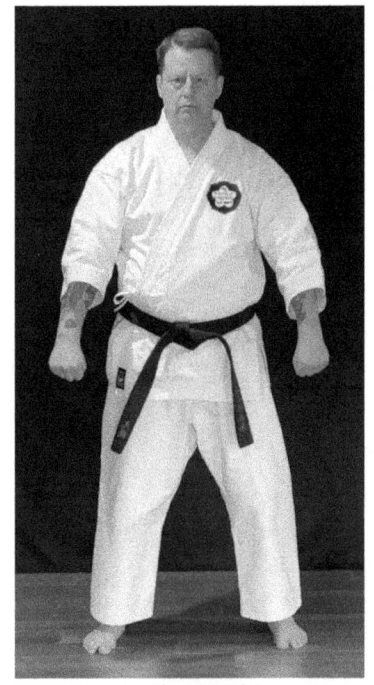
Heiko Dachi

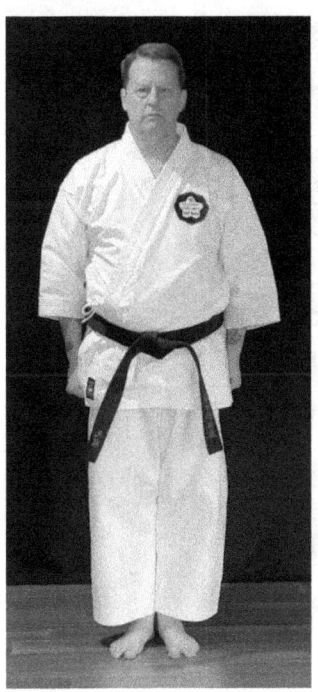
Musubi Dachi

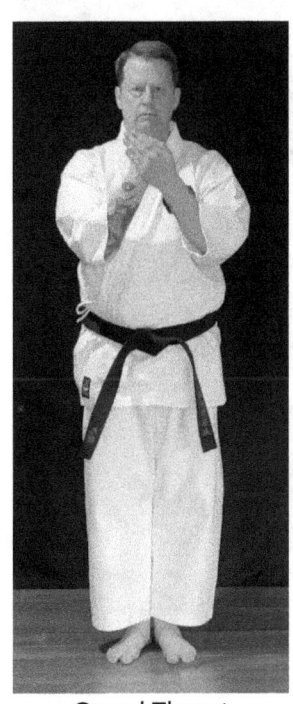
Guard Throat

Genshin

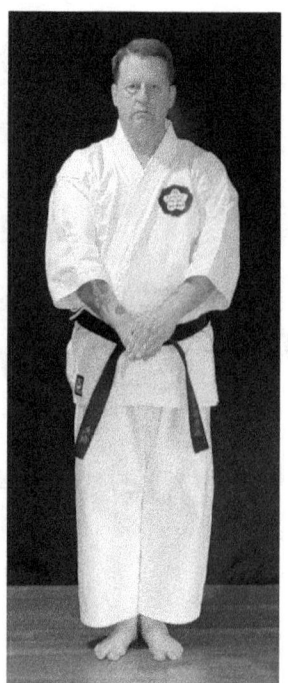

Turn Hands Down to Guard Groin

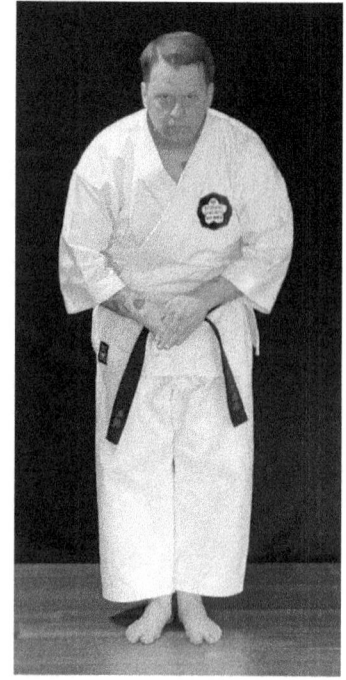

Rei

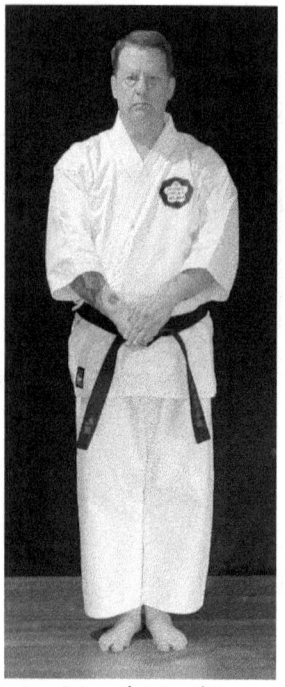

Musubi Dachi

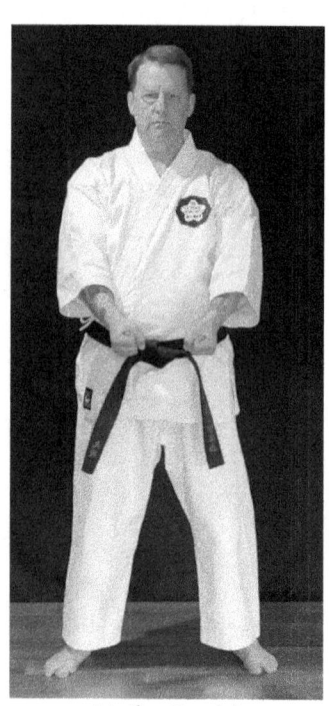

Heiko Dachi

Isshoni San

Isshoni San means "together three." Described in more details below, this was Shodai's original 3rd kata and follows much of the same patterns of the Gekisai series. It was changed when Gekisai San was created to a slightly more difficult version with tai sabaki head blocks. As one of the first katas Shodai created, it was created with open hand head blocks and other moves not contained in Gekisai Ichi and Ni. Eventually he would create a new introductory kata, Kihon Ichi and his own version of Gekisai San. When Gekisai San was created, he transferred some of the basic moves from Isshoni San to Gekisai San and made Isshoni San slightly more advanced.

Below is the method by which Ketsugo Goju-Ryu performs Genshin kata. Complete details about each move are not included, as this is simply a demonstration.

These are the Japanese terms used for this kata. Bear in mind, karate terms are not completely streamlined. There are terms that were used in the middle of the 20th Century that are no longer used today. Oftentimes there are more than one term that can be used for the same technique. The important thing is not what it is called, but the technique itself.

Barai - Sweeping Block	**Neko Ashi Dachi** - Cat Leg Stance
Chudan - Middle	**Nukite** – Spear Hand
Dachi – Stance	**Oshi** - Push
Fumikomi Geri – Stamping Kick	**Otoshi** - Dropping (Downward)
Gedan – Low	**Rei** – Bow (Respect)
Hajime – Command to Begin	**Shiko Dachi** - Straddle Leg Stance
Hari Uke – Open Hand Block (Palm Up)	**Shotei** - Palm Heel
Heiko Dachi - Parallel Stance	**Shuto Uchi** – Chop Strike
Hiki Uke – Open Hand Block (Palm Down)/Pulling Block	**Tettsui Uchi** – Hammer Fist Strike
	Tsukami Hiki – Grab and Pull
Jodan – High	**Tsuki/-Zuki** - Punch

Juji Uke – X Block **Kake Uke** - Hook Block **Kokutsu Dachi** – Rear Leaning Stance **Kosa Dachi** – Crossed Stance **Ko Uke** - Back of Wrist Block **Mae Keage Geri** – Front Snap Kick **Morote** – Double **Musubi Dachi** - Attention Stance, Toes Out	**Uchi** – Strike **Uke** – Block (Receive) **Ura Zuki** – Inverted Punch **Uraken Uchi** - Back Fist Strike **Yoi** – Ready Command **Yoko** - Side **Zenkutsu Dachi** - Forward Leaning Stance

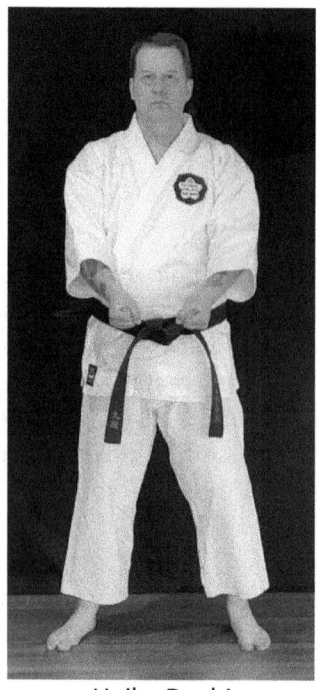

Heiko Dachi

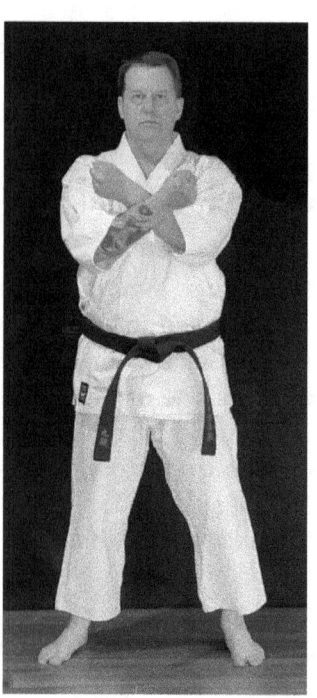

(Yoi) Brings Arms Up, Crossed at the Wrist

Isshoni San

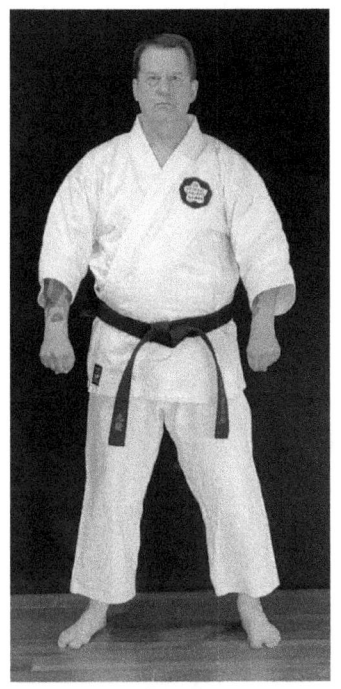

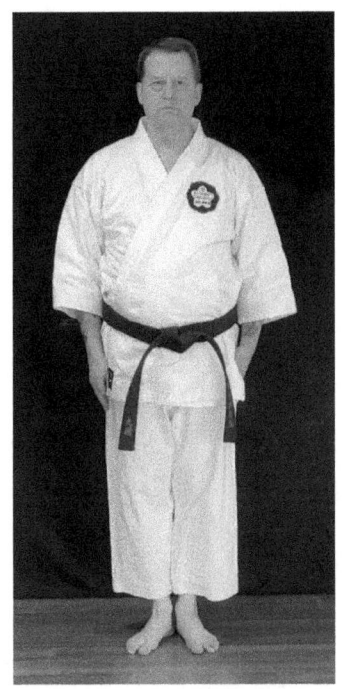

Hajime (Begin)

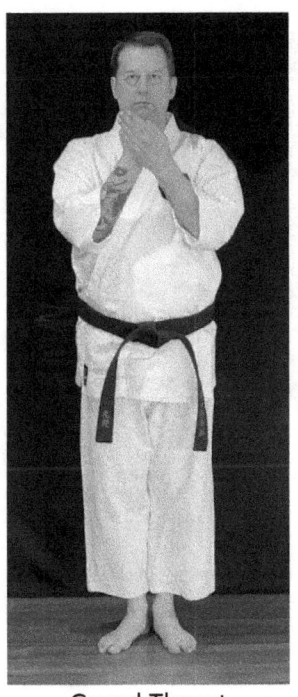

Guard Throat

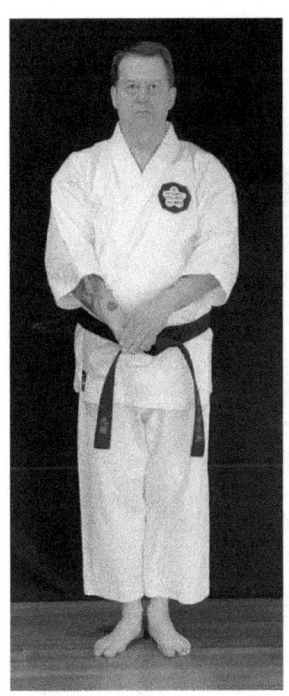

Turn Hands Down
to Guard Groin

Isshoni San

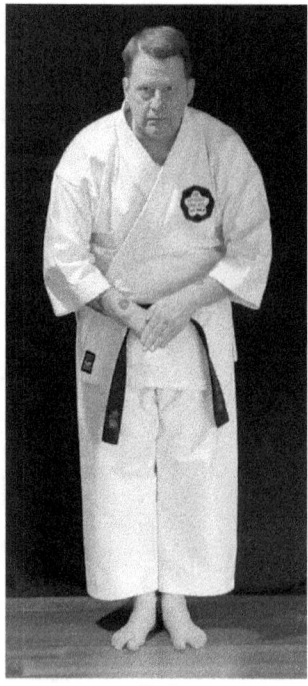
Rei

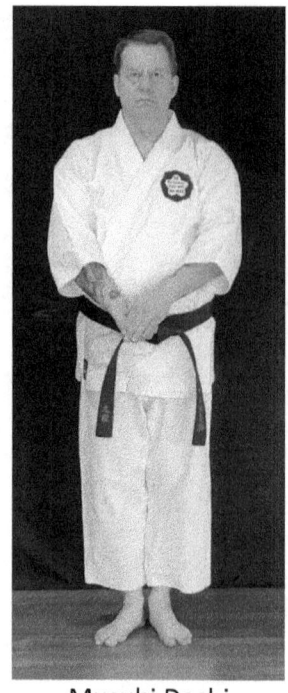
Musubi Dachi

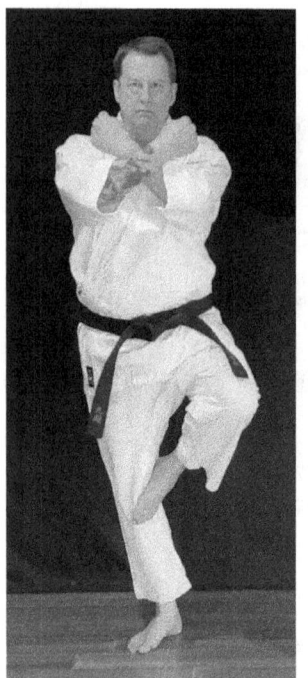
Bring Left Foot Up and Cross Arms

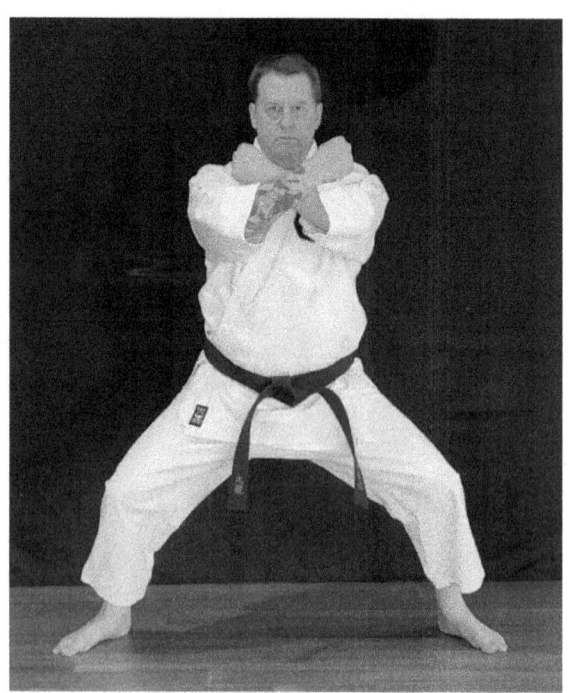
Come Down into Shiko Dachi

Isshoni San

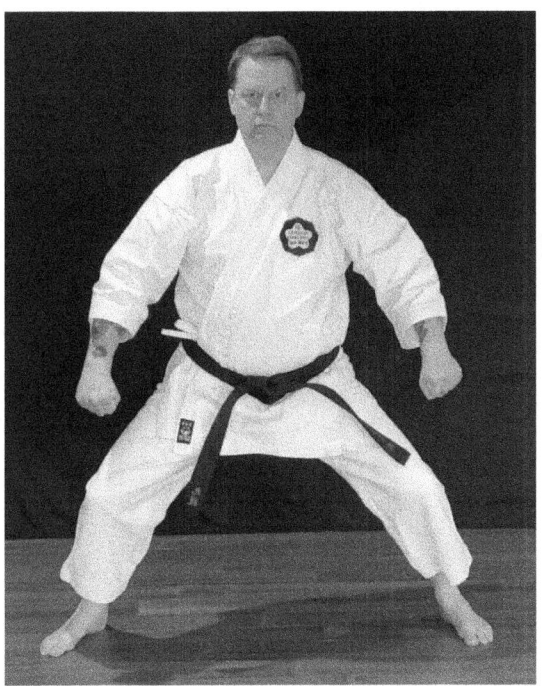

Complete Morote Gedan Barai Slowly

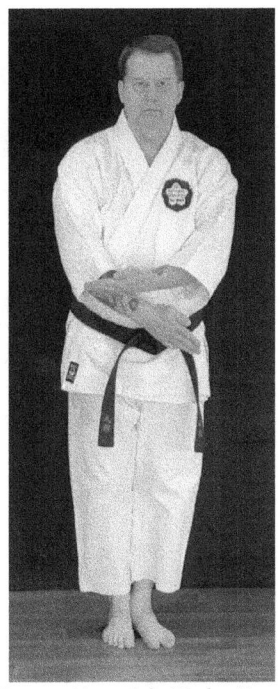

Come Up with Right Foot to Left Foot, Stepping Forward, Complete Chudan Hari Uke

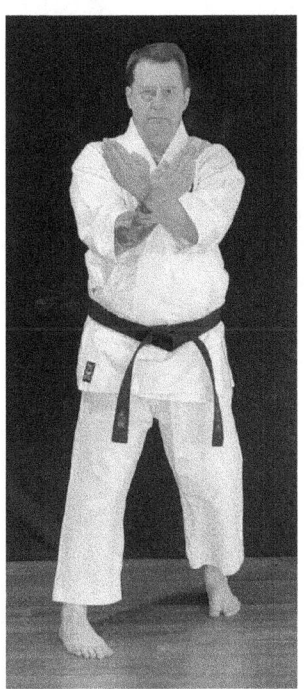

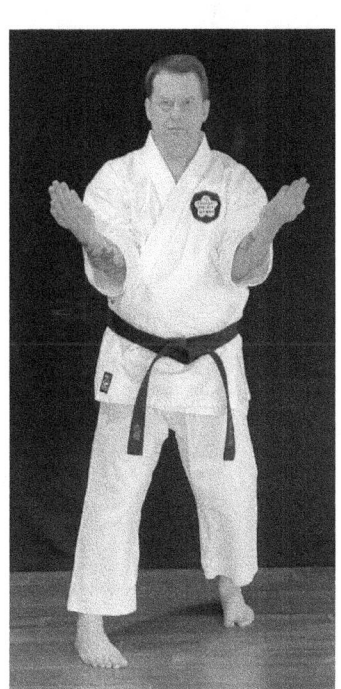

Morote Hari Uke (cont.)

Isshoni San

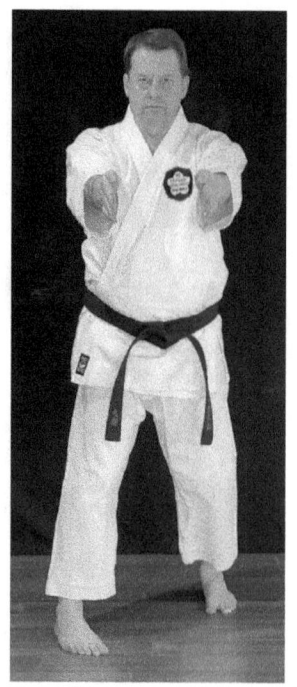 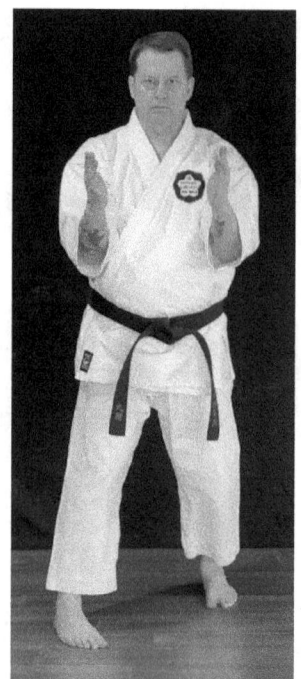

Set with Open Hands

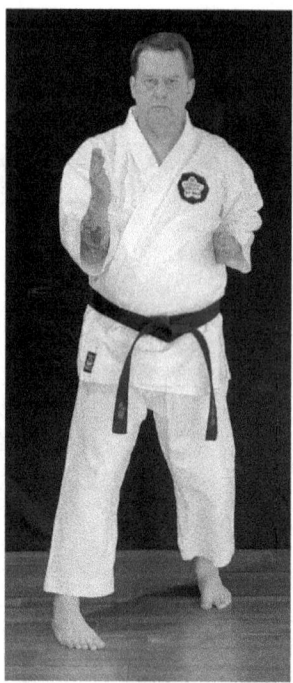 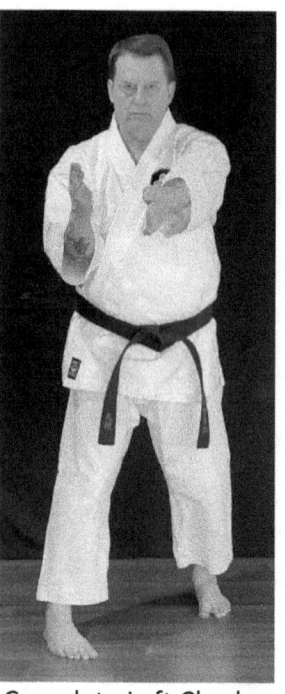

Chamber Left Hand

Complete Left Chudan Nukite Uchi

Isshoni San

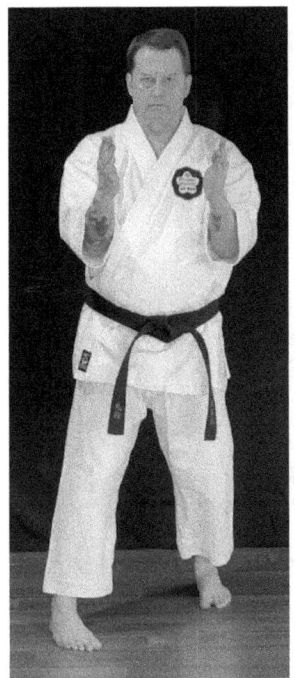

Set

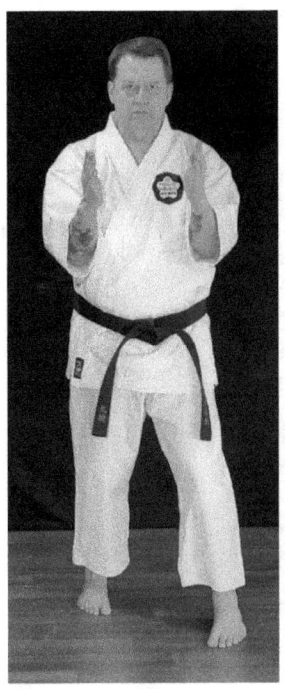

Step

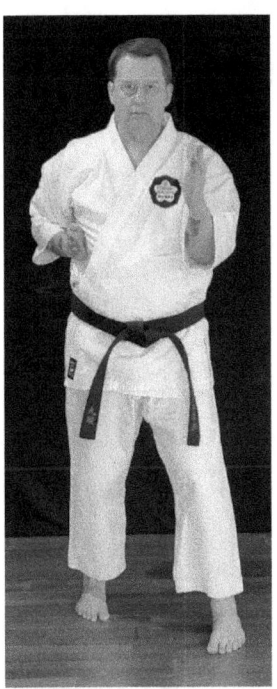

Chamber Left Hand

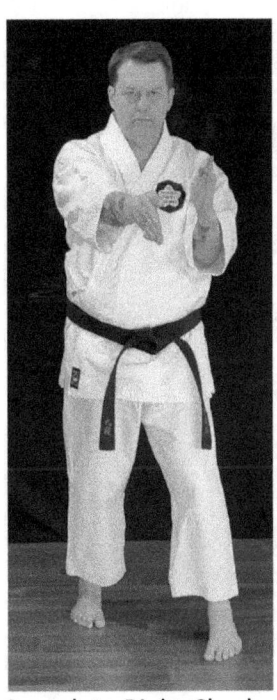

Complete Right Chudan Nukite Uchi

Isshoni San

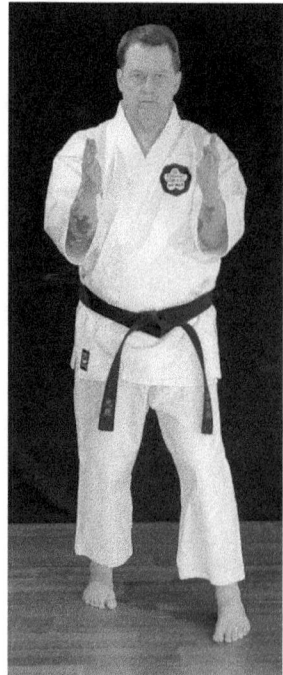

Set

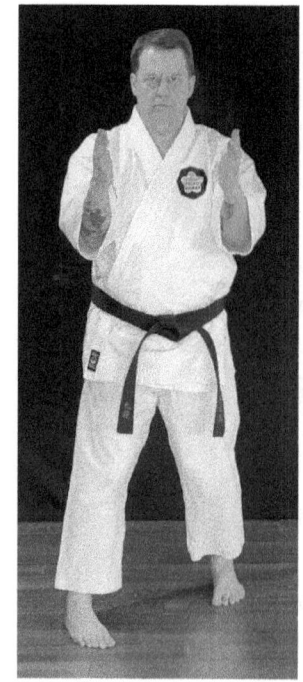

Step

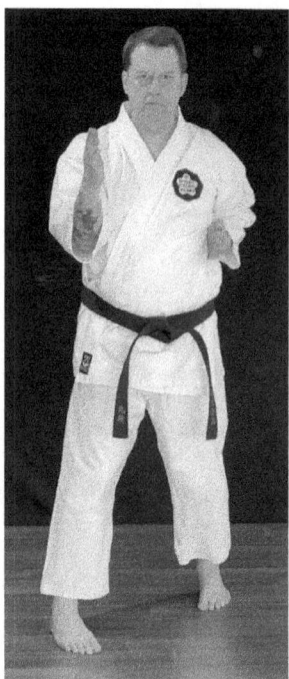

Chamber Left Hand

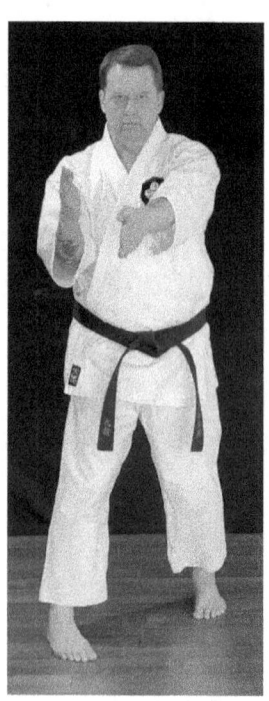

Complete Left Chudan Nukite Uchi

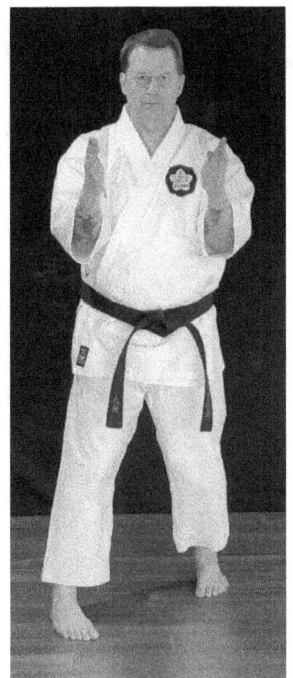

Set

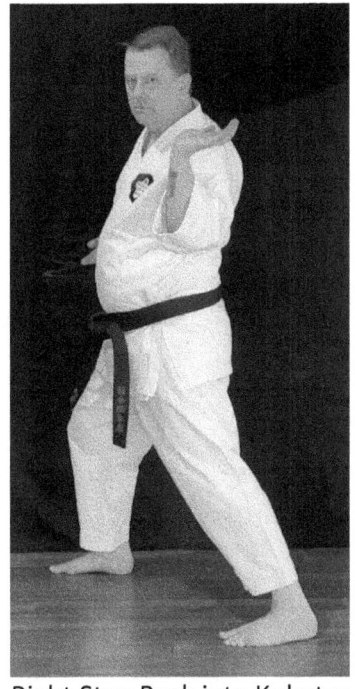

Right Step Back into Kokutsu Dachi at 225° Prepare Left Gedan Shotei Barai

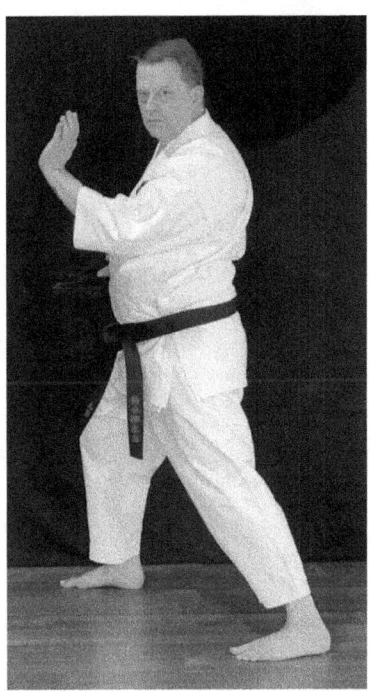

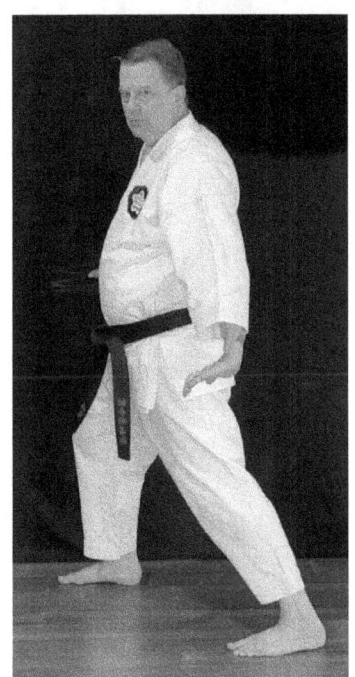

Left Gedan Shotei Barai (cont.)

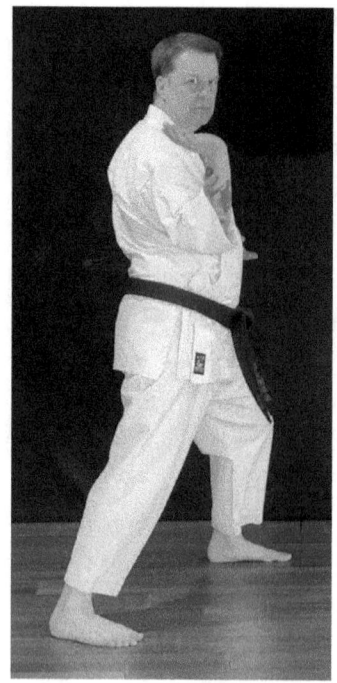 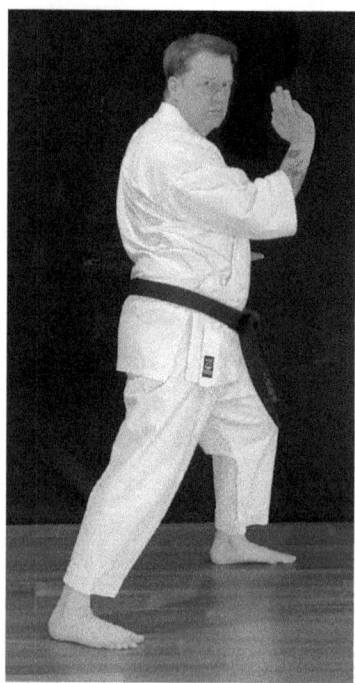

Right Step Back into Kokutsu Dachi at 135°,
Complete Right Gedan Shotei Barai

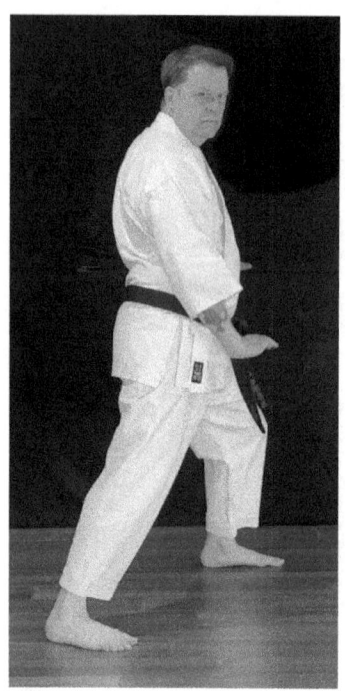 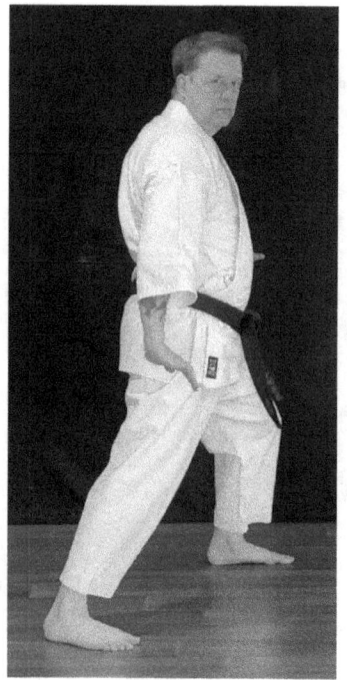

Right Gedan Shotei Barai (cont.)

Isshoni San

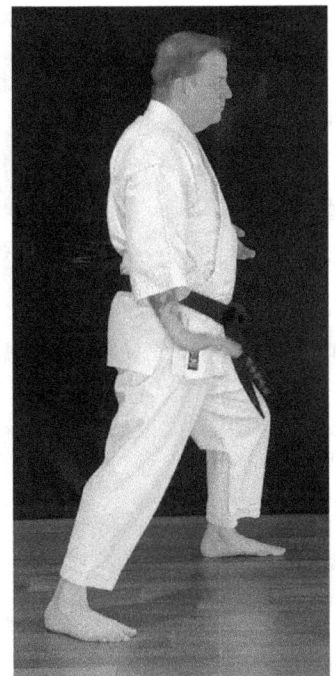 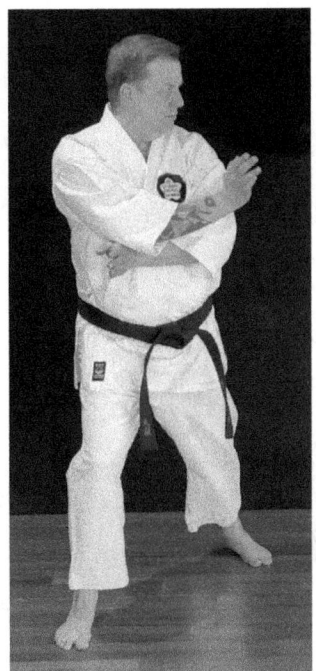

Look Left, Pivot Right, Prepare Left Jodan Yoko Ko Uke

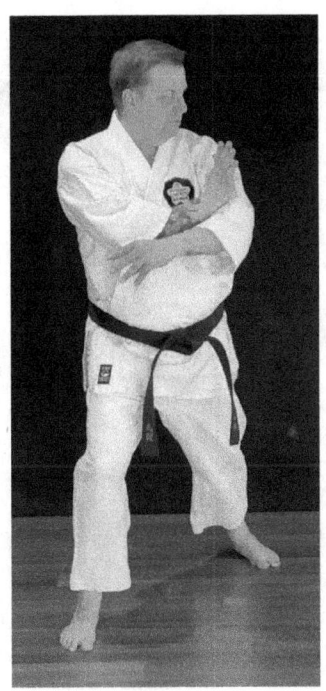 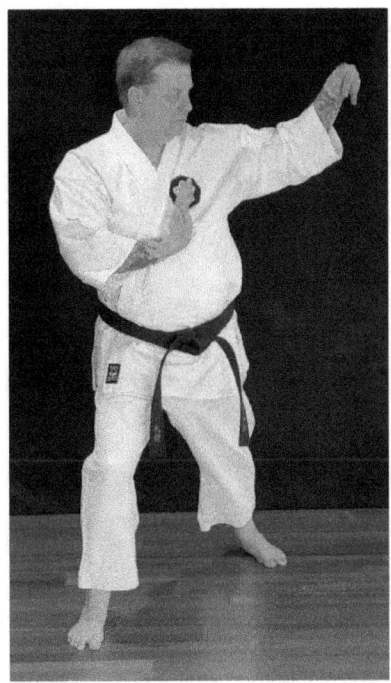

Jodan Yoko Ko Uke (cont.)

Isshoni San

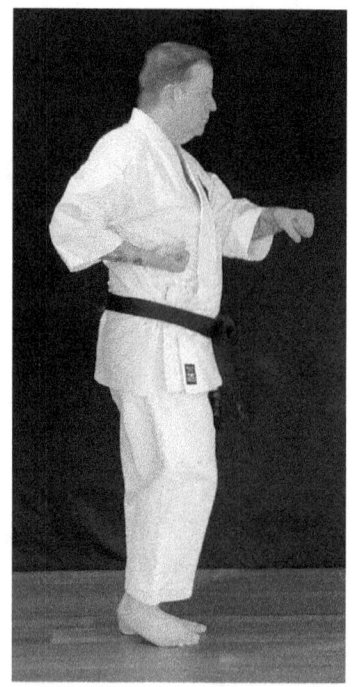 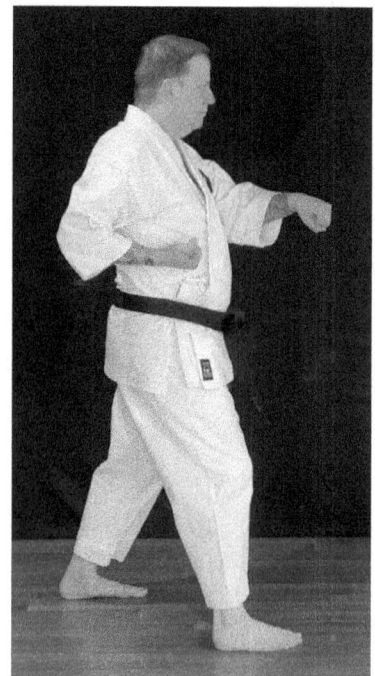

Step Up with Right Foot

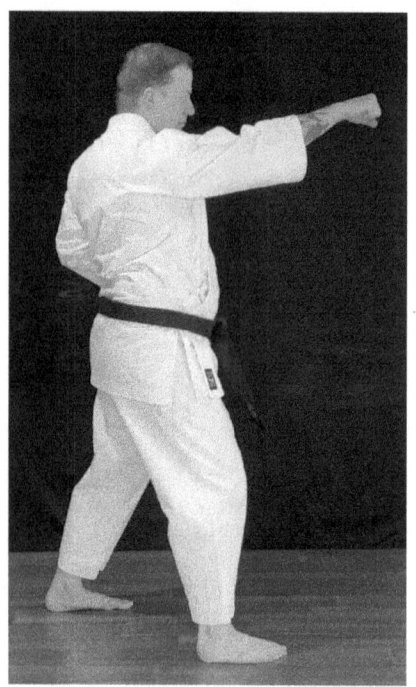 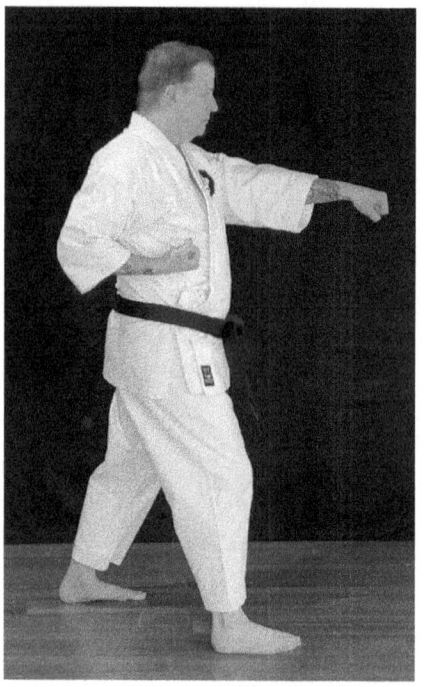

Complete Right Jodan Zuki (pause one beat), then…

…Complete Left Chudan Zuki

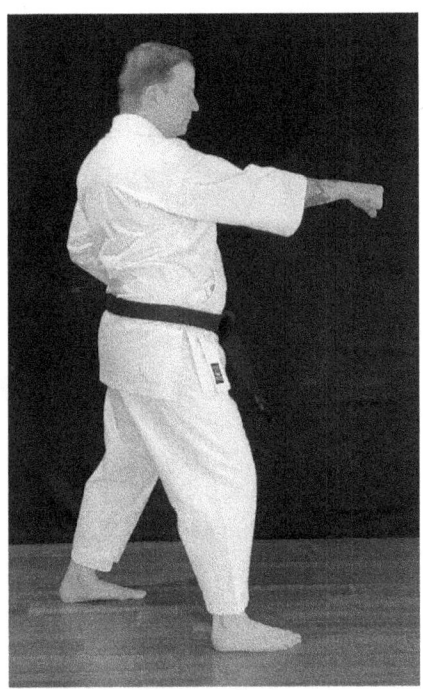

...then Immediate Right
Chudan Zuki

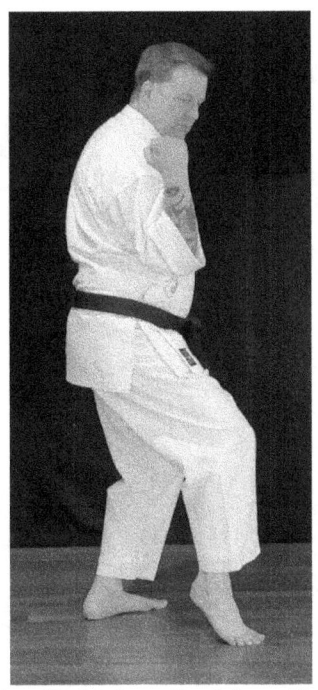

Bring Right Foot Back into Neko
Ashi Dachi, Prepare for Right
Gedan Yoko Barai

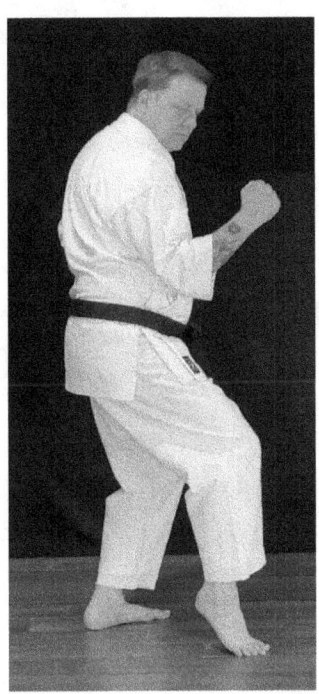

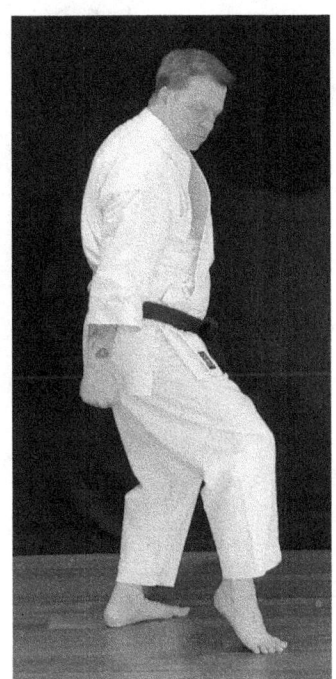

Complete Right Gedan Yoko Barai

Isshoni San

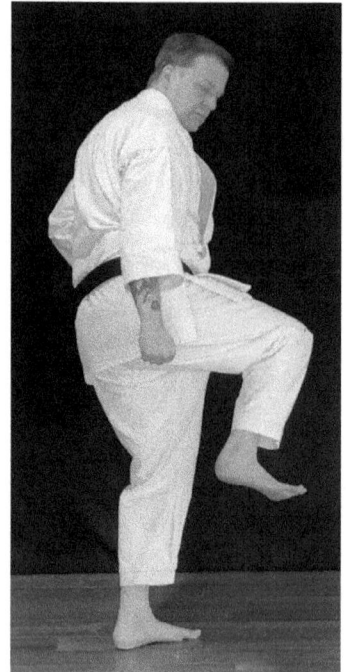
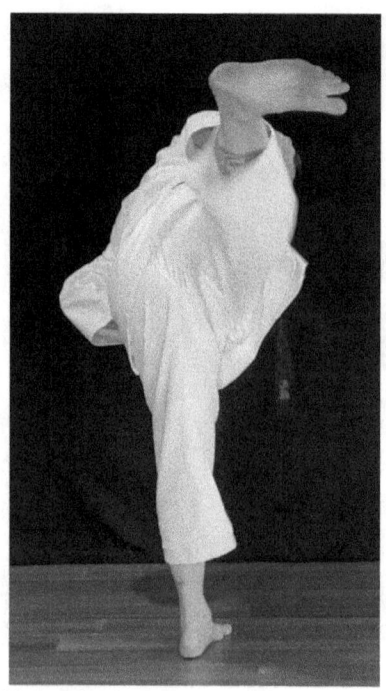

Complete Right Jodan Yoko Geri

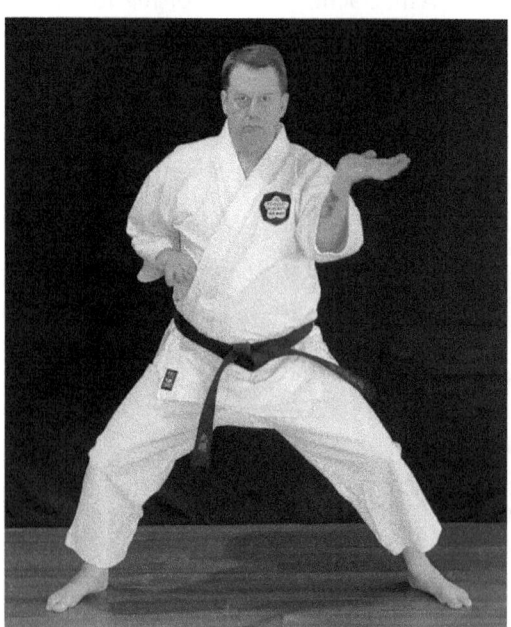
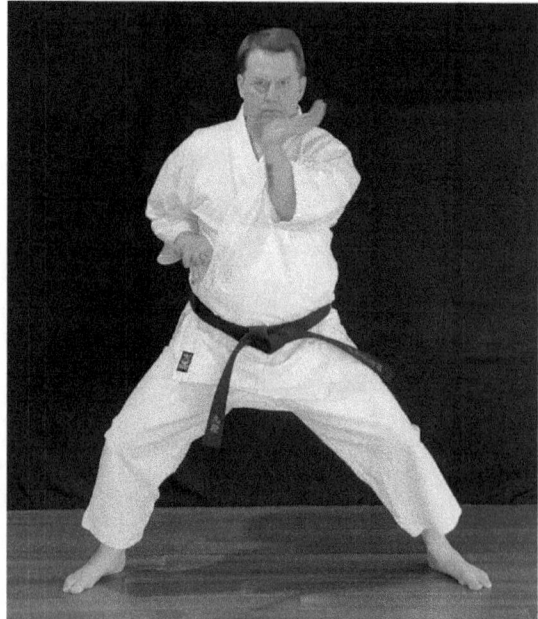

Without Putting Right Foot Down After the Kick, Step into Shiko Dachi, Complete Left Gedan Shotei Barai

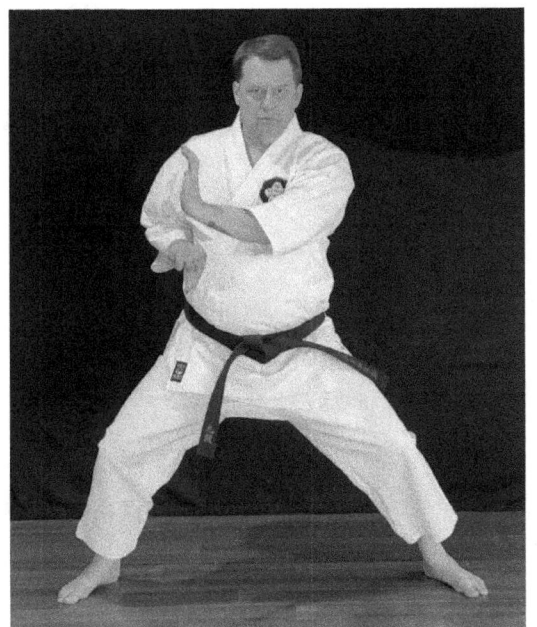 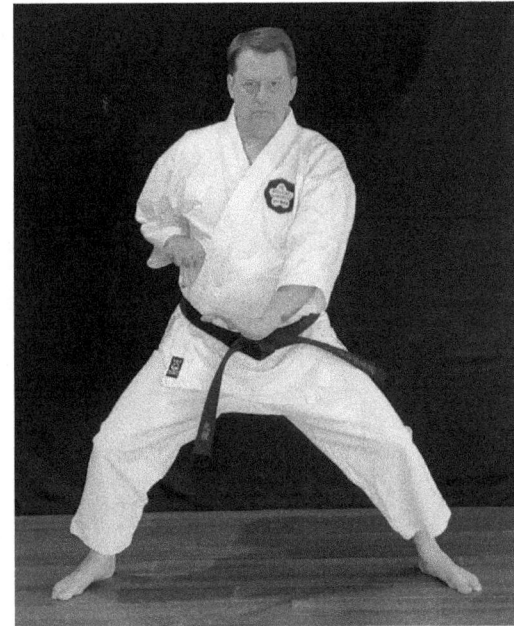

Gedan Shotei Barai (cont.)

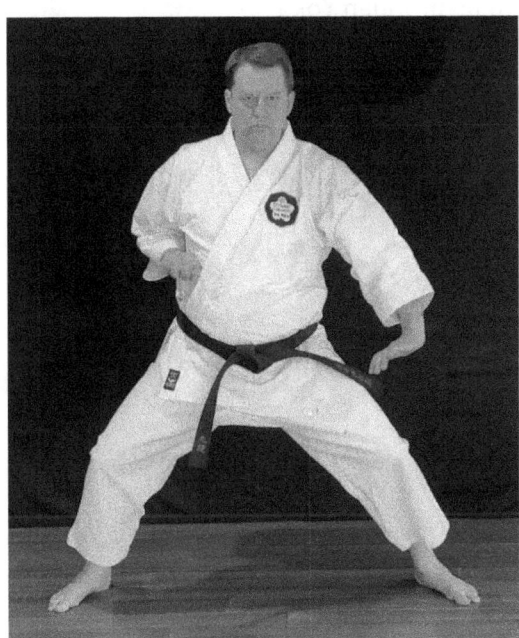 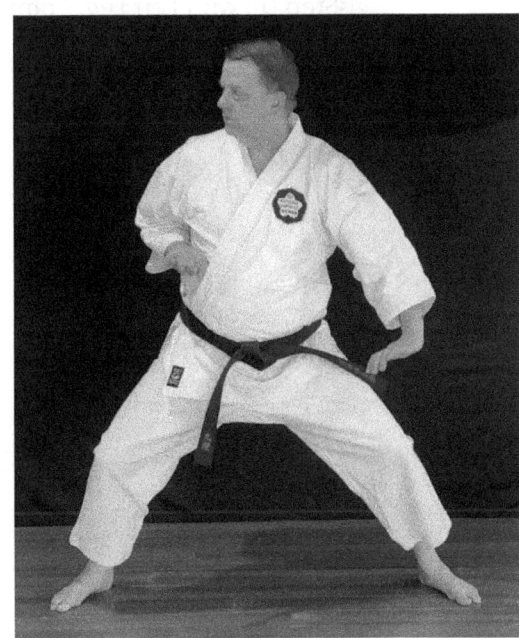

Gedan Shotei Barai (cont.) Look Right

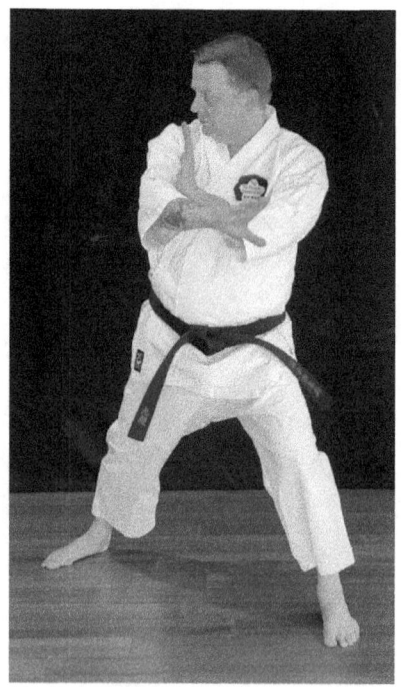 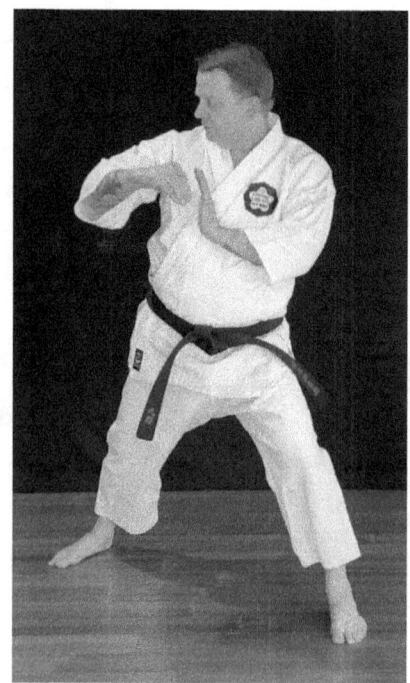

Step Up with Left Leg, Complete Right Jodan Yoko Ko Uke

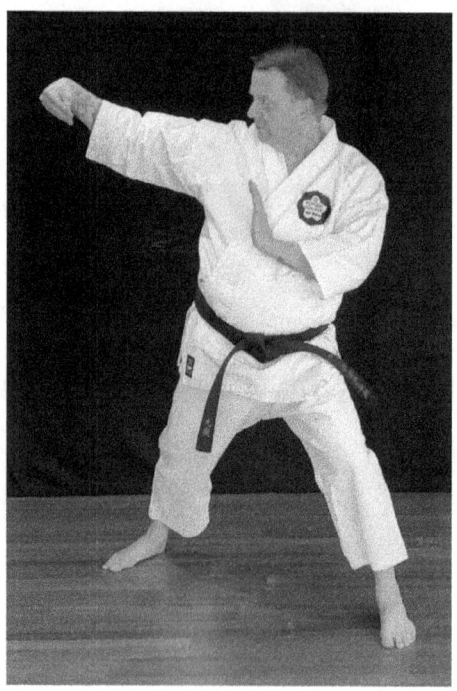 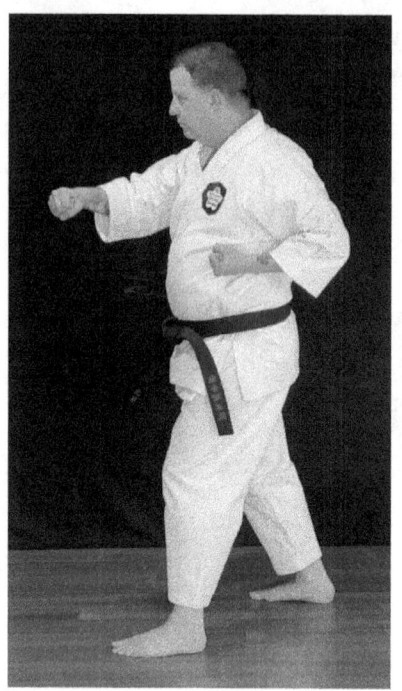

Jodan Yoko Ko Uke (cont.)   Step Up with Left Foot

Isshoni San

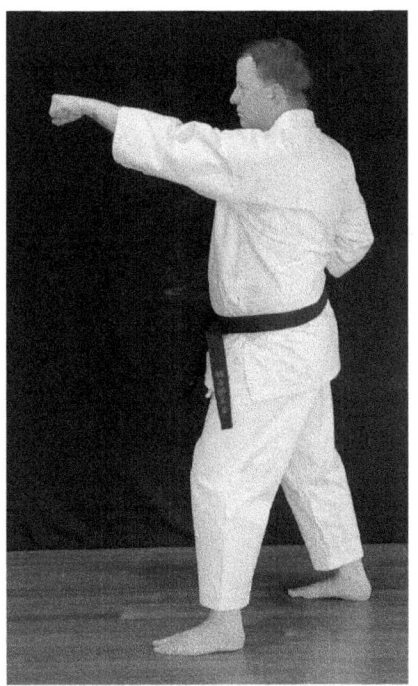

Complete Left Jodan Zuki (pause one beat), then

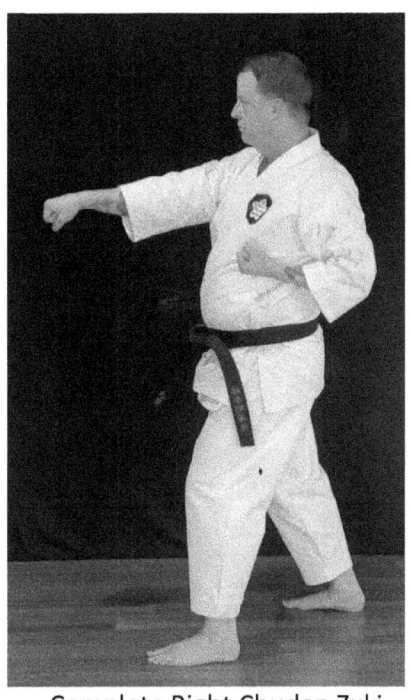

...Complete Right Chudan Zuki

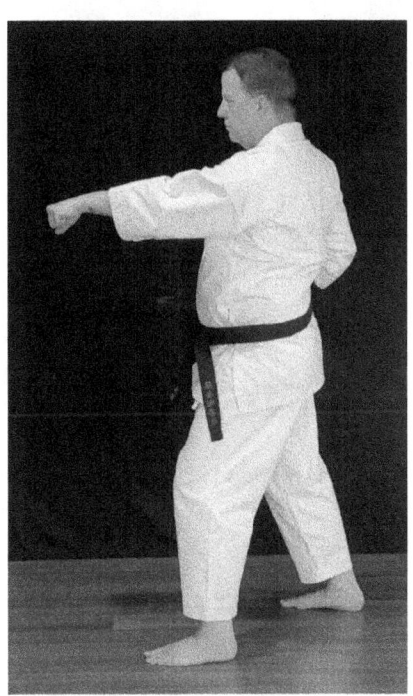

...then Immediate Left Chudan Zuki

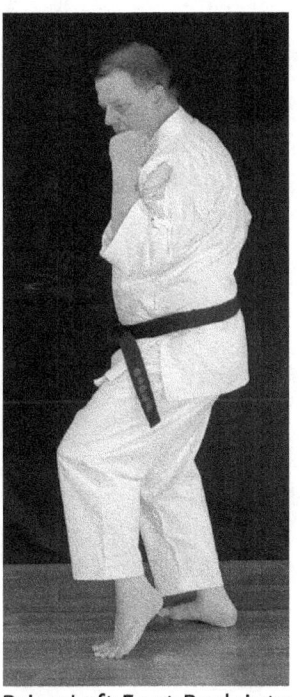

Bring Left Foot Back into Neko Ashi Dachi, Prepare for Left Gedan Yoko Barai

Isshoni San

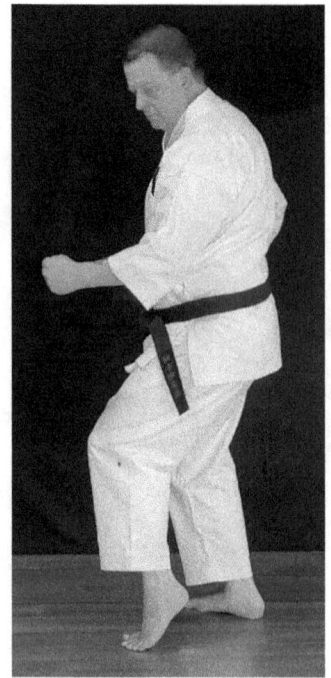 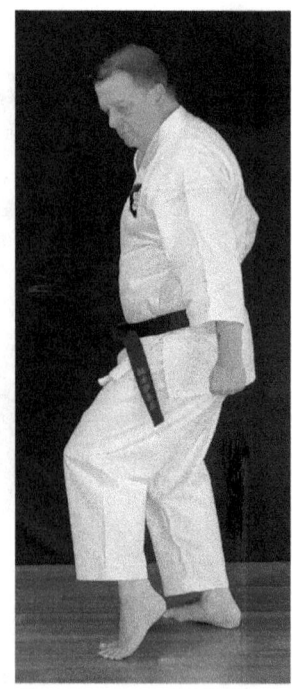

Complete Left Gedan Yoko Barai

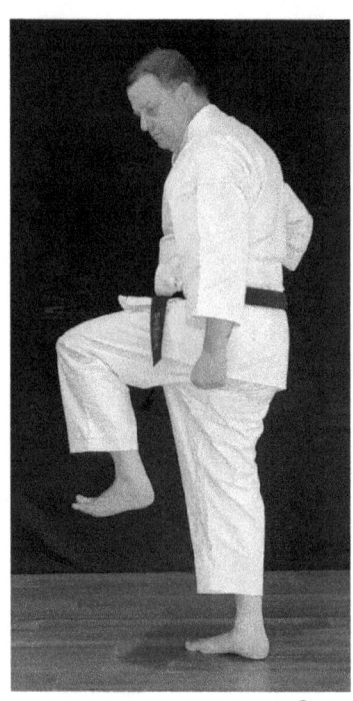 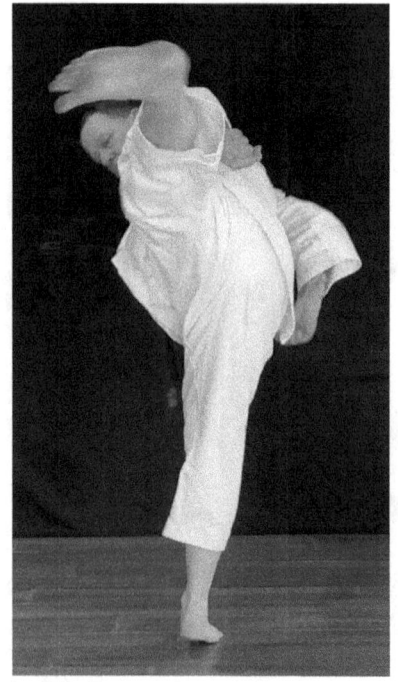

Complete Jodan Yoko Geri

Isshoni San

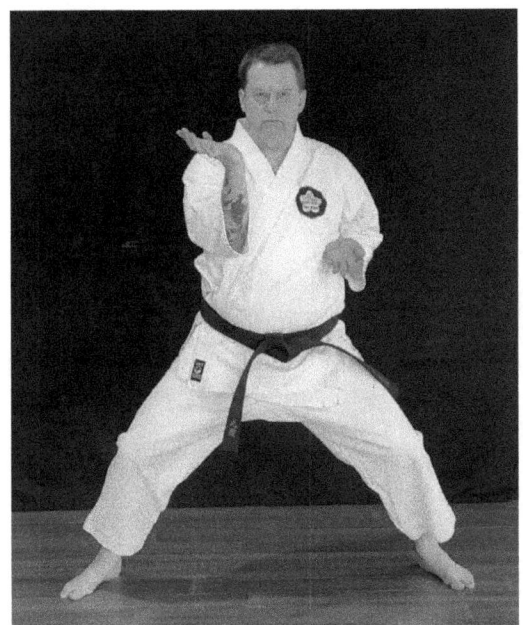
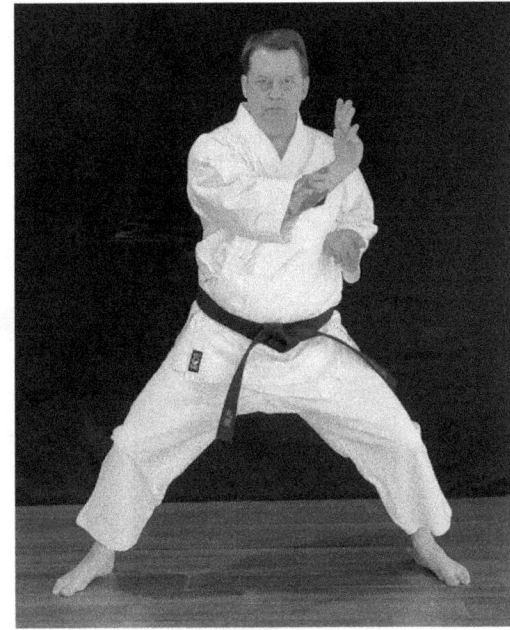

Without Putting Left Foot Down After the Kick,
Step into Shiko Dachi, Complete Gedan Shotei Barai

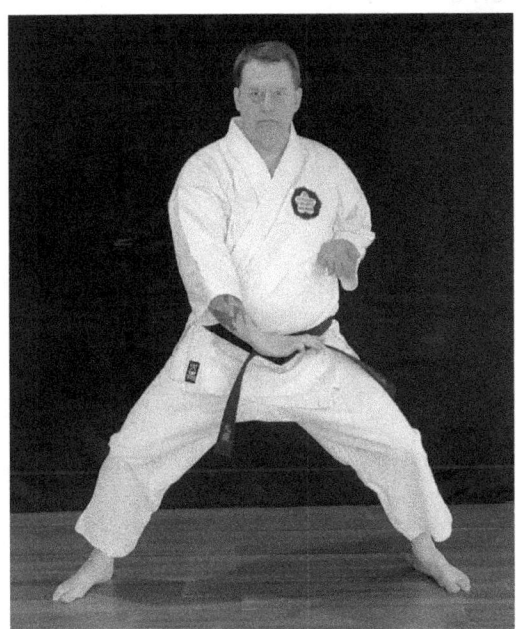
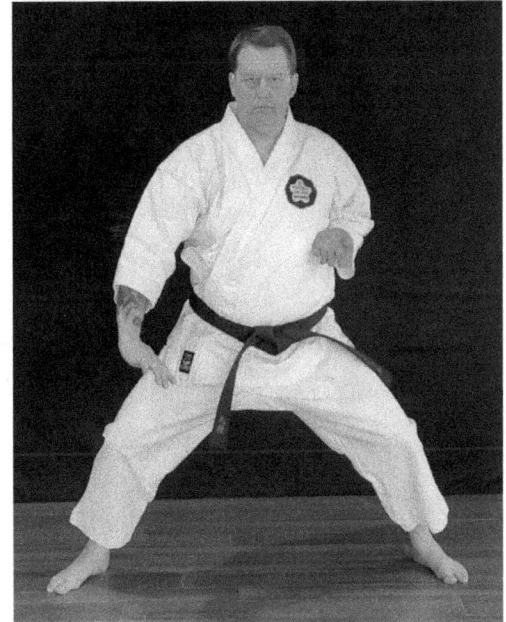

Gedan Shotei Barai (cont.)

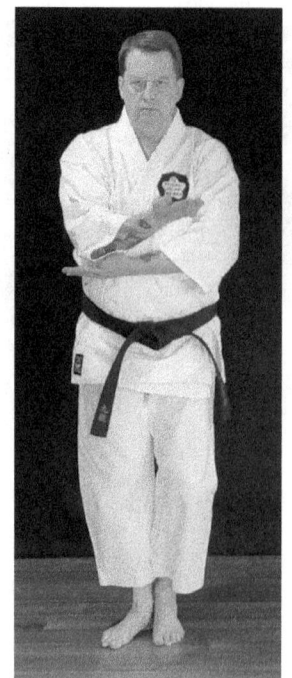 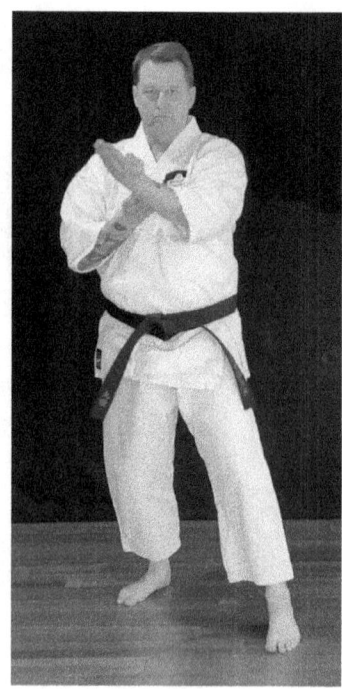

Come Up with Left Foot to Right Foot, Stepping Forward,
Complete Left Chudan Hari Uke into Hiki Uke

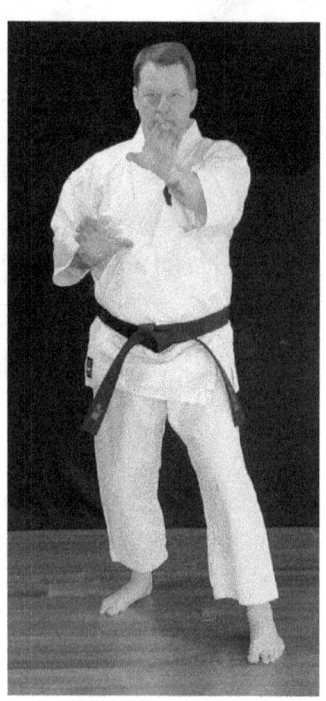 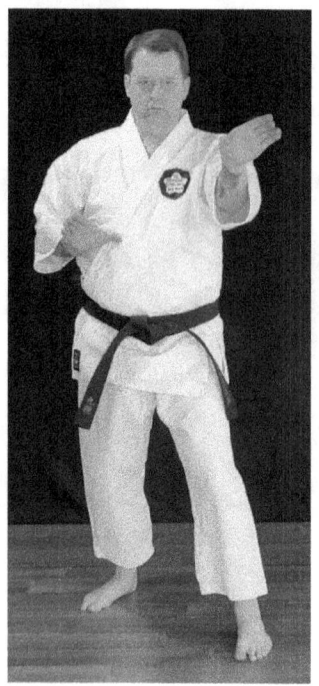

Left Chudan Hiki Uke (cont.)

Isshoni San

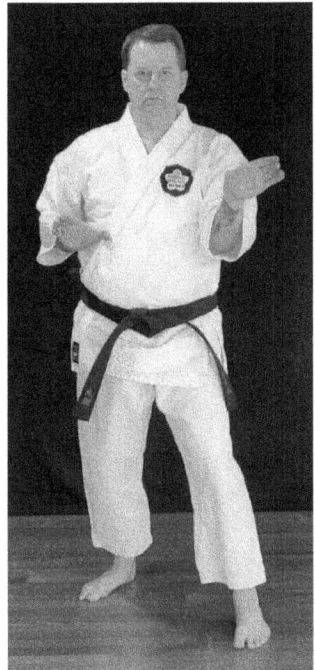
Set

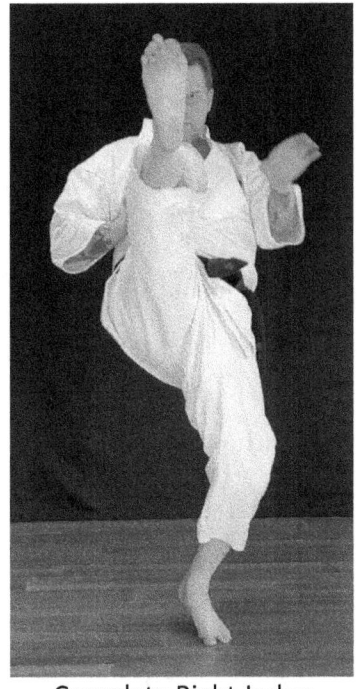
Complete Right Jodan Mae Keage Geri

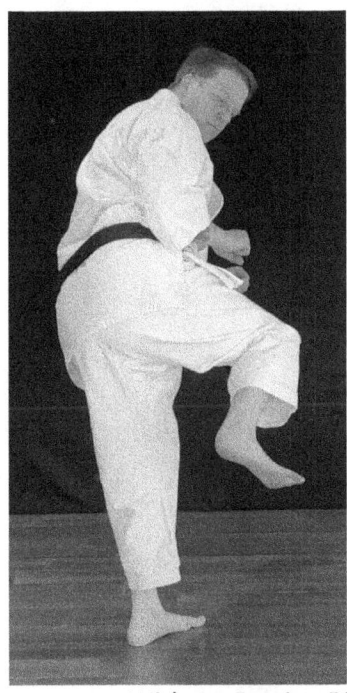
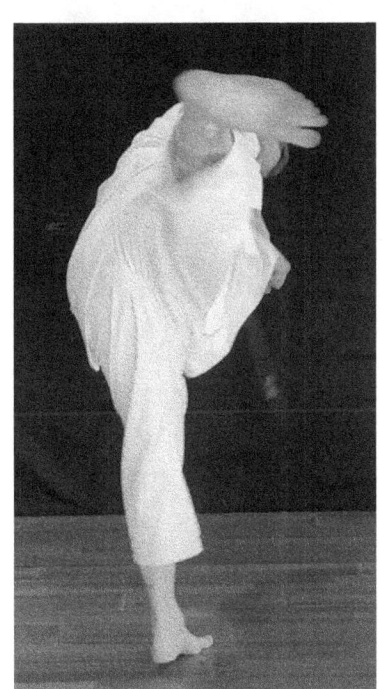
Without Putting Right Foot Down After the Kick, Pivot Right and Complete Right Jodan Yoko Geri (kiai)

Isshoni San

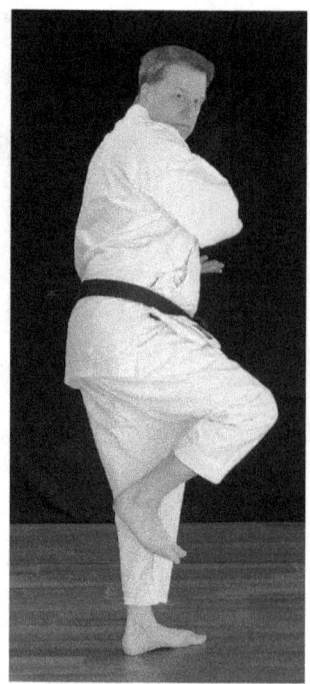
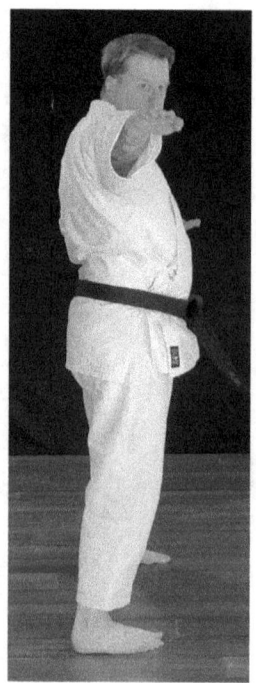

Come Down with Right Yoko Shuto Uchi

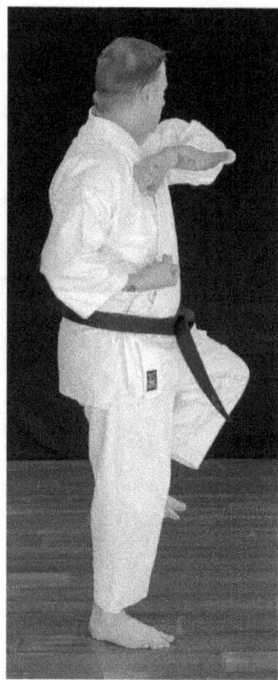

Bring Left Foot and Left Hand to Chamber Looking Rear and Facing Left

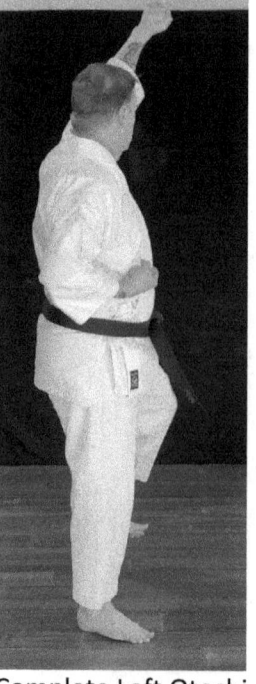

Complete Left Otoshi Tettsui Uchi with Fumikomi Geri

Isshoni San

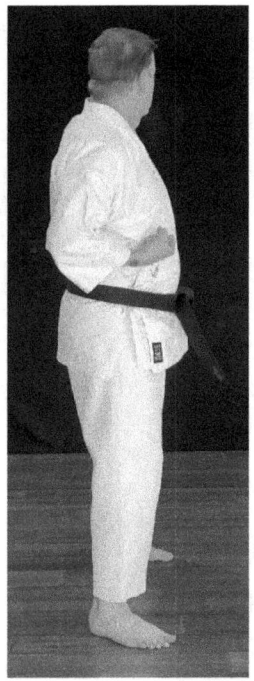
Complete Tsukami Hiki

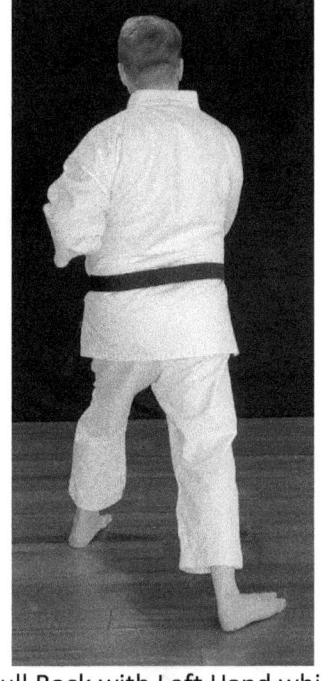
Pull Back with Left Hand while Completing Right Ura Zuki

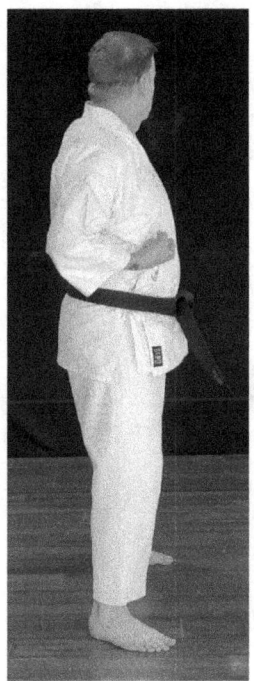
Bring Right Foot Back into Heiko Dachi, Oshi

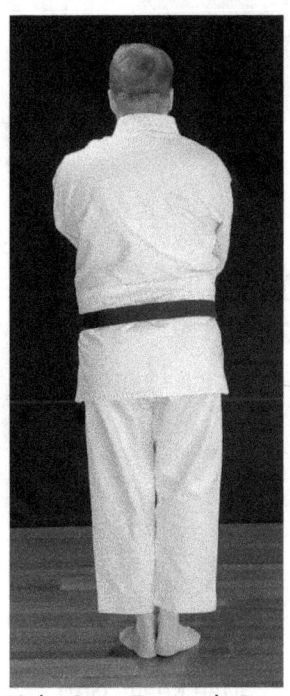
Right Step Towards Rear

Isshoni San

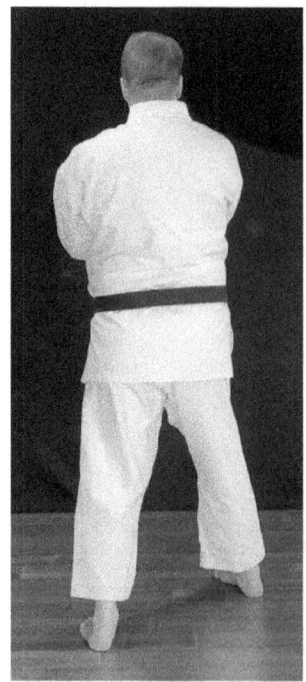 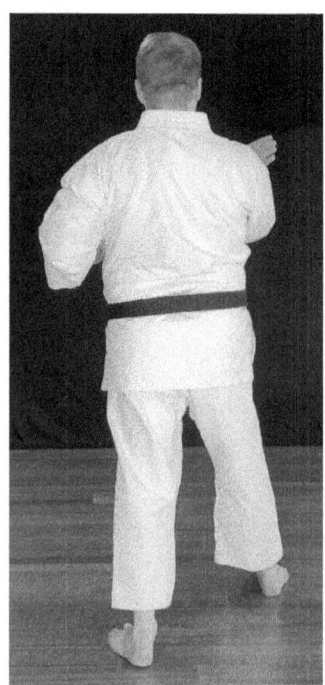

Complete Right Chudan Hari Uke into Hiki Uke

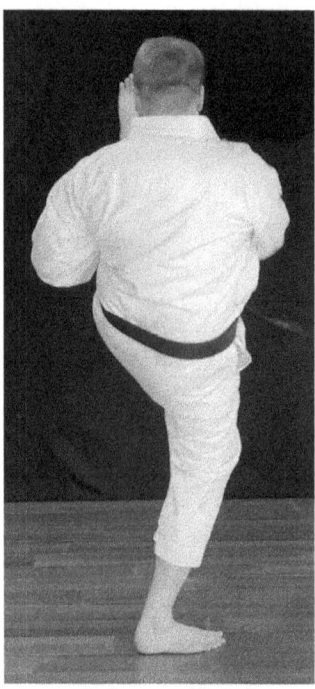 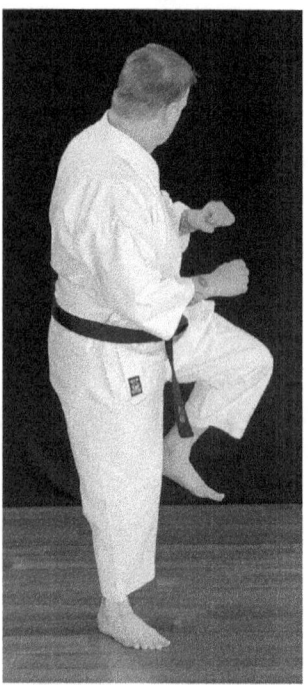

Complete Left Jodan Mae Keage Geri   Without Putting Left Foot Down After Kick, Pivot Right

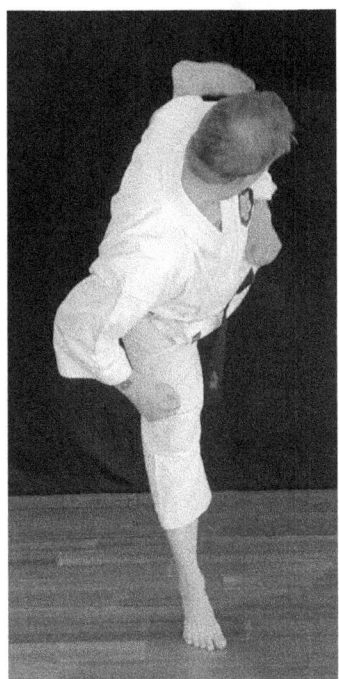

Complete Left Jodan
Yoko Geri (kiai)

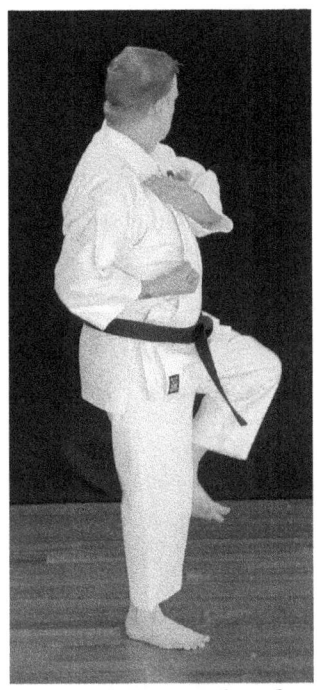

Come Down with Left
Yoko Shuto Uchi

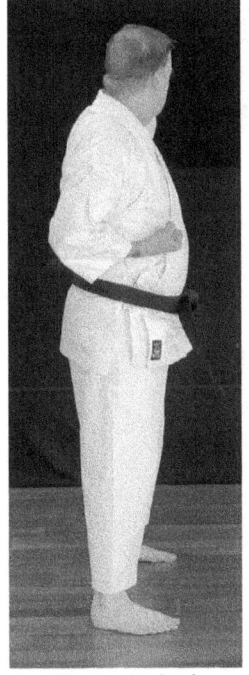

Yoko Shuto Uchi (cont.)

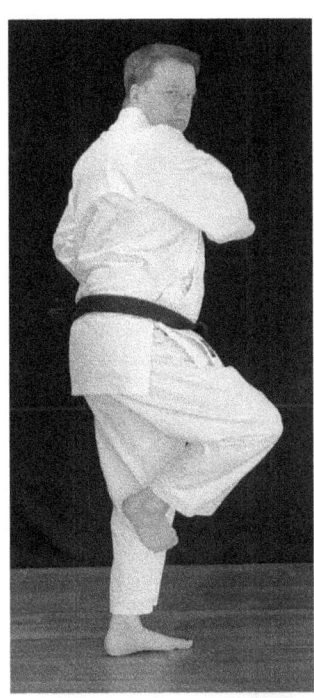

Bring Right Foot and Right Hand
to Chamber Looking Forward
and Facing Left

Isshoni San

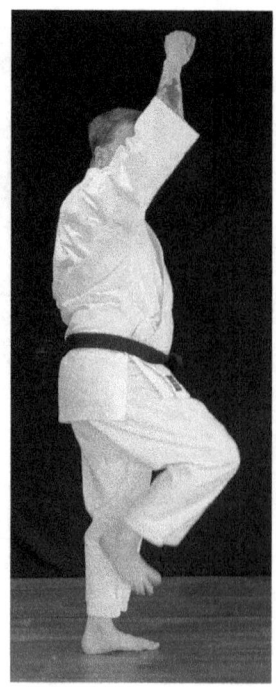 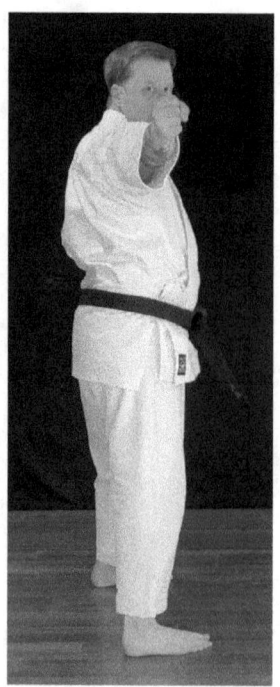

Complete Right Otoshi Tettsui Uchi
with Fumikomi Geri

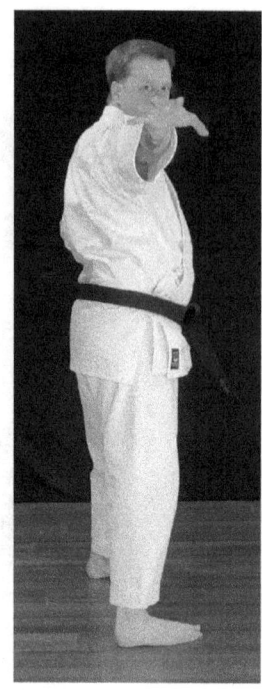 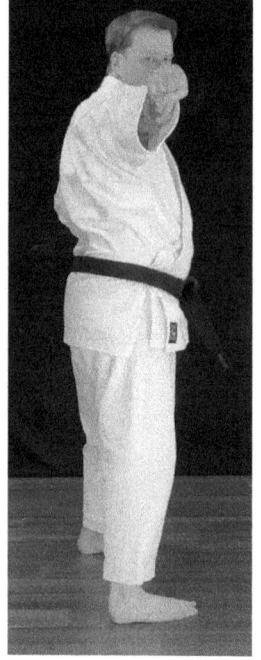

Complete Tsukami Hiki

Isshoni San

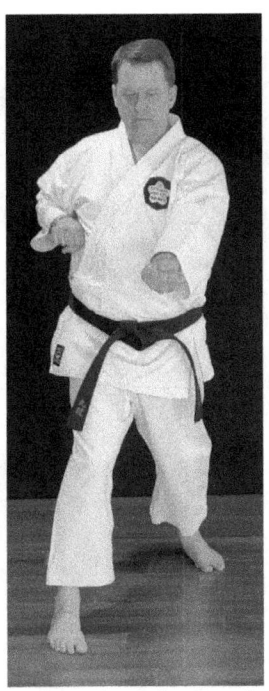

Pull Back with Right Hand while
Completing Left Ura Zuki

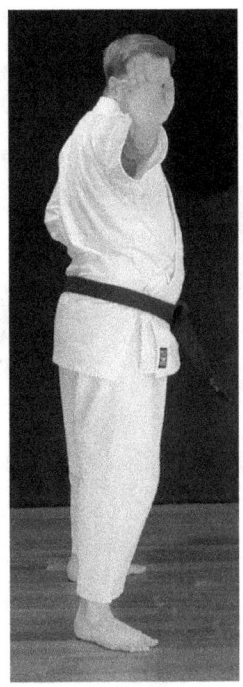

Bring Left Foot Back into
Heiko Dachi, Oshi

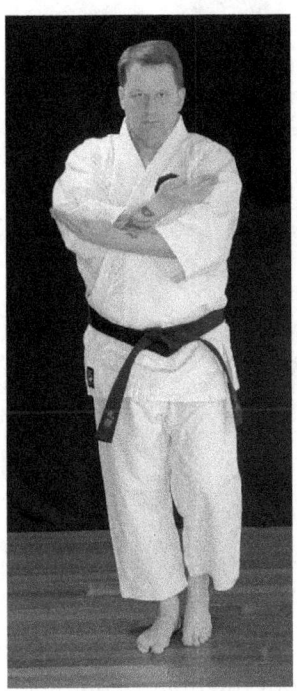

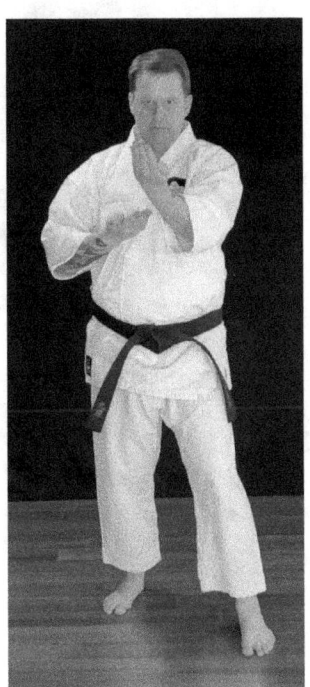

Come Up with Left Foot to Right Foot, Stepping Forward,
Complete Left Chudan Hari Uke into Hiki Uke

Isshoni San

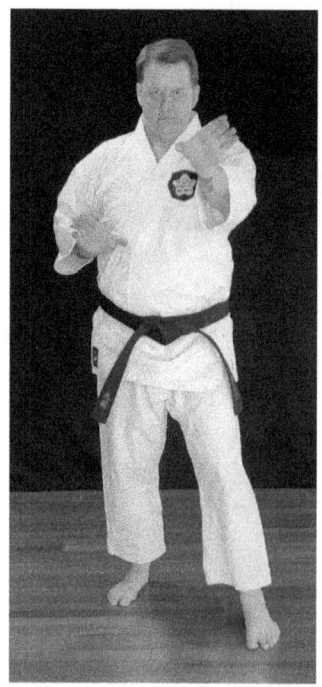
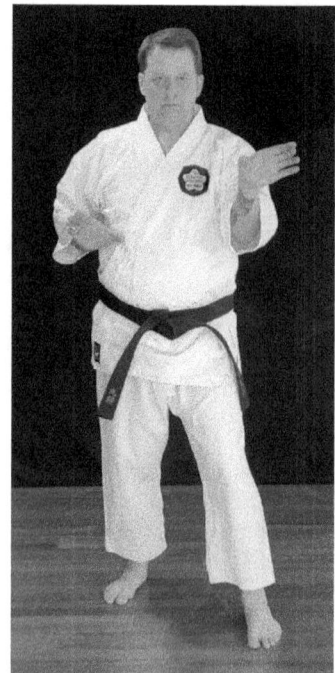

Left Chudan Hiki Uke (cont.)

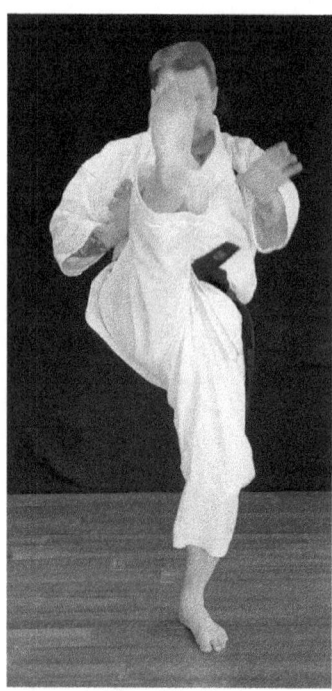

Complete Right Jodan Mae Keage Geri

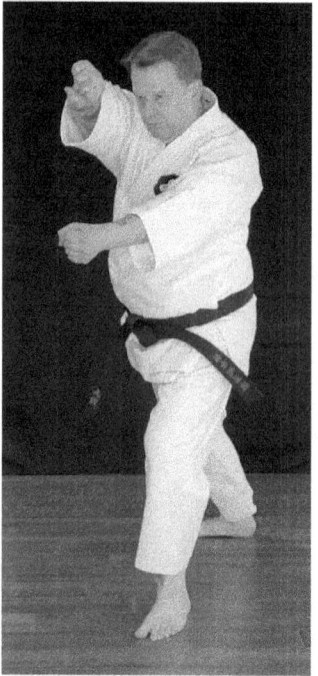

Step Back on 315° Angle, Fists in Front (Right at Head Height, Left at Chest Height)

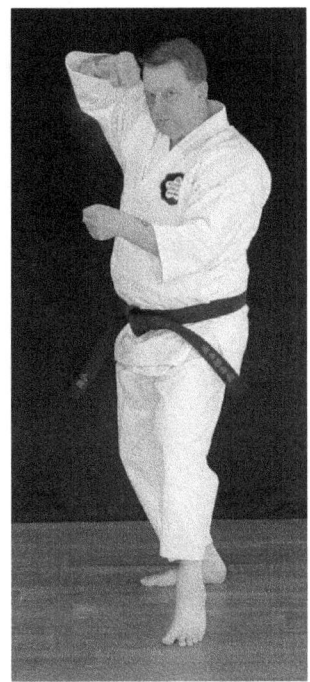

Pull Right Hand to Head, Left Hand in Front of Chest, Landing in Neko Ashi Dachi

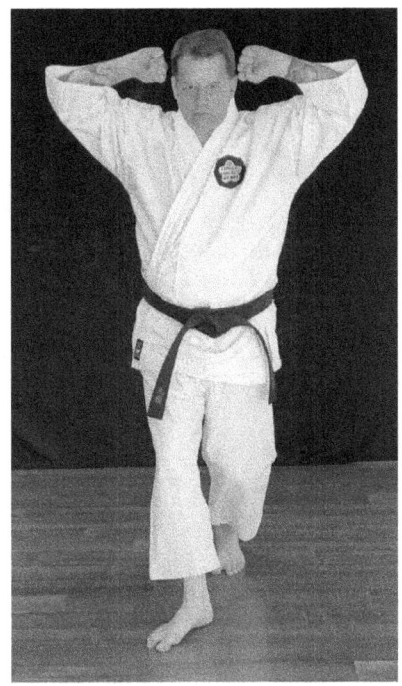

Step Up with Right Foot Facing Forward, Chamber Both Hands

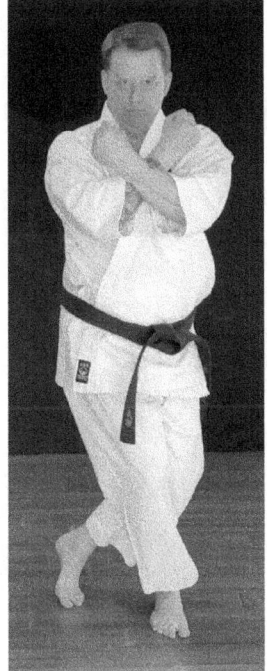

Bring Left Leg Behind Right into Kosa Dachi, while Completing Chudan Juji Uke

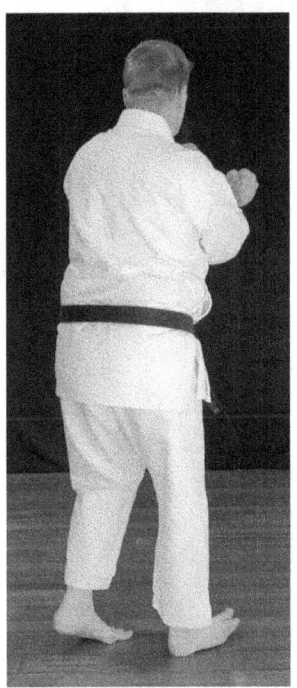

Spin Around 360° on Right Foot

Isshoni San

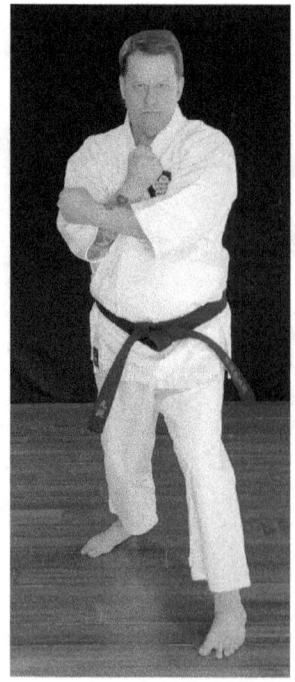 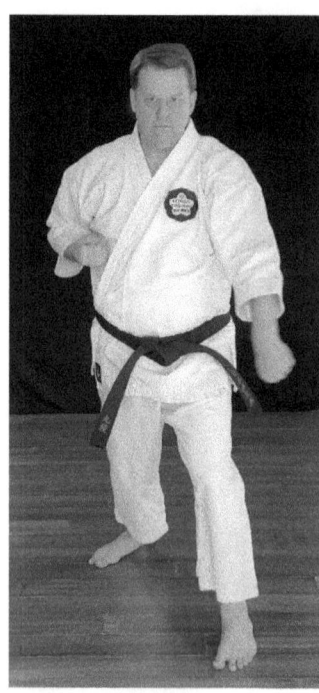

Land with Left Foot in Front, Complete Left Gedan Barai

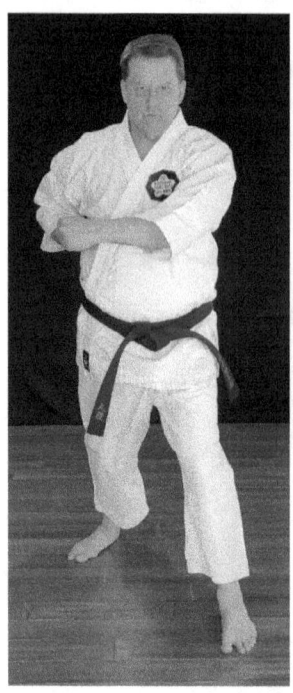 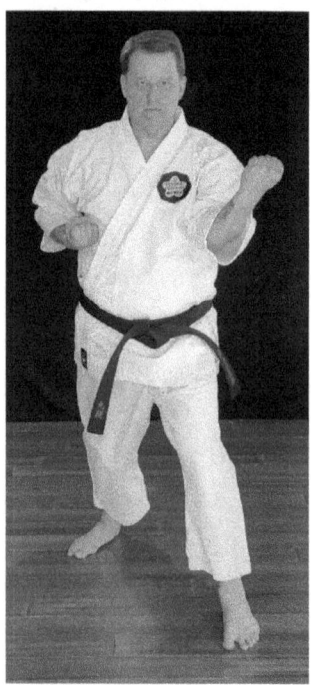

Bring Left Hand Up into Left Chudan Uke

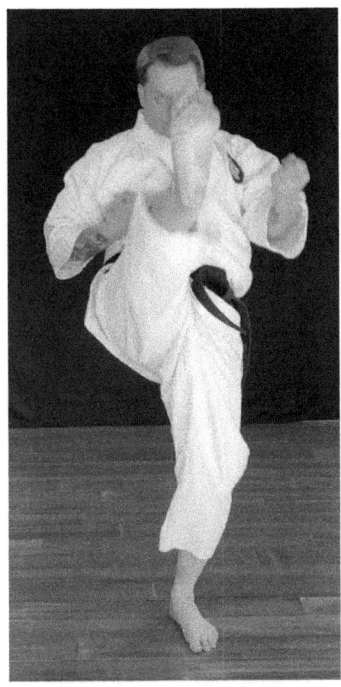

Complete Right Jodan
Mae Keage Geri

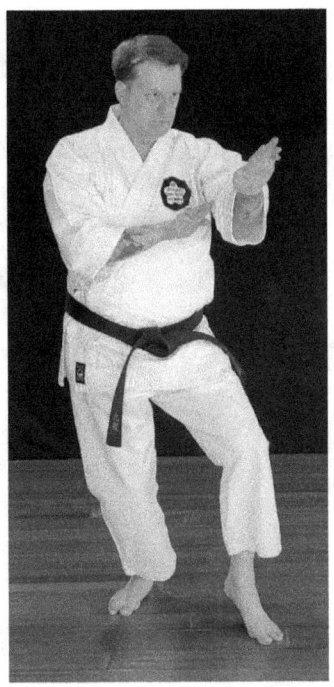

Set Back into Neko Ashi
Dachi on 45° Angle

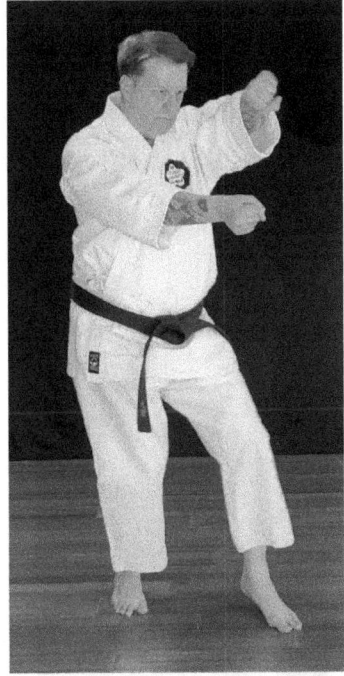

Left Step Back on Same Angle,
Fists in Front (Left at Head
Height, Right at Chest Height)

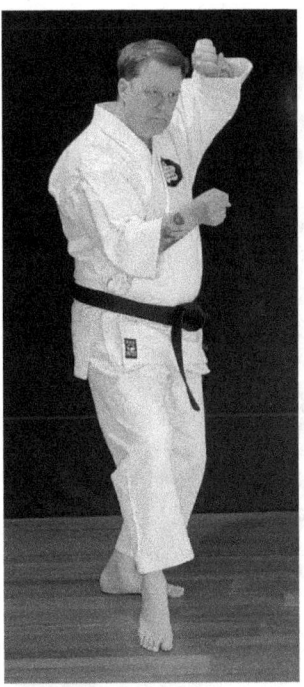

Pull Left Hand to Head,
Right Hand in Front of Chest,
Landing in Neko Ashi Dachi

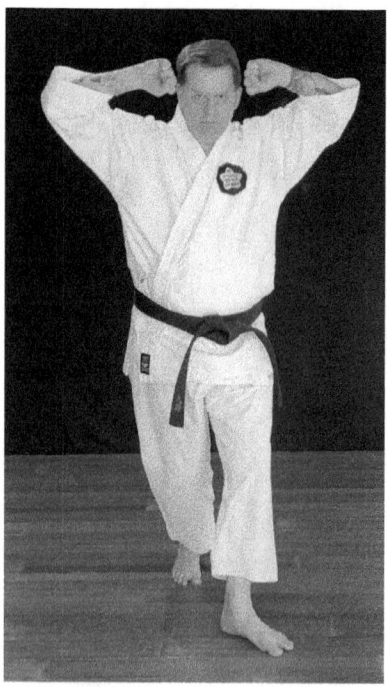

Step Up with Left Foot
Facing Forward,
Chamber Both Hands

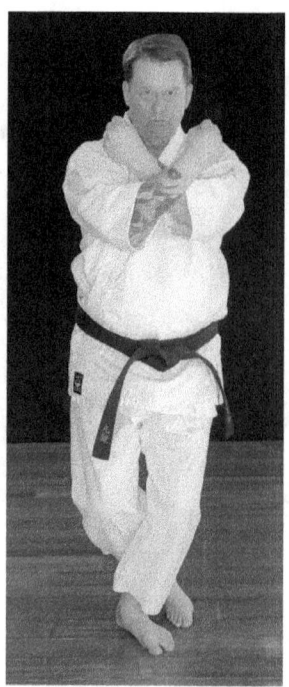

Bring Right Leg Behind Left
into Kosa Dachi, while
Completing Chudan Juji Uke

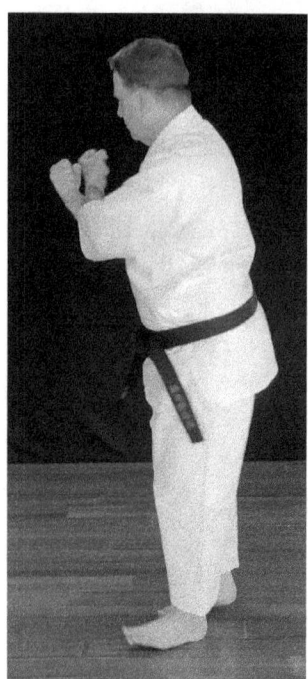

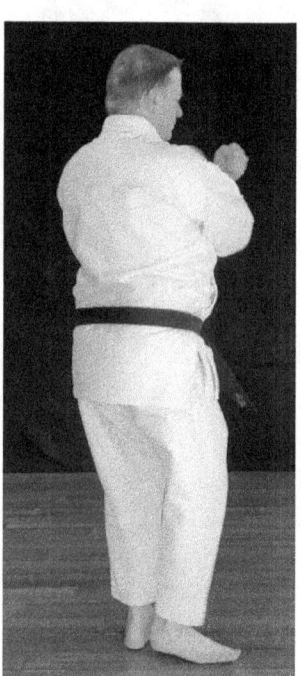

Spin Around 360° on Left Foot

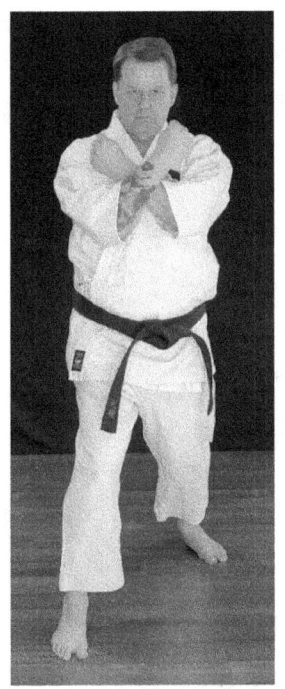 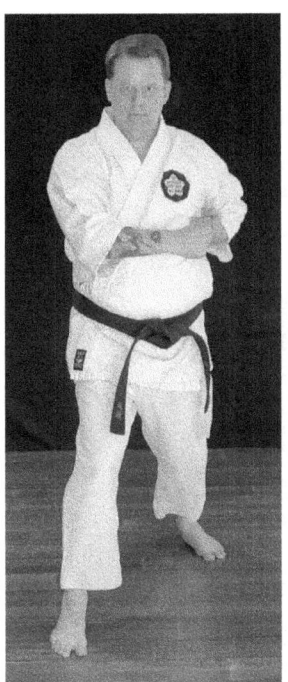

Land with Right Foot in Front, Complete Right Gedan Barai

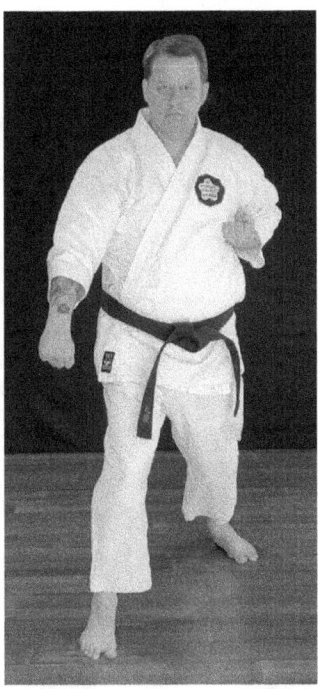 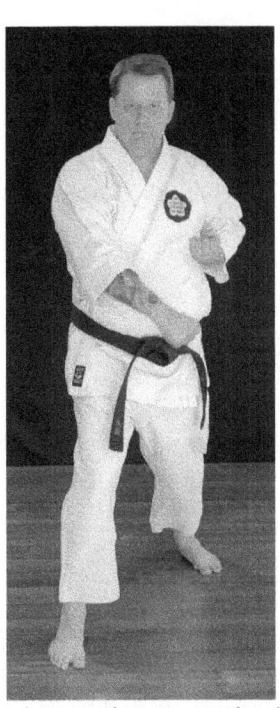

Right Gedan Barai (cont.)   Bring Right Hand Up into Chudan Uke

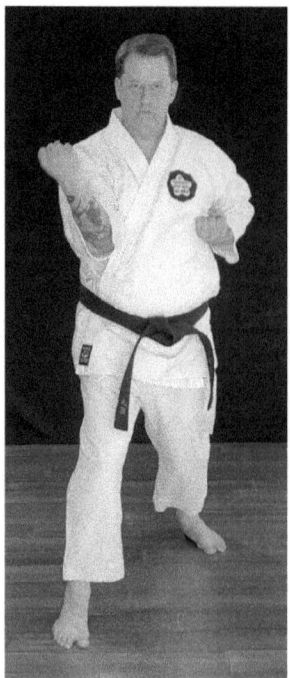
Chudan Uke (cont.)

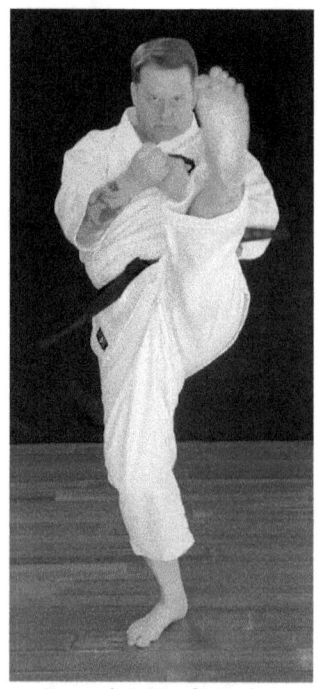
Complete Left Jodan Mae Keage Geri

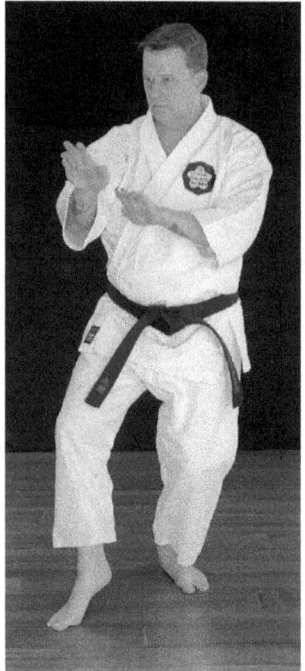
Step Back Left into Neko Ashi Dachi on 315° Angle

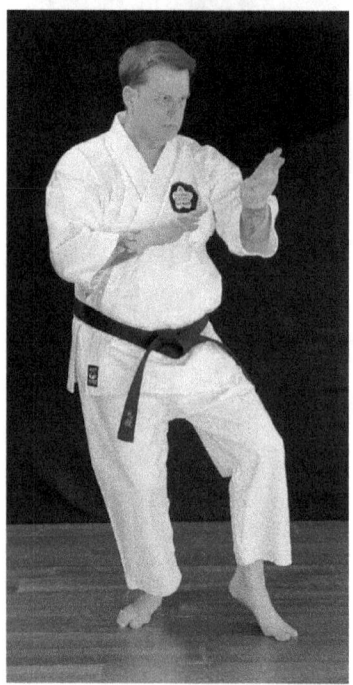
Step Back Right into Neko Ashi Dachi on 45° Angle

Isshoni San

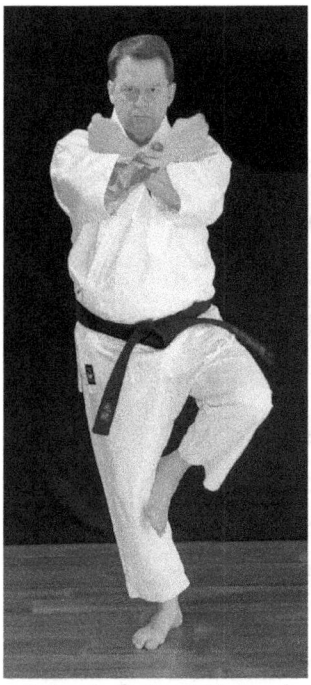
Bring Left Foot Up and Cross Arms

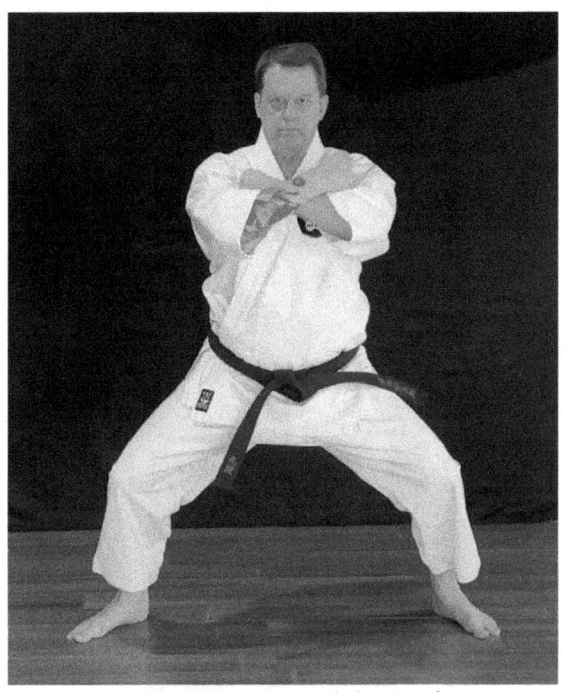
Come Down into Shiko Dachi

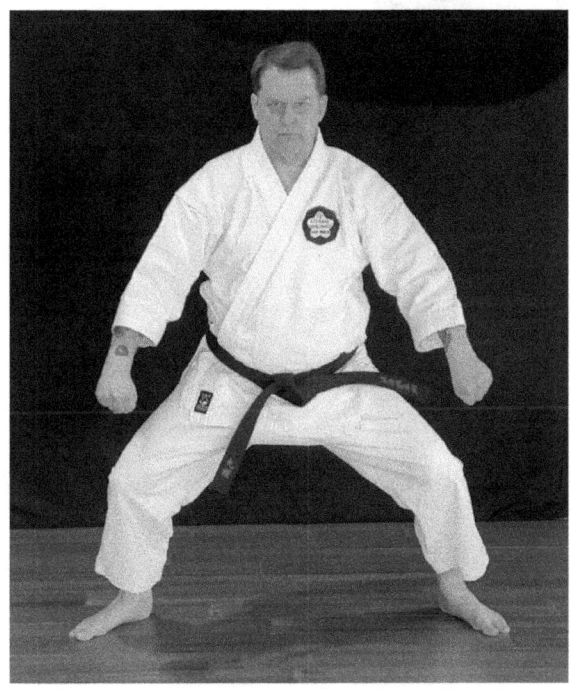
Complete Morote Gedan Barai Slowly

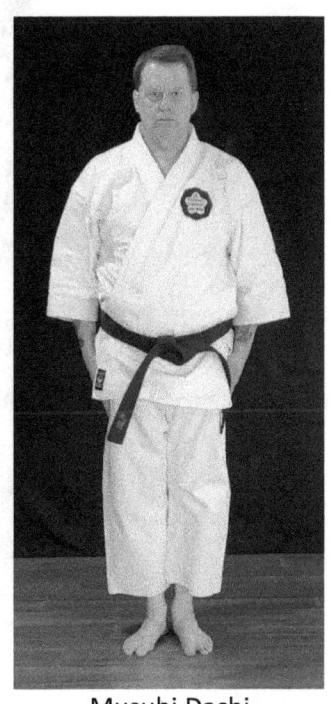
Musubi Dachi

Isshoni San

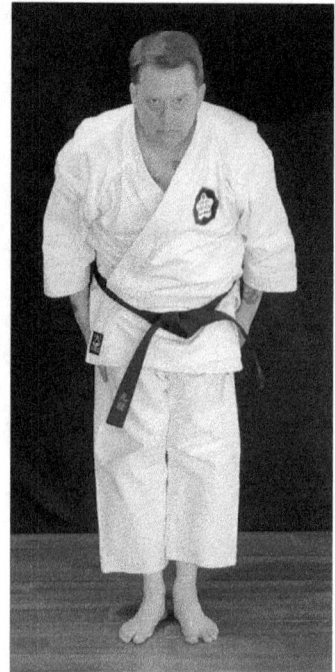
Rei

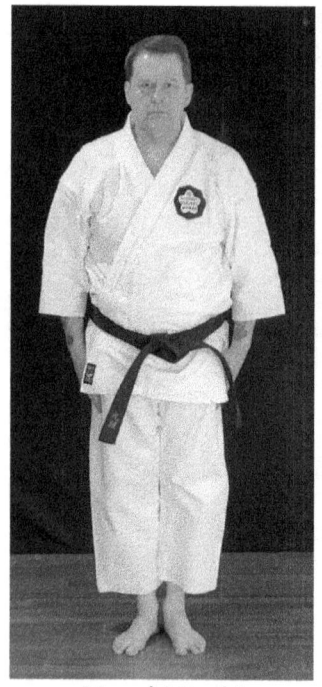
Musubi Dachi

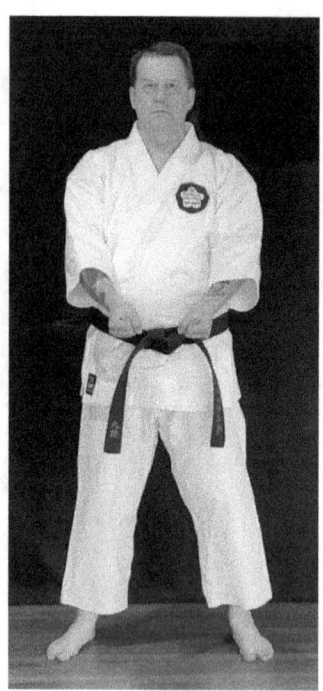
Heiko Dachi

Self-Defense

The core of karate is self-defense. Much of the criticism levied at karate is how realistic or unrealistic it is; preparation for a fight that may or may not happen. In other words, "if I take karate, will I be able to defend myself if I get into a fight?" The answer should always be yes, but confidence is a tricky subject. A person can be confident enough to live without being in a constant state of fear, but one should also be smart about the way one goes about their day and not be cocky about what they think they can do. Therefore, while remaining cautious, one should also practice self-defense and get comfortable with it. Realistic self-defense training should improve a person's confidence significantly. Realism, however, is often denigrated to the type of sparring one does; but true realism in the martial arts lies in the depth of study and practice of self-defense. If there is any value in karate, or any martial art, it should be in its emphasis of self-defense.

When Shodai was learning karate in Okinawa, on weekends he and his fellow Marine dojo mates spent time practicing self-defense moves from katas. He loved kata, but was somewhat skeptical about what techniques would work on Americans, who, in his experience were taller and bigger than most of the Okinawans that he witnessed. He knew there was more to self-defense than just kata. To be fair, if bunkai (analysis) is taught and studied along with kata, there is plenty of deliberate self-defense in kata. And while some karate styles only teach kata and sparring, some dojos will spend time practicing kata moves with a partner. In Ketsugo Goju-Ryu, we use many methods to practice self-defense with a partner, one is within an exercise called kiso kumite and another called bunkai kumite. These drills will be explored in other volumes of the Ketsugo Goju-Ryu series, but they involve either practicing offensive techniques as counters (kiso kumite) or practicing offensive and defensive techniques together (bunkai kumite), typically taken from a kata or several katas. When Shodai left Okinawa and was teaching in Jacksonville Beach, Florida, he met a jiu-jitsu practitioner Bill Beach, who soon taught Shodai what he called "takeaways." Shodai loved them and wanted to include takeaways in his curriculum. When devising the Ketsugo Goju-Ryu system, he created drills to practice particular self-defense moves (separate from kiso kumite and bunkai kumite that is) with a partner that focuses solely on escaping a hold or a grab.

A few things about self-defense practice; first, it is always good to test self-defense as realistically as possible. It will not do a student any good if the aggressor simply lays hands on the student's neck. The student must have some sense of danger to escape from. This can be a little jarring at first to someone with a background of being attacked, but it is important in the learning process to turn that fear into action. After all, this is why many people take martial arts in the first place, and it does no good to hide from it.

Second, one must have an open mind when it comes to self-defense, both on the instructing side and the receiving side. There is no perfect defense any more than a perfect attack. Circumstances will always vary, as do body sizes, strengths, etc. In the beginning, students need to learn what their bodies can do and control. Control of one's body is key to why it is inadvisable to rely purely on theoretical self-defense, seminars, or watching a video as a guide for self-defense preparation. Not that the information is necessarily bad, incorrect, or ineffective, but without the right frame of mind, it can give a false sense of security. Once a modest amount of bodily self-control is reached, students should stretch their minds when it comes to self-defense. They should think about adaptability and improvisation. But that comes with time.

Next, the student must develop a strength of will that is ultimately more important than any technique or technical knowledge a person may possess. The question is, can the student ignore intimidation while doing what needs to be done in a self-defense situation? Or will fear take over and a person freezes up, despite having a library of self-defense knowledge? For example, my mother watches every true crime story she can watch, and knows exactly what she should do if she was ever attacked, but would she have the will to really hurt someone if she had to? Hopefully she will never have to find out, but for most people it takes diligent training, not just of the mind, but in the controlling of one's emotions, to defend themselves. When people go to seminars or read a book about self-defense, it is purely academic until it is practiced, again and again and again.

Situational awareness, staying away from danger, is an instinct that most people try to follow, but sometimes a person has no choice and danger finds them. It would be obvious to say that no one should drive around alone in the middle of the night with an empty gas tank in a rough part of town, but what if a person is attacked by someone they know, in their own home, during the day? The fact is, we simply do not know if, when, or where we may be attacked. We can use experience and general caution as a guide, not paranoia, but when it comes down to it, we must try to conquer our fear of others. This starts with confidence through regular training.

Another important point is not to allow a would-be attacker to get within a certain range of your body if it can be helped. Putting out a hand as a barrier combined with a stern voice may quell someone who is not sure he or she wants to truly engage in a fight. But if all attempts to keep a fight from happening fail, action must be performed with serious intentions. If a life is at stake, nothing is off limits. However, consider the different levels of self-defense – suppression or life/death. Dealing with a bully is different than someone on the street who is really trying to cause serious harm

Self-Defense

or kill. Recognizing the attacker's degree of intention is extremely important. Staying calm and not letting emotion get in the way is the key to accurately assessing a situation. Overreaction to an attack may land a person in jail, whether in the right or not.

Considering the myriad self-defense possibilities, this book will focus on a few basic attacks, their escapes, and some alternatives. The keys to these escapes are commitment and speed. A defender must react as if he or she is weaker than their attacker; the student must react quickly for self-defense to work. Some of these attacks, like the front choke, without a quick reaction, could end a life in a matter of seconds. There is simply no time to think about a reaction; it will happen, or it will not. The last point is that when we train in self-defense, we practice with the intention of getting away, not prolonging the confrontation.

Warning #1: always practice self-defense with a qualified instructor who will watch for any safety concerns and make sure the techniques are performed correctly.
Warning #2: there are probably hundreds of ways to get out of the holds presented here. These are only sample methods that we practice in Ketsugo Goju-Ryu, not the only methods possible.

Front choke escape (2 variations)

The two handed front choke does a few things: it cuts off the blood flow to the brain with the fingers on both sides of the neck, and the thumbs crush the windpipe. Reaction time is critical and obviously it is never advisable to let someone put their hands around your neck. This demonstration would be a case when a choke happens without warning. For a sense of realism, even when practicing, the choke should be performed with reasonable force but be careful of the thumbs on the trachea (directly in front of the throat).

The first defense method is the most basic. Once choked, take a step back with one leg and simultaneously bring both hands up in a double chest block. A quick step back will help loosen the grip on the throat. Combined with a good solid stance and quick double arm block, this should allow the defender to break free. To keep the attacker's forward momentum at bay after blocking their arms, immediately after the block, put one hand out towards the attacker's body while chambering the other hand for a punch or a shotei uchi to the face. Strike the attacker twice, ideally in the face, then the solar plexus, but use whatever target is in reach.

Self-Defense

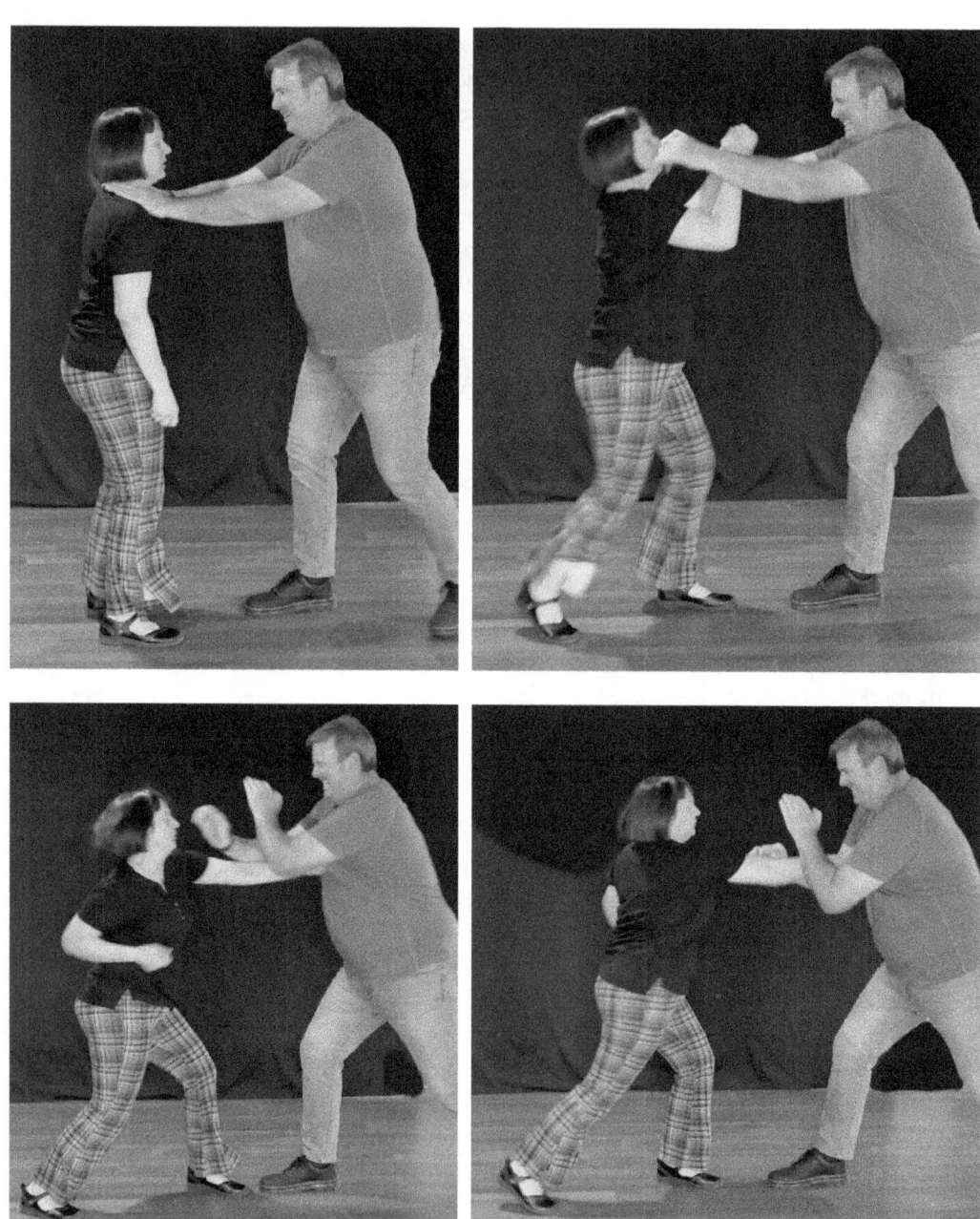

Self-Defense

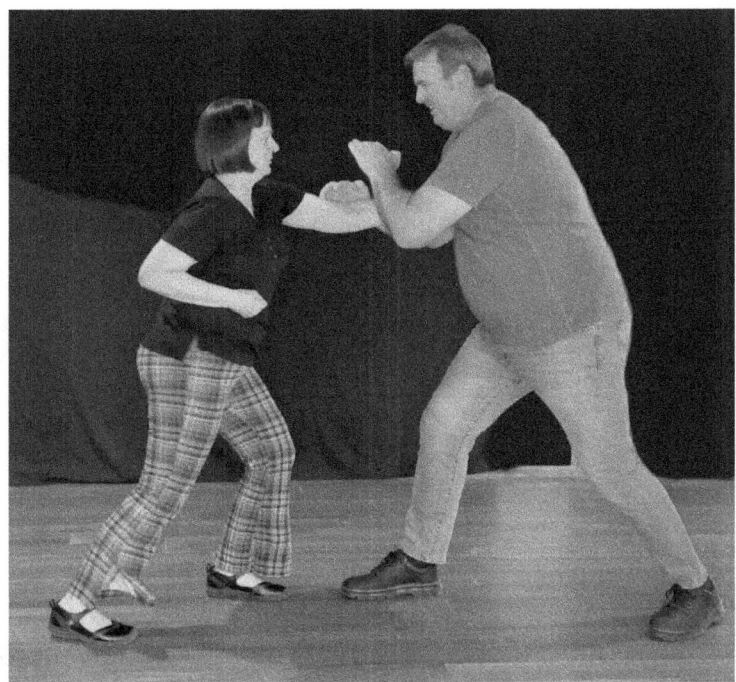

An alternative involves going over the top with your arms instead of coming up from the middle. Take the same step back with one leg like the other example and strike the attacker's arms with either a double shuto uchi or double tettsui uchi. See below.

If the attacker is still holding on, using the back leg, kick the attacker to the groin, or use a shin or knee depending on how close the attacker is. At that point if the attacker is still holding on, turn to the side and slap down hard on their arms with one hand while chambering the other hand into a tettsui uchi (hammer fist strike), pivot back towards them and strike the attacker's head. Alternatively, this could be shuto uchi (chop strike) under the ear or neck.

Self-Defense

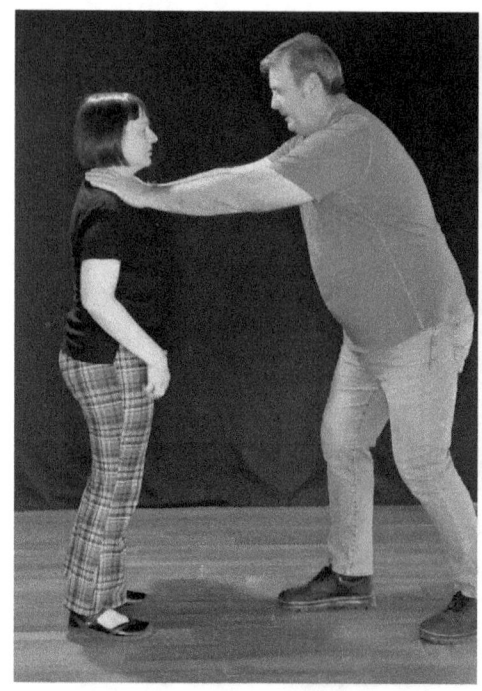
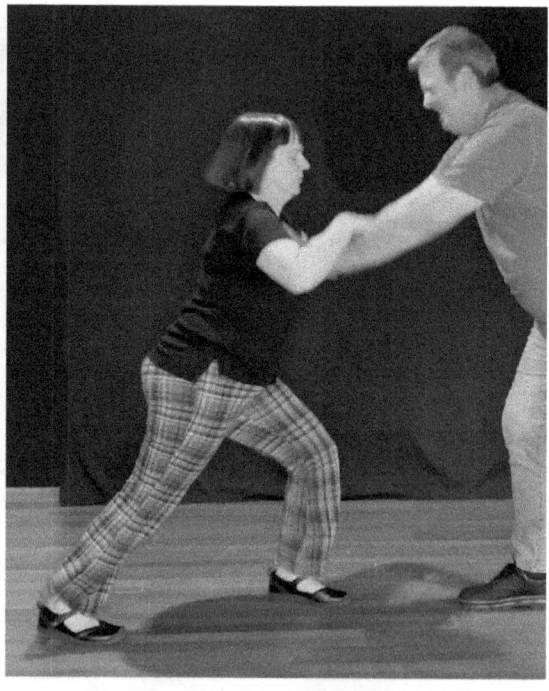
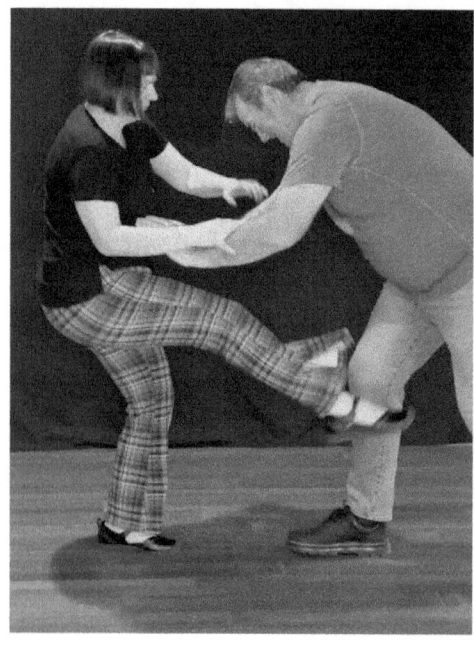
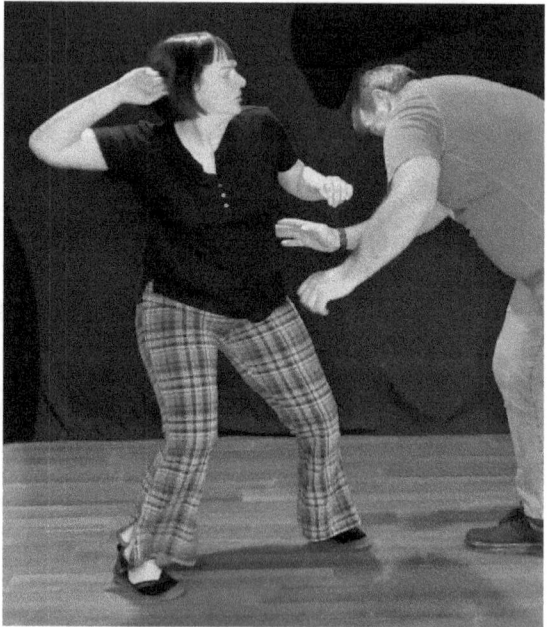

Self-Defense

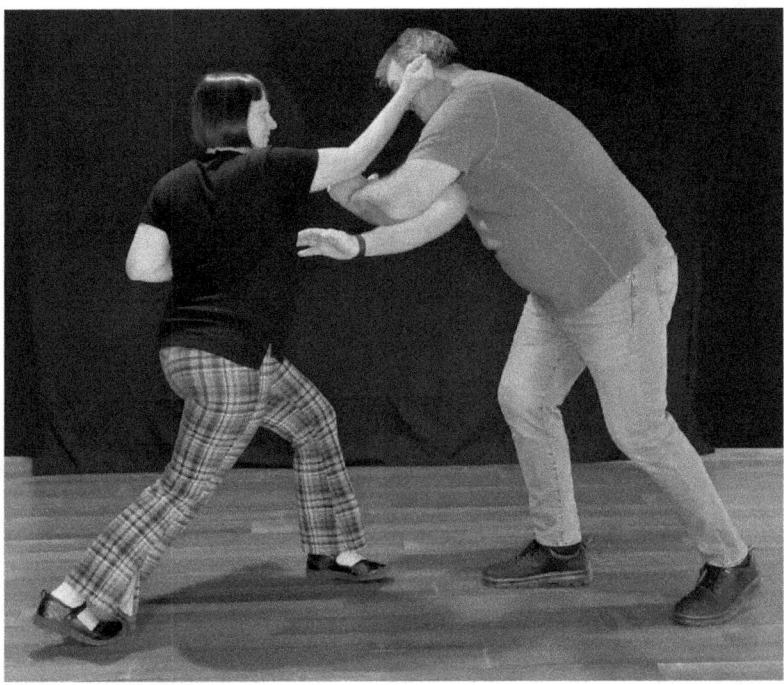

Shoulder grab defense (2 variations)

With a shoulder grab, it should be assumed that the attacker has something in his other hand, a weapon perhaps or a clenched fist ready to punch. There are a few options. For a basic response: step in towards the attacker while doing a side block. Immediately strike with the free hand, and then with the other hand. This is a good method to learn first, to get used to stepping into an attack, but realistically, defending against one arm when the attacker has two may only delay the attacker's actual intention.

Self-Defense

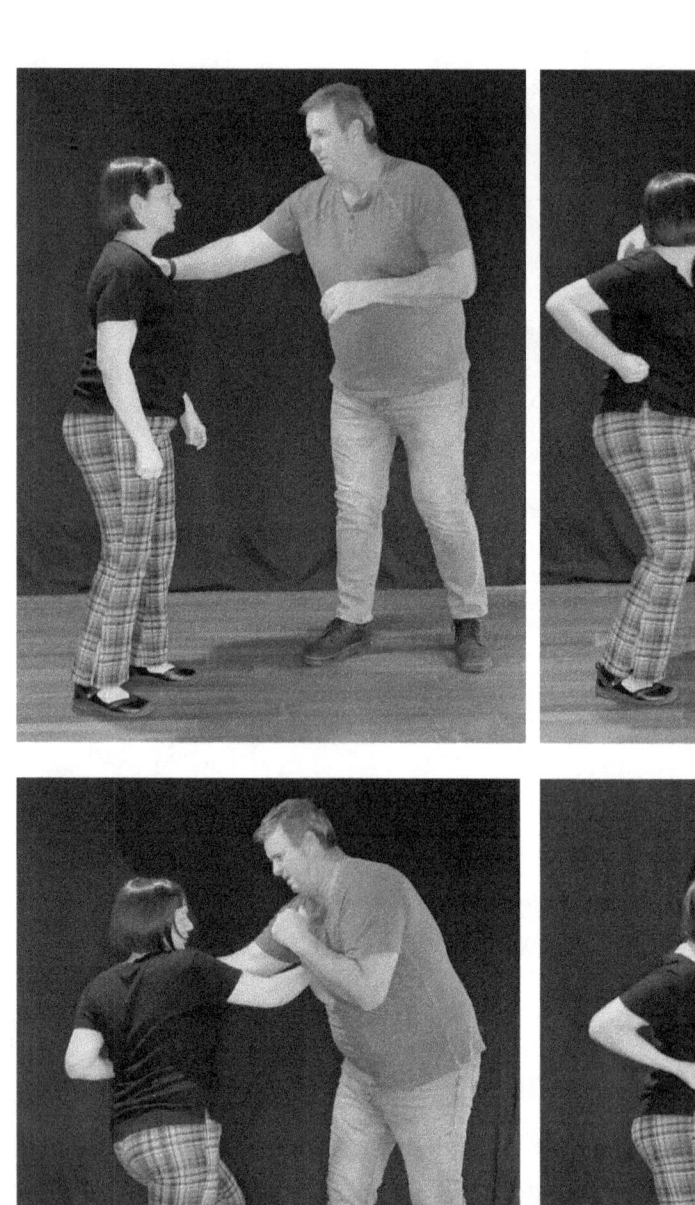
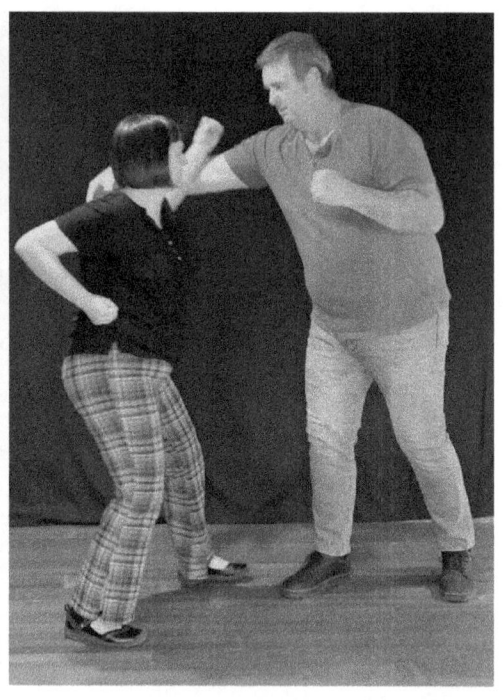
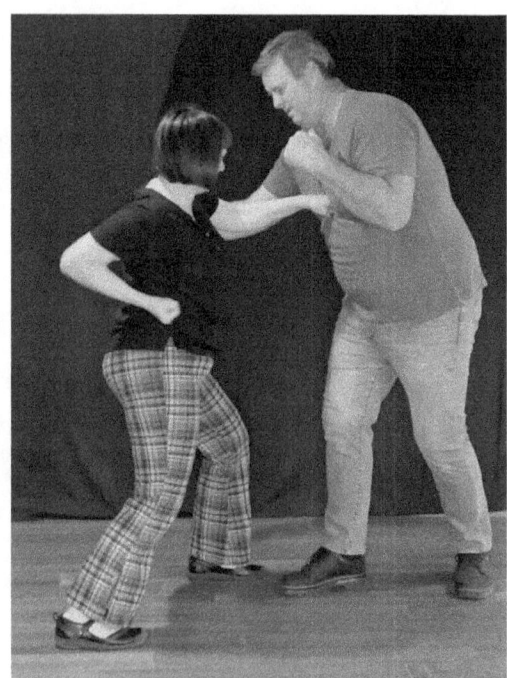

Self-Defense

As an alternative, particularly if the non-grabbing hand is actively striking, ignore the shoulder grab and do a hooking chest block to the second strike, catching both arms. Follow up with a hook punch to the ribs, then to the head.

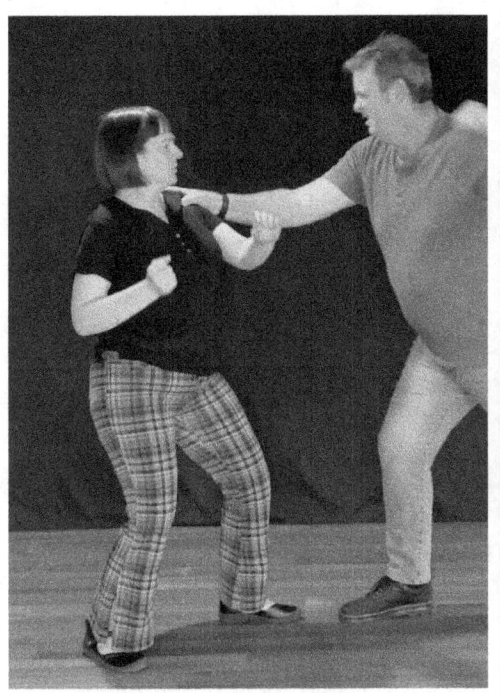
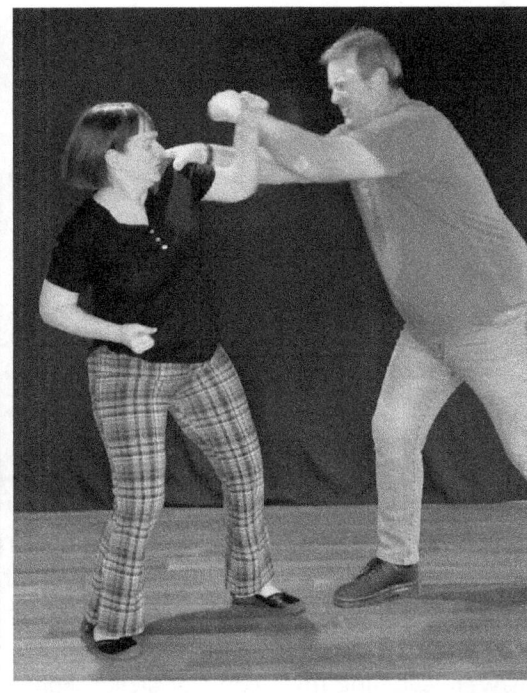
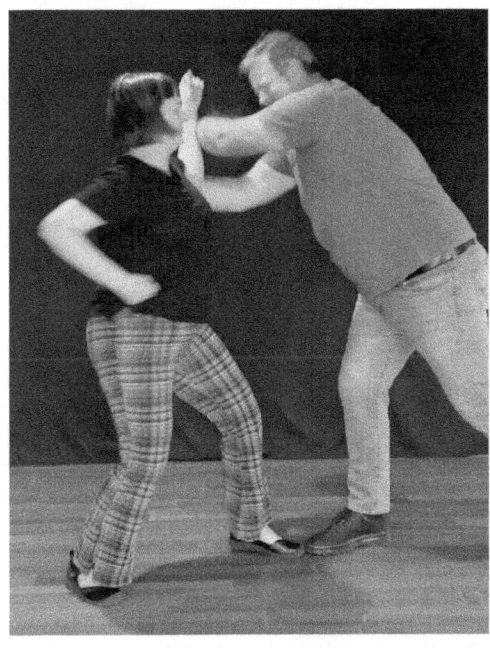
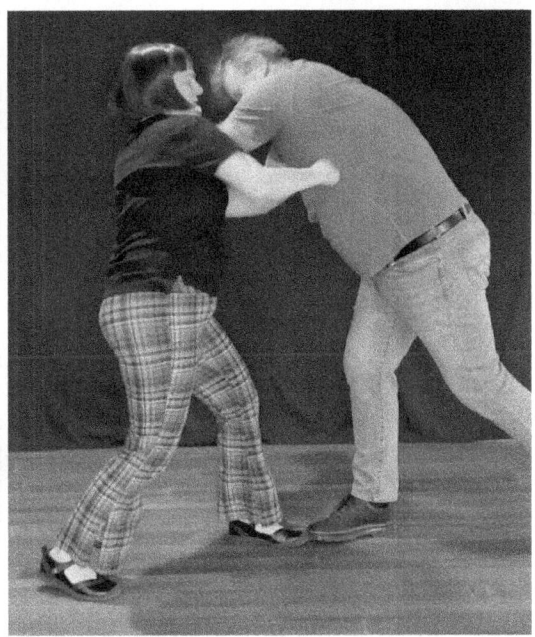

Self-Defense

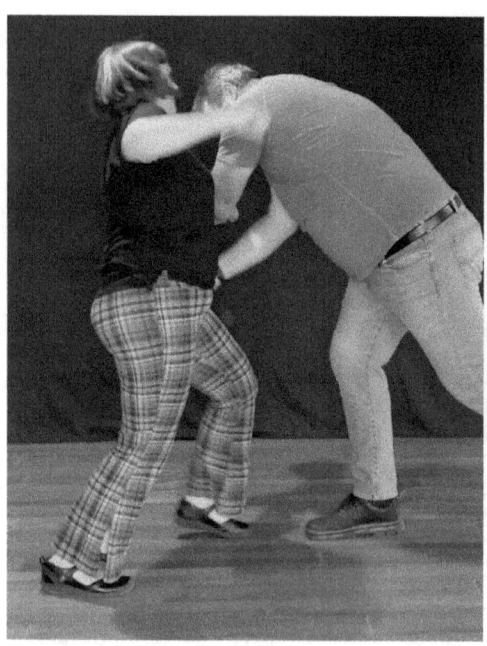
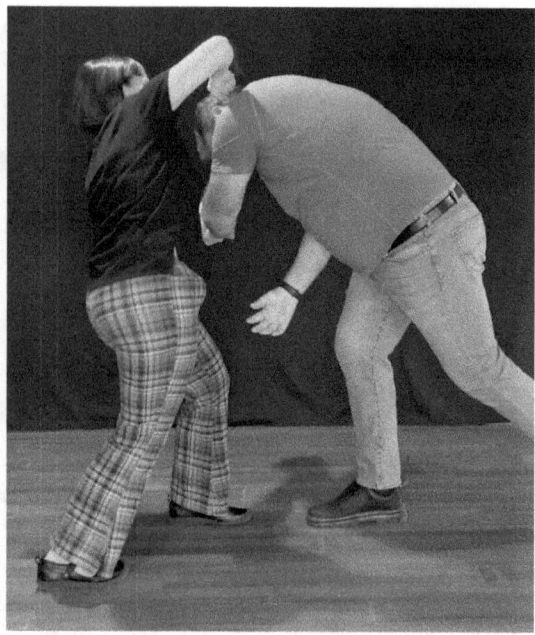

As another alternative, step in towards the attacker and simultaneously lift the arm being grabbed over the attacker's grabbing arm, preferably above their elbow. Once the arm is locked, bring the elbow in and lift it for better control. This type of armbar could dislocate the attacker's elbow and perhaps damage their pectoral muscle as well, allowing for a counter strike. Follow up with a haito uchi (ridge hand) to the groin. Finally, grab the head and hiza uchi the attacker in the face, then push away.

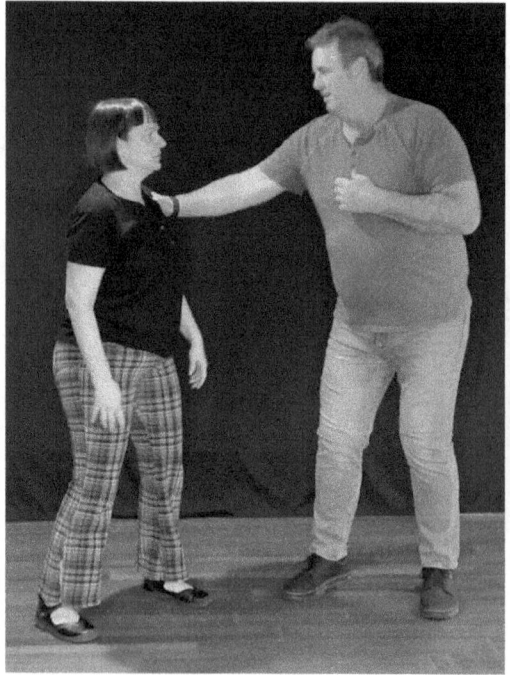
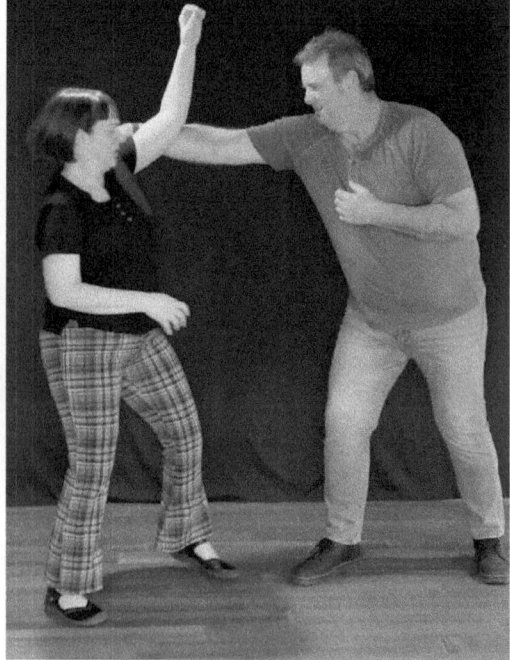

Self-Defense

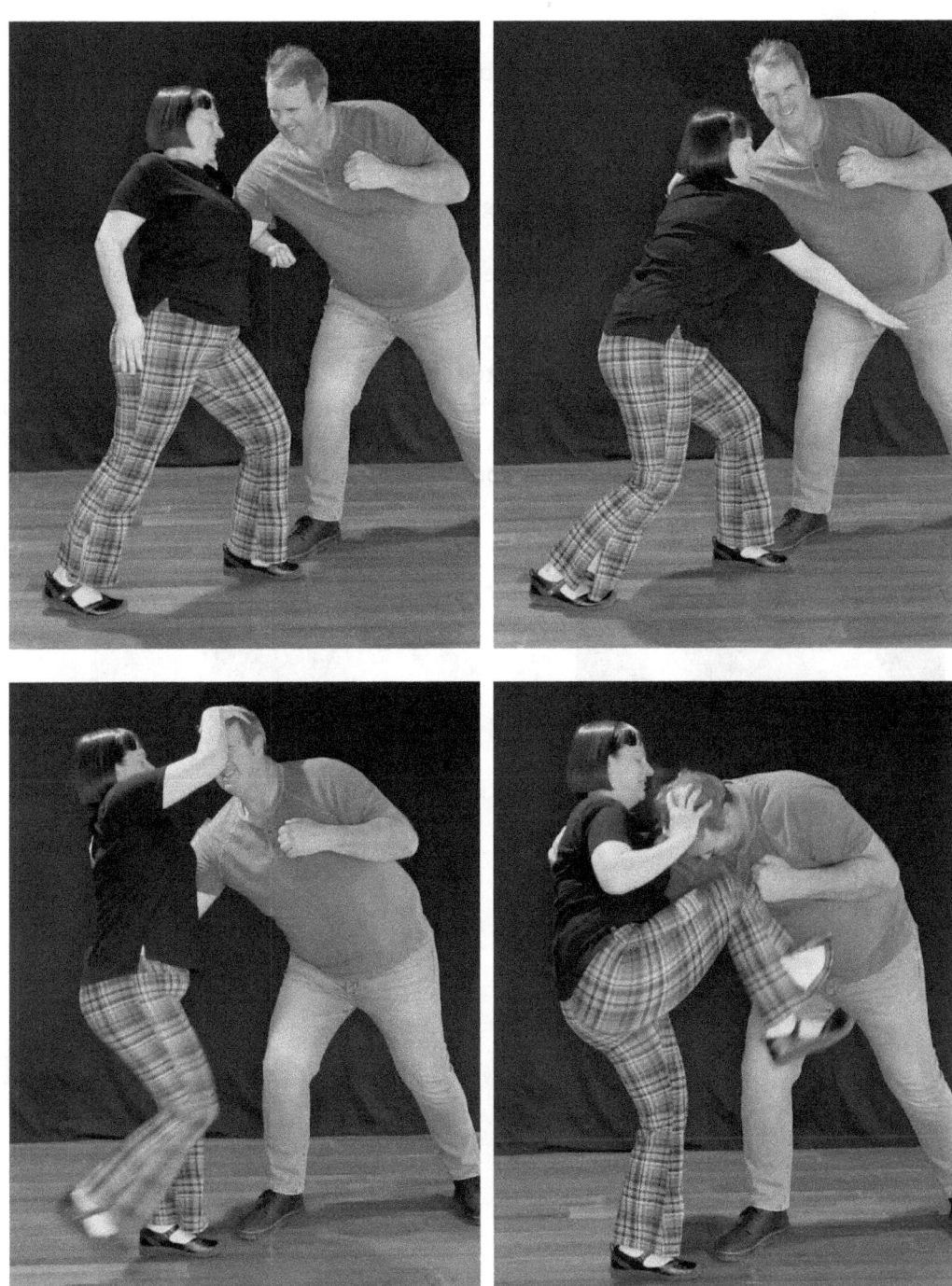

Self-Defense

Double lapel grab defense (3 variations)

An attacker grabs the top of someone's jacket or shirt from the front with both hands, the defender can: slap down on the arms to loosen the hold. Next, step into one side close, hip to hip, bringing the opposite hand between the arms to the chin and the back hand behind the attacker's head. Grab the head or hair and pull towards the shoulder, then quickly swing the back leg around, dropping to one knee. Strike the attacker.

Attempting to muscle the attacker's head to the ground is unlikely to work unless the defender is considerably stronger than the attacker. For this reason, the body should do most of the work for the takedown. The defender should also remember to get hip to hip with the attacker when attempting the takedown. The more distance between the attacker and defender, the harder it will be to do. The attacker, when practicing, should remember to perform a proper breakfall when going to the ground. The arm going to the ground should absorb the shock of going to the ground. Never land directly on the shoulder, elbow, wrist, or palm.

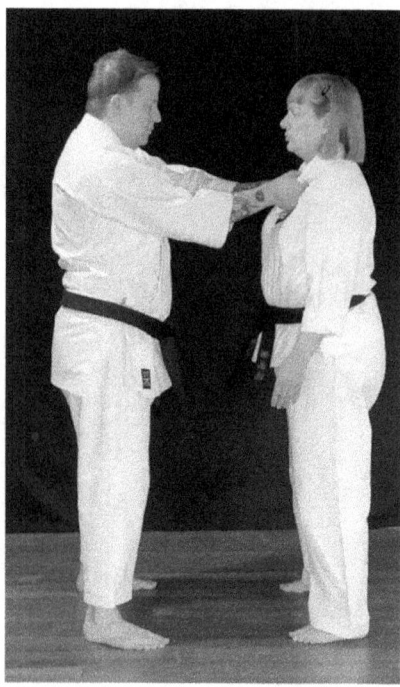
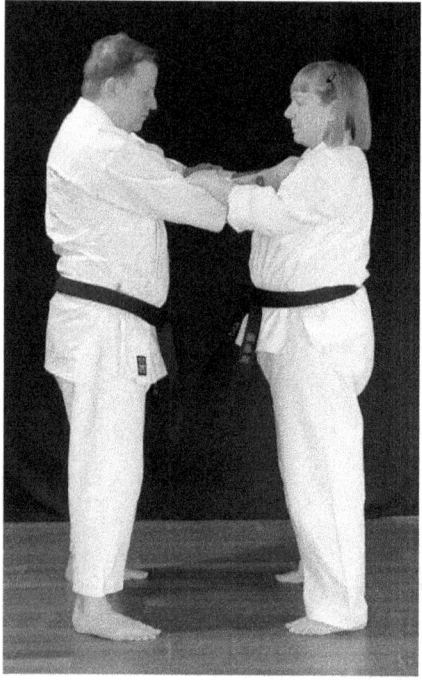

Self-Defense

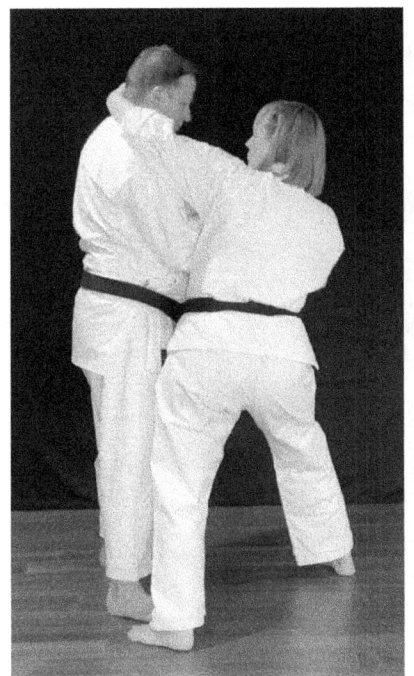
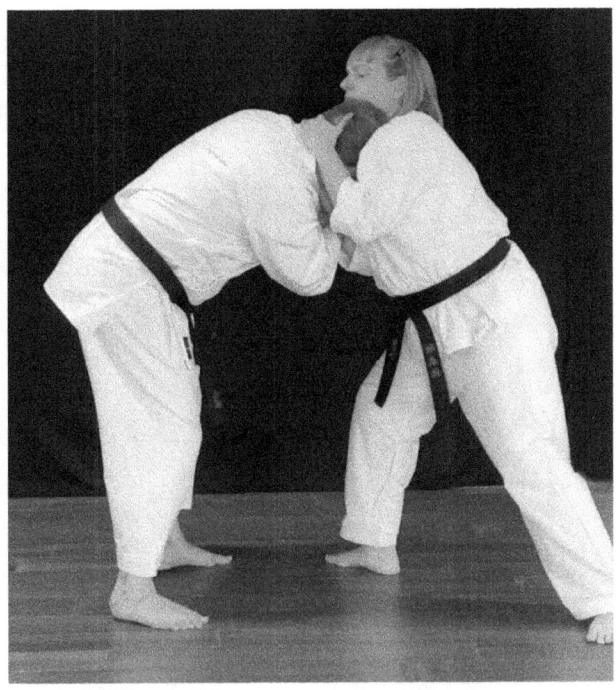
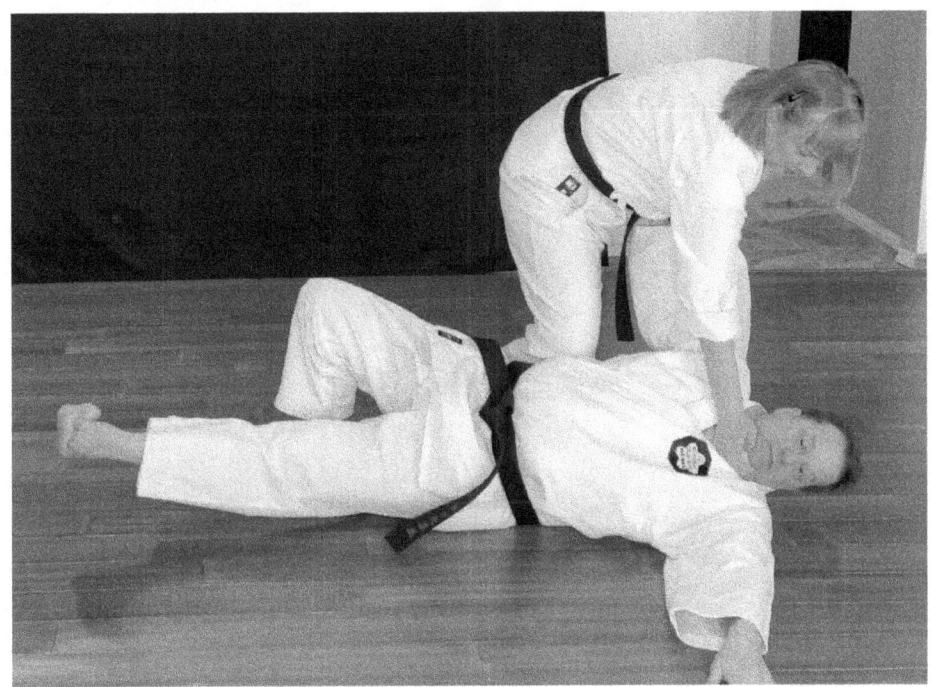

Self-Defense

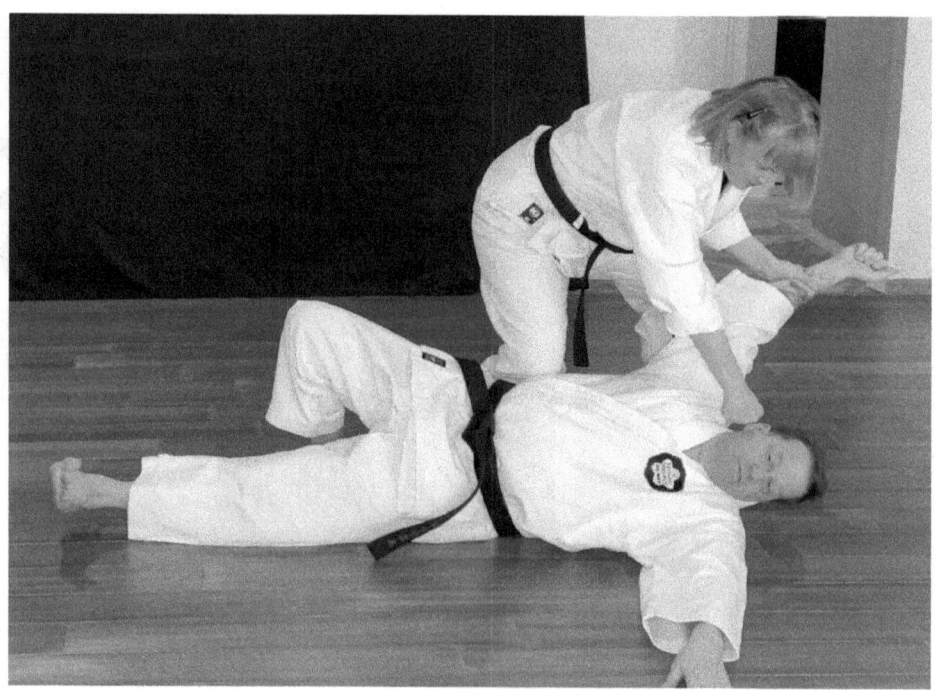

An alternative to the hair takedown is the hand grab. Once grabbed, the defender reaches over with one hand and supports with the other hand. Immediately after grabbing the attacker's hands, twist the hands while stepping over into shiko dachi, using the elbow to bring the attacker down. Follow up with an elbow to the temple.

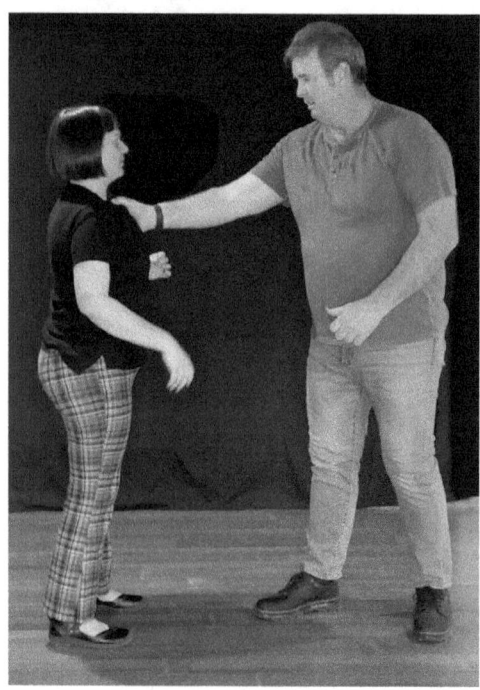 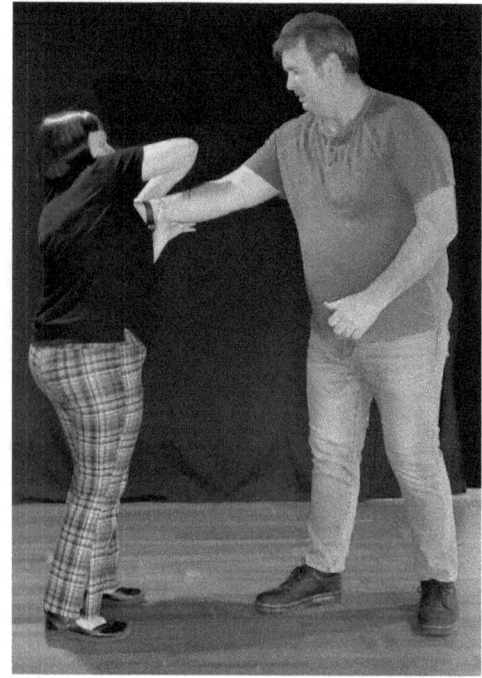

Self-Defense

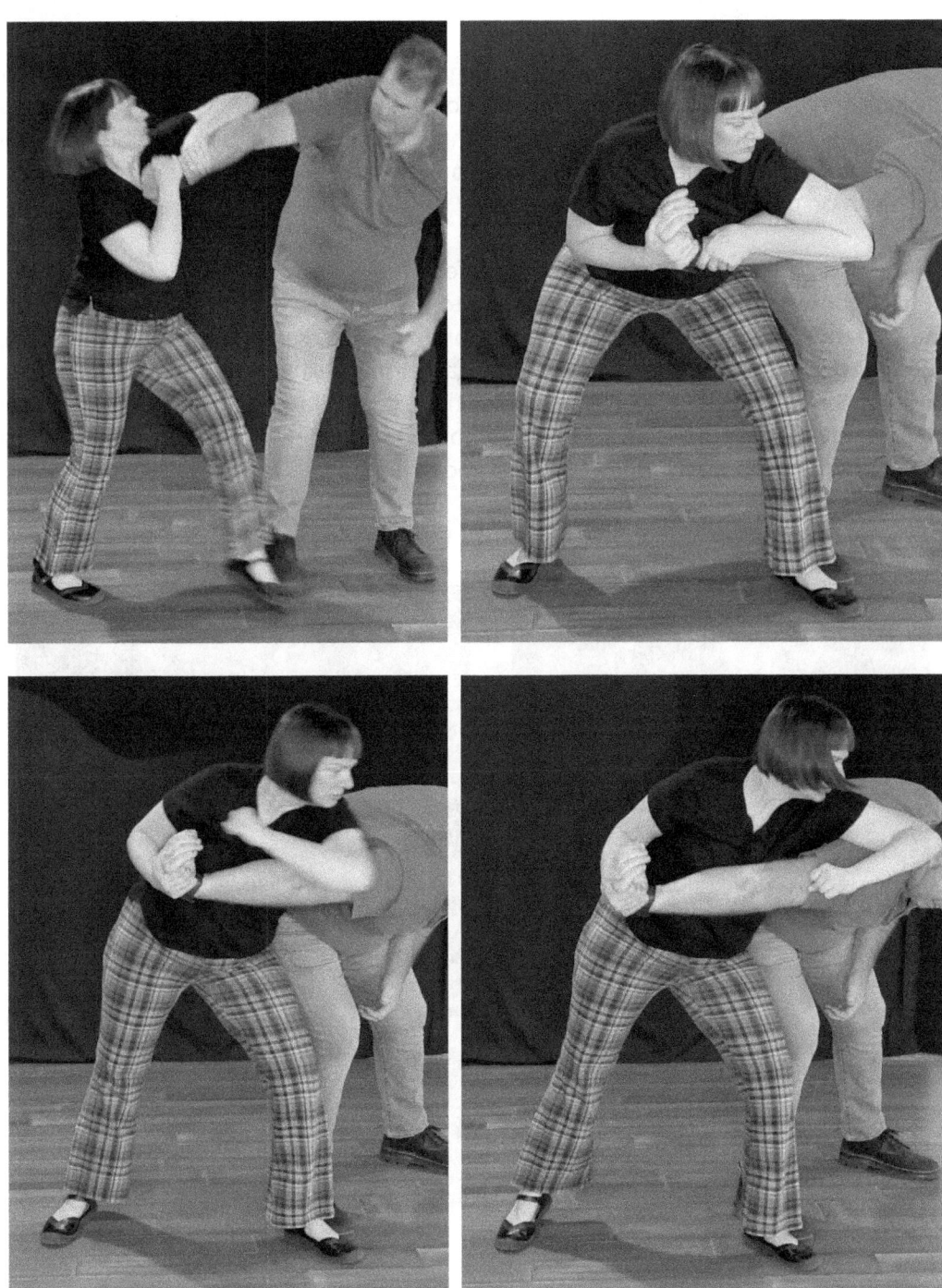

385

Self-Defense

Hammer lock escape (2 variations)

The hammer lock itself is easy enough to do, pull someone's arm behind their back, generally to push them somewhere. For the attacker, if he wants the best hold, he will pull up on the arm, palm up. The non-grabbing hand is going to hold on to the opponent's opposite shoulder. This will help with stability and steering the person in the direction desired.

On the other end of the hammer lock, to defend it:

Loosen the grip on the arm first by stomping on the attacker's foot, specifically the side that's holding the arm. In that second, the attacker may loosen his grip long enough to use the free arm to elbow the attacker in the jaw. When the elbow is used, simultaneously move the leg (same side as the free arm) in the same direction as the elbow to the outside of the attacker. The elbow arm should wrap around, trapping both the attacker's arms. Follow that up with a gedan hiza uchi.

To summarize: stomp foot, elbow face, knee to groin.

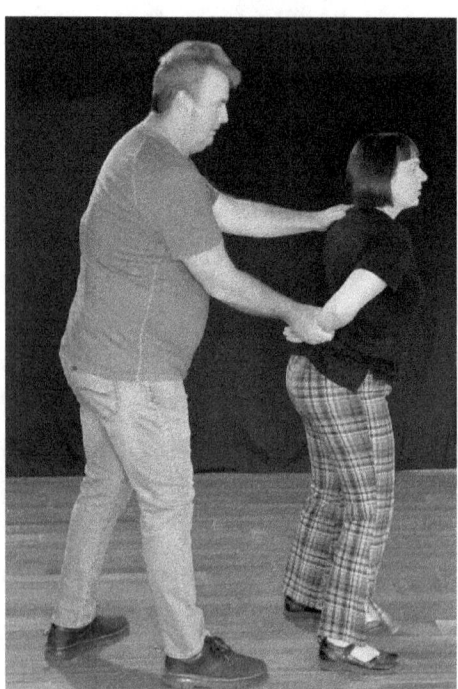 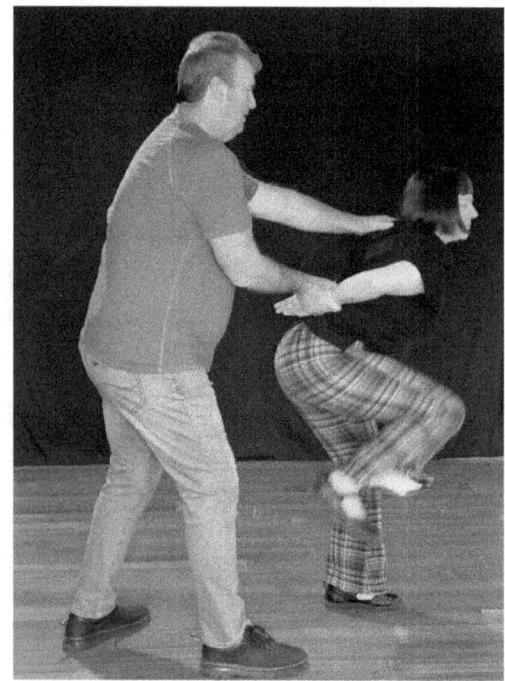

Self-Defense

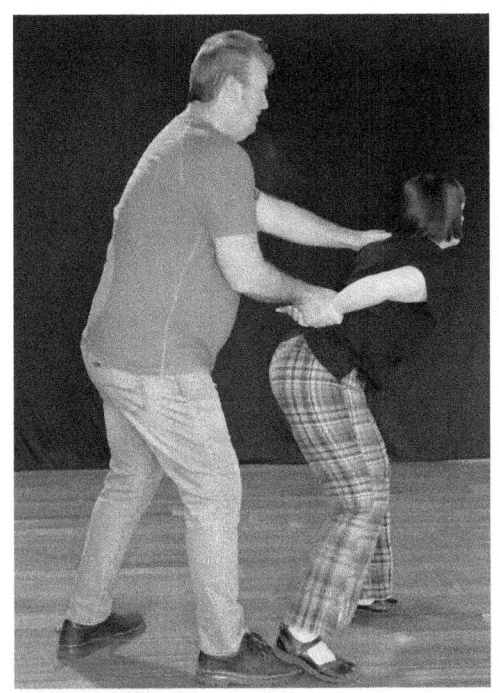
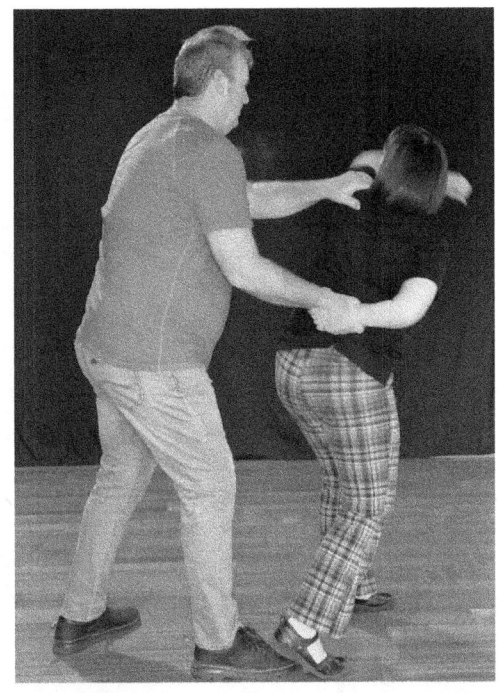
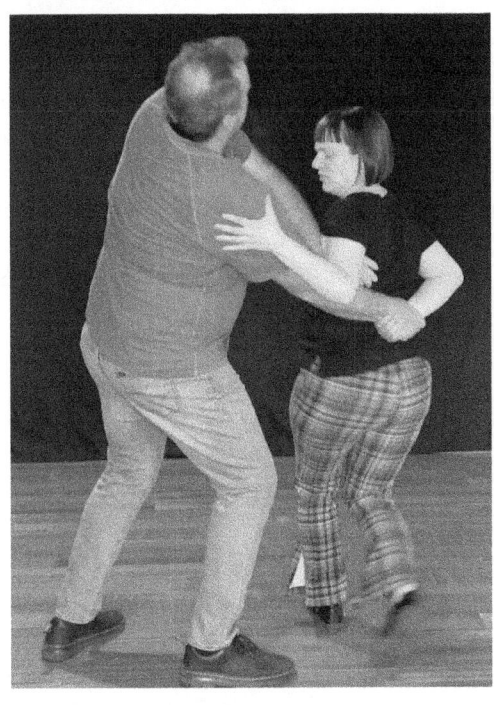
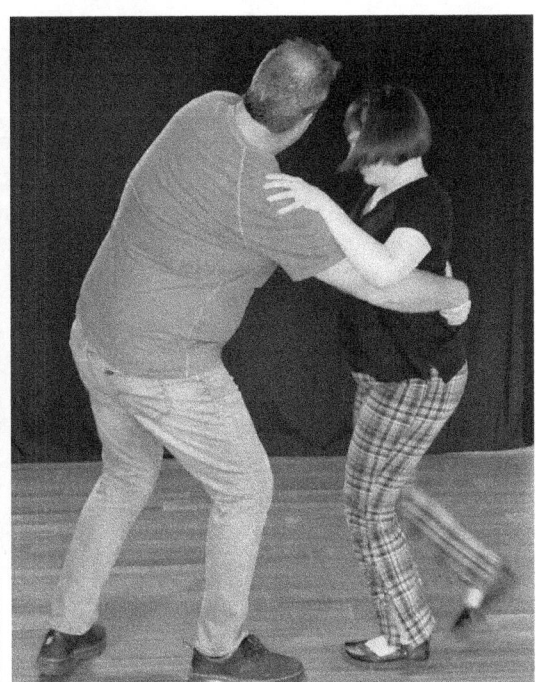

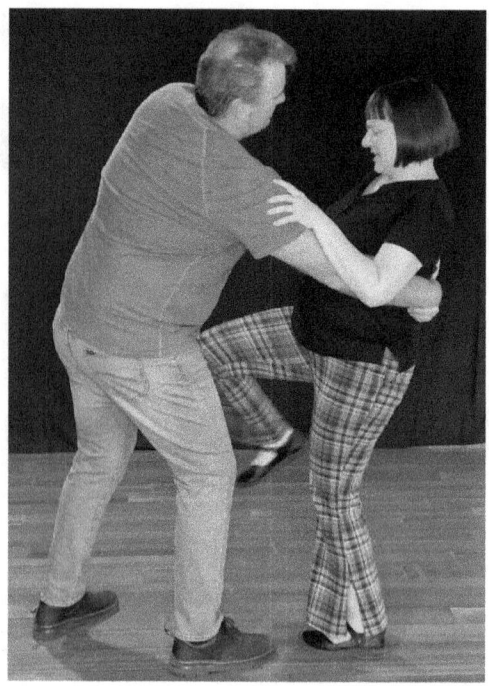

An alternative is:

When attempting the elbow strike, if the attacker blocks the elbow, grab the attacker's wrist with the arm that's being held. Hold onto their wrist while spinning in the opposite direction, then pull their arm up from the wrist while pushing down at the top of the arm just under the socket, bending their head forward. Kick the attacker in the face (or use the knee if too close to kick), then break the attacker's arm with a forearm strike to the top of the elbow.

Self-Defense

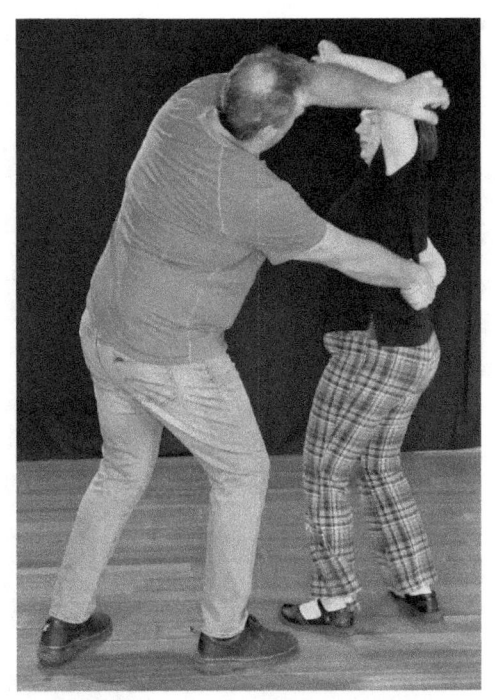
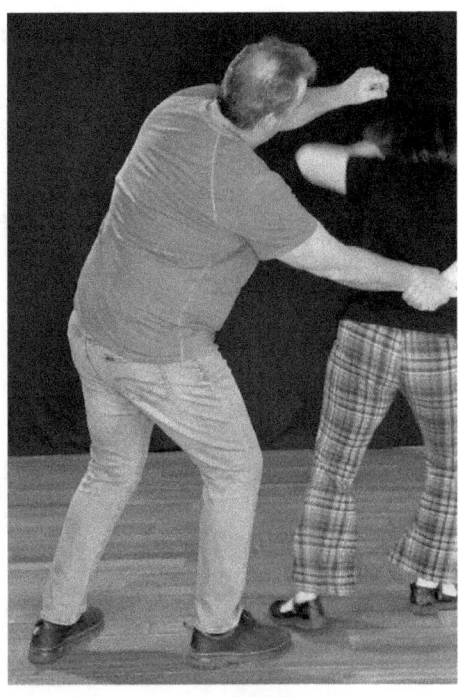
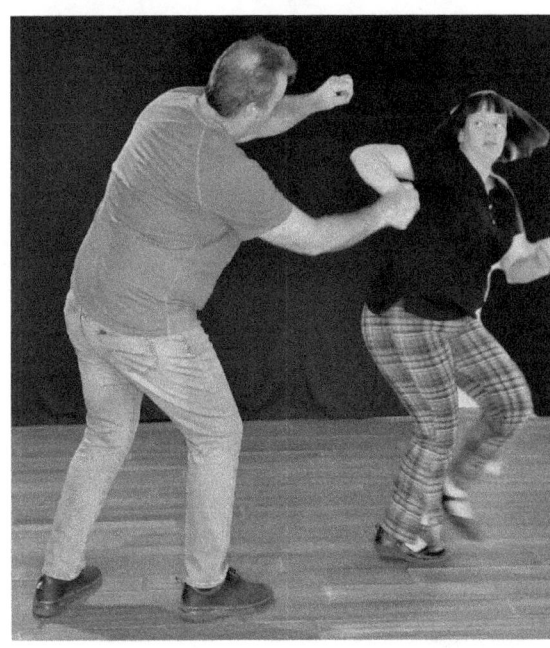
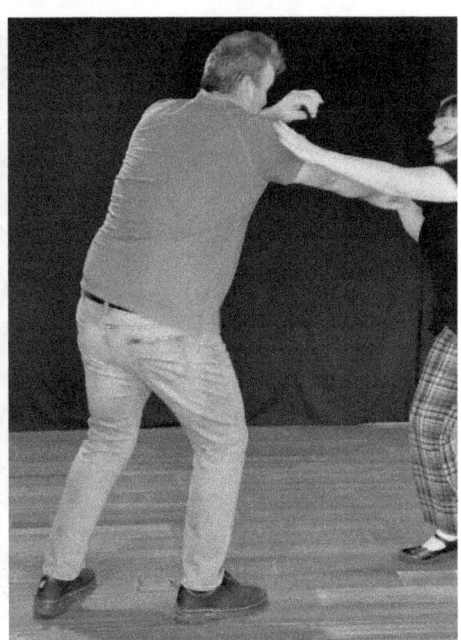

Self-Defense

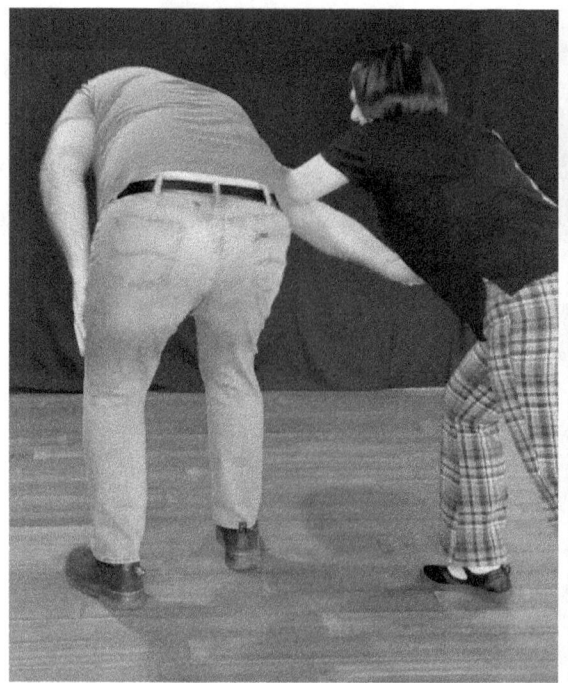
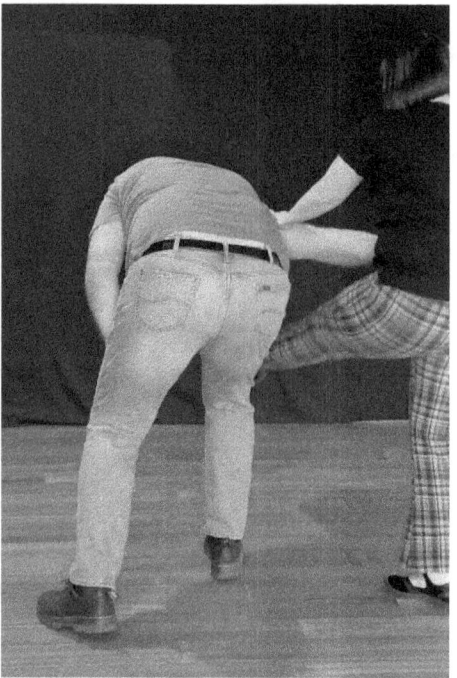
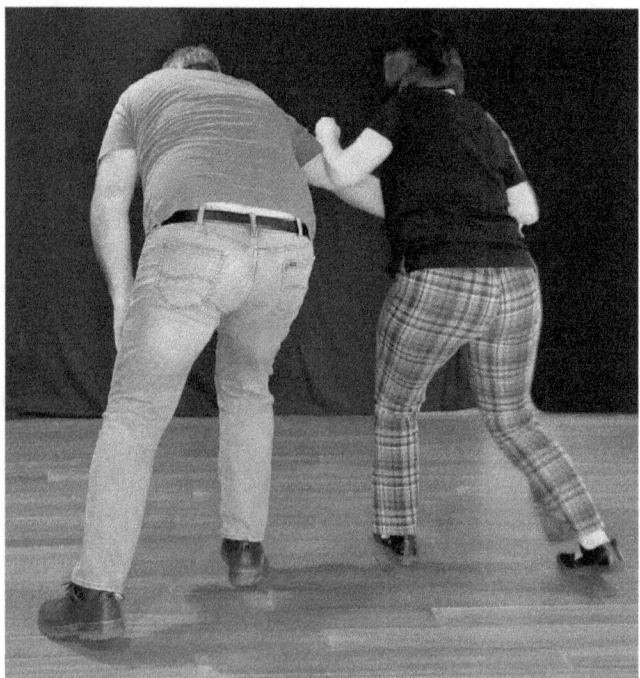

Full Nelson escape (2 variations)
 A full nelson is done from a rear position. Putting someone in a full nelson involves getting behind someone, putting the arms up between the opponent's arms and their body (up near the arm pit), then placing hands behind their neck, pushing down to keep leverage. This is used sometimes to break up a fight.

Self-Defense

To defend against the full nelson, consider that the arms are locked up high. Throw the head back in case the attacker's face is right behind. This could loosen the hold, but the attacker may be smart enough to keep their head down for this very reason.

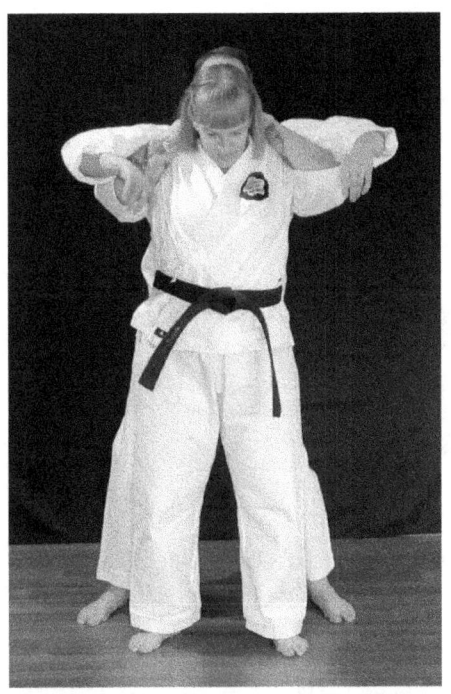
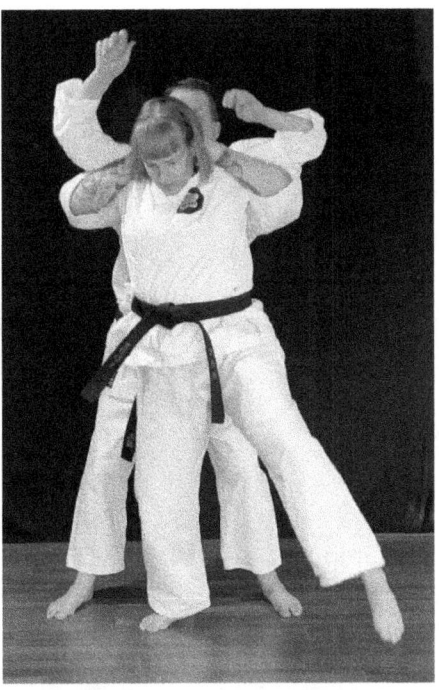
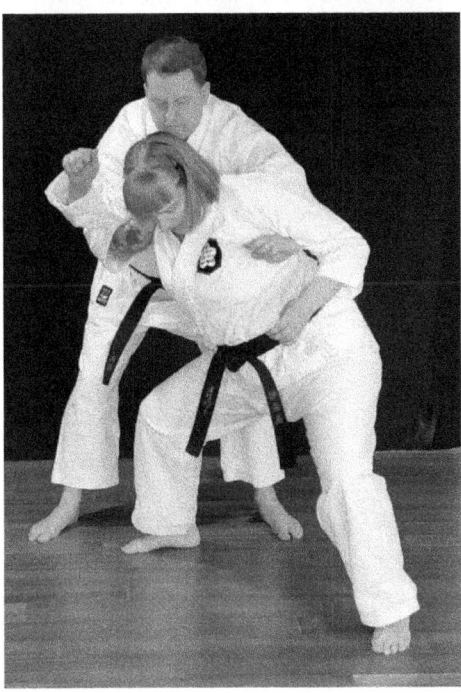
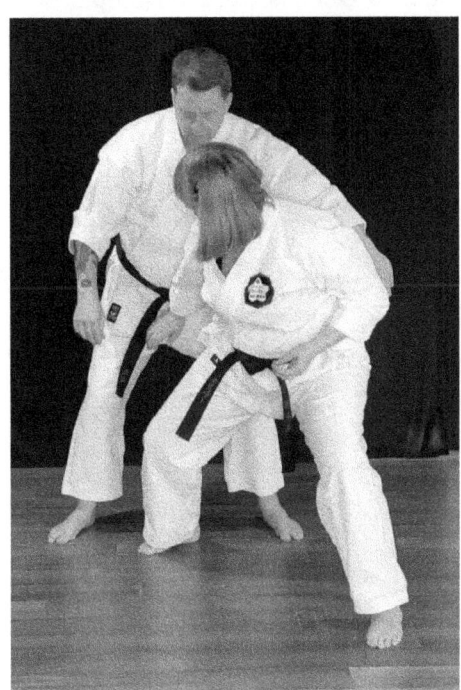

Self-Defense

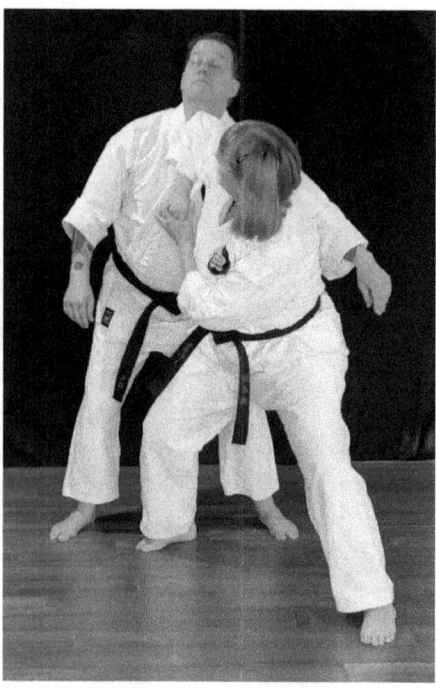

Step out at a forty-five degree angle into a low shiko dachi stance while simultaneously throwing the arms down to break the hold. If the hold breaks, pivot away from the attacker, shuto uchi to the groin, then elbow the face.

If the hold is still not broken, step around behind the attacker, planting the inside knee behind the attacker's thigh. Grab the attacker's legs and pull back hard, flipping them onto their back while the inside elbow drives into the attacker.

Self-Defense

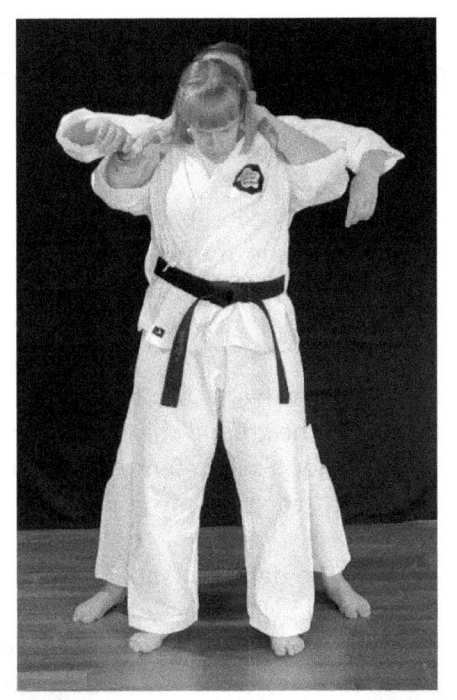
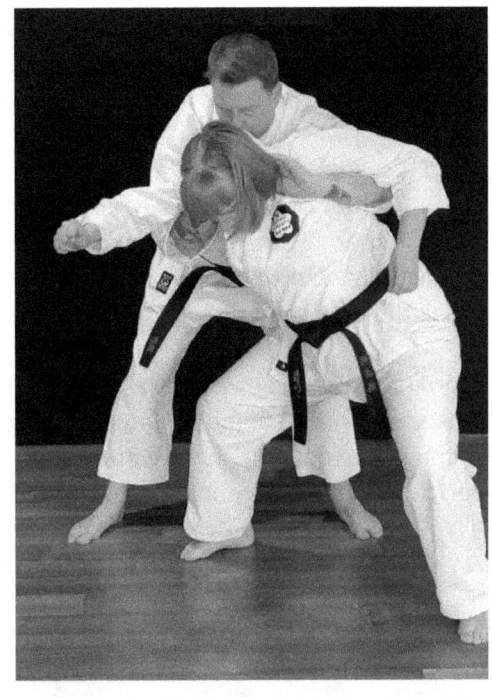
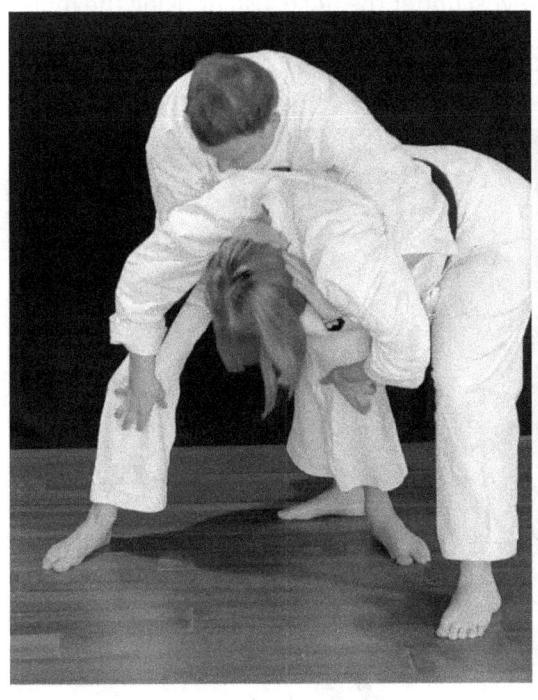
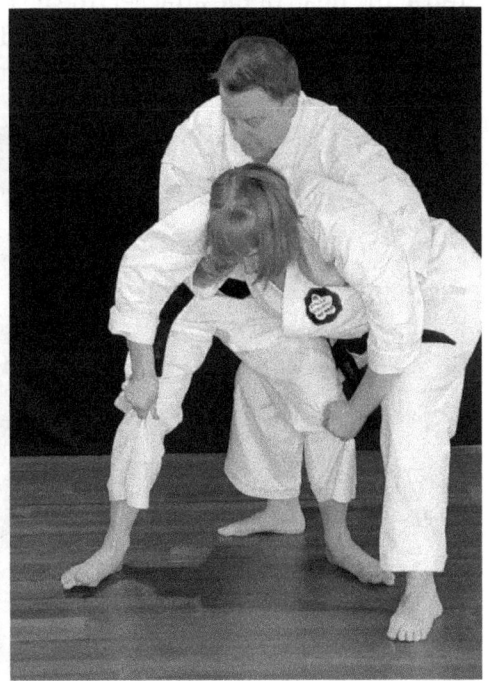

Self-Defense

If you have nowhere to step, (pushed up against a wall, perhaps) reach behind and attempt to grab and pull the ears, eyes, or hair of the attacker. Even pinching the attacker's skin on the arms can be effective.

Head lock escape

A headlock involves wrapping an arm around someone's head and holding it in place, either by the throat, neck, or jawline, then grabbing the opposite wrist and pulling tight. Using the throat as a target, the defender can choke; using the jaw can break the neck, and directly on the neck can cut the blood flow to the head.

Word of caution - be very careful practicing the headlock. If an attacker, even practicing, puts someone in a headlock and then suddenly drops to the ground still holding on, the training partner can be severely injured. The head lock self-defense is simple to perform, but like defending against many other attacks, reaction time is critical.

The defender should put the chin down first. The defender should protect his throat first and foremost. If standing up, the defender will likely get pulled down, bending over at the waist. If on the ground, the defender's body is likely twisted. Either way, the defender will have a hand behind and a hand in front. Use the hand behind to grab at the head of the attacker: the hair, eyes, under the nose, fish hooking the mouth, anything that can be grabbed and pulled. At the same time, use the front arm and pull behind the knee closest. This should lift them backwards and release the hold.

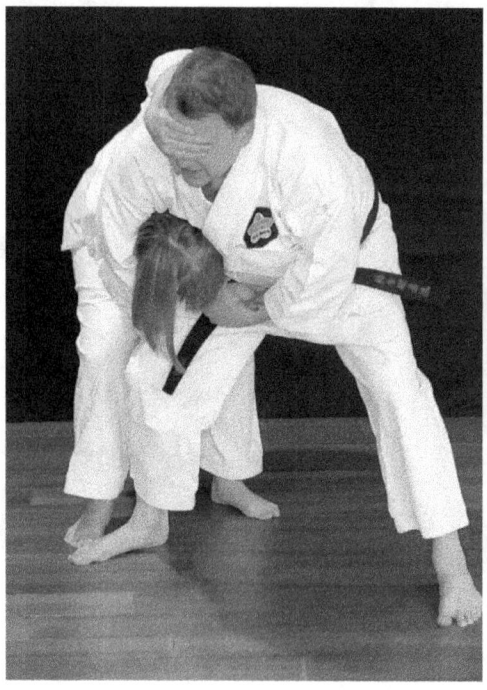
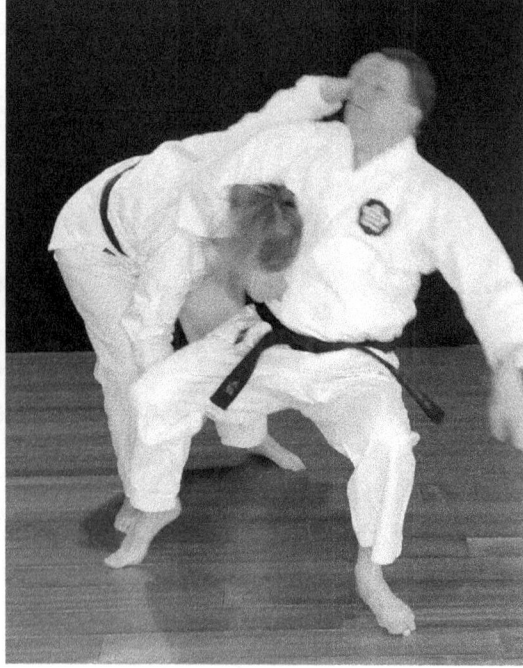

Self-Defense

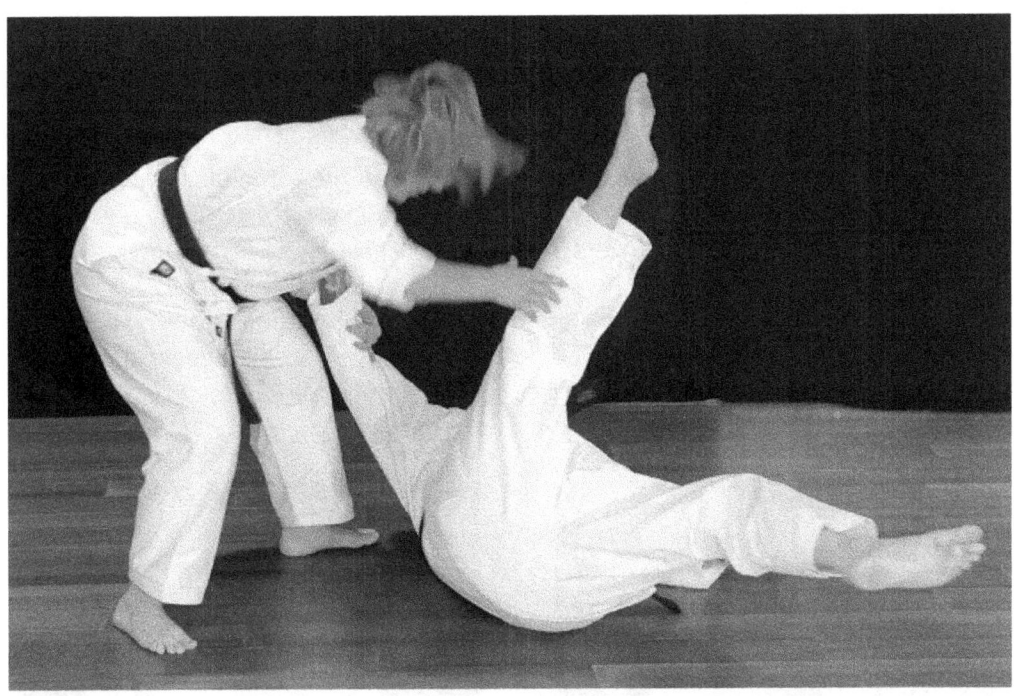

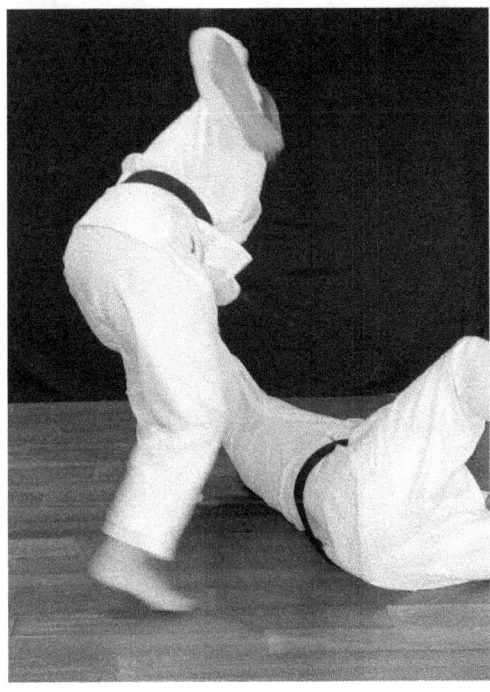

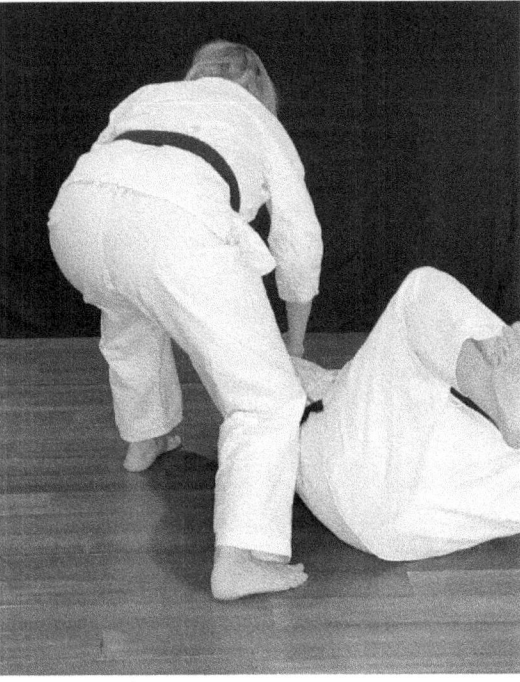

Self-Defense

Front Bear Hug & Rear Bear Hug (2 variations)

A bear hug involves someone wrapping their arms around someone, pinning his arms to the sides. This may be an attempt to crush someone, or they may try to throw the person to the ground. For defense, like the full nelson, throwing the head back to headbutt the attacker's face (or using the top of the forehead to head butt the attacker's nose in the case of a front bear hug) is a good start. The defender may also be able to reach down and grab the attacker's groin area. Twisting and pulling will certainly deter an attack.

For demonstration purposes, and if the first two methods do not work or are not possible, step out at a forty-five degree angle into a low shiko dachi stance while simultaneously throwing the hands straight out in front to break the hold. If the hold breaks, pivot away from the attacker, shuto uchi the groin, then elbow the face.

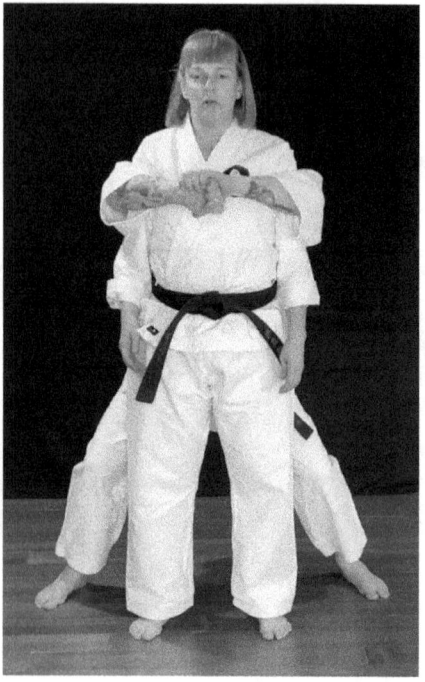
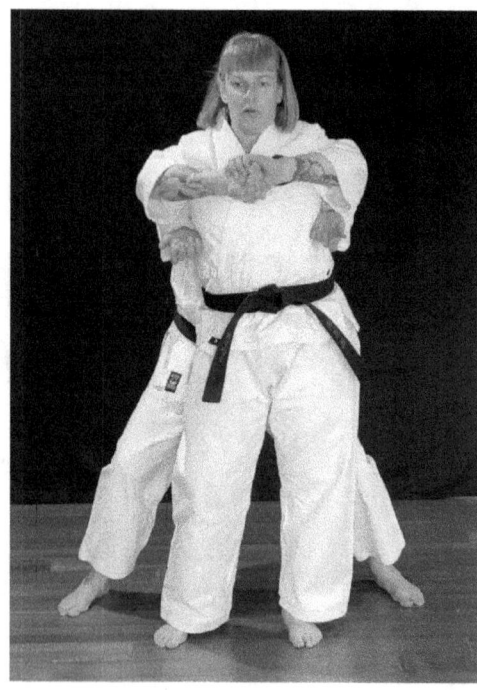

Self-Defense

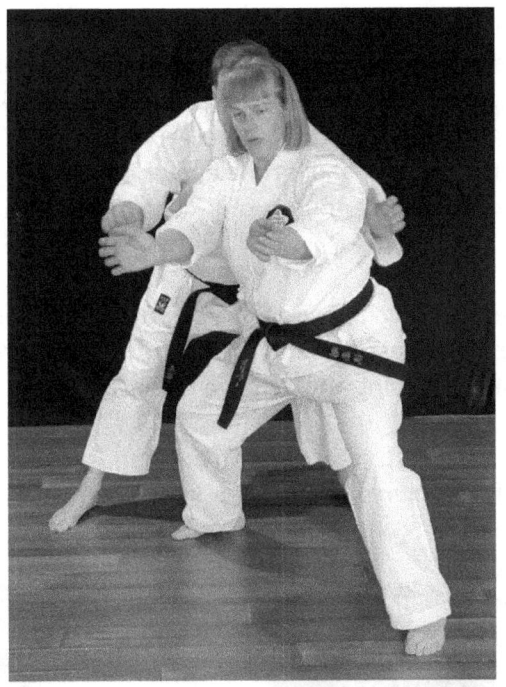
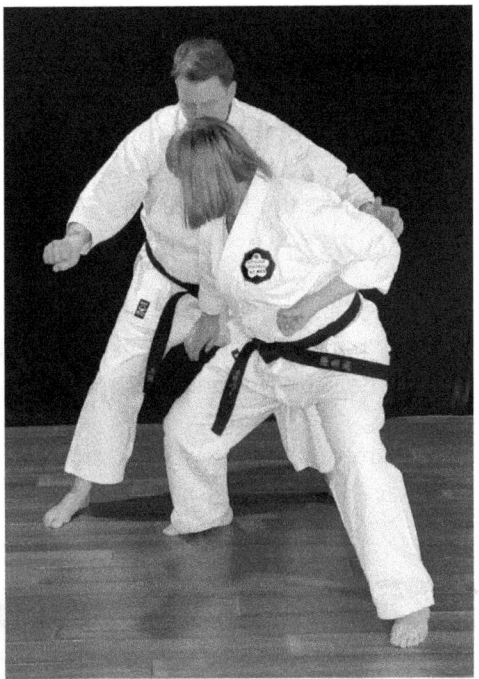
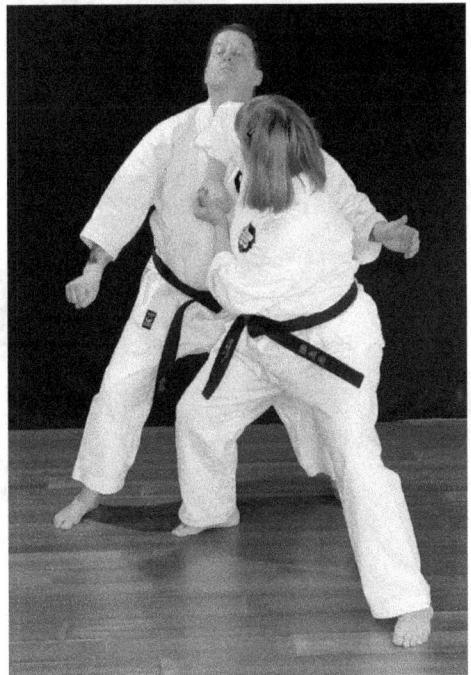

And like the full nelson defense, if this doesn't work, step around behind the attacker, planting the inside knee behind the attacker's thigh. Grab the attacker's legs and pull back hard, flipping them onto their back while the inside elbow drives into the attacker.

If the attacker approaches from the front, first, do not let an attacker get close enough to perform a front bear hug. If reaction time is too slow, the options are limited to either a knee to the groin or a head butt to the face. While these options may work, it is always better to keep from being fully grabbed in the first place. As the attacker's arms start to go around, take a step back with one foot and lift the elbows to block the attacker's arms up. Immediately after blocking, use the thumb knuckles* to strike the attacker's ribs.

* Instead of thumb knuckles, using a double shuto uchi, haito uchi, or tettsui uchi can also work here. Ideally the target should be the lowest ribs, the floating ribs. These are the most delicate ribs and the smaller the striking point, the damage is concentrated.

After the double strike (both sides of the ribs), reach up with one hand and claw at the face (the eyes or hair) and pull the face down while using a knee strike to the groin.

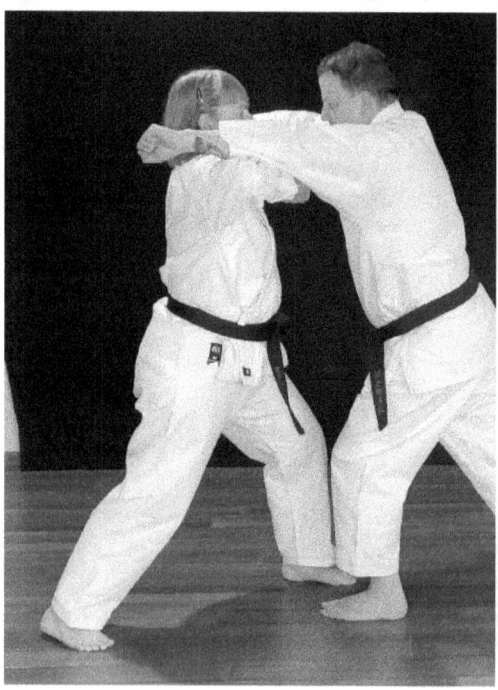
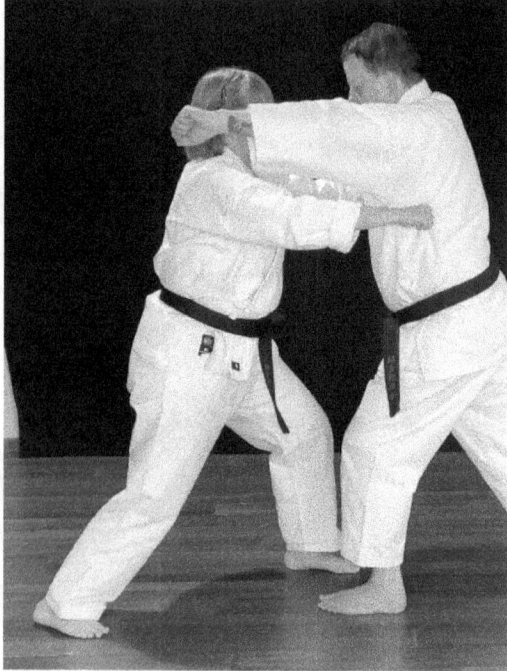

Self-Defense

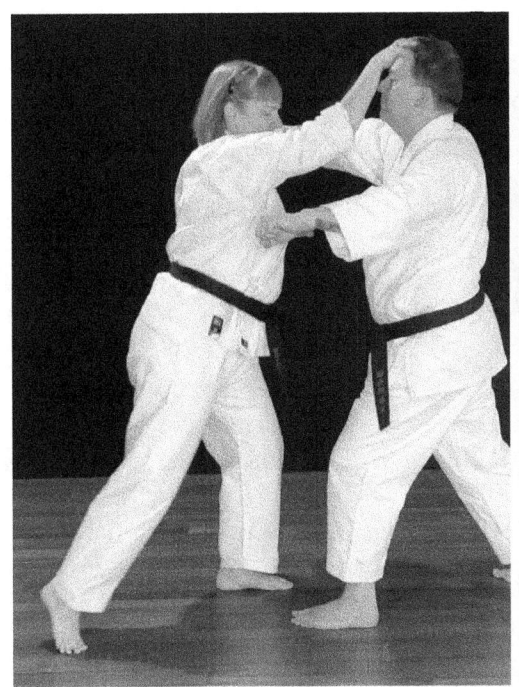
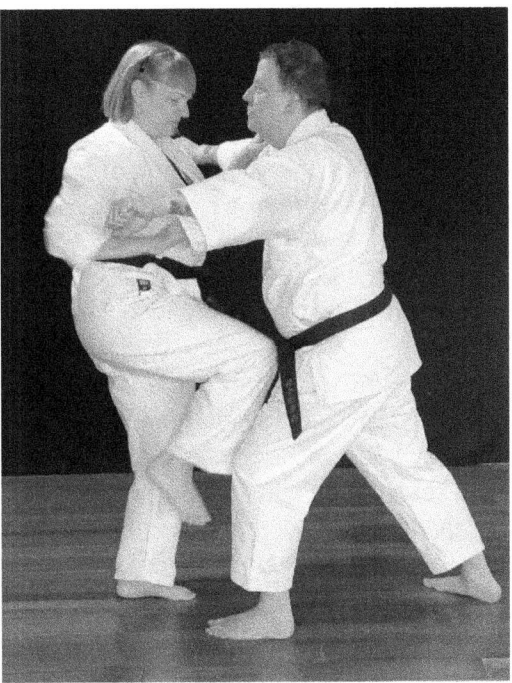
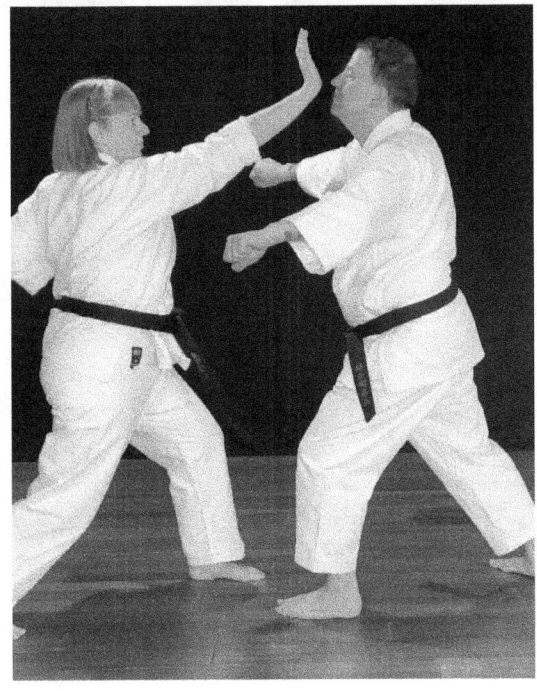

Self-Defense

Wrist grab defense

If someone reaches for your wrist, generally a strike to the face, body, or a kick will get the person to release. As most people are right handed, if they grab the wrist closest to them it will be the defender's left wrist. A turn of the wrist will loosen the grip and depending on the intention of the grab, it may be worth just turning yourself loose. But if the attacker has a clenched opposite fist or a weapon, that's different.

Same side wrist grab: complete the moves of a chest block, turning into a grab, bending the attacker's arm away. Break arm at or just above the elbow.

The defense for someone grabbing the opposite wrist is very simple because the attacker is already in a compromised position. First, put the free hand on top of the attacker's hand (the one grabbing the wrist). This seems counterintuitive but the idea is to keep the attacker's hand trapped.
Using the trapped hand, wrap it around the attacker's wrist and tighten the grip between the radius and ulna (forearm bones), or attempt to spiral the two bones together, pushing down.

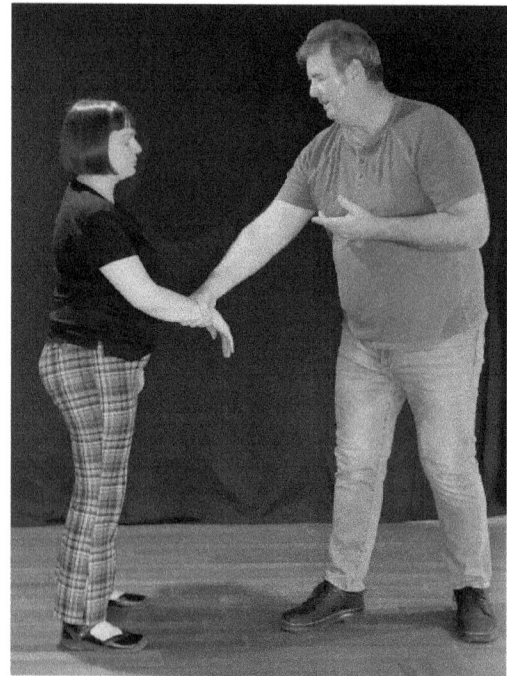 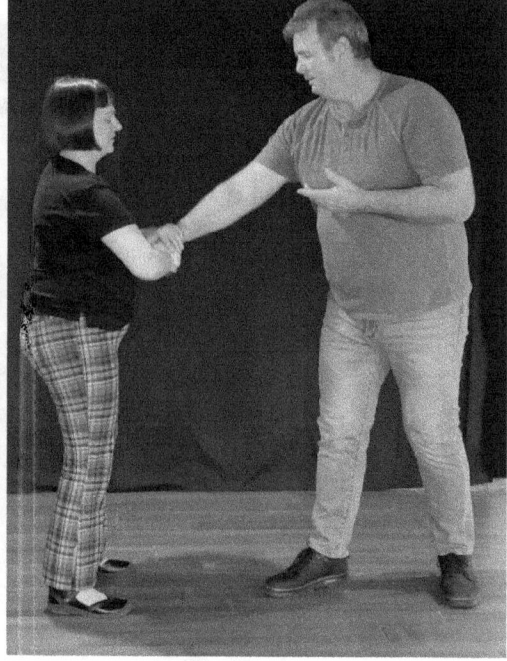

Self-Defense

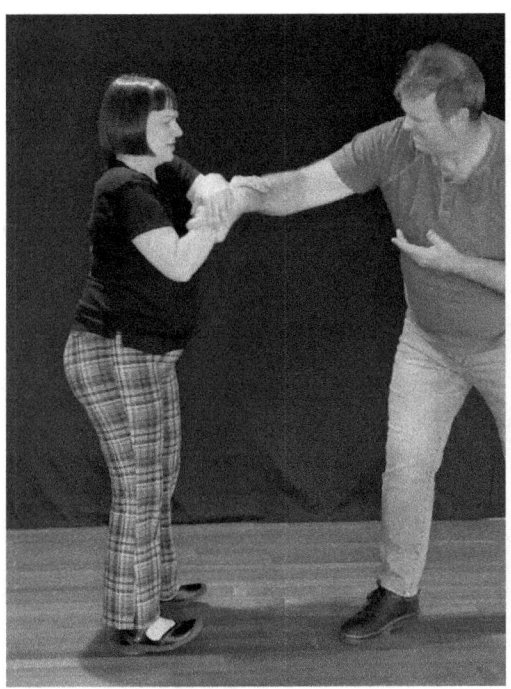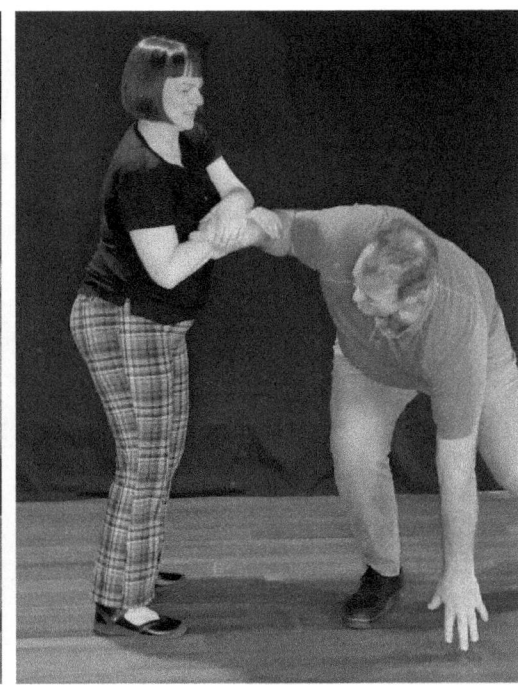

Rear choke escape

The rear choke involves wrapping an arm around someone's neck from behind, almost like a head lock. The attacker is directly behind the opponent and will use the choking arm to grab the opposite bicep muscle, then use the other hand to push behind the neck.

Like the head lock, the first step to defending against the rear choke is breathing. The defender should first turn the head into the crook of the attacker's elbow, giving a chance to breathe. Use one elbow to strike the attacker in the ribs. This will hopefully loosen the attacker's grip somewhat. Go down to one knee and use the other arm to pull the attacker down from the back of their shoulder. The goal is to put the attacker's armpit down over the defender's shoulder with no space between. While dropping to one knee, extend the other leg out for stability and throw the attacker around front, over the shoulder. This should be performed very quickly and followed by an immediate strike at the downed attacker.

Self-Defense

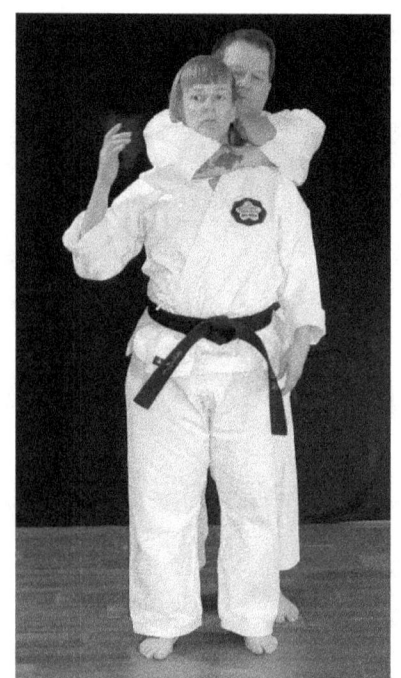
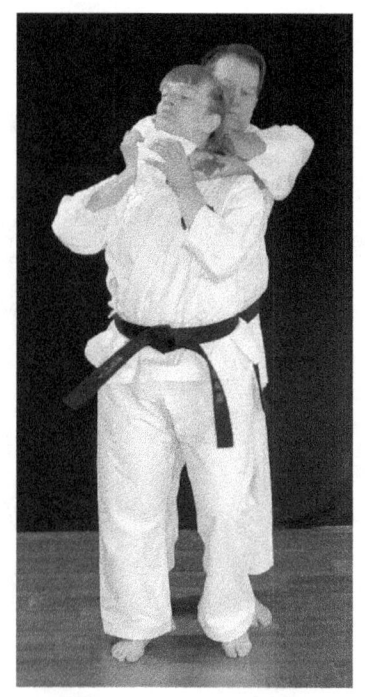
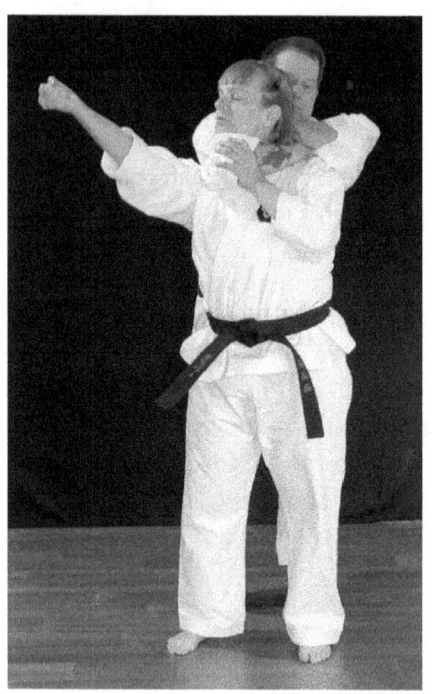
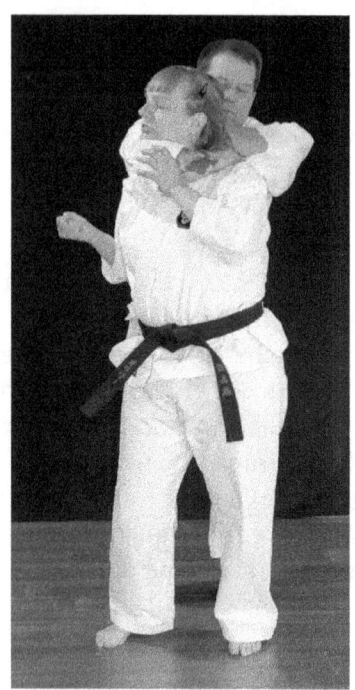

Self-Defense

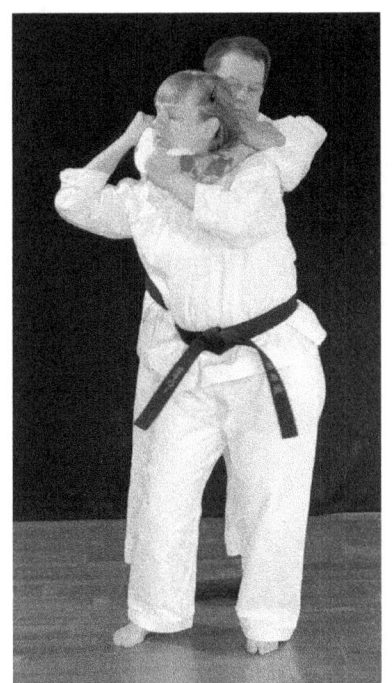
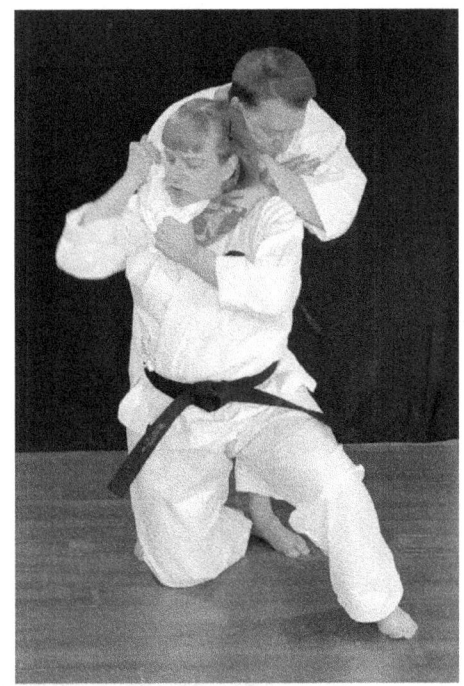
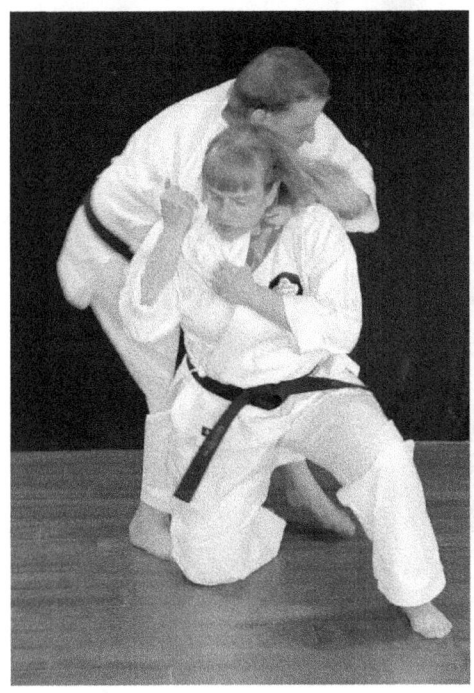
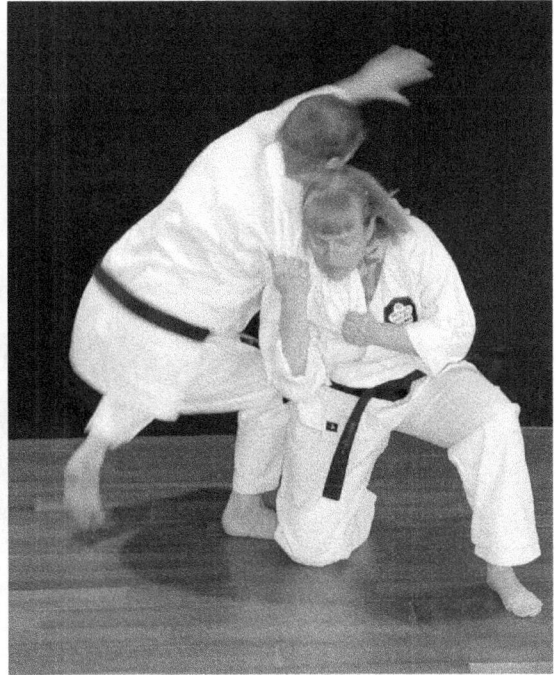

Self-Defense

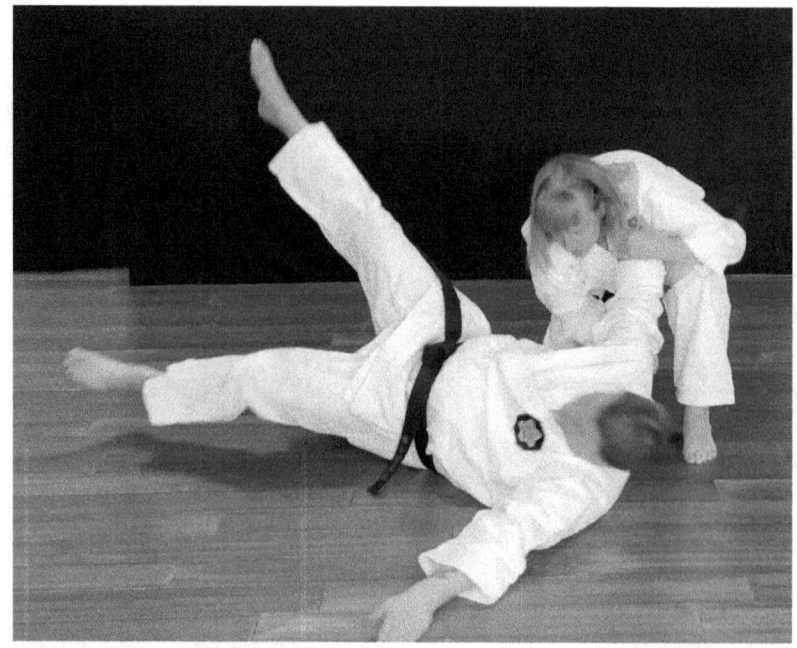

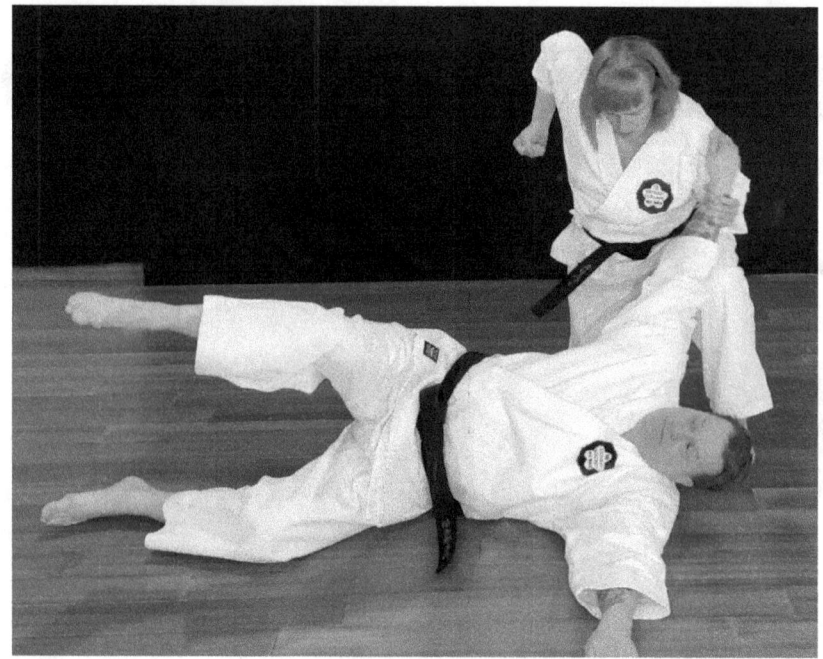

Self-Defense

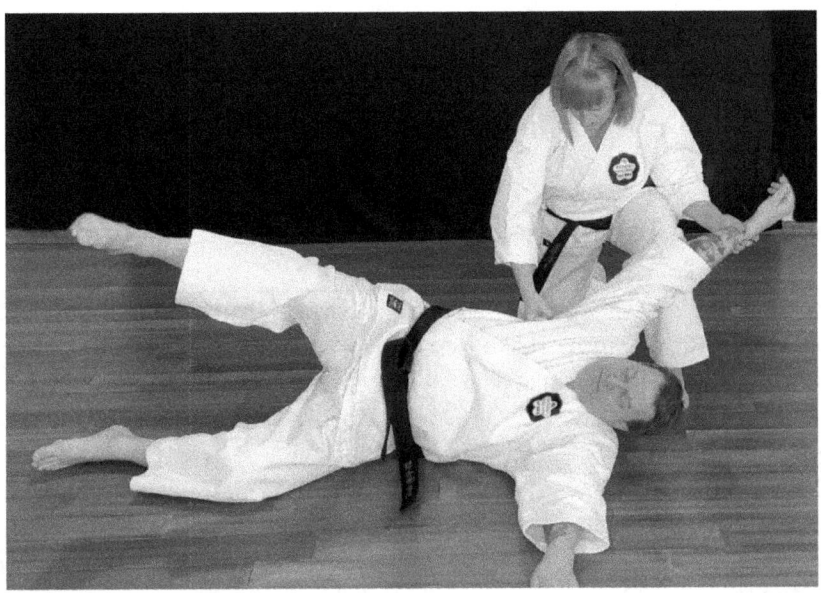

Remember that there are an infinite number of ways to escape from holds and locks. The methods shown here are just a few ways to consider. When a student practices self-defense, just like with kata or bunkai, he is practicing technique. That is only the beginning. A real fight is never going to be exactly how a person practices because there is no way to account for every possibility. But that does not mean a student should not practice. With a calm mind, when put in a bad situation, a person must draw on his training and apply it to what is happening, adjusting as need be.

The defender, in a split second, must identify as much as possible and rely on several things. Is there an escape route? How many people are there? Is there a weapon or weapons? Is it a public place? Is there a wall or a door, a low ceiling? Do I have a weapon? Is there a police officer in sight? Is anyone else in sight? Am I alone or with friends? Am I with friends who can help or would help? Am I going to need to put my glasses down? Am I in a public place? How big is the person right in front of me? Where are his hands? Is his hands in a fist or in his pockets? What are his friend's hands doing?

Without living in constant fear and paranoia, just being watchful, especially with people, is much like defensive driving.

Appendix

Japanese Karate Terms

Age - Rising
Age Empi Uchi – Rising Elbow Strike
Age Hiji Ate – Rising Elbow Strike
Age Uke - Rising Block
Ashi Barai – Leg Sweep
Barai - Sweeping Block
Bunkai - Analysis
Chudan - Middle
Dachi – Stance
Dojo – Training Hall
Embusen – Footwork Pattern One Follows When Practicing Kata
Empi – Elbow
Fumikomi Geri – Stamping Kick
Furi Uchi - Swinging or Hook Punch
Gedan – Low
Geri – Kick
Goju-Ryu – Hard-Soft Style
Gyaku Zuki - Reverse Punch
Haisoku - Instep
Haito Uchi – Ridge Hand Strike
Hajime – Command to Begin
Hari Uke – Open Hand Block (Palm Up)
Heiko Dachi - Parallel Stance
Heisoku Dachi - Traditional Stance, Feet Together
Hiki Uke – Open Hand Block (Palm Down)/Pulling Block
Hiraken - Second Knuckles Fist
Hiza Geri – Kick (To the Knee)
Hiza Uchi – Strike (Using the Knee)
Hojo Osae Uke – Augmented Pressing Block
Hojo Oshi – Augmented Push
Hojo Uke – Augmented Block
Ippon Ken – Single Knuckle Fist
Jodan – High
Josokutei - Ball of Foot

Mawashi Geri – Roundhouse Kick
Mikazuki Geri – Crescent Kick
Morote – Double/Augmented
Morote Chudan Uke – Double Chest Block
Morote Gedan Barai – Double Down Block
Morote Heiko Uchi – Double Parallel Strike
Morote Hiraken Zuki – Double Fore Knuckle Punch
Morote Nakadakaken Uchi – Double Middle Knuckle Fist Strike
Morote Shotei Uchi – Double Palm Heel Strike
Morote Sukui Uke – Double/Augmented Scooping Block
Morote Zuki – Double Punch
Musubi Dachi - Attention Stance, Toes Out
Neko Ashi Dachi – Cat Leg Stance
Nihon Nukite – Two Finger Spear Hand
Nukite – Spear Hand
Odeko Ate – Head Butt
Oshi - Push
Otoshi - Downward (Dropping)
Otoshi Tettsui Uchi – Down Hammer Fist Strike
Rei – Bow (Respect)
Sanchin Dachi – Hourglass Stance
Seiza – Formal Sitting
Shiko Dachi - Straddle Leg Stance
Shomen – The Front Wall of a Dojo
Shotei – Palm Heel
Shuto Uchi - Chop Strike
Soto Uke – Outside Block
Suihei Osae – Horizontal Pressing
Sukui Uke – Scooping Block

Juji Uke – X Block	**Tenchi no Kamae** – Position with One Palm Up and One Palm Down
Kagi Zuki – Hook Punch	
Kakato - Heel	**Tettsui Uchi** - Hammer Fist Strike
Kake Geri - Hook Kick	**Tora Guchi** – Wheel Block
Kake Uke - Hook Block	**Tsukami Hiki** – Grab and Pull
Kamae – Posture, Basic Defensive Stance	**Tsuki/-Zuki** - Punch
Karate – Empty Hand	**Uchi** – Strike
Karateka – Karate Student	**Uchi Uke** – Inside Block
Kata - Form	**Uke** – Block (Receive)
Keage Geri – Snap Kick	**Ura Mawashi Empi Uchi** – Spinning Elbow Strike
Keri/-Geri - Kick	
Ketsugo - United	**Ura Zuki** – Inverted Punch
Ko Uke - Back of Wrist Block	**Uraken Uchi** – Back Fist Strike
Kokutsu Dachi – Rear Leaning Stance	**Ushiro** – Rear (Back)
Koryu – Traditional School (Refers to Traditional Kata)	**Ushiro Empi Uchi** – Rear Elbow Strike
	Ushiro Mawashi Geri – Spinning Hook Kick
Kosa Dachi – Cross Leg Stance	
Kote Uchi – Forearm Strike	**Yoi** – Ready Command
Kumite – Fighting	**Yoko** - Side
Mae – Front	**Zenkutsu Dachi** - Forward Leaning Stance
Mae Keage Geri – Front Snap Kick	

Appendix

More stories from the dojo:

In the book, Shodai Jay Trombley, many former students of Shodai wrote their own impressions of him and what he and karate meant to them, stories, etc. Since that book came out, several people submitted to me the following:

Christine Landmon

Shodai loved stories. He loved telling them, hearing them and reading them. You were suspicious if you didn't have stories. So, I would be remiss not to tell mine. I was in my late twenties when I first stepped into the dojo. I was getting out of an abusive marriage that left me completely broken. That's why I was there, because I was so consumed with fear and anxiety, that I couldn't go into a grocery store by myself, and I had excruciating headaches, for which I was taking medicine. I knew I had to do something; I couldn't live like this. I was so impressed by what I saw in the dojo. The tradition, the discipline, the respect, the confidence. My dad (who was with me) and I checked out a couple of other schools, nothing like this! I wanted all of that, so I joined! I had a problem as I trained, a lot of the time my head would hurt so bad that I would have to bow out and go to the back room and lay down (or throw up) and I would be perfectly still and breathe and be calm! Well, I knew I couldn't go on like this and most likely it wouldn't be tolerated. It was also embarrassing and made me feel weak. So, one night after this happened once again, I went into Shodai's office. I explained that I loved karate, but I was gonna have to quit because I couldn't get through a workout without bowing out, from my head. He looked at me and said, "you can quit if you want, doesn't matter to me, but if you leave those headaches will never go away." I was so taken back by his lack of sympathy, that I vowed that day, my head would explode all over his floor before I quit!

It was so hard. I remember my first tournament; Mr. Johnson came up to me as I was stretching and asked if I was ok! I know my eyes were bugged out and I said, "no I can't do this!" He said, "nobody is expecting anything, just get through it!" They called my name and before I knew it, I took first in Kata and first in fighting. Two six foot trophies! No one could believe it, most of all me! I knew that day that I was on the right path!

Once I got hit between the eyes by Mr. Madison, who you didn't want to get hit by, and the next day I had two black eyes. I was proud. I had some extremely great successes with Shodai, that I would have never thought I was capable of, including making it to Sandan (third Black) but there is not a day that goes by that I can't apply something I learned from karate, like "courage is not the absence of fear but the conquest of it." I am so eternally grateful for every day I spent in Shodai's dojo. The training, the relationships, the pain, the joy, the knowledge, but most of all, everything combined, I haven't had a headache in over 30 years. After 11 years I stopped training to be a mom (something else I thought was not going to happen, if you believe doctors) but Shodai would still call me back to sit on tests and important things, so we stayed in contact, laughed and told stories! Thanks to Shodai and his love karate, I became a version of myself I couldn't have dreamed would be possible and will never forget it.

Cliff Knudson

Appendix

Shodai was without a doubt one of the most influential people in my life and I owe him far more gratitude than mere words can ever express. To the best of my knowledge, I am the only student of Shodai's that has had the unique experience of effectually making black belt in Ketsugo Goju-Ryu twice, and at two vastly different stages of my life.

The first time was as a kid. I trained under Shodai from 1987-1997 and earned my junior black belt in 1996 at the age of 14. At the time, I was the youngest junior black belt that Shodai had ever had. (As a kid my last name was Brunken. I changed it as an adult for personal reasons.) I returned to the dojo as an adult in 2010 and resumed my training under Shodai until he retired in 2016. Upon his retirement I joined Hanshi Oliver's dojo, where Shodai would occasionally stop by to visit or attend high ranking belt tests. I continued training there until 2020.

With very rare exceptions, once someone has earned a senior black belt from Shodai, they retain that rank indefinitely. Junior black belts however do not. So, when I returned to the dojo as an adult I started over from the beginning as a white belt. Returning to the dojo as an adult felt like returning home. Both Shodai and I were a little older, and the dojo had moved to Watauga, but other than that, it felt like nothing had changed. I was a little rusty at first, a bit out of shape, and far less flexible, but thanks to my previous training I progressed my way back through the system in record time and became Shodai's 29th black belt in 2012 when I earned my 1st Dan, followed by my 2nd Dan in 2014, and my 3rd Dan in 2019.

Having spent the majority of my childhood training in Ketsugo Goju-Ryu, there is no doubt in my mind that my experiences growing up in the dojo and the lessons I learned from Shodai, and the other black belts are all a fundamental part of who I am today. Together they taught me far more than just the skills to defend myself. Their lessons instilled within me a sense of self-confidence, discipline, and perseverance that extended far beyond the dojo walls and have remained with me ever since. As such, along with Shodai, I owe a special thanks to the following black belts: David Griffin, Ken Johnson, Bob Lowenstein, Mark Ashraf, Allen Crowley, Christine Landmon, Andrew Smith, Marvin Madison, Kyle Brown, Russell Dare, and Chris Collins. They may not have thought much of it at the time, but I will be forever grateful to each and every one of them.

I first started training in Ketsugo Goju-Ryu when I was 5 years old. The year was 1987 and I was totally hooked on the most "radical" new show on TV, Teenage Mutant Ninja Turtles. My parents had been trying to find an outlet for my energy and had previously tried signing me up for several of the typical sports such as soccer, tee-ball, and basketball, none of which I was all that enthusiastic about. But that year when they asked me what I wanted to do, I boldly declared "I want to do karate like the Ninja Turtles!" The following week they enrolled me at the Pipeline Rd. dojo in Hurst and thus set me on an unexpected path that will forever be a part of my life.

When I first joined the dojo, I was part of the "mighty-mites" class which was specifically for 5-6 year old's. Shodai was never all that fond of working with really young kids and though he was occasionally involved, most of my early training was left to other back belts as well as some intermediate and advanced kyu ranks. I particularly remember working with Sensei Ken Johnson the most, as well as Sensei Christine

Appendix

Landmon, though she was not yet a black belt at that time. Nevertheless, Shodai's influence was always present in the dojo, even if he wasn't.

As I progressed both in rank and age, I eventually graduated to the all ages beginner class and soon came to realize that when Shodai was at the dojo, his presence was palpable. Don't get me wrong, the other back belts exuded an undeniable and serious aura that without a doubt commanded everyone's respect. And they always ran classes in the same no-nonsense way, regardless of whether Shodai was there or not. But whenever Shodai was at the dojo, something was just different. His presence didn't just command respect, it demanded it! Everyone was affected by it, black belts included. Make no mistake, classes were always serious business, and students were expected to give nothing less than their best efforts at all times, regardless of who was running the class or if Shodai was there or not. But whenever he was there, something in the air changed and everyone seemed to hold themselves to a slightly higher standard. Everyone's movements became a little crisper, strikes and blocks grew a little stronger, and stances just got a little deeper. Even if you were already giving 100%, somehow you managed to find a little more and you'd push yourself to 105%. All of this happened for two reasons. The first was in the hope that he might offer some sort of praise or approval of your efforts, which was both a rare and proud moment as he had extremely high standards and was not easy to impress. The second was that to do otherwise would risk incurring potentially unwanted attention and possibly even his wrath, which is exactly what you could expect if he thought you were slacking off. Ironically, both of these reasons were often simultaneously motivating. And it didn't help that as he always had the same serious look on his face, making it next to impossible to tell what he was thinking or what sort of mood he was in. I can't count how many times he would be watching me during a class with that signature look on his face and I would all but drive myself crazy wondering if I was about to be corrected or if he liked what he saw. It was truly nerve-racking, and I would never want to play poker with him, but I knew I wasn't the only one to feel it. If you weren't careful those thoughts would make you lose focus and start making mistakes. But I eventually realized that was the whole point. He liked to test his students to see if they could perform under pressure. But regardless of his mood, or if he was offering praise or criticism, the aura he projected in the dojo was nothing less than formidable and always intense. Even when he was just casually sitting and watching class from the audience section of the dojo, his gaze had a weight that could be felt.

Combined with his reputation of being less than gentle with his corrections and criticisms, the overall effect he had on some students was often profound and many students found his presence to be nothing less than intimidating. So much so that occasionally some students would even skip classes if they thought Shodai was going to be there. This was especially true on fight nights. Shodai took no offence to this though. He was well aware of the effect he had on some of his students, and likely a little proud of it too.

The funny part was that for Shodai, it became a bit of a game to surprise students with his attendance. In the early to mid 90's, there were more than enough black belts to run classes without Shodai needing to be involved all the time, so he was not at the dojo on a fixed schedule. However, he always kept tabs on student attendance by regularly looking at the class sign-in sheets with which he could easily tell who was coming to class and when. Since most students had predictable schedules and attendance, it wasn't hard to see patterns. Occasionally he noticed certain students were not showing up to class on days he was there. Back in those days, Shodai was driving a giant conversion van that when parked in front of the Hurstview dojo, could not be missed. It didn't take much for him to connect the dots. So from time to time, he would park in back of the building, out of sight from the road, or he would have one of the black belts open the school and wait until after class had started to make his entrance and surprise unsuspecting students – some of whom might have otherwise skipped class that night. One day while reminiscing with him as an adult, I recounted to him my memory of these times. He laughed pretty hard and told me that the look of surprise on some of the students' faces were priceless! Especially the ones that thought they had cleverly avoided him.

The fact that they had tried to avoid him in the first place is not entirely shocking though. Regardless of age or rank, Shodai's approach to teaching was not for the faint of heart. Though I have never been in the military myself, I often felt classes resembled what one might expect at a clichéd boot camp and I think it's safe to say that his time in the marines definitely influenced his style of teaching. Shodai's dojo was a no-nonsense place reserved for serious training only. There was no goofing-off or horseplay allowed, and traditional etiquette and respect was expected at all times. Classes were physically and mentally demanding, even for the beginners and intermediate classes, and especially so in the advanced class. He was strict, had high expectations of his students, demanded nothing less than their best efforts, regardless of their rank, and he was completely unsympathetic to excuses. If you had a rough day at work or problems at home – too bad – leave your problems at the door. If you'd suffered minor injuries like broken fingers or toes – use some tape and suck it up – "Fingers and toes don't count!" If you were the type to need constant pats on the back for a job well done, you were in the wrong place. He rarely offered praise other than an occasional subtle nod, and his silence indicated that you had done well enough to satisfy his expectations. He was a stickler for details and was quick to correct even the smallest mistakes. If you failed to fix those mistakes, he would quickly grow impatient. Repeated corrections would grow increasingly less pleasant, sometimes to the point of being harsh, which many students would often mistake for a personal affront. Bottom line: If you showed up for class, you had better be ready to give 100% every time! If you didn't, you would come to regret it very quickly.

If you only knew Shodai's personality while class was in session, it would be easy to make the mistake of taking his verbal lashings personally. But those who persevered through his training and got to know him better, especially outside of class, usually came to realize that his abrasive approach to teaching was not something that should be taken too personally because despite appearances, there was a method to his madness.

Shodai's whole approach to teaching could be summed up in two words, tough love! And he was not reserved when it came to dishing it out, to the point that his intentions were often misunderstood. Shodai didn't just want his students to be physically tough, skilled only in the mechanics of karate, he wanted to teach them to be mentally tough as well. Shodai loved to tell students that the "secret" to karate came down to 3 things: "Renshū, Renshū, Renshū!" (*Practice, Practice, Practice!*). He often reminded his students of this, especially when they were struggling to learn something new. It took me a long time to realize that this "secret" not only applied to the mechanics but to the mental aspect of karate as well. To that end, I think Shodai truly believed that an occasional ass-chewing was good for a person. Although he never said it outright, I believe he saw it as a form of mental conditioning and a method to help students develop a "thick skin," which was a quality I know he valued in both himself and in others.

This became abundantly clear to me one day after witnessing an incident that occurred between Shodai and one of his intermediate students at the time. I will spare the details of who and why, they are inconsequential, and to be honest I don't remember verbatim exactly what was said and will have to paraphrase, but here's the gist: The student was an adult and Shodai was chewing him out pretty hard. You could tell that the student's pride and ego were taking offense as his expression made it clear that his emotions were starting to get the better of him as Shodai continued to chew him out. The student managed not to argue, but he the audacity to tell Shodai "...I don't appreciate you speaking to me like that." This enraged Shodai further and he sent the student home for the day. (To his credit though, the student returned to class the next day and said nothing further about it.) As I was a Sensei at the time, I believe that what Shodai said to me afterwards was not only to vent his frustrations with the student, but also to provide me some insight on his approach to teaching. Shodai's rhetorical question to me was something to the effect of, "How does he expect to handle himself in a real fight when he can't even handle a few words? They're just words! What's he going to do when someone's really trying to hurt him?" I chose contemplative silence and a thoughtful nod as my response at the time, but I did give it some thought. And though the situation could have been handled more gracefully, I had to admit that he had a point. Anyone who has spent enough time in the ring can tell you that getting emotional during a fight does not help. In fact, it's quite the opposite. Everyone's heard of a blind rage. There's a reason they call it that. Your emotions can effectually blind you if you let them, and going "blind" in a fight is the last thing you want to do. If you can't control your emotions and think with a clear head just because of a few harsh words, chances are you won't be able to control them if someone punches you in the face. It was just another of Shodai's tactfully indirect but clear lessons.

Because of his often abrasive demeanor, his rigorous approach to training, and the fact that he didn't seem to care about his students struggles outside of the dojo, it's not all that surprising that the majority of students that joined didn't last very long. Especially considering that society has largely grown to shun those who callously speak their mind and practically criminalizes those who dare to verbally offend or hurt the feelings of others. All of which Shodai was notoriously guilty of. Truth be told, he rarely filtered his thoughts and often spoke harshly to people. Because of this I think it's safe to say that at one point or another, everyone who trained under Shodai eventually reached a point where they began to question why they voluntarily continued to subject themselves to Shodai's rigorous and often unpleasant manner of training. For me that answer was simple. One look at any of Shodai's black belts and it was clear to me that anyone who made through his training came out the other side tough as nails and a force to be reckoned with. Shodai's black belts weren't just "good" at karate, they were badass! I knew from an early age that I wanted to reach that level too. Obviously

Shodai never made it easy, but I can honestly say it was worth it. Like the saying goes, nothing good comes easy.

What I most respected about Shodai was his unwavering commitment to martial arts, to his dojo, and his students, as well as the fact that he refused to change with the times or compromise his values for money despite ample opportunities and changes of society's expectations. A sad truth of the vast majority of karate dojos today is that over time they have become mere shells of what they once were and have since become mostly profit focused businesses. Many of them are even franchised and are often owned or operated by individuals with little to no personal training in martial arts. As such they typically have little to no expectations of students and effectually sell rank to anyone willing to pay. Some even offer black belt "packages" complete with upfront timelines so their customers will know exactly how long it will take them to receive a black belt. Like so many others, Shodai could have easily compromised his principles and values to follow the money as well. Had he done so, he probably would have become a very wealthy man. But to him, that would have been like selling his soul.

For Shodai, karate was far more than just his passion, it was his life. He charged his students dues in order to pay the bills and keep the lights on, and while I'm sure he wasn't opposed to making a profit, his goal in running a dojo was never to become wealthy. All he really wanted was to train strong, dedicated, and loyal students who loved karate as much as he did. Rank from Shodai could not be bought, it had to be earned. He didn't make it easy either. As such, every time you advanced in rank it was an accomplishment you knew you could be proud of. He believed that to be a black belt truly meant something special. In fact, his standards and expectations of what it took to earn a black belt were so high that although he trained hundreds of students over his life, only a handful of his students actually managed to earn a black belt in Ketsugo Goju-Ryu. Without a doubt, being able to count myself among them is one of my proudest achievements and greatest honors of my life.

Bibliography

Gekisai Ichi
1: Nagamine, Shoshin. The Essence of Okinawan Karate-Do. C.E. Tuttle Books. 1976. Pg. 104

Saifa
2: Warrener, Don. Traditional Goju-Ryu Karate. Masters Publication. 1982. Pg. 134
3: Opdam, Lex. Karate Goju Ryu Meibukan. Empire Books. 2007. Pg. 98

Sanchin
4: Bishop, Mark. Okinawan Karate: Teachers, Styles and Secret Techniques. 1990, ci.nii.ac.jp/ncid/BB10175635.
5: St Mark's Hospital Nursing Team. "Exercising Your Sphincter Muscles to Help Improve Bowel Control." *University Hospitals of Leicester*, Jan. 2023,yourhealth. leicestershospitals.nhs.uk/library/chuggs/ general-surgery/pelvic-floor-and-bowel-function/2425-exercising-your-sphincter-muscles-to-help-improve-bowel-control/file. Accessed 26 Oct. 2024.

Seiunchin
6: "Kata Dictionary." *Alan Godshaw*, 5 Nov. 2021, alangodshaw.com/photos/%E7%9B%AE%E9%8C%B2%E3%81%AE%E5%BD%A2.

Sepai
7: Opdam, Lex. Karate Goju Ryu Meibukan. Empire Books. 2007. Pg. 101

Appendix

Ketsugo Goju-Ryu Schools

Honbu Dojo (Home School)
Oliver Karate Academy
Colorado Springs, Colorado
(719) 581-3161
www.oliverkarate.com

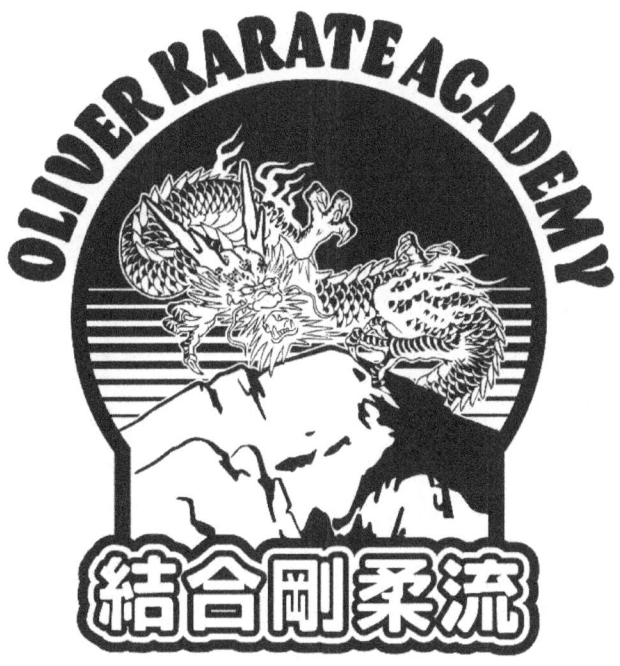

Branch Dojo
Bryant Karate Academy
North Richland Hills, Texas
(682) 325-9755
www.bryantkarateacademy.com

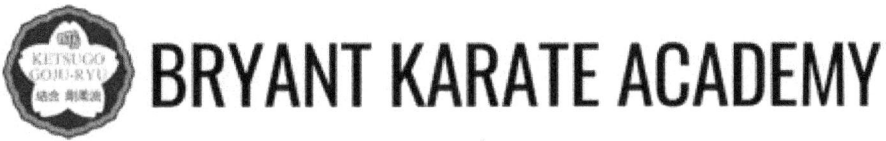

Appendix

Appendix

www.ingramcontent.com/pod-product-compliance
Lightning Source LLC
Chambersburg PA
CBHW081206170426
43198CB00018B/2873